UNITED NATIONS SCIENTIFIC COMMITTEE
ON THE EFFECTS OF ATOMIC RADIATION

1986 REPORT

GENETIC AND SOMATIC EFFECTS OF IONIZING RADIATION

United Nations Scientific Committee on the Effects
of Atomic Radiation
1986 Report to the General Assembly, with annexes

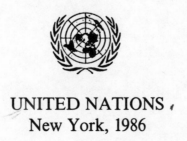

UNITED NATIONS
New York, 1986

NOTE

The report of the Committee without its annexes appears as Official Records of the General Assembly, Forty-first Session, Supplement No. 16 (A/41/16).

The designations employed and the presentation of material in this publication do not imply the expression of any opinion whatsoever on the part of the Secretariat of the United Nations concerning the legal status of any country, territory, city or area, or of its authorities, or concerning the delimitation of its frontiers or boundaries.

UNITED NATIONS PUBLICATION

Sales No. E.86.IX.9

ISBN 92-1-142123-3

004800P

CONTENTS

Report of the United Nations Scientific Committee on the Effects of Atomic Radiation to the General Assembly

CONTENTS

INTRODUCTION

1. This is the ninth substantive report of the United Nations Scientific Committee on the Effects of Atomic Radiation (UNSCEAR)[a] to the General Assembly.[b] As anticipated in its 1982 report, UNSCEAR had been planning to conduct detailed studies on selected subjects, together with comprehensive assessments of the type normally issued. This report contains reviews of three special topics in the field of biological effects of ionizing radiation that are among those presently under consideration by the Committee: genetic effects of radiation (annex A), dose-response relationships for radiation-induced cancer (annex B), and biological effects of pre-natal irradiation (annex C).

2. The preparation of this report with its scientific annexes took place essentially from the thirty-first to the thirty-fifth sessions of the Committee, although the preparation of annex B started much earlier, its publication being delayed pending the dosimetric revision on the survivors of Hiroshima and Nagasaki. Most of the scientific work for this report was done at meetings of groups of specialists, which considered working papers prepared by the Secretariat that were modified and amended from one session to the next, according to the Committee's requests. The report itself was drafted at the thirty-fifth session. Mr. Z. Jaworowski (Poland), Mr. D. Beninson (Argentina) and Mr. T. Kumatori (Japan) served as Chairman, Vice-Chairman and Rapporteur, respectively, at the thirty-first session. The following members of the Committee acted in such capacities at subsequent sessions: Mr. D. Beninson (Argentina),

Mr. T. Kumatori (Japan) and Mr. A. Hidayatalla (Sudan) at the thirty-second and thirty-third sessions; and Mr. T. Kumatori (Japan), Mr. A. Kaul (Federal Republic of Germany) and Mr. A. Hidayatalla (Sudan) at the thirty-fourth and thirty-fifth sessions. The names of those experts who attended the thirty-first to the thirty-fifth sessions of the Committee as official representatives or members of national delegations are listed in appendix I.

3. The Committee was assisted in the preparation of the report by a small scientific staff and by consultants appointed by the Secretary-General. That group, whose members are listed in appendix II, was responsible for the preliminary review and evaluation of the technical information received by the Committee or published in the open scientific literature. In approving the report, the Committee itself assumes full responsibility for its content; it wishes, however, to acknowledge the help and advice given by the group.

4. Representatives of the World Health Organization (WHO), the International Atomic Energy Agency (IAEA), the International Commission on Radiological Protection (ICRP) and the International Commission on Radiation Units and Measurements (ICRU) attended the sessions of the Committee held during the period under review. The Committee wishes to acknowledge their contribution to the discussion. Representatives of the United Nations Environment Programme (UNEP), to which the secretariat of the Committee is attached, were also present at all the sessions. The Committee would like to express its appreciation for the special attention and the support given to its activities by this organization.

5. The reports received by the Committee from States Members of the United Nations and members of the specialized agencies and of the IAEA, as well as from those agencies themselves, during the period from 27 March 1982 to 18 April 1986 are listed in Appendix III. Reports received before 27 March 1982 were listed in earlier reports of the Committee to the General Assembly. The information received officially by the Committee was supplemented by, and interpreted in the light of, other data available in the current scientific literature or, in some rare cases, from unpublished communications of individual scientists.

6. In the following, the Committee summarizes the main conclusions from the three specialized studies already mentioned, also in the light of previously released substantive documents.

7. Following past practice, only the main text of the report is submitted to the General Assembly, while

---

[a] The Committee was established by the General Assembly at its tenth session in 1955. Its terms of reference are set out in resolution 913 (X). It was originally composed of the following Member States: Argentina, Australia, Belgium, Brazil, Canada, Czechoslovakia, Egypt, France, India, Japan, Mexico, Sweden, Union of Soviet Socialist Republics, United Kingdom of Great Britain and Northern Ireland and United States of America. The membership of the Committee was subsequently enlarged by the General Assembly in its resolution 3154C (XXVIII) to include Germany, Federal Republic of, Indonesia, Peru, Poland and Sudan.

[b] For the previous substantive reports of the Committee, see *Official Reports of the General Assembly, Thirteenth Session, Supplement No. 17* (A/3838); *ibid., Seventeenth Session, Supplement No. 16* (A/5216); *ibid., Nineteenth Session, Supplement No. 14* (A/5814); *ibid., Twenty-first Session, Supplement No. 14* (A/6314 and Corr.1); *ibid., Twenty-fourth Session, Supplement No. 13* (A/7613 and Corr.1); *ibid., Twenty-seventh Session, Supplement No. 25* (A/8725 and Corr.1); *ibid., Thirty-second Session, Supplement No. 40* (A/32/40); *ibid., Thirty-seventh Session, Supplement No. 45* (A/37/45). These documents will be referred to in this context as the 1958, 1962, 1964, 1966, 1969, 1972, 1977 and 1982 reports, respectively. The 1972 report with appendices and scientific annexes was also made available as: *Ionizing Radiation: Levels and Effects, Volume I: Levels* (United Nations publication, Sales No. E.72.IX.17); and *Volume II: Effects* (United Nations publication, Sales No. E.72.IX.18). The 1977 report with appendices and scientific annexes appeared as: *Sources and Effects of Ionizing Radiation* (United Nations publication, Sales No. E.77.IX.1). The 1982 report with appendices and scientific annexes appeared as: *Ionizing Radiation: Sources and Biological Effects* (United Nations publication, Sales No. E.82.IX.8).

the full report, together with the scientific annexes mentioned above, will be issued as a United Nations sales publication. This practice is intended to achieve wider dissemination of the findings to the international scientific community, which makes use of the Committee's assessments as a source of independent and authoritative information. The Committee wishes to draw the attention of the General Assembly to the fact that separation of the main text of the report from its scientific annexes is simply for reasons of convenience. It should be borne in mind that the scientific data given in the annexes are very important and form the basis for the main conclusions contained in this report.

I. GENETIC EFFECTS OF RADIATION

8. The Committee reviewed recent advances in various areas relevant to the evaluation of genetic radiation hazards in man. The most important areas are: the identification of the prevalence of naturally occurring monogenic, chromosomal and other disorders; the use of recombinant DNA technology for the analysis of human genetic material in normal individuals and in those with genetic disease; the relationships between gene mutations, chromosomal aberrations and cancer; the role of movable genetic elements in the production of spontaneous mutations and their implications for the estimates of the genetic risk; and other data directly or indirectly bearing on the quantification of genetic hazards and detriment in man. As a result of this extensive analysis, the Committee believes that the assessment of radiation-induced genetic risk contained in its 1982 report remains broadly valid.

9. The considerations that determined the choice of the major themes listed above can be briefly summarized as follows: (a) a precise knowledge of the prevalence of Mendelian and chromosomal disorders and those with a strong genetic predisposition constitutes an essential framework for perceiving the impact of such disorders in human populations and for placing the radiation risk estimates into perspective; (b) the advances in recombinant DNA technology that have occurred during the last few years have imparted a level of precision hitherto not possible to the study of the human genome for unravelling the action of specific genes in health and disease, including cancer, for analysing the mutation spectra and the nature of spontaneous and radiation-induced mutations and for formulating new approaches to the management of heritable disorders; (c) the recent convergence of ideas and techniques from viral oncology, cell genetics and molecular biology has resulted in major breakthroughs in knowledge on the molecular genetic basis of several spontaneously arising and mutagen-induced cancers; (d) the demonstration that there are movable genetic elements (mobile DNA sequences) in a number of species (and presumptive evidence for their occurrence in humans), and that a sizeable proportion of spontaneous mutations (in bacteria, yeast and drosophila) are due to these movable genetic sequences, is raising questions concerning the extent to which they may be causing spontaneous mutations in humans and whether there is a difference in nature between radiation-induced and spontaneous mutations; and (e) new data from human studies on detriment associated with certain spontaneously arising disorders of complex aetiology, as well as information from mammalian and other studies on genetic effects of radiation, illustrate the validity of the Committee's earlier views and conclusions.

10. New data on the prevalence of certain specific monogenic disorders in humans essentially confirm the Committee's earlier assessments. Likewise, a re-analysis of data bearing on the contribution of chromosomal anomalies to spontaneous abortions and still births suggests that at least 40% of the spontaneous abortions that occur in the period from the fifth to the twenty-eighth week of gestation and about 6% of still births are associated with chromosomal anomalies. Recent results from cytogenetic surveys of new-borns carried out using banding methods show that the frequencies of spontaneously occurring reciprocal translocations and inversions are higher than those detected in studies in which banding methods were not used.

11. The frequencies of chromosomal anomalies in patients with mental retardation and multiple congenital anomalies vary from about 2.5% to 20% with a mean of about 12%. In sub-fertile males, the prevalence of such anomalies is an order of magnitude higher than in new-borns (6.0% versus 0.6%), but the frequencies of specific anomalies show considerable variation.

12. A substantial amount of information has now become available on fragile sites on human chromosomes. These are chromosomal regions exhibiting fragility (as evidenced by abnormal chromosomal configurations in metaphase preparations), which can be made visible under specific tissue culture conditions. The fragile site is always at exactly the same point on the chromosomes in all individuals or kindred, but is never seen in all cells examined. About 40 fragile sites are currently known, including one on the long arm of the X-chromosome. The latter is associated with X-linked mental retardation and is the most common genetically determined cause of mental handicap, next only to trisomy-21 (Down's syndrome). There are indications that certain fragile sites on chromosomes other than the X may predispose chromosomes to breakage. There is evidence, furthermore, that several non-random chromosomal changes involved in certain cancers have breakpoints that coincide with the fragile sites.

13. A systematic comparison of three studies of the estimated live-birth prevalences of congenital anomalies (a prospective study in the United States and two retrospective studies in British Columbia and in Hungary) shows that the prevalences vary from 8.5% in the United States to 6.0% in Hungary and to 4.3% in British Columbia. Among the reasons for the differences between those estimates are geographical and ethnic variations and differences in ascertainment efficiencies. Particularly noteworthy is the finding that musculoskeletal anomalies constitute about 50% of all congenital anomalies in Hungary, about 45% in the United States and about 30% in British Columbia. Anomalies of the integument constitute, furthermore, about 10% of the total in the United States, and about 1% in Hungary and British Columbia. The Committee

has used the live-birth prevalences from Hungary (6.0%) as a basis for making detriment estimates for spontaneously arising congential anomalies.

14. Preliminary data suggest that the prevalence of other disorders with a strong genetic predisposition, which are disorders primarily of adulthood, may be at least about 60% in Hungary. Each of these disorders has a population prevalence of not less than 1 per 10,000. The values for the individual conditions in Hungary are well within the ranges reported for other countries. These conditions are both aetiologically and clinically heterogeneous. The estimated population prevalence of 60% is an order of magnitude higher than the 4.7% for British Columbia. It should, however, be stressed that: (a) since many individuals have more than one disorder, the actual proportion of the Hungarian population that suffers is probably less than 60% although still far more than the 4.7% in British Columbia; and (b) the value of 4.7% applies only to disorders appearing before the age of 21, whereas the value of 60% applies to those appearing up to age 70.

15. During the last few years, the application of recombinant DNA technology to the study of the human genome has revolutionized the field of human genetics. By using a variety of enzymes specifically active on the cells' genetic material, it has become possible to make direct analyses of normal and mutant genes. Several findings emerging from these studies have applications in the detection of carriers of serious genetic disorders, in pre-natal diagnosis and in the typing of tumours and lymphomas. Molecular approaches are increasingly being used to study mutation and DNA repair in mammalian cells.

16. Exciting advances have also been made during the last few years in understanding the genetic basis of cancer. Among these, the following deserve mention: (a) the discovery that mammalian and other genomes contain nucleotide sequences related to viral oncogenes (i.e. genes responsible for the production of tumours in a number of avian and mammalian species) and that these sequences, termed cellular proto-oncogenes, have oncogenic potential; (b) the identification of activated forms of proto-oncogenes in tumour cells and the discovery that such activations can occur through point mutations or specific chromosomal aberrations in which the breakpoint may involve the cellular oncogene itself; and (c) the probable participation of proto-oncogenes in the regulation of cell proliferation.

17. The conceptual foundations for dealing with movable genetic elements, one of the most active areas of current genetic research, were laid by McClintock over three decades ago. From genetic studies with maize, she postulated the existence of what are now called movable genetic elements. Such elements have since been discovered in a number of species, including bacteria, blue-green algae, yeast and drosophila. There are several lines of evidence suggesting that they are also present in mammalian (including human) genomes, and some of these have been characterized at the molecular level. In the organisms studied, these transposable genetic elements have been shown to be capable of inducing chromosome breaks, duplications and a variety of other structural alterations, as well as gene mutations and changes in gene expression at many gene loci.

18. The finding that a sizeable proportion of spontaneous mutations in experimental organisms studied in this respect can be caused by movable genetic elements, and that the rate of transposition is either not affected or only minimally so by exposure to mutagens, could have implications for the evaluation of genetic radiation hazards. For instance, if the majority of spontaneous mutations in humans is a by-product of the dynamics of transposable genetic elements and if the nature of these spontaneous mutations differs from that of mutations induced by mutagens, the use of the doubling dose method in hazard evaluation may need to be re-examined. There is, however, no evidence at present for the thesis that a majority of spontaneous mutations in humans is due to movable genetic elements.

19. A number of recent studies on mammalian somatic cells have shed further light on the nature of the lesions in DNA that lead to chromosomal aberrations and the process of DNA repair associated with the formation of these aberrations. Particularly interesting are the new data obtained by the use of restriction endonucleases. These are enzymes that recognize specific sequences in the DNA and cleave them, producing fragments that are either blunt ended (both strands cleaved at the same position) or cohesive ended (each strand cleaved at a different position). Although the absolute frequencies of chromosomal aberrations were found to depend on the restriction enzyme used, those producing blunt-ended DNA breaks were much more efficient than those producing cohesive-ended breaks. Since these enzymes are known to produce only double-strand DNA breaks, these data provide further direct evidence that double-strand breaks in the DNA are the principal lesions involved in the production of chromosomal aberrations.

20. New data obtained on lymphocytes (white blood cells) of patients with chromosome instability syndromes show that, except in one case, the spontaneous rates of mutation relative to those of blood cells from normal individuals are higher by factors ranging from three to ten. The newly developed T-lymphocyte cloning technique has been successfully used in studies on radiation induction of 6-thioguanine mutants in human lymphocytes. The data show dose-dependent increases in mutation frequency and these frequencies are of the same order of magnitude as those determined in experiments with established fibroblast cell lines.

21. The results of an international collaborative study on the x-ray induction of chromosomal aberrations in human lymphocytes in vitro show that at low doses (from 0.004 to 0.3 grays) there is no increase in aberration yields up to 0.05 grays, beyond which the increase is linear with dose. Furthermore, according to the authors' analysis, the frequencies of all types of aberrations at 0.004 grays are significantly lower than the control values.

22. Data from direct cytological analysis of spermatozoa from normal human males have shown that the frequencies of chromosomal abnormalities in these cells vary between individuals (0-28%) with a mean of about 9.0%. Both numerical and structural anomalies have been found, the frequencies of the former in different individuals ranging from 0.6% to 5.0% and those of the latter from 1.5% to 15.8%. The frequencies of chromosomally abnormal spermatozoa in men who had undergone radiotherapy were higher (averaging over 20% but ranging from 6% to 67%, with a significant correlation between the frequencies of abnormal sperm and testicular dose) than before radiotherapy and were also higher than in non-irradiated men; again, both structural and numerical chromosomal anomalies were present.

23. The frequencies of spontaneously arising chromosomal anomalies in Chinese hamster oocytes and early zygotes have been determined using an improved chromosome preparation technique. The data suggest that the incidence of aneuploidy of maternal origin (2.1%) is three times higher than that of paternal origin and first division meiotic errors are about three times more frequent than second division errors.

24. Further data on the x-ray induction of nondisjunction in young and old female mice have become available. In one set of experiments, the frequencies of eggs having more than the haploid number of chromosomes (hyperhaploidy) were higher in old (1.5%) than in young (0.2%) non-irradiated mice. After x irradiation, the frequencies of hyperhaploid eggs from both young and old mice showed a linear relationship with dose, but there were no differences between the young and old mice in this regard. In another set of experiments with young female mice and eggs, sampled at various intervals after irradiation, significant and greater-than-linear increases in hyperhaploidy were found, as the eggs sampled at shorter intervals after irradiation were found to be less sensitive than those sampled at other time intervals. In a further set of experiments, it was shown that the use of gonadotropin to induce ovulation had no effect on the sensitivity of the oocytes to the radiation induction of either numerical or structural anomalies.

25. Further genetic evidence on the x-ray induction of heritable reciprocal translocations in male mice (following spermatogonial irradiation) has been obtained. This shows that there is a dose-dependent increase in frequency up to 6 grays, the average rate being $(3.9 \pm 0.3) \times 10^{-3}$ per gray. The frequencies of translocations after 1.5 grays are consistent with expectations based on cytogenetic studies, whereas at higher exposures the frequencies appear to be lower than expected, in line with previous findings.

26. A comparison of the cytogenetic data on the x- or gamma-ray induction of reciprocal translocations in a number of non-human primate species (including the data reviewed in the 1982 report) show that the spermatogonia of one marmoset species, Callithrix jacchus, have a sensitivity similar to that of the Rhesus monkey. However, both these species are much less

sensitive than another marmoset, Saguinus fuscicollis. The crab-eating monkey, Macaca fascicularis, is intermediate between Rhesus monkey and Callithrix jacchus, and Saguinus fuscicollis, which was studied over 10 years ago. Changes in technique may be partly responsible for these differences. The recently studied crab-eating monkey, Macaca fascicularis, is about twice as sensitive as the Rhesus monkey to acute irradiation, but the most recent data suggest that the former species may be less sensitive to chronic gamma irradiation.

27. Data on the induction by x rays of congenital anomalies in the offspring of irradiated mice show that the incidence of these anomalies (detected by in utero examination) is significantly higher following irradiation of post-meiotic germ cells in males. The frequencies of these anomalies also tended to rise after spermatogonial exposure.

28. Further data have become available on the radiation induction of heritable tumours in mice. Spermatids in males and maturing oocytes in females seem to be the most sensitive stages for the induction of genetic changes that lead to tumours in the progeny; spermatogonia are also affected. The pattern of transmission of these tumours is consistent with a dominant mode of inheritance and a penetrance of about 40%; they also have a low expressivity.

29. In order to estimate the radiation risks associated with the induction of reciprocal translocations in human germ cells, model studies using x-irradiated blood lymphocytes and fibroblasts have been carried out. The location of the translocation break points, lengths of segments involved etc., were determined in banded chromosome preparations. The information so derived was used: (a) to inquire into the minimum possible imbalance that each of these translocations will generate, should they occur in germ cells; and (b) to compare these estimates with those available from studies reported in the literature of cases of partial monosomies and trisomies (i.e. loss or addition, respectively, of small chromosome segments). The main conclusion was that about two fifths of these translocations could generate viable imbalances in terms of abnormal progeny. More data are required before these figures can be used within the framework of risk assessment.

30. On the basis of limited data then available on the incidence of unbalanced structural rearrangements in new-borns and in spontaneous abortuses, the Committee estimated in its 1972 report that about 6% of all human conceptions with a structurally unbalanced chromosome complement could result in live births with congenital anomalies. This value was also used in the Committee's 1977 and 1982 reports. Recently, the Committee's attention was drawn to an error in these calculations, which when corrected gave a value of 3.5%. However, a further re-calculation using the more extensive data currently available led to a revised estimate of 9% of imbalanced products of balanced reciprocal translocations surviving to birth and resulting in congenitally malformed children.

31. In its 1982 report, the Committee estimated that the risk for the irradiation of males from the induction of dominant mutations (leading to genetic disease in the first generation progeny) lies in the range of one to two cases of affected individuals per million live-borns per milligray of sparsely ionizing, low-dose-rate, irradiation; the rough estimate of risk for the irradiation of females under similar conditions was 0-1 case per million live births. These estimates were based on the induction of dominant skeletal and cataract mutations in mice. New information from radiation-induced reduction of litter size in mice following exposure of parental males to x or gamma rays suggests the induction of genetic changes having dominant effects in the first generation and manifesting after birth at a stage earlier than that under scrutiny in the skeletal and cataract studies. The rate of induction of these changes appears to be about one half of that mentioned above for males. It seems probable that in the human species these lethals would act at some stage in early life.

32. In its 1977 and 1982 reports, the Committee estimated that the risk from the induction of autosomal recessive mutations (i.e. mutations in genes located on chromosomes other than the X) leading to recessive genetic disease was negligible, and it made no further attempts to quantify this risk. A recent study has shown that it is possible to provide a quantitative estimate for this class of disorders. These calculations, based on a combination of data from observations on human populations and from mouse experiments, show that a one-time exposure to a dose on the order of 1 milligray of sparsely ionizing, low-dose-rate, irradiation of the parental generation is not associated with any risk of induced recessive genetic disease in the first generation, thus confirming the earlier conclusion of the Committee. However, in the following ten generations, such an exposure may result in about one extra case per million live-borns by the tenth generation.

33. In 1982, the risk associated with the induction of structural chromosomal aberrations (predominantly reciprocal translocations) in males and females was estimated to lie between 0.03 and 1, and 0 and 0.3 cases, per million, respectively, of congenitally abnormal children per milligray of sparsely ionizing, low-dose-rate, irradiation. Using all the currently available data on primates, the Committee now estimates that the expected number of congenitally abnormal children ranges from 0.1 to 1.5, and 0 to 0.5, following irradiation of males and females, respectively (all rates expressed per million live births per milligray).

34. The risk estimates discussed so far are arrived at by using the so-called direct methods and pertain to effects expected in the first generation following a one-time radiation exposure of the parents. In contrast, the doubling dose method is primarily used to quantify risks under conditions of continuous radiation exposure. With this method, the expected risks are related to, and expressed as a fraction of, the spontaneous prevalence of Mendelian and chromosomal disorders as well as those of a more complex aetiology. The Committee sees no reason for any alteration of its 1982 estimates for autosomal dominant, X-linked and chromosomal disorders. These estimates are briefly recapitulated in the following (all estimates per milligray of continuous sparsely ionizing, low-dose-rate, irradiation of the parental generation and on a population of one million live births): (a) autosomal dominant and X-linked disorders, 10 cases of affected individuals at equilibrium and 1-2 cases in the first generation; and (b) chromosomal disorders (mainly those arising as a consequence of unbalanced structural anomalies), 0.4 case at equilibrium and 0.3 case in the first generation. In these calculations, the spontaneous prevalence figures assumed are: 1.0% dominant and X-linked disorders; 0.25% autosomal recessive; and 0.3% chromosomal disorders. The doubling dose was, furthermore, assumed to be 1 gray.

35. New data on congenital anomalies and other disorders of complex aetiology suggest that their spontaneous prevalence (especially of the latter) is higher than the estimates considered in the 1982 report (see paragraphs 13-14). This difference is mainly due to the inclusion of data on individuals up to 70 years of age in the recent studies, whereas an earlier one only contained data on individuals up to 21 years of age (the estimates from the latter were used in the 1977 and 1982 reports). Considerable uncertainties still remain on the following problems: (a) whether the doubling dose estimate of 1 gray (this is based on mouse data on clear-cut genetic end-points such as specific locus mutations, dominant visibles and reciprocal translocations) is valid for disorders of complex aetiology; and (b) whether the estimate of 5% mutational component used in the 1977 and 1982 reports is realistic for these disorders. In the absence of further information, particularly on the mechanisms of maintenance of these disorders in the population, and thus a basis for predicting a possible radiation-induced increase in their prevalence, the Committee is not in a position to provide risk estimates for these disorders.

36. The Committee continued to focus attention on detriment (handicap, years of life lost, years of handicapped life) associated with spontaneously arising genetic and partially genetic disorders, with the hope of eventually formulating an adequate framework to view the increases in such detriment at the individual and societal levels as a result of radiation exposures. Some limited information from the follow-up of children with sex chromosomal anomalies and autosomal balanced structural rearrangements shows: (a) that no individual with sex chromosomal anomalies has had any serious mental retardation; and (b) that balanced structural rearrangements are probably not as harmful as previous reports (based on cytogenetic studies of mentally retarded individuals and inmates of penitentiaries) have implied.

37. The results of a study on the estimation of detriment associated with spontaneously arising congenital anomalies in humans have been published. In this study, the authors used the live-birth prevalence

values derived in Hungary for these anomalies (about 60,000 per million live births) to estimate detriment in terms of years of life lost, years of potentially impaired life and years of actually impaired life. For the period and the population for which these estimates apply, the mean life expectancy is 70 years. Calculations show that, with a total prevalence of 60,000 per million live births (i.e. 60,000 individuals per million affected with one or another type of isolated or multiple congenital anomalies), about 480,000 years of life are lost, 2.0-3.7 million years of life are potentially impaired and, of the latter, 450,000 years of life are actually impaired per million live births.

38. In terms of the average number of years of life lost (an index of detriment at the individual level), the central nervous system anomalies cause the greatest amount of detriment (55 years), followed by anomalies of the respiratory and cardiovascular systems and chromosomal anomalies (about 25 years for each of these) and others. Anomalies of the ear, face and neck (including cleft lip, with or without cleft palate), of genital organs and of the musculo-skeletal system have a small or negligible effect in this regard.

However, when the ranking is done according to the total number of years of life lost (an index of detriment at the population level), anomalies of the cardiovascular system are associated with the highest amount of detriment (about 180,000 years per million live births), followed by those of the central nervous system (about 120,000 years per million live births), of the alimentary system (43,000 years per million live births) and others.

39. One possible crude way of expressing detriment is in terms of the number of years of actually impaired life. Expressed in this way, anomalies of the cardiovascular system are associated with the greatest amount of detriment (98,000 years per million live births), followed by those involving the genital organs (72,000 years per million live births), chromosomal anomalies (56,000 years per million live births) and others.

40. On the basis of the above analysis, a comparison of the detriment caused by congenital anomalies with that caused by monogenic disorders (the latter is discussed in the 1982 UNSCEAR report) reveals that detriment is much higher for congenital anomalies.

II. DOSE-RESPONSE RELATIONSHIPS FOR RADIATION-INDUCED CANCER

41. The Committee examined the nature of the dose-response relationships for a variety of cellular and sub-cellular radiobiological effects in vitro and in vivo. Under a number of simplifying assumptions, the quantitative information derived was used to fit various models of radiation action to cancer induction data in experimental animals and in humans, in an attempt to predict the possible shape of the dose-induction curves for cancer, at low doses and dose rates that, although most interesting for practical purposes, cannot be studied directly. These procedures enabled the Committee to suggest the most probable form that the relationships for several types of cancer would take under these conditions and the type of bias that might affect the estimates of risk coefficients at low doses and dose rates, if one or the other model should apply. This exercise is seen as an important preliminary step towards a re-evaluation of the risk estimates for radiation-induced cancer, which the Committee is planning to release in the near future.

42. In order to estimate the risk coefficient, i.e. the frequency, of radiation-induced cancer or the relative increase of tumour frequency per unit dose over the natural incidence at low doses and dose rates, two types of information are required: firstly, empirical data on the incidence of various forms of malignancy at relatively high doses where observations have actually been made; and, secondly, a knowledge of the form of the relationships linking the incidence of cancers with the radiation dose. Such data would allow predictions to be made of the cancer incidence at doses, and perhaps also at dose rates, very much lower than those at which direct observations are available in humans.

43. When the incidence of a given tumour in exposed animal or human populations is followed as a function of increasing dose, several findings are apparent. At relatively low doses (about 0.1 gray of sparsely ionizing radiation), only seldom (and then mostly in controlled animal experiments) can a statistically significant increase of cancer or leukaemia be shown. At higher doses (from a few to several grays, with considerable differences between different tumours), the incidence of such malignancies may be shown statistically to exceed the level observed in non-exposed control populations, the excess increasing as some function of the dose. At still higher doses (many grays) the incidence gradually starts to fall off, owing to cell killing. Dose-response relationships of this type, passing through a maximum at some intermediate dose, are often found in experimental animals.

44. The usual interpretation of such a shape postulates the concurrent presence of two different phenomena: (a) a dose-related increase of the proportion of normal cells that are transformed into malignant ones; and (b) a dose-related decrease of the probability that such cells may survive the radiation exposure. Both of these phenomena are normally operating in the region of doses where data are available, but to a different degree for various doses and different types of cancer. With this interpretation, some of the cells that would otherwise show transformation are killed, so that the fraction actually seen as transformed is reduced at high doses. What happens at the low doses, where direct information is lacking, may only be inferred from a combination of empirical data and theoretical assumptions, linked together into some models of radiation action.

45. The models referred to are simplified semi-quantitative representations of complex biological phenomena. Present knowledge of the mechanisms of carcinogenesis, including radiation carcinogenesis, is not adequate to design comprehensive models accounting for all physical and biological factors known to influence the induction of cancer. To avoid some of the complications involved, the Committee suggests that the range of doses over which extrapolations may meaningfully be performed should be limited to low and intermediate doses, below about 2 grays of sparsely ionizing radiation. Under these conditions, it seems likely that no serious distortions would result from non-stochastic radiation effects, which are observed when doses exceed fairly high thresholds, characteristic for each tissue and each effect.

46. The formulation and analysis of models of radiation carcinogenesis must rely on a few basic assumptions, as follows:

(a) The observed dose-response relationships for clinically visible tumours in vivo approximately reflect the relationship between dose and cancer initiation at the cellular level, despite host reactions and the effect of latency, which may modify this relationship to some degree. This assumption is based on the overall similarity of the dose-response curves for cancer induction with those of various other cellular effects of radiation. The Committee postulates this concept simply as a working hypothesis;

(b) Cancer initiation is believed to be a uni-cellular process occurring at random in single cells. This is also a working hypothesis that has not yet definitely been proved. However, evidence to the contrary, i.e. that cancer initiation takes place in several cells, is less convincing, although some limited evidence supports the idea. The uni-cellular theory of cancer induction is compatible with the notion that some, still ill-defined, influences resulting from irradiation of neighbouring cells or other organs may modify the probability that an initiated cell will develop into an overt malignancy. Firm biological evidence in favour of this last notion is very fragmentary;

(c) The absence of a dose threshold for induction is characteristic of many, if not all, tumours. For some animal tumours (e.g. tumours of the ovary or thymic lymphoma of the mouse), threshold-type dose-response relationships are observed. In other cases (e.g. tumours of the skin), cancer is only induced with great difficulty, i.e. after high doses of radiation. In still others (i.e. epidermoid lung cancer in humans), the data are unclear, owing perhaps to a short follow-up of the patients. In spite of these exceptions, however, the absence of a threshold dose is assumed by the Committee as a working hypothesis for the moment;

(d) The susceptibility of an irradiated animal or human population to tumour induction is assumed to follow a bell-shaped distribution. Although genetic predispositions to the development of some forms of malignancy are well documented, efforts to show that such phenomena apply also to radiation-induced human cancer have not been successful so far. Therefore, pending further studies, the same distribution of susceptibilities to the induction of cancer in irradiated and non-irradiated populations is also provisionally accepted as a working proposition.

47. On the above assumptions, it is possible to infer likely shapes for the dose-response relationships of radiation-induced cancer. Such inferences rely on the analysis of various other radiation effects observed at the cellular level. These effects involve the cells' genetic material, which is also thought to be the primary target for cancer initiation. The production of mutations and chromosomal aberrations in somatic and germinal cells and the oncogenic transformation in vitro of mammalian cell lines are examples of such effects. If cancer induction in vivo involves mechanisms similar to, or related to, those underlying the effects listed above, it is expected that all these phenomena will respond similarly with respect to changes in dose, dose rate and fractionation. As such similarities have actually been observed, it may be possible to extrapolate the shape of dose-response relationships between the effects mentioned above and the phenomenon of cancer induction.

48. Three basic non-threshold models of radiation action as a function of dose have been reviewed with respect to such cellular effects and to cancer initiation: the linear, the linear-quadratic and the pure quadratic models. Notwithstanding some exceptions, these may provide a general envelope for the dose-response curves of a variety of radiation-induced end-points at the cellular level, as well as for tumour induction in experimental animals and human populations.

49. The vast majority of dose-response curves for induction of point mutations and chromosomal aberrations by sparsely ionizing x rays and gamma rays can be described by a linear-quadratic model. For the same end-points, when cell killing is accounted for, a linear model usually applies to densely ionizing radiations, such as alpha particles or neutrons. As a rule, for a number of chromosomal structural abnormalities, curvilinearity (upward concavity) is observed for sparsely ionizing radiation. For the same effects and a wide range of doses, linearity prevails for densely ionizing particles. Linearity of the dose-response for somatic mutations and terminal chromosomal deletions has been found in some cell lines, even for sparsely ionizing radiation, although this is rare.

50. Approximate estimates of proportionality constants linking the chromosomal effects with the dose or its square may be obtained experimentally; they allow the frequency of such effects to be predicted at low doses and dose rates from observations at higher doses. For cancer induction, however, only fragmentary information supports the notion that similar quantitative relationships with the dose might apply. The Committee has estimated that, if the risk of tumour induction at 1 or 2 grays of sparsely ionizing radiation (at high dose rate) were extrapolated linearly down to zero dose, this procedure would overestimate the risk by a factor of up to five in typical situations.

51. Over the last few years, much information on radiation-induced oncogenic transformation of mammalian cells has become available. The cancerous nature of the transformed cells is shown by the fact that after transformation in vitro they are able to form malignant tumours upon transplantation back into animals, under appropriate conditions. Transformation in vitro is therefore regarded as a model, albeit a simplified one, of radiation carcinogenesis at the cellular level. Cells exposed in vitro to sparsely ionizing radiation 24 hours after seeding are transformed according to complex kinetics that cannot be fitted to models used for other cellular effects, such as cell killing. Moreover, fractionation of the dose (below 1.5 grays total) has in some instances appeared to enhance transformation, which is contrary to what would be predicted by a linear-quadratic model; in other instances, however, it has clearly not enhanced transformation.

52. Further research is needed to reconcile such conflicting observations on the nature of the response after fractionation at low doses. Several experiments indicate that anomalous results can arise from atypical conditions of cellular growth soon after establishment of the culture. In fact, irradiation of non-dividing cells or cells under exponential growth conditions (which are thought to be more representative of an asynchronously dividing cell population in vivo) produces results that are compatible with those obtained for other cellular effects; thus, for example, high-dose-rate gamma irradiation results in a greater frequency of transformation than low-dose-rate exposure.

53. There are indications that, when cells are irradiated with neutrons, low dose rates or dose fractionation may increase the rate of transformation, even at low doses. However, whereas some observations on tumour induction in experimental animals clearly support these findings, others do not. In other experiments,

enhanced transformation by neutron fractionation or protraction was seen only at intermediate and high doses. In view of the paucity of such data and of the uncertainties involved, further research is needed before enhancement of cancer induction by neutron fractionation and protraction (relative to single or high-dose-rate exposure) can be accepted for the purposes of risk assessment. Such a possibility should, however, be kept in mind, even though the theoretical basis to explain these phenomena is uncertain at present.

54. Recent experimental findings on radiation-induced tumours in experimental animals have not substantially changed the main conclusions reached in annex I of the 1977 UNSCEAR report. Most data support the notion that dose-response relationships for x rays and gamma rays tend to be curvilinear and concave upward at low doses. Under these conditions, tumour induction is dose-rate dependent, in that a reduction of the dose rate, or fractionation, reduces the tumour yield. A linear extrapolation of the risk from high doses delivered at high rates to zero dose would thus, as a rule, overestimate the real risk at low doses and dose rates. However, in one experimental mammary tumour system (matched by epidemiological data on human breast cancer), irradiation with x rays and gamma rays produced a linear dose response with little fractionation and dose-rate dependence.

55. For densely ionizing neutron irradiation, tumour induction in animals follows in general a very nearly linear curve at the lower end of the dose scale and shows little dependence on dose rate. In some cases, however, enhancement upon fractionation (and possibly protraction) has been noted. Above about 0.1 gray, the curve tends to become concave downward, markedly so in some cases. Under these conditions, a linear extrapolation of the risk down from intermediate or high doses and dose rates would involve a variable degree of underestimation.

56. The Committee reviewed existing data on dose-response relationships for radiation-induced tumours in man. This whole matter must be treated with caution because, at present, observations are very fragmentary, those for neutrons totally absent, and definitive data for atomic bomb survivors at Hiroshima and Nagasaki are still not available. For example, dose-response data for sparsely ionizing radiation have not been reported for lung and bone tumours, while data for densely ionizing radiation have not been reported for thyroid and mammary cancer. For sparsely ionizing radiation, the data available in some cases (lung, thyroid and breast) are consistent with linear or linear-quadratic models. For breast cancer, linearity may, however, predominate, as the incidence is little affected by dose fractionation. The linearity of the response for lung cancer after exposure to alpha particles from radon daughters does not contradict the above statement, because the dose-squared component with alpha particles is minimal. Some doubts still remain, however, as to osteosarcoma induced by bone-seeking alpha- or beta-emitting radionuclides. Thus, in spite of the fragmentary character of the data from humans, a general picture is emerging from which several tentative conclusions can be derived.

57. For sparsely ionizing radiation, linear extrapolation downwards from about 2 grays would not overestimate the risk of breast and possibly thyroid cancer, would slightly overestimate the risk of leukaemia, and would definitely overestimate the risk of bone sarcoma. A lack of direct evidence does not permit any assessment to be made of the magnitude of the overestimate for lung cancer.

58. For densely ionizing radiation, the risk of lung cancer from accumulated exposures to radon decay products at low dose rates from dose levels roughly corresponding to 20-50 sieverts would neither be overestimated nor underestimated by linear extrapolation to very low doses. However, extrapolation from observations made at higher cumulative exposures might result in a significant underestimation owing to observed flattening (saturation) of the dose-response curve in this region. It should be stressed that the absolute risk coefficients derived for male miners, of whom a high proportion are smokers, should not be applied to the general public without due corrections for various factors (intensity of smoking, lung ventilation rate, presence of other contaminating pollutants etc.) that are thought to increase the risk in miners.

59. The incidence of bone sarcoma after alpha-particle internal irradiation by long-lived bone-seeking radionuclides is distorted by the existence of a pronounced inverse relationship between accumulated dose and latent period, resulting in an apparent threshold at low doses. If this is a correct explanation for the upward concavity of the dose-response relationship, a linear extrapolation from a mean skeletal dose of a few tens of grays down to the milligray region would grossly overestimate the risk.

60. No data on the induction of breast cancer and leukaemia in humans by densely ionizing radiations are available at present and therefore no direct inferences can be made about risk extrapolation to the low-dose domain. On the basis of general knowledge, if the risk at intermediate doses could be derived from data on sparsely ionizing radiation (suitably corrected for the greater effectiveness of the densely ionizing particles), a linear extrapolation down to low doses might either underestimate or correctly estimate the real risk in these cases.

61. For radiation-induced cancers of other organs, only data on experimental animals are available. For sparsely ionizing radiations, upward concave curvilinear dose-response relationships with pronounced dose-rate and fractionation effects are usually found. If similar curves apply to cancers in humans, a linear extrapolation of risk coefficients (obtained at the intermediate dose region after acute irradiation) to the low dose and low dose rates would very likely overestimate the real risk, possibly by a factor of up to five. For densely ionizing radiation, should relevant values become available, a linear extrapolation from high to intermediate doses would probably underestimate the risk.

62. Upon close inspection of the data, some regularities seem to emerge that may indirectly help in assessing the character of dose-response relationships

in humans. A similarity in the shape of the relationships was noted between humans and experimental animals for tumours of several organs for which reasonably good information exists: mammary and thyroid cancer (sparsely ionizing radiations) and lung and bone cancers (densely ionizing radiations). Should this pattern be confirmed, knowledge derived from epidemiological studies in humans at intermediate or high doses, and from the shape of the dose-response relationships in several animal species, would make it possible to assess the bias introduced by linear extrapolation of the risk coefficients to low doses.

III. BIOLOGICAL EFFECTS OF PRE-NATAL IRRADIATION

63. **The Committee reviewed the following: modern knowledge of developmental events, particularly in the brain of mammalian embryos and fetuses; recent data on effects induced by irradiation of animals in utero; and findings concerning children exposed to radiation in the mother's womb during the atomic bombings at Hiroshima and Nagasaki. These, and a large body of older data, were used to derive quantitative estimates of risk for a number of radiation effects in utero, such as the induction of death, malformations, severe mental retardation and cancer. For the small doses and dose rates of radiation likely to be encountered in practice, the risk is judged to be relatively small in comparison with the natural incidence of congenital anomalies in non-irradiated individuals.**

64. The consequences of pre-natal radiation exposure have attracted much attention since the last review of this subject by the Committee in 1977. New information from experimental animals irradiated in utero, recent findings of human embryology (particularly in the central nervous system) and a review of dosimetric and clinical data on children exposed before birth during the atomic explosions of Hiroshima and Nagasaki, called for a new study of this subject. There was also a need for a detailed re-assessment of effects such as the induction of malignancies following irradiation in utero, which had not been covered in depth in the 1977 report.

65. The Committee had already identified and described the main consequences of pre-natal exposure in mammals and had roughly classified them as follows: (a) lethal effects, induced by relatively small doses before or immediately after implantation of the embryo into the uterine wall, or induced after increasingly higher doses during all stages of intra-uterine development, to be expressed either before or after birth; (b) malformations, characteristic of the period of major organogenesis when the main body structures are formed, and especially of the most active phase of cell multiplication in the relevant structures; (c) growth disturbances without malformations induced at all stages of development, but particularly in the latter part of pregnancy; and (d) miscellaneous effects on various body structures and functions. The Committee had concluded, on the basis of considerable experimental evidence available at that time, that killing of cells, mainly through the induction of chromosomal aberrations, was the common mechanism underlying all these effects; any differences were particularly related to the time during development when the radiation insult was applied.

66. It should be realized that congenital anomalies arise in all animal species even in the absence of any radiation beyond that received from natural sources. Human malformations may be classified, according to their cause, into: those that can be traced back to the mutation of single genes (representing about 6% of all malformations scored at birth); those originating from the incorrect interplay of numerous genetic factors (about 50%); those due to the presence of chromosomal anomalies (about 5%); and those caused by some known environmental teratologic agents (about 6%). There is no apparent cause for about one third of all malformations. The incidence of congenital anomalies depends to a large extent on the time at which they are scored. If a level of about 6% incidence of malformed babies at birth (birth prevalence) is taken as an average value for the human species, a higher value applies to embryos and fetuses before birth, because the malformed new-borns are only the carriers of the relatively milder forms, which are compatible with life. Some malformations disappear after birth, although more become evident that are not scored at birth. Thus, the global incidence of malformations roughly doubles if grown-up children, rather than new-born babies, are examined. The global incidence figures are, however, highly dependent on a large variety of factors and so are the figures pertaining to the various classes of malformations. Any assessment of the radiation's effectiveness in inducing damage in utero must be viewed against this natural level of inborn defects and its variable expression.

67. The Committee reviewed much information derived from human specimens and experiments in non-human primates, establishing to an increasing degree of detail and precision the developmental events that are important for their radiobiological consequences. Morphological embryology is gradually providing an accurate description of the stages in embryonic human growth, in good agreement with the results of non-invasive clinical measurements. The newest findings are increasingly pointing to the cerebral cortex as an extremely sensitive structure in human development, particularly (but not exclusively) in early pre-natal life, from the eighth to the fifteenth week after fertilization. At the same time, the microscopic study of the brain cortex is providing a very detailed picture of the cellular events leading to the formation of this structure as development proceeds. Such morphological analyses are integrated by biochemical studies, which help to provide an overall description of the structure and function of the developing brain.

68. These studies show the formation of the cerebral cortex as a carefully programmed and unique sequence of events in which cell division, migration and maturation are taking place concomitantly. Numerical, spatial and temporal relationships between various types of cells must be maintained with a high degree of precision in order for the brain cortex to be correctly assembled and its function normally developed. Disruption of this programme of cellular and tissue phenomena by radiation, coupled with the

limited capacity for repair of neurons, the functional brain cells, may cause irreversible damage. Whether radiation impinges on the reproductive capacity of the primitive brain cells, interferes with the orderly migration to their ultimate position in the cortex, or inhibits establishment of the appropriate cellular connection, the net result of the radiation insult is manifested in a loss of cerebral, particularly mental, function. This is the picture, albeit very schematic, emerging from the available data. However, the morphological and functional complexity of the developing brain cortex defies any simple interpretation of radiation effects, on the basis of the criteria applying to other self-renewing tissues of the body.

69. Pre-natal development of mammals in utero may be roughly divided into three periods: the pre-implantation, extending from fertilization to settling of the embryo into the uterine wall; the major organogenesis, characterized by the formation of the main body structures; and the fetal period, during which growth of the structures already formed takes place. There is a very large variability in the relative duration of these periods between animal species, as well as in the total duration of intra-uterine life. Also, at any given stage of development, the state of differentiation or maturation of any one structure, with respect to all the others, varies considerably in different species.

70. There have been no new findings in humans on the effects of radiation during the pre-implantation phase, owing presumably to the difficulties of obtaining information during this stage. In animals, however, many new data have been produced by analyses in vitro and in vivo. These data have mainly confirmed the special sensitivity of the pre-implantation embryo to killing and a decreasing sensitivity with increasing developmental complexity, with ample oscillations of the responses as a function of time, particularly during the earliest phases of embryonic development. In the rodent, doses on the order of one-tenth of a gray or less have been reported to increase mortality significantly for irradiation during pre-implantation.

71. For irradiation during the phase of major organogenesis, new data on experimental animals have added details to the previously known picture, but have not substantially altered its main features. At this stage, malformative effects emerge as the most prominent consequences of irradiation, sometimes accompanied by growth disturbances of various structures or of the whole body. The presence of maximum sensitivity periods at the time of the main differentiation of the various structures results in a marked time dependence for the appearance of various types of malformation. Some malformations, particularly those of the skeleton, have been very well studied as a function of dose, generally confirming a curvilinear trend; others, especially those of the central nervous system, have been carefully analysed in terms of cellular events and reactions leading to their formation.

72. Contrary to what is observed in experimental animals, radiation-induced malformations of body structures other than the central nervous system are uncommon in humans. The Committee has discussed the reasons for such a difference. Beyond any explanation, however, the discrepancies between different species must be taken as a warning against indiscriminate attempts to project findings across species, without due consideration of the embryological characteristics of each species; short of this, any extrapolations, particularly the quantitative ones, would be unwarranted.

73. Radiation-induced damage to the central nervous system in humans is first observed at the conventionally assumed end of organogenesis (eight weeks post-fertilization) and extends well into the fetal period (up to 25 weeks). A re-examination of the dosimetric and clinical findings in individuals irradiated in utero at the time of the atomic explosions in Japan has allowed an important step forward to be made in the analysis of effects and the establishment of a risk estimate in man. At the same time, morphological and biochemical studies on human samples have established a clear-cut correlation between the time of maximum sensitivity of the brain structures and the time of most intense division and migration of the neurons in the brain cortex, thus extending to man a concept found to be valid for experimental animals.

74. A study of about 1600 children exposed in utero at Hiroshima and Nagasaki to various doses and at various developmental stages has confirmed that about 30 of them have shown clinically severe mental retardation, an incidence far higher than would normally be expected. When the occurrence of this condition was studied as a function of developmental stage at the time of the bombing, it was found that mental retardation was not observed before 8 weeks from conception, was at a maximum between 8 and 15 weeks when neuronal proliferation in the cortex is most active, and then was somewhat lower between 16 and 25 weeks, when the supporting tissues in the brain develop and connections between neuronal cells are established. The incidence of mental retardation as a function of dose is reported to be apparently linear without threshold at 8-15 weeks, with a risk coefficient of 0.4 per gray. The incidence is about four times lower at 16-25 weeks. There is an indication that, in addition to these extreme mental handicaps, other less prominent functional brain deficits might be present in children irradiated in utero, and it is expected that this cohort will eventually yield more useful information. While some aspects of these findings may not yet be explained on available radiobiological knowledge, there is no doubt as to their overall interest, particularly with respect to the quantification of the attendant risk.

75. A variety of effects have been documented in the experimental animal following irradiation during the fetal stages, including effects on the haemopoietic system, the liver and the kidney, all occurring, however, after fairly high radiation doses. The effects on the developing gonads have been particularly well documented, both morphologically and functionally. There appears to be at present little correspondence between the cellular and functional damage as a function of dose, but doses of a few tenths of a gray as

a minimum are necessary to produce fertility changes in various animal species.

76. Data on effects in utero following the uptake of radioactive subtances by the mother and their passage to the developing fetus are very fragmentary, particularly in view of the many variables that may influence the dose eventually delivered to the conceptus. Among the most important variables, the following should be mentioned: the physical and chemical characteristics of the radionuclides; the route and schedule of administration; and the kinetics of transfer and metabolism in the mother, through the placenta and into the fetus. Only for some nuclides of practical importance (tritium, plutonium, iodine) is the amount of information slightly more extensive, but there is clearly a need to enlarge the data base in a systematic way to other nuclides and to investigate an adequate range of concentrations and tissue doses.

77. A number of physical and chemical factors have been reported that appear to modify the response of the developing mammals, but here again the information is insufficient for broad generalizations. Among the physical factors, both the type and energy of the radiation, with values of the relative biological effectiveness (RBE) on the order of five for neutrons at intermediate doses, have been examined in some detail. Fractionation and protraction of the dose have also been investigated for both sparsely and densely ionizing radiations and have consistently produced a reduced effect in comparison with singly administered doses. The picture emerging from these data is sketchy, however, and leaves conspicuous gaps in our knowledge. Among the chemical factors, oxygen and a variety of radio-protective and radio-sensitizing drugs have been proved (at least qualitatively) to have modifying effects in developing tissues similar to those seen in adult tissues. There have also been some scattered results from combined treatments of radiation with other agents, although much more systematic work would be required to substantiate some claims, particularly those of synergistically active treatments.

78. The Committee has reviewed in some depth the data available on the induction of tumours in animals irradiated pre-natally, in an attempt to compare their susceptibility with that of animals irradiated after birth. Such comparisons are rendered particularly difficult, however, owing to variations in species, strain and sex, the lack of extended time- and dose-response analyses, and the interplay of various biological end-points. In the Committee's opinion, the available evidence fails to substantiate the existence of a higher susceptibility to radiation-induced carcinogenesis of animals in utero, and points, on the contrary, to a lower susceptibility. Differences in tumour types arising in animals irradiated before or after birth are probably the most consistent finding in the work analysed, a finding that is not unexpected in view of the different developmental stages of the animals at irradiation.

79. In humans, evidence on tumour induction by pre-natal irradiation comes essentially from two major sources: firstly, children that survived in utero irradiation at Hiroshima and Nagasaki, and that have continued to show no evidence of excess cancer in the studies conducted so far; secondly, two large retrospective studies of children exposed in utero for medical reasons. The latter children have consistently shown an excess of tumour and leukaemia cases over the first 10-15 years of their post-natal life, to a level roughly 50% above the natural incidence for the low (but not very well known) doses involved. Correction of the data for a number of social and medical factors that might have distorted the association between irradiation and incidence of tumours in those children was insufficient to cancel the correlation entirely. The Committee has reviewed and discussed several inconsistencies between the experimental and the human findings, as well as between the epidemiological findings themselves.

80. Beyond the existence of the association itself, which appears to be sufficiently well established, the most significant issue in this respect concerns the causality of the pre-natal radiation treatment in increasing the post-natal incidence of leukaemia and cancer. The Committee believes that the important consideration in these matters is the existence of the association. Denying the causal relationships on the basis of the overall inconsistency of the experimental and epidemiological findings would mean emphasizing scientific considerations over the practical need of allowing for any possible risk. The Committee has therefore decided to accept provisionally the causal nature of the association for practical purposes, while emphasizing that this is simply on account of prudence and not on any firmly established scientific grounds.

81. At the end of its review, the Committee attempted to derive quantitative risk estimates for a number of radiation-induced effects in utero (mortality, induction of malformations, mental retardation, tumours and leukaemia) and to attribute the risk to the periods of pregnancy over which it applies. Under a number of qualifying assumptions, it is possible to conclude that, for the small doses likely to be encountered in practice, the overall risk is relatively small (no more than 0.002 for the live-born at 0.01 gray) in relation to the natural incidence of malformations in non-irradiated individuals, which is on the order of 0.06 in the human species.

LIST OF MEMBERS OF NATIONAL DELEGATIONS

List of experts attending the thirty-first to the thirty-fifth sessions
as official representatives or members of national delegations

ARGENTINA

D. Beninson (Representative), D. Cancio, A.J. Gonzalez

AUSTRALIA

K.H. Lokan (Representative)

BELGIUM

M. Errera (Representative), J. Maisin (Representative),
J.B.T. Aten, F.H. Sobels, A.D. Tates

BRAZIL

L.R. Caldas (Representative), E. Penna Franca (Representative)

CANADA

E.G. Letourneau (Representative), A.M. Marko (Representative), W.R. Bush, G.C. Butler, D.K. Myers

CZECHOSLOVAKIA

M. Klímek (Representative)

EGYPT

S. El-Din Hashish (Representative), M. El-Kharadly

FRANCE

H. Jammet (Representative), P. Pellerin, A. Bouville,
R. Coulon, B. Dutrillaux, J. Lafuma, R. Masse

GERMANY, FEDERAL REPUBLIC OF

A. Kaul (Representative), F.E. Stieve, U. Ehling, W. Jacobi,
H. Kriegel, C. Streffer

INDIA

K. Sundaram (Representative)

INDONESIA

A. Baiquni (Representative), M. Ridwan (Representative),
O. Iskandar (Representative)

JAPAN

T. Kumatori (Representative), J. Inaba, R. Ichikawa,
Y. Kameyama, A. Kasai, A. Yamato

MEXICO

J.R. Ortiz Magaña (Representative)

PERU

M. Zaharia (Representative), L.V. Pinillos Ashton (Representative)

POLAND

Z. Jaworowski (Representative)

SUDAN

A. Hidayatalla (Representative), A.A. Yousif

SWEDEN

B. Lindell (Representative), K. Edvarson, L.-E. Holm,
K.G. Lüning, S. Mattsson, J.O. Snihs, J. Valentin,
G. Walinder

UNION OF SOVIET SOCIALIST REPUBLICS

L.A. Ilyin (Representative), A. Guskova (Representative),
E. Golubkin, D.F. Khokhlova, A.A. Moiseev, Yu.I. Moskalev,
V. Pavlinov, O. Pavlovsky, V.V. Redkin, V.A. Shevchenko

UNITED KINGDOM OF GREAT BRITAIN AND NORTHERN IRELAND

J. Dunster (Representative), J.H. Edwards, K.E. Halnan,
P.S. Harper, A. Searle

UNITED STATES OF AMERICA

R.D. Moseley (Representative), R.E. Anderson, R. Baker,
C. Edington, J.H. Harley, H.H. Rossi, W.L. Russell,
P.B. Selby, W.K. Sinclair, J.W. Thiessen, H.O. Wyckoff

Appendix II

LIST OF SCIENTIFIC STAFF AND CONSULTANTS WHO HAVE CO-OPERATED WITH THE COMMITTEE IN THE PREPARATION OF THIS REPORT

A. Czeizel
A.M. Kellerer
J. Liniecki
K. Sankaranarayanan
G. Silini
F.D. Sowby

Appendix III

LIST OF REPORTS RECEIVED BY THE COMMITTEE

1. Listed below are reports received by the Committee from Governments between 11 November 1982 and 14 April 1986.

2. Reports received by the Committee before 11 November 1982 were listed in earlier reports of the Committee to the General Assembly.

Document No.	Country	Title
A/AC.82/G/L.		
1673	Czechoslovakia	The values of strontium-90 concentration in vertebrae
1674	Union of Soviet Socialist Republics	Ingestion of global strontium-90 and caesium-137 with the food ration of the population of the Soviet Union 1976-1979
1675	Germany, Federal Republic of	Environmental radioactivity and radiation levels—annual report 1979
1676	United Kingdom of Great Britain and Northern Ireland	Radioactive fallout in air and rain: results to the end of 1981
1677	United Kingdom of Great Britain and Northern Ireland	Environmental radioactivity surveillance programme: results for the UK for 1981
1678	Switzerland	25th report of the Federal Commission on radioactivity for the year 1981
1679	Union of Soviet Socialist Republics	Combined effects of radionuclides and external irradiation on the organism of rats
1680	Union of Soviet Socialist Republics	Studies on the radiation health in the Russian Soviet Socialist Republic (RSFSR) following the stratospheric fallout of strontium-90 and caesium-137 1963-1978
1681	Union of Soviet Socialist Republics	Calculations of microdosimetry characteristics for heavy charged particles with energy levels of 2-10 MeV/nucleon
1682	Czechoslovakia	The values of stable strontium in vertebrae, femoral diaphyses, and their ratio in different age groups (1970-1973)
1683	Germany, Federal Republic of	Environmental radioactivity and radiation levels—annual report 1980
1684	Union of Soviet Socialist Republics	Combined effects of radiation and chemical factors
1685	France	Surveillance de la radioactivité en 1981
1686	Belgium	Radioactivity measured at Mol 1980
1687	United States of America	Environmental Measurements Laboratory: Environmental report, 1 May 1982
1688	United States of America	Environmental Measurements Laboratory: Worldwide deposition of strontium-90 through 1981
1689	United Kingdom of Great Britain and Northern Ireland	Radioactive fallout in air and rain: results to the end of 1982
1690	New Zealand	Environmental Radioactivity Annual Report 1982
1691	Czechoslovakia	Lung cancer in exposed human populations and dose-effect relationship—July 1983

Document No.	Country	Title
1692	United Kingdom of Great Britain and Northern Ireland	Environmental radioactivity surveillance programme: results for the UK for 1982
1693	Union of Soviet Socialist Republics	Brief results of a study into the combined effect of ionizing radiation and other environmental factors in the Ukrainian SSR
1694	Union of Soviet Socialist Republics	Relative biological effectiveness of protons and heavy ions
1695	Union of Soviet Socialist Republics	Study of the vertical migrations of radionuclides in the bottom deposits and soil of a body of water with no through current
1696	United States of America	Environmental Measurements Laboratory: Graphic presentation of strontium-90 fallout data 1954-1982
1697	Switzerland	26th report of the Federal Commission on radioactivity for the year 1982
1698	France	Surveillance de la radioactivité en 1982
1699	Union of Soviet Socialist Republics	Mechanisms of the competitive effect of iron on the exchange processes of plutonium-239 in the organism
1700	New Zealand	Environmental Radioactivity Annual Report 1983
1701	United States of America	Strontium-90 in the U.S. diet, 1982
1702	United States of America	Worldwide deposition of strontium-90 through 1982
1703	Japan	Radioactivity Survey Data in Japan, Number 65, June 1983
1704	Switzerland	27th report of the Federal Commission on radioactivity for the year 1983
1705	United Kingdom of Great Britain and Northern Ireland	Environmental radioactivity surveillance programme: results for the UK for 1983
1706	United Kingdom of Great Britain and Northern Ireland	The radiation exposure of the UK population— 1984 review
1707	United States of America	The high altitude sampling program: radioactivity in the stratosphere
1708	Germany, Federal Republic of	Environmental radioactivity and radiation levels in the years 1981/82
1709	United States of America	Strontium-90 in the human bone in the US, 1982
1710	United States of America	Annual report of the surface air sampling program (EML-440)
1711	United Kingdom of Great Britain and Northern Ireland	Radioactive fallout in air and rain: results to the end of 1983
1712	Japan	Radioactivity Survey Data in Japan, Number 68, March 1984
1713	Japan	Radioactivity Survey Data in Japan, Number 69, June 1984
1714	Union of Soviet Socialist Republics	Radiation doses of workers using radio-isotope devices in industry
1715	Union of Soviet Socialist Republics	Justification of assessments of the carcinogenic risk associated with low-dose radiation
1716	Union of Soviet Socialist Republics	Assessment of the possibility of using an iron preparation for optimal monitoring of the plutonium-239 content in the human body
1717	Union of Soviet Socialist Republics	Radiation loads from pharmaceutical preparations marked by radioactive iodine isotopes

Document No.	Country	Title
1718	Union of Soviet Socialist Republics	The effect of differences in the radiosensitivity of cells in certain persons to the accuracy of the extrapolation of dose ratios to low-dose values
1719	Union of Soviet Socialist Republics	Quantitative evaluation of the diagnostic informativeness of the test for the absorption of radioiodine by the thyroid gland in various forms of thyroidal pathology
1720	Union of Soviet Socialist Republics	Radiation exposure of the population of the USSR during 1981-1982 as a result of the use of ionizing radiation sources for medical diagnostic purposes
1721	Union of Soviet Socialist Republics	Site approach in the simulation of survival curves as a function of radiation quality
1722	Union of Soviet Socialist Republics	On the assessment of the effect of incorporated radionuclides and external radiation on the basis of non-stochastic effects
1723	New Zealand	Environmental Radioactivity Annual Report 1984
1724	Union of Soviet Socialist Republics	The influence of non-radiation factors on the kinetics of radioactive iodine metabolism in the thyroid
1725	Union of Soviet Socialist Republics	Some problems of biological effects under the combined action of nitrogen oxides, their metabolites and radiation
1726	United States of America	Occupational exposure to ionizing radiation in the United States—a comprehensive review for the year 1980 and a summary of trends for the years 1960-1985
1727	United States of America	Environmental Measurements Laboratory: Worldwide deposition of strontium-90 through 1983
1728	United Kingdom of Great Britain and Northern Ireland	Radioactive fallout in air and rain: results to the end of 1984
1729	Switzerland	28th report of the Federal Commission on radioactivity for the year 1984
1730	Japan	Radioactivity Survey Data in Japan, Number 70, September 1984
1731	Japan	Radioactivity Survey Data in Japan, Number 71, December 1984

Scientific Annexes

ANNEX A

Genetic effects of radiation

CONTENTS

28

Introduction

1. The 1982 UNSCEAR Report [U1] presented a comprehensive review of data on the genetic effects of ionizing radiation in eukaryotes together with quantitative estimates of genetic risks in man. Since then, some advances have been made in a number of areas relevant to the work of the Committee. The purpose of this review is to cover these advances, focusing attention on the following main themes: (a) the prevalence of naturally occurring Mendelian and chromosomal disorders and those of complex aetiology in humans; (b) the application of recombinant DNA technology to the analysis of the human genome and genetic disease; (c) further data on genes, chromosomes and cancer in man; (d) movable genetic elements and their relevance to the estimation of spontaneous mutation rates and evaluation of genetic risks using the doubling dose method; (e) basic studies on the mechanisms of induction of chromosomal aberrations in eukaryotic systems including mammalian and human somatic cells; and (f) other data that bear, either directly or indirectly, on the evaluation of genetic radiation hazards in humans and on the quantification of genetic detriment.

I. THE PREVALENCE OF NATURALLY OCCURRING MENDELIAN AND CHROMOSOMAL DISORDERS AND THOSE OF COMPLEX AETIOLOGY

A. CONCEPTS AND DEFINITIONS

2. Under the heading Mendelian disorders are included autosomal dominant, X-linked and autosomal recessive conditions, inherited in a simple Mendelian fashion. Different genotypes are thus due to two or more alleles at a single locus (so-called unifactorial or unilocal inheritance). The chromosomal disorders are those that are associated with structural or numerical changes of chromosomes. Disorders of complex aetiology include: (a) congenital anomalies (which are present at birth irrespective of whether they are detected at that time or not); and (b) other disorders, most of which are not manifest at birth but have variable ages of onset, many manifesting late in life. A major proportion of disorders of complex aetiology do not show a simple Mendelian pattern of inheritance. Twin and family studies suggest that their aetiology is multifactorial, depending on polygenic genetic pre-

disposition and environmental factors, which may also be multiple. Among the features common to these disorders are, firstly, the proportion of first-degree relatives affected is much larger than in the general population and, secondly, there is a sharp decrease in the proportion affected on passing from first- to second- to third-degree relatives. The terms irregularly inherited, polygenic, and multifactorial are often used to denote these disorders. In this document, the term multifactorial disorders is used here synonymously with disorders of complex aetiology and, for convenience, is considered under two headings: (a) congenital anomalies; and (b) other multifactorial disorders.

B. MENDELIAN DISORDERS

3. Some new data on the prevalence of certain Mendelian disorders have become available since the publication of the 1982 UNSCEAR report [G20-G22, G61-G63, H22, Y6]. These, however, do not require any revision of the Committee's earlier overall prevalence estimates to be made for these disorders (1.0%, autosomal dominant and X-linked, 0.25%, autosomal recessives). Similarly, the review of Matsunaga [M1] on this subject is based essentially on the same material that was extensively reviewed in the 1977 [U2] and 1982 [U1] UNSCEAR reports and will not be gone into here.

4. The findings of Altukhov [A10] (subsequently published by Dubinin and Altukhov [D23]) on the frequencies of rare (non-polymorphic) electrophoretic variants in normal healthy new-borns (500 children), and in premature infants and babies with multiple congenital anomalies (227 infants) were briefly alluded to in the 1982 UNSCEAR report. These data showed that: (a) the frequencies of these variants (at over 20 genetic loci coding for the synthesis of enzyme proteins and erythrocyte antigens) were about an order of magnitude higher in premature infants and in babies with congenital anomalies than in the healthy new-born controls; and (b) a sizeable proportion of the variants in the study group was due to de novo mutations, suggesting that mutations of this type could play an important role in the genesis of congenital defects and/or prematurity.

5. In order to confirm these results, Neel and Mohrenweiser [N40] conducted a study to determine rare electrophoretic variant frequencies (haemoglobin and a set of serum proteins and erythrocyte antigens) in blood samples derived from 178 children who were either born prematurely or had congenital anomalies (31 premature, 27 with chromosomal abnormalities and physical defects and 120 with congenital anomalies not known to be associated with chromosomal anomalies). Similar data (the placental cord blood series) from new-born infants in Ann Arbor provided information on control frequencies of these variants (see also [N17]). A total of 5341 determinations (10,603 locus tests) involving 45 proteins were made in the study group and 108,963 determinations (215,609 locus tests) in the control. There were 15 rare variants in the study group (0.00141 per locus tested) and 236

in the control (0.00109 per locus tested). Thus, there was no strong evidence for an excess of rare variants in the study group; furthermore, all these variants were present in one or the other parent, indicating no new mutational events.

C. CHROMOSOMAL ANOMALIES

6. New data on chromosomal anomalies in man have come from cytogenetic studies involving spontaneous abortions and still births, new-born babies, amniocentesis programmes, mentally retarded or otherwise handicapped individuals, infertile males, direct analysis of human spermatozoa and of fertilized eggs and heritable fragile sites. These data will be discussed in the following paragraphs.

1. Chromosomal anomalies in spontaneous abortions and still births

7. The cytogenetics of pregnancy wastage has recently been reviewed by Boué et al. [B78]. Hook [H1] re-examined the available data [H2, H62, S1, W1] on the contribution of chromosomal anomalies to spontaneous abortions and still births from the standpoint of gestational age. His analysis, summarized in Table 1, shows that 40% of spontaneous abortions occurring in weeks 5-28 are associated with chromosomal anomalies. In the weeks 5-7 the rate is lower (17.5%), rising to nearly 50% in weeks 8-15, decreasing to about 30% at 16-19 weeks and dropping to 10% at 20-27 weeks. The overall rate estimated by Hook of 40% of spontaneous abortions associated with chromosomal anomalies is lower than the 50% commonly assumed. The latter figure, however, allows for developmental arrests that probably occur before the fifth week of gestation (although in these cases, the pregnancy might be unrecognized and such early specimens are seldom received for examination). In still births (those born dead at or after 28 weeks), the overall rate is 5.7% [K1, S1].

8. Hook used the results of the above analysis to obtain approximate estimates of cytogenetic abnormalities for all embryonic and fetal deaths, including still births. These estimates, summarized in Table 2, show that about 15.5% of all conceptuses recognized from the fifth week of gestation onwards do not survive to live birth. The proportion of all recognized pregnancies associated with both embryonic or fetal death and a cytogenetic abnormality is 4.5%. Thus 4.5/15.5 or roughly 30% of all embryonic and fetal deaths recognized after the fourth week of gestation are associated with a chromosomal abnormality. Since about 0.6% of new-born babies carry chromosomal anomalies [U1], the proportion of recognizable conceptions with a chromosomal anomaly can be estimated as 4.5 + (0.6% × 84.5%) = 5.0%.

9. The 1982 UNSCEAR report discussed data on the delineation of the parental origin of the extra chromosome in individuals with trisomy-21, using cytologically detectable heteromorphism of chromosome 21. Those results, from over 300 informative families, showed that,

while there were considerable variations between studies with respect to the proportion of cases attributable to maternal or paternal non-disjunction, most trisomy-21 resulted from non-disjunction occurring in maternal meiosis-I (65-80%); the contribution of errors in spermatogenesis and maternal meiosis-II was small, but significant (20-35%).

10. Hassold et al. [H23] have extended this approach to trisomies involving chromosomes 3, 4, 9, 13, 14, 15, 16, 21 and 22 in spontaneous abortions. Chromosome heteromorphisms of the parents and trisomic fetuses were compared using either QFQ-banding or Q-banding with dichloromethoxyacridine/spermine for evaluation of trisomies-3, -4, -13, -15, -21 and -22 and either CBG-banding or distamycin/DAPI staining. Their material consisted of 204 single trisomies mentioned above (66 informative cases), 9 mosaic trisomies (3 informative cases) and 9 double trisomies (5 informative cases). The results demonstrate that non-disjunction at maternal meiosis-I is the most likely source of the additional chromosome for all trisomies studied and this was the case at all maternal ages. In 61 of the 66 single trisomies, all 3 mosaic trisomies and 3 of the 5 double trisomies, the extra chromosome was of maternal origin. The proportion of paternally derived cases varied considerably among the trisomies; thus, for instance, the frequency of paternal non-disjunction was 22% (2/9) for both trisomies-13 and -21, but only 2% (1/48) for the remaining trisomies.

11. When these data were pooled with similar ones published in the literature, giving a total of 338 (137 informative) cases of single trisomies, the evidence for the increased contribution of paternal non-disjunction to trisomy-21 relative to other trisomies remained strong, i.e., in spontaneous abortions, trisomy-21 is more likely than other trisomies to be paternally derived. The maximum-likelihood estimate for paternally derived trisomy-21 was about 0.25, twice that for any other individual trisomy and approximately three times that for all trisomies other than 21. However, the pooled data did not bear out the high rate of paternal non-disjunction observed for chromosome 13.

12. It is worth pointing out that the technique of using chromosomal heteromorphism to identify the origin of extra chromosomes in trisomies is currently being supplemented by that involving restriction fragment length polymorphisms (RFLPs). This aspect is considered later.

13. In another study, Hassold and Chiu [H43] examined the effect of maternal age on the incidence of chromosomally normal spontaneous abortions and of different categories of chromosome abnormality (sex-chromosomal monosomy, trisomies and polyploids) among all clinically recognized human pregnancies. The data on 2264 spontaneous abortions karyotyped from 1976 to 1983 were used for this purpose. The main findings were as follows: (a) the overall rate of spontaneous abortions was 8.3%, although this varied significantly with maternal age, namely, the rate was relatively constant from age 20 to 30 years (6-8%), but from the mid-30-year-old on-

wards there was a marked increase, with more than 25% of all registered pregnancies terminating in spontaneous abortion by age 40 years; (b) the hospital-based value of 8.3% is probably an underestimate of the real level of fetal wastage; (c) the overall rate of chromosome abnormality was 50.4%, with trisomy accounting for nearly 30% of the abortions and sex-chromosome monosomy and polyploidy for approximately 10% each; (d) the relative proportions of the four different categories of abortion (chromosomally normal, sex-chromosome monosomy, trisomy and triploidy) changed significantly with maternal age, trisomy accounting for 20% of abortions involving women under 25 years of age, for approximately 33% of those occurring in the 30-35 year age-group and for 67% in women aged 40 years and older; correspondingly, the relative proportions of the other three categories of abortion declined with increasing maternal age; and (e) the authors estimated that, for women aged 35-39 years, about 10% of all recognized conceptions were trisomic and for those 40 years and older, this figure was around 30%; they also found that their data are in general agreement with those published by Aymes and Lippman-Hand [A15] and Warburton et al. [W36].

2. Chromosomal anomalies in fetuses diagnosed pre-natally in amniocentesis programmes

14. Schreinemachers et al. [S50] analysed the results of 19,672 pre-natal cytogenetic diagnoses reported to the New York State Chromosome Registry and to the United States Interregional Chromosome Register System for the period 1977-1980 and arrived at estimates of numerical sex-chromosomal and autosomal anomalies. The data pertain to women who were 35 years or older, for whom there was no known cytogenetic risk for a chromosomal abnormality except maternal age. The overall frequencies were the following: 47,XYY: 10 (0.051%); 47,XXY: 25 (0.127%); 47,XXX: 20 (0.102%); 45,X: 5 (0.025%); 47,+21: 179 (0.910%); 47,+18: 49 (0.249%) and 47,+13: 12 (0.061%). Taking maternal age into account, the authors estimated expected rates at amniocentesis from a regression analysis on the observed rates, using a first-degree exponential model.[a] The expected rates were compared with estimated rates by maternal age in live births, which were derived from various studies carried out in the late 1960s and early 1970s, summarized earlier by Hook [H24].

15. The main findings are the following: (a) the rates at amniocentesis for XXX and XXY increase with maternal age, with those for XXY being almost identical to those in live births, suggesting no late fetal mortality for this condition; the rates for XYY show a slight decrease with maternal age, which is also consistent with a low late fetal mortality; (b) the rates for 47,+21 at amniocentesis and at live birth are approximately parallel, with the latter being about 80% of the former; (c) those for 47,+18 at amnio-

[a] $y = \exp(a + bx)$ where x is the maternal age at the time of expected live birth and y is the rate of the cytogenetic defect at age x; x is on the average 0.4 years higher than the age at the time of amniocentesis.

centesis and live birth are also parallel, but the latter are only about 30% of the former, which is consistent with the high fetal mortality associated with this condition; and (d) the rates of 47,+13 at amniocentesis show an increase with maternal age, which is not as marked as that estimated from data on live births.

16. Similar results on structural chromosome abnormalities have been recently published by Hook et al. [H24] on the basis of data reported to the registries mentioned above (New York State Chromosome Registry, for the period 1977-1981 and the US Interregional Chromosomal Register System, up to the middle of 1980). The primary indication was, again, advanced maternal age. There were, in these series, 27,225 fetuses among which 61 (0.224%) had one or another kind of structural abnormality, detected using banding techniques (non-mosaic and mosaic cases). The breakdown was the following: balanced reciprocal translocations, 14 (0.051%); balanced Robertsonian translocations, non-Robertsonian translocations and supernumeraries etc., 35 (0.129%); and inversions, 4 (0.015%). Among these were 33 non-mosaic de novo rearrangements (2 inversions, 9 balanced reciprocal translocations, 6 balanced Robertsonian translocations and 16 unbalanced rearrangements). Of interest was the finding that the frequency of supernumerary markers and fragments (0.07%) was about threefold higher than that expected on the basis of live birth studies (about 0.02%; ref. [J10]). For these abnormalities, there was a trend for an association with advanced maternal age. The frequency of Robertsonian translocations, however, was only about one-fifth of that in new-borns.

17. Van Dyke et al. [V1] published the results of chromosome analyses carried out in amniocentesis programmes at the Henry Ford Hospital in Detroit, incorporating the data from two similar studies [G23, C28]. These data pertain to balanced autosomal rearrangements recorded in 8158 amniocenteses for which advanced maternal age was the principal indication. Analysis with banding techniques revealed that 33 fetuses (0.40%) carried such rearrangements. Of these, 14 (0.17%) carried balanced reciprocal translocations, 9 (0.11%) carried balanced Robertsonian translocations and 10 (0.12%) carried inversions (involving chromosomes 2, 3, 4, 6, 10, 11, 16, 18). Among these were 7 de novo rearrangements (4 reciprocal translocations, 2 Robertsonian translocations and 1 inversion), which give a mutation rate estimate of 4.3×10^{-4}/gamete/generation. This rate is higher than the figure of 1.88×10^{-4}/gamete/generation estimated by Jacobs [J10] on the basis of data from surveys of new-borns involving 59,452 babies. Van Dyke et al. [V1] suggest that: (a) while maternal-age amniocentesis series would provide a biased sample with respect to the frequencies of trisomy-21 or dominant mutations, this is not likely to be true with regard to the frequencies of balanced structural rearrangements; and (b) the higher frequencies, as well as the higher mutation rates, recorded in their work reflect the efficiency of detecting inversions and reciprocal translocations in banded chromosome preparations.

18. It is worth noting that the frequencies of balanced structural rearrangements in the work of Van Dyke et al. [V1] are all higher than those in the series of Hook et al. [H24], in spite of the fact that banding methods were used in both. The reasons for this discrepancy are not clear.

3. Chromosomal anomalies in new-born children

19. In its 1982 report, UNSCEAR summarized the results of 10 cytogenetic surveys on the prevalence of chromosomal anomalies in new-born children. In 7 of these surveys (59,465 babies) conventional Giemsa staining procedures were used, while in the other three (7549 babies) banding methods were used. Among the 67,014 babies screened, 424 (0.63%) were chromosomally abnormal, the breakdown being as follows: 158 (0.24%) sex-chromosomal anomalies, 95 (0.14%) autosomal numerical anomalies, 134 (0.20%) balanced autosomal structural rearrangements, and 37 (0.06%) unbalanced structural rearrangements and supernumerary chromosomes. With the sample sizes involved, there were no striking differences between the banding and conventional staining methods in the efficiency of detection of the chromosomal anomalies, except for inversions.

20. Recent results from cytogenetic surveys of new-borns carried out in Norway [H13] and Denmark [N1], in addition to results from some pre-natal genetic studies (e.g., ref. [V1]) (banding methods were used in all these), suggest that earlier studies of new-borns (without banding methods) have underestimated the frequencies of inversions and of reciprocal translocations. In the Norwegian survey [H13], chromosome analyses were made in blood lymphocytes derived from umbilical cord blood of 1830 consecutively born infants. Two G-banded cells were karyotyped from each individual. When one or both of these cells showed chromosome aberrations, at least another 20 cells were studied and supplemented with C-, Q- and R-banding methods when necessary. The Danish survey of Nielsen et al. [N1] is essentially a continuation of their earlier work [N11]. Five BrdU-treated cells from each of 3658 children were photographed and analysed; from 20 to 50 cells were analysed when one or more of these cells showed a chromosome aberration and further cells were examined when mosaicism was suspected. The Q- and/or C-banding methods were used for structural chromosome aberrations for chromosomal variants where further analyses with other staining methods were indicated.

21. Table 3 compares the main results of these two surveys with the earlier Danish survey (the ethnic background is fairly similar for these two populations) and with the pooled results of the earlier cytogenetic surveys in which no banding methods were employed. It can be seen that the total frequencies in the Norwegian and the new Danish surveys (1.97 and 2.02%) are substantially higher, relative to the earlier Danish survey (0.83%) and to the one based on the pooled results of earlier surveys (0.63%). Particularly noteworthy is the much higher rate of detection of inversions (most of these, however, involve chromosome 9 and are currently regarded as variants) and of reciprocal translocations in the two new surveys.

4. Chromosomal anomalies in mentally retarded or otherwise handicapped individuals

22. Rasmussen et al. [R1] presented data on the prevalence of chromosomal abnormalities among mentally retarded persons in Arhus, Denmark. In this area there were 2157 patients, both institutionalized and living at home, and chromosome analysis was possible in 1905 cases. Of these, 359 (18.8%) had a chromosomal abnormality: 281 (14.7%) with Down syndrome (260 cases due to trisomy-21, 14 due to translocations[b] and 7 mosaics), 45 (2.4%) with one or another kind of autosomal anomaly other than Down syndrome (7 cases of autosomal numerical anomalies, 20 cases of autosomal structural anomalies, including unbalanced translocations, deletions, duplications etc., 12 cases of inversions predominantly of chromosome 9, and 6 cases of balanced reciprocal translocations) and 35 cases (1.8%) of sex-chromosomal anomalies including mosaics. In comparison with similar data summarized in the review of Jacobs et al. [J1], and other data subsequently published [A1, F1, K2], the Danish results show that the prevalence frequencies in each of the different subgroups (Down syndrome, autosomal anomalies other than Down, and sex-chromosomal), are higher (Table 4). The authors attribute these differences to the use of banding methods in the Danish study, which was not the case in the other surveys.

23. Coco and Penchaszadeh [C1] published a cytogenetic study of 200 children with mental retardation and three or more major or minor congenital anomalies. These cases were selected from the population of patients referred to the Genetics Unit of the Children's Hospital of Buenos Aires for diagnostic evaluation because of mental retardation and multiple congenital anomalies. Patients with a clinical diagnosis of Down, Turner or Klinefelter syndromes were excluded, but a clinical suspicion of any other chromosomal syndrome was not considered adequate reason for exclusion. In all cases, the chromosomes were studied with conventional staining methods and with at least one of the banding techniques. The age of the patients varied from new-born to 18 years, roughly one-half being under one year old.

24. Of the 200 patients, 42 (21%) had chromosome anomalies. The breakdown is as follows: 11 cases (5.5%) of autosomal (chromosome 9, 13, 18, 22) trisomes; 5 cases (2.5%) of sex-chromosomal aneuploidies (XYY, XXY and mosaics); 19 cases (9.5%) of de novo structural rearrangements (deletions, rings, unbalanced rearrangements and extra marker chromosomes), 2 cases (1%) of unidentifiable supernumerary chromosomes and 5 cases (2.5%) of unbalanced genomes originating from a balanced structural rearrangement in one of the parents.

25. Table 5 compares the results of similar studies in which chromosome analyses were made of patients with mental retardation and multiple congenital anomalies. It can be seen that the frequencies of chromosome anomalies in such patients vary from 2.5% to

20%, with a mean of 11.0%. These variations in the frequencies are due to several factors, including the following: (a) the lack of strict comparability of the populations (some studies sampled institutions for the retarded, others investigated hospitalized patients); (b) differences in age distributions; (c) the degree of care taken to exclude known or recognizable syndromes; and (d) the particular cytogenetic techniques used.

26. Dykes [D3] presented the results of what is perhaps the most extensive survey of severely handicapped children. Included in this survey are over 10,000 severely handicapped children under the age of 16 in New South Wales, Australia. It showed that 7228 children, representing 71.7% of the total, were handicapped by one or more of the following diseases or disabilities: mental retardation, 6758; Down syndrome, 1162; and cerebral palsy, 1419. The total number of chromosomal abnormalities in the survey was 1214, with 1162 of these (95.7%) being in children with Down syndrome. The anomalies detected in the other 52 (4.3%) children were sex-chromosomal aneuploidy including mosaicism, autosomal trisomies, balanced and unbalanced translocations, ring chromosomes, partial deletions and duplications of chromosomes. All these children, besides being mentally retarded (the degree of severity ranging from mild to profound), had one or more congenital malformations.

5. Chromosomal anomalies in subfertile males

27. Dutrillaux et al. [D24] compiled the results of chromosome studies (in blood lymphocytes) on 958 patients who attended two male infertility clinics in Paris. Of these, 150 were studied without chromosome banding and the remainder with banding techniques. On the basis of sperm analysis, the patients were classified into those with azoospermia (absence of live spermatozoa in semen, 278 cases), predominantly oligospermia (scarcity of spermatozoa in the semen, specifically, less than 20 10^6/ml, 486 cases), predominantly asthenospermia (weakness or loss of vitality of the spermatozoa) and/or teratospermia (abnormal sperm morphology) and a much less defined category, namely unknown and miscellaneous (97 cases). A total of 58 chromosome anomalies were detected (6.1%), the frequencies being different in the different groups (azoospermics, 37/278 or 13.3%; oligospermics, 15/486 or 3.1%; astheno/teratospermics, 2/97 or 2.1% and the unknown and miscellaneous group, 4/97 or 4.1%). The details of these chromosome anomalies are given in Table 6. Not shown in the Table is the finding that among the sex-chromosomal anomalies, all but 3 cases (of inversion of the Y chromosome) were found in the azoospermic males (33/278 or 11.8%); among the autosomal anomalies, 4 were observed in azoospermic males (4/278 or 1.4%) and 12 among oligospermic males (12/486 or 2.5%). Thus, there is a clear correlation between sex-chromosomal anomalies and azoospermia, mostly, although not exclusively, due to cases of Klinefelter syndrome.

28. The authors compared their results with similar ones published in the literature, taking into account

---

[b]Nine 14/21, one 15/21, four 21/23 translocations and one involving chromosome 21 and an unidentified chromosome.

the fact that there were heterogeneities in patient selection (in particular, the proportion of azoospermic males among all infertiles) and differences in methods of chromosome analysis and of data reporting. In these studies, the overall frequencies of chromosomal anomalies ranged from 2.2 to 29%, with the proportion of azoospermics in the range 7-100% (some authors did not report on the latter).

29. Reliable estimates of the prevalences of chromosomal anomalies in subfertile men are hampered by a lack of similar data for an unselected population of adult males. Dutrillaux et al. [D24] therefore made a comparison with the frequencies recorded in surveys of new-borns and the results are summarized in Table 7. The general conclusion is that the prevalence of chromosomal anomalies in subfertile males is about an order of magnitude higher than in new-borns, although the frequencies of specific abnormalities show a great deal of variation.

30. Results similar to those of Dutrillaux et al. [D24] have also been published by Micic et al. [M51]. In the latter study, lymphocyte chromosomes of 820 infertile men were examined in banded preparations. The data are summarized in Table 8, where it can be seen that the frequency of infertiles with chromosomal anomalies is 7.3% (60/820), i.e., similar to that reported by Dutrillaux et al. Of these males, 77 (9.4%) had chromosomal variants, the significance of which is not clear, although a similar high frequency of variant D and G group chromosomes has also been reported by Moreau and Teyssier [M52] (10% among infertiles versus 4% in fertile men). As in the study of Dutrillaux et al., all patients with sex-chromosomal anomalies were azoospermic, the most frequent among them being those with an XXY constitution. Other interesting aspects of the data of Micic et al. include: (a) the relatively high incidence of pericentric inversions in chromosome 9 among infertiles (2.8%) who were either oligo- or azoospermic (this frequency is still higher than those recorded by Hansteen et al. [H13] and Nielsen et al. [N1] in studies of new-borns discussed earlier); (b) the finding of 1.1% of balanced autosomal translocations, a figure that is in agreement with that of Dutrillaux et al. (1.6% or 15/958); and (c) the absence of structural aberrations of the X or Y chromosomes (in contrast to the finding of such aberrations by Dutrillaux et al.) [D24].

6. Direct chromosome analyses of human spermatozoa and of fertilized eggs: further results

31. The data of Rudak et al. [R7], representing the first direct analyses of the chromosome constitution of human spermatozoa after fertilization of hamster (Mesocricetus auratus) eggs, were presented in the 1982 UNSCEAR report [U1]. These authors analysed 60 spermatozoa from one normal male and found a 5% frequency of aneuploidy. These studies have now been extended by Martin et al. [M11] and Brandriff et al. [B22, B38]. In the work of Martin and colleagues, chromosome analyses of 1000 spermatozoa from 33 normal men (21 of proven fertility and 12 of

unproven fertility; age range, 22-50 years) were performed. Of the spermatozoa analysed, 8.5% were abnormal (range, 0-28%), of which 5.2% were aneuploid and 3.3% had structural aberrations. About half of the aneuploid sperms were hypohaploid; the rest were hyperhaploid with a very small proportion (0.1%) having double aneuploidy. All chromosome groups were represented among the aneuploid complements, but there were none with 24, YY constitution. This finding is at variance with other studies in which fluorescent Y bodies were used as markers (in those, which were reviewed in the 1982 UNSCEAR report, the frequency of sperm with 2 Y bodies ranged from 1 to 5%). Most structural anomalies were chromosome breaks (22/33), but the anomalies were not equally distributed among the sperm of the 33 males: 2 males had 11 of the 33 structural anomalies.

32. The paper of Brandriff et al. [B22] reports data on 2468 spermatozoa from 11 males (repeat sampling was carried out for 2 individuals after 14 or 16 months) and includes data published earlier [B38]. The males were between 21 and 49 years of age. The overall frequency of abnormal spermatozoa was 9.4% (1.7% were aneuploid, with a frequency range of 0.6-3.1%, and 7.7% had structural abnormalities, with a range of 1.5-15.8%). Again, as in the work of Martin et al. [M11], aneuploid chromosome complements involved all groups, and the majority of structural anomalies, in order of frequency, were chromosome breaks, followed by acentric fragments, chromatid exchanges, chromatid breaks, deletions, dicentrics, translocations and duplications. The repeat sampling of spermatozoa from two males did not reveal any significant changes in the frequencies of abnormal sperm. Parallel studies with lymphocytes showed that, in six individuals, the percentages of structurally abnormal cells were significantly higher in sperm than in lymphocytes by factors of up to 8, but there were no correlations between lymphocyte and sperm data.

33. The subsequent work of Martin et al. [M53, M81] was focused on the analysis of sperm complements of 13 cancer patients before radiotherapy and at regular intervals thereafter. The men were from 19 to 47 years of age and the estimated doses to the testes ranged from 0.4 to 5 Gy. Before radiotherapy, the frequency of chromosomal abnormalities in sperm was zero in all men. After radiotherapy, the majority were azoospermic for two years. Analysis of chromosomes of 4 men at 12 and 24 months showed high frequencies of abnormal sperm (12.5% and 12.7%); after 36 months (during which time sperm production was recovered in most men), the frequency of abnormalities in 8 men was 20.9%, which was significantly higher than in control donors (8.5%). For individual men, the range of abnormalities was from 6 to 67% and there was a significant correlation between testicular dose and the frequency of abnormalities. Both numerical and structural abnormalities were present.

34. Angell et al. [A9] reported on studies dealing with in vitro fertilization of human oocytes by human sperm. Oocytes were removed from ovaries of 7 women (aged between 31 and 39) at laparoscopy and sperm was collected from 7 healthy males aged between 27

and 39, all with informed consent. Fertilization was carried out in small petri dishes under carefully controlled conditions. Complete chromosomal analysis was possible in only 3 embryos (8-cell stage). Two of these were chromosomally abnormal (22,X,−15; 47,XY,+D). The haploid embryo contained only maternal chromosomes and in the diploid embryo, the extra D chromosome could not be more precisely identified. Of the further 8 embryos that were analysed for their DNA content (microfluorimetric methods), 2 appeared to be haploid (excluding the one mentioned above that was chromosomally analysed). The authors emphasize that over 100 babies have now been born after in vitro fertilization without any apparent chromosomal abnormality and that the abnormalities of the kind found in their study would clearly lead to early embryonic loss, and probably contribute to the high failure rate after embryo transfer.

7. Fragile sites

(a) General aspects and classification

35. In the 1982 UNSCEAR report, some of the properties of the heritable fragile sites then known in human chromosomes and the association between the fragile site on the X chromosome with macroorchidism and mental retardation were discussed. Since then, considerable progress has been made (e.g., [B2, C10, G1, G25, H3, H13, K10, O9, S2, S24-S27, S55-S57, T3, T4]). Well over 40 fragile sites have now been discovered and are currently subdivided into two major groups, the rare (or relatively so) and the common or constitutive. The rare fragile sites have been classified, according to the conditions of tissue culture under which they are expressed, into folate sensitive, distamycin-A inducible and BrdU requiring. Nineteen rare fragile sites are currently known.

(i) Rare fragile sites

36. Group 1: Folate-sensitive fragile sites. There are 16 of these at 2q11, 2q13, 6p23, 7p11, 8q22, 9p21, 9q32, 10q23, 11q13, 11q23, 12q13, 16p12, 19p13, 20p11, 22q13 and Xq27. They are termed folate sensitive because removal of folic acid (and thymidine) from the culture medium was the first factor found to be essential for their demonstration in lymphocyte cultures, i.e., they are invisible in complete media but can be seen in deprived media (such as medium 199) deficient in folic acid and thymidine. The recently discovered fragile site at 19p13 [T30] was found to be expressed in medium containing low folate and by addition of FdU, whereas high folate, thymidine and thymidine analogues inhibited its expression.

37. Group 2: Distamycin-A inducible fragile sites are those at 16q22 and 17p12. These are not dependent upon conditions of tissue culture but are enhanced by the addition of distamycin A to lymphocyte cultures [C10]. The site at 17p12 was not originally accepted as a fragile site but is now included in this group in view of the finding that it fulfils the definition of a fragile site [S55, S58, S59].

38. Group 3: BrdU-requiring fragile site. The fragile site at 10q25 was independently discovered by Scheres and Hustinx [S60] and by Sutherland et al. [S61]. It is expressed only if BrdU or related compounds are present in the culture medium some hours prior to harvest of cell cultures for chromosome studies.

(ii) Common fragile sites

39. Paradoxically, less is known about these than about the rare ones. The common fragile sites were initially regarded as hot spots or autosomal lesions and not as fragile sites, because until recently they were not known to be inducible, did not appear to be heritable and were usually seen in only a small proportion of the metaphases [S55].

40. Group 1: Aphidicolin-inducible fragile sites. Glover et al. [G25] showed that fragile sites at 2q31, 3p14, 6q26, 7q32, 16q23 and Xp22 (a total of six) are weakly induced by the same conditions as those that induce folate-sensitive sites, but are more strongly induced by aphidicolin (a specific inhibitor of DNA polymerase alpha) and most effectively by these conditions together.

41. Group 2: 5-azacytidine-inducible fragile sites. Discovered recently by Sutherland et al. [S57], these fragile sites in bands 1q42 and 19q13 are induced by 5-azacytidine, an analogue of cytidine; maximum induction is observed when the inducing agent is added 5-8 hours prior to harvest.

42. Group 3: BrdU-inducible fragile sites. Also discovered by Sutherland et al. [S57], these occur at 6q13, 9p21, 10q21 and maximum induction is observed when BrdU is added 4-6 hours prior to harvest. (Note that band 9p21 contains a common fragile site and a rare folate-sensitive site; a detailed comparison of these by high resolution banding has not yet been performed and hence it is unknown whether they are coincident.)

(iii) Properties of rare and common fragile sites

43. The cytological appearance of fragile sites is variable, but there are several essential properties of rare fragile sites: (a) there is a non-staining gap of varying width that usually involves both chromatids; (b) the fragile site is always at exactly the same point on the chromosomes in all individuals or kindred; (c) the fragile site is inherited in a Mendelian codominant fashion; and (d) the fragile site exhibits fragility under conditions of induction, as evidenced by acentric fragments, deleted chromosomes, triradial figures, etc. [S53]. The triradial (or multiradial) is the most spectacular cytogenetic manifestation of the fragile site and is essential for distinguishing fragile sites from other phenomena causing chromosome breakage.

44. The common fragile sites have the following properties [D27]: (a) they occur in cells of all individuals tested with the particular set of conditions

at the same chromosomal location; (b) they are detectable in both homologues and are homozygous in a proportion of cells; (c) they usually occur within G-positive bands (most of the rare ones occur in G-negative bands); and (d) they do not seem to exhibit specific triradial formation characteristic of most of the rare fragile sites. The common fragile sites are presumably heritable, but family studies have not yet been performed [S57] because of the low frequency at which some of these are expressed and the problem of identifying the separate homologues of chromosomes without C-band or fluorescent variants.

45. The fragile sites mentioned above are the confirmed ones. Other possible rare fragile sites (at 1q32, 2p11, 5q35, 22q, Xq26 and Yq12) and common fragile sites (at 1p22, 1p32, 1p36, 1q25, 2p13, 2q33, 3p24, 3p27, 5q31, 7p31, 7q22, 8q22, 9q32, 11p13, 14q24, 22q12, Xq22, and probably many others) reported in the literature and discussed by Sutherland and Hecht [S53] need confirmation.

46. There are some suggestions that the expression of the fragile site at Xq27 is decreased in blood specimens delayed in transit to the laboratory [J11, B26], and Fonatsch [F18] reported a marked decrease in the frequency of expression of fragile-X in blood that had been stored for five days prior to culture compared to freshly cultured blood. Daniel et al. [D27] noted that when the blood was stored for 2-4 days at 4°C or at 25°C prior to culture, there was a decline in the expression of fragile-X relative to unstored samples and this decline was less pronounced in the samples stored at 4°C. Storage of the samples for 1-5 days and at 4°C, 25°C, 37°C and 39°C prior to culture revealed that the per cent expression of the fragile-X was inversely related to the temperature and duration of storage, the decline being more pronounced at temperatures higher than 4°C and with longer storage periods.

(b) The fragile site on the X chromosome and its association with mental retardation

(i) Localization

47. It is now firmly established that the X-linked fragile site (associated with mental retardation) is near the end of Xq. There has been some uncertainty, however, regarding its exact location, i.e., whether the site is in band Xq27, Xq28 or at the Xq27-Xq28 interface. In a scanning electron microscope study, Harrison et al. [H63] localized the fragile site at Xq27.3. In their preparations, the fragile site appeared as an isochromatid gap in the majority of cases, confirming light microscopy observations. Utilizing high resolution banding, Brookwell and Turner [B23] assigned the fragile site to band Xq27, close to the Xq27-Xq28 interface. A more recent study by Krawczun et al. [K34], in which high-resolution banding was also used confirmed the localization to band Xq27.3.

48. In genetic linkage studies in Sicilian families, Filippi et al. [F15] reported that the G6-PD locus at

Xq28 and the fragile site are linked (see also [H26]). The recent success in cloning and mapping of the human coagulation factor IX gene to the region from Xq26 to Xq28 by several laboratories and the identification of a common TaqI restriction fragment length polymorphism (RFLP) [C57, C58, J19, J20, K35] catalyzed the search for linkage between the fragile X gene and the factor IX TaqI RFLP. In the work of Camerino et al. [C29], out of 17 informative meioses in two families, recombination between these genes was not observed, resulting in an estimate of the genetic distance of less than 12 centimorgans (cM). Warren et al. [W37] carried out linkage analyses with a factor IX cDNA probe in a family[c] with the fragile-X-linked mental retardation and were able to identify a recombinant individual (among two affected brothers), suggesting that the linkage between these two genes is not as close as the data of Camerino et al. [C29] might suggest. Recombination between these genes has also been observed in the work of Choo et al. [C59]. (See also Davies et al. [D43] and Mulligan et al. [M60].)

(ii) Expression and relation to age and IQ

49. Herbst et al. [H4] considered that over 1% expression of fra(X) was necessary to identify the carrier status with certainty. Age further complicates the expression of fra(X) in lymphocytes and there are reports suggesting that fra(X) is more difficult to detect in older carriers [J11, C30, B24]. In the absence of serial studies over time in carriers, it is difficult to be certain whether an age effect might explain why there are problems in detecting the fra(X) in carrier females.

50. Chudley et al. [C31] studied eight Saskatchewan families (37 affected males and 22 carriers) and showed a significant inverse relationship between age and the frequency of fra(X) expression; they also found that in carrier females the frequency of fra(X) expression and IQ were inversely related and that in affected males this relationship was less pronounced. Fishburn et al. [F16] observed that mildly retarded fra(X) heterozygotes had a significantly higher percentage of fra(X) expressing lymphocytes, compared with intellectually normal heterozygotes.

51. In 28 heterozygotes from the same families as those studied by Chudley et al. [C31] (one-third of these were mentally retarded), Knoll et al. [K18] investigated the frequency of fra(X) expression and fra(X) replication pattern. The retarded carriers had a higher frequency of early replicating fra(X), in addition to higher overall frequencies of fra(X) expression than did normal carriers, i.e., mental retardation in females heterozygous for fra(X) may be largely a function of the proportion of cells with an early replicating, active X-chromosome possessing the fragile site. The early replicating fra(X) accounted for more of the variability in IQ than the late replicating one, a finding in accordance with the results of Uchida and Joyce [U5] and Uchida et al. [U6]. When the data were adjusted

---

[c]The family consisted of 2 grandparents, 2 parents, 2 affected sons (brothers), 1 affected and 1 normal daughter and 1 son unavailable for study.

for age, the nature of the relationships between IQ and proportion of early replicating fra(X), between IQ and proportion of late replicating fra(X) and between IQ and frequency of fra(X) did not change, suggesting that age had a minimal effect.

52. In the work of Brondum-Nielsen et al. [B24] involving 63 obligate and potential carriers of fra(X), a difference was found between normal and mentally retarded carriers in the expression of fra(X), in that the mean percentage of positive cells was 8% in the former versus 31% in the latter. Furthermore, there was an inverse relationship between the percentage of positive cells and age in normal carriers, whereas retarded carriers generally showed high percentages at all ages (see also Fryns [F29]). Fra(X) carriers of normal intelligence with low fra(X) expression had a tendency towards higher frequencies of late replicating fra(X), whereas those with high fra(X) expression had a tendency towards early replication of fra(X). These findings are at variance with those recorded by Knoll et al. [K18]: fra(X) carriers of normal intelligence expressing fra(X) in relatively high frequency showed a tendency towards an excess of late replicating fra(X) chromosomes as did the normal intelligent carriers with a low frequency of fra(X).

53. The results of studies on fra(X) replication patterns and their relationship to IQ do not allow unambiguous statements to be made on whether X-inactivation plays an important role in determining the intelligence of carriers of fra(X). Furthermore, as Sutherland notes (see [O9]), the use of BrdU labelling to study fra(X) expression is questionable, since this compound is known to inhibit fra(X) expression; late replicating fra(X) chromosomes are less likely to express the fragile site than early replicating ones, leading to an apparent excess of early replicating fra(X) chromosomes. Additionally, there is the question of whether X-inactivation as seen in lymphocytes reflects X-inactivation within the central nervous system, an aspect more likely to be relevant to intellectual function.

54. The results of cytogenetic analyses of individuals in 110 pedigrees of fra(X) syndrome presented by Sherman et al. [S54] show that: (a) mentally retarded males have a higher frequency of fra(X) positive cells than mentally impaired females and the latter have higher frequencies of these cells than normal females; (b) there is no effect of marker expression on IQ in affected males, but there is a significant inverse relationship between IQ and the expression of fra(X) in females; and (c) there is a small but significant effect of age on fra(X) frequency (a decrease in fra(X) positive cells) in both males and females, but in females it is restricted to those of normal intelligence, retarded females showing no significant effect.

(iii) *Prevalence and mutation rate estimates*

55. Currently, about 25% (58/243) of the X-linked mutations listed in McKusick's catalogue [M21] lead to, or are associated with, mental retardation [O9]. Herbst and Miller [H14] estimated that the minimal

prevalence of non-specific X-linked mental retardation in British Colombia was 18.3 per 10^4 males and that about one-half of this (9.2 per 10^4 males) was due to fra(X). The latter estimate was arrived at using cytogenetic data (on the prevalence of males with fra(X) chromosome among families with X-linked mental retardation) published in the literature [J11, J13, H30, T20]. They argued that, if the latter estimate is valid, fra(X) would be, next to trisomy-21, the most common chromosomal abnormality associated with mental retardation.

56. Again, based on literature data, Turner and Jacobs [T19] arrived at a lower estimate of 4-5 per 10^4 males for the prevalence of fra(X)-linked mental retardation. In a subsequent paper on segregation analysis of data from 110 families of fra(X) mental retardation (using the programmes SERGAN and POINTER developed by Morton and colleagues), Sherman et al. [S54] found that: (a) there was a deficit of at least 20% of affected males,[d] the most plausible explanation for which was, in their opinion, incomplete penetrance of the gene in some affected males, such males being indistinguishable from normal on both psychometric and cytogenetic tests (cases of apparently asymptomatic males transmitting the gene to their daughters have in fact been reported in the literature [C29, D26, F17, F19, J12, M29, N18, R29]); (b) the penetrance of mental retardation in carrier females was about 30% and of mental impairment and/or fra(X) expression, 56%; (c) there was no evidence for the occurrence of sporadic cases among affected males, i.e., all the males had received the fra(X) gene from their carrier mothers; and (d) assuming normal segregation, the data were consistent with a prevalence of fra(X)-linked mental retardation in females of 4.1 per 10^4 (which is nearly the same as that for males) and a mutation rate estimate in male germ cells of $7.2 \ 10^{-4}$/locus/generation, or, in relation to germ cells of both sexes, of $2.4 \ 10^{-4}$/locus/generation (their analysis provided no evidence for mutations in females).

57. In a further segregation analysis of the fra(X) syndrome in 96 pedigrees, Sherman et al. [S85] found that: (a) the segregation pattern for any degree of mental impairment was similar to that in the 110 pedigrees discussed above; (b) for the combined data, the best estimate of penetrance of mental impairment was 79% in males and 35% in females; and (c) there was little evidence for sporadic cases among affected males.

(iv) *Prevalence of fra(X) among mentally retarded individuals*

58. Kähkönen et al. [K10] made a cytogenetic study of 150 male patients with mental retardation of

[d]Such a deficit of affected males was not observed in the study of Fryns [F29]. In his study, 55 carrier females gave birth to 299 children, 171 males and 128 females. Thirteen boys died early in infancy and the majority of them were said to be mentally subnormal. Of the total of 171 males, only 56 were mentally normal. The ratio of mentally retarded (102) to mentally normal (56) males was 1.82 : 1 (even with the exclusion of the 13 boys who died).

unknown origin in Finland. Six of these patients (4%) had the fragile-X; one of them had no family history of mental retardation, four had one or more mentally retarded first-degree relatives and one had a family history suggestive of X-linked mental retardation. In other similar studies, the proportion of those with fragile-X has varied from 2% in Australia [S28] to 6% in Sweden [B2] to 16% in South Africa [V3]. In their review of published cases of non-specific X-linked mental retardation (n = 187 males), Tariverdian and Weck [T3] found that the fragile-X was present in a majority (170) of cases. The range of lymphocytes showing the fragile site, however, varied widely (3-61%). The results with obligate female carriers have been disappointing. Of 85 such cases discussed by the above authors, only 45 showed the fragile-X in 0.5-38% of cells.

59. In an earlier study on the prevalence of fra(X) positive males among an unselected series of severely mentally retarded boys (IQ < 50) born during the years 1959-1970 in the northern Swedish county of Västerbotten, Blomquist et al. [B2] found that 6 out of 96, or 6%, were fra(X) positive (subsequently, one more case was found). In an extension of this work to less severely mentally retarded children of both sexes, Blomquist et al. [B25] recorded that 5 out of 110 boys (4.5%) and none of 61 girls had the fra(X). Thus, the fra(X) was seen in 2.9% of the total series of 171 children. Relating the total number of severely and less severely mentally retarded fra(X) positive children so far found (12) to the total number of births for the period 1959-1970 and alive at one year of age (40,871), the authors estimated that the prevalence of fra(X) syndrome in that Swedish county was about 1 per 3000 new-borns.

60. Sutherland [S86] published the results of his continuing population cytogenetic studies carried out in Australia on unselected neo-nates, retardates in mental institutions, special schools for the retarded, sheltered workshops for the mentally handicapped and in hospital referral patients. This paper also incorporates the data from his earlier [S5] studies. Among 3558 neo-nates, there were no cases of fra(X) and this was also true of those in sheltered workshops (0/128). Among institutionalized retardates, 1.6% of the males (7/444) and none of the females (0/80) were fra(X) positive. In hospital referral patients, the frequencies were 5.3% in males (13/2283) and 1.6% in females (3/1890).

61. By far the highest frequency of fra(X) among institutionalized retardates has been recorded in the study of Fryns [F29], in which 57 of the 354 males (16.1%) and 1 of 30 females (3.3%) were fra(X) positive. These 58 patients were found to belong to 37 different families. These and other data bearing on the prevalence of fra(X) are summarized in Table 9, which shows that the frequencies are generally higher among males in mental institutions and in those referred for cytogenetic examinations than among females.

(v) *Prevalence of fra(X) among autistic children*

62. In 1970, Sivasankar [S87] reported an increase in the rate of chromosomal breakage in leucocyte cultures from autistic children.[e] Subsequently, Turner et al. [T20] described the fragile-X syndrome in an autistic boy and this association was later reported by several others [B40, B41, B44, G37, G38, L21, L22]. In a recent Swedish multicentre study, 102 cases (83 boys and 19 girls) of infantile autism (age range, 2-24 years) were examined for fra(X) [B39]. Thirteen of the 83 autistic boys (15.7%) had the fra(X) expressed in 1-70% of their lymphocytes, but none of the 19 girls was fra(X) positive. Of the 13 boys who were fra(X) positive, 1 was classified as having normal intelligence (IQ > 85), 1 was subnormal (IQ = 70-84), 7 had mild mental retardation (IQ = 50-69) and 4 were severely mentally retarded (IQ = 0-49).

(c) *Autosomal folate-sensitive fragile sites: prevalence estimates and effects*

63. Sutherland's recent paper [S86] summarizes the results of screening for folate-sensitive rare autosomal fragile sites, including those he published earlier [S5], those of Turner et al. [T31] and those of some studies carried out in France [R48, G39, Q1]. His own results show that in unselected neo-nates, the frequency is quite low (5/3438 or 0.15%) and significantly higher in all the other groups: referral patients, 0.38% (16/4173); institutionalized retardates, 0.95% (5/524); those attending special schools, 1.0% (5/502); and those in sheltered workshops, 1.6% (2/128). Of the 28 autosomal folate-sensitive fragile site ascertainments in his laboratory, where both parents have been studied, the mother was the carrier parent 22 times and only once was the father the carrier (in the remaining five instances neither parent could be shown to be a carrier). The figure for referral patients cited above (0.38%) is higher than those reported by Raoul (0.14%, 11/8000) [R48], Quack et al. (0.14%, 14/10,000) [Q1], and Guichaoua et al. (0.21%, 17/7786) [G39].

64. The results of Sutherland's other study [S6] on the prevalence of BrdU-requiring fragile site at 10q25 in 1026 unselected neo-nates, 901 patients referred to for chromosomal studies and 87 institutionalized retardates showed no differences between these groups. Apart from one homozygote (found in the group of neo-nates), all the rest were heterozygotes for the 10q25 site. The frequencies were as follows: neo-nates, 2.3% (24/1026); patients, 2.4% (22/901); and retardates, 3.4% (3/87).

65. The distamycin-requiring fragile sites at 17p12 and 16q22 are the ones about which least is known from a population point of view. Although they were detected in all the groups studied, it is only recently

---

[e]Autism is a form of behaviour and thinking observed in young children, in which the child seems to concentrate upon himself or herself without regard for reality. It often appears as excessive shyness, fearfulness or aloofness and later as withdrawal and introspection. It may be an early manifestation or part of a childhood type of schizophrenia.

that the conditions required for their expression have been delineated [S56]. In Sutherland's [S86] study, the fragile site at 17p12 was seen in 1 out of 368 neo-nates (0.27%) and the one at 16q22 was not detected in this group; 8 out of 491 patients had the 16q22 (1.6%) and 1 in 491 had the 17p12 (0.02%). Sanfilipo et al. [S87] induced the fragile site at 16q22 with 15 mg/1 BrdU added 7 h prior to harvest and found it in 4/155 institutionalized retardates (2.6%) and 14/1444 patients (1.0%) referred for diagnostic cytogenetics.

66. Apart from the fragile site at Xq27, for which the evidence of association with one form of mental retardation is strong, the question of whether other fragile sites may be associated with adverse phenotypic effects is not entirely resolved. Sutherland and Hinton [S51] recorded the presence of fra(12q13) in a kindred involving six members of five generations, but without clinical abnormalities. Giraud et al. [G24], however, reported two cases of fra(12q13), one in a boy with severe mental retardation and the other in the mother of a malformed infant with a normal karyotype (no clinical details were given). The reports of Donti et al. [D25] and of Moric-Petrovic and Laca [M28] show that the fra(12q13) may be associated with phenotypic abnormalities (round head, small chin, low set ears, abnormally long fingers and considerable psychomotor retardation). The only difference between these cases is the presence of a Robertsonian translocation (13q; 14q; familial) in the case described by Moric-Petrovic and Laca (in addition to the fra(12q13)). In neither case was the fragile site familial. Moric-Petrovic and Laca speculate that the phenotypic abnormalities may not be a consequence of the presence of the fragile site per se, but could be due to a loss, in some cells, of a large part of 12q.

(d) Fragile sites and propensity to chromosome breakage

67. There are indications that certain autosomal fragile sites may predispose the chromosomes to breakage [S52, C30]. Hecht and Hecht [H28, H29] made a systematic study to explore this possibility. From the data recorded in the New York State Chromosomal Registry, they extracted information on the location of break-points leading to constitutional chromosomal anomalies (deletions, duplications, inversions and non-Robertsonian translocations) found in amniocentesis studies and in those on spontaneous abortions, still births and new-borns.

68. The break-points were individually compared with the location of 44 known fragile sites [S53]. Based on a haploid karyotype of 400 bands [I6] and the assumption that each band has the same probability of breakage, it would be expected that, by chance alone, 11.0% of the breaks would be coincident with the fragile sites (44/400). In the rearrangements recorded in the amniocentesis studies, there was a total of 278 break-points of which 59 (21%) were observed to be in bands containing the fragile sites, compared to an expectation of 11.0%. In those recorded in the abortions, still births and new-borns,

165 (18.5%) of the total of 894 break-points were found in the bands with fragile sites, again a significant excess, compared with the expected 11.0%; in this work, no break-points in rearrangements were found in 8 bands containing the fragile sites (2q11, 3p14, 6q26, 9q32, 16p12, 16q23, Xq26 and Xq27).

69. The total data with the separation of the break-points according to the origin of the rearrangements (maternal, paternal or unknown) are given in Table 10. It is clear that these data are in line with the concept that certain fragile sites may predispose the chromosomes to breakage and formation of rearrangements in meiosis. The authors caution that in view of the heterogeneity of the data base from which the pertinent information was extracted, more evidence is required to provide convincing proof that fragile sites are regions in the chromosomes predisposed to breakage in meiosis.

70. Braekeleer [B42] raised some objections on the methodology used by Hecht and Hecht [H28, H29] in their analysis, the principal points being that: (a) the latter authors considered only the total number of bands; (b) all chromosome bands do not have the same length; and (c) the chance of having a break in a band is dependent on its length. Therefore, it would be more accurate to consider the probability of a relationship between fragile sites and predisposition to chromosome breakage according to the relative lengths of the bands. On this hypothesis, Braekeleer re-analysed the data of Hecht and Hecht using Monte Carlo simulation methods. He found that there was indeed a significant relationship between fragile sites and rearrangements scored at amniocentesis as well as in spontaneous abortions, still births and new-borns, but the levels of statistical significance were lower than those of Hecht and Hecht. Braekeleer stressed that further studies are needed to assess whether fragile sites are predisposing to meiotic chromosome breakage and structural rearrangements per se.

71. At the experimental level, Yunis and Soreng [Y11] tested whether the expression of the common fragile sites could be enhanced by specific culturing regimes and whether at such sites there would be more chromosome breaks. Lymphocytes were grown in modified Eagle's medium (MEM) lacking in folic acid and thymidine (FTD medium). In one set of cultures, FdU was added during the last 24 h in culture; and in a second set, FdU and caffeine were added (the latter during the last 6 h in culture). Chromosome preparations were made by appropriate procedures to reveal 670-850 bands per haploid set. The results showed that: (a) 51 common fragile sites could be delineated;[f] (b) in the FTD + FdU + caffeine regime, there was a 10-fold enhancement (as a minimum) in the expression of fragile sites over the FTD + FdU regime; (c) there were more breaks in the FTD + FdU + caffeine group (519/100 cells) than in the other group (45.6/100 cells), most of the breaks expressed in the presence of caffeine being represented in the 51 common fragile

---

[f]The fragile sites were distributed in the different chromosomes as follows (the number of sites given in parentheses): 1 (5), 2 (6), 3 (3), 4 (2), 5 (1), 6 (3), 7 (5), 8 (3), 9 (2), 10 (3), 11 (4), 12 (1), 13 (2), 14 (2), 16 (2), 17 (1), 18 (2), 20 (1), 22 (1) and X (2).

sites (74-82%) and the rest being scattered among the other bands (frequently in Giemsa-negative ones); (d) the relative distribution of breaks among the 51 fragile sites was similar in the presence or absence of caffeine, indicating that the expression of these fragile sites is not elicited but only enhanced by caffeine; and (e) triradial configurations, typically observed at the rare (heritable) fragile sites were also observed at sites 3p14.2, 6q25.3, 8q24.1, 16q22.1, 16q23.2 and Xq22.1.

(e) *Fragile sites and break-points of certain specific chromosomal changes in cancer*

72.   Evidence is rapidly accumulating [B43, L11, Y4, Y11] to suggest that some non-random chromosomal changes involved in certain cancers have break-points that coincide with the fragile sites (Table 11). Six other chromosomes (2, 7, 12, 17 and 20) that are consistently involved in rearrangements or numerical changes in malignant cells also contain fragile sites, although localized to different chromosome bands. In addition, 10 of the 12 autosomes carry both a cellular oncogene and a fragile site, but they coincide only in the case of chromosome 8 (fragile site and c-mos at 8q22). The cellular oncogenes of chromosomes 6, 8, 9 and 11 are in the same regions as the cancer-related break-points with c-myb on 6q15-q24, c-myc on 8q24, c-abl on 9q34 and c-ras^{H1} on 11p15. On the basis of all these findings, it has been suggested [B43, L11, Y4, Y11] that fragile sites may act as predisposition factors for certain chromosomal rearrangements in human neoplasias and that some of them may represent oncogenic sites.

D.   CONGENITAL ANOMALIES

73.   In its 1982 report, UNSCEAR used a prevalence figure of $430/10^4$ live births for congenital anomalies (CAs) in man, one that was estimated by Trimble and Doughty [T9] for the population of British Columbia, Canada. Although the data of Myrianthopoulos and Chung [M12] for the United States of America, and some of the data of Czeizel [C11, C12] for Hungary, were mentioned, no systematic comparisons were made between these three sets of data. Czeizel and Sankaranarayanan [C13] have now published extensive data on the prevalence of CAs in Hungary and have also made the comparisons mentioned above with the aims of: (a) examining the extent to which the prevalences of different CAs in Hungary agree with those in the other two studies; and (b) using the Hungarian prevalences to estimate detriment due to spontaneously arising CAs. Since such comparisons are useful both in the context of assessing the load due to spontaneously arising CAs and of estimating possible risks due to radiation exposures, the general problems inherent in such comparisons, the nature of the three sets of data and the kinds of comparisons made by these authors are summarized below.

74.   The difficulties involved in comparing prevalences of CAs in different parts of the world have been discussed in a number of publications (e.g., [C25, C32,

L20, L23, N35, S84, W35]; see also section I.C. in Annex C to the present report). Among the various factors that are responsible for the differences in prevalences that have been recorded in the different studies are: the source of data (epidemiological studies, registries), study design (prospective, retrospective), the efficiency of ascertainment (dictated by the size of the material, the available expertise, whether the screening included still births and live births, whether autopsy was performed on stillborn babies, the period of follow-up, if any, in the case of live births), definition, diagnostic criteria and classification schemes adopted, geographical, regional, ethnic and other differences. It is thus obvious that an average figure (from different studies), either for the total prevalence or for individual conditions, is unlikely to reflect the situation in a global context and is admittedly crude. Such a figure will undoubtedly mask the existence of real differences—sometimes large—between studies or countries, for which there may be a genetic basis.

75.   The large-scale collaborative study of Stevenson et al. [S84] is illustrative in this regard. In this study, which involved a series of consecutive births in 24 centres in 16 countries and the outcomes of 421,781 pregnancies, the summed frequency of all major CAs was $127/10^4$ total births with a range between $31/10^4$ and $225/10^4$ in the different centres located in various parts of the world. Among the major conclusions that emerged from this study are: (a) CAs recognized at birth are predominantly of types that are suspected to have complex genotypic as well as environmental contributions to their aetiology; (b) the frequency of the CAs present at birth, if all children were followed up for a few years, would be increased by about 50%, although the numbers missed at birth depend on the type of CA and vary from zero upwards; and (c) there are large and sometimes real geographical, regional and ethnic differences in the estimates of several specific CAs (e.g., neural tube defects, cleft lip with or without cleft palate, hip dislocation or dysplasia). These findings lend support to many views based on previous evidence, have been amply documented in a number of subsequent studies and need to be taken into account when international comparisons of prevalences are made.

76.   When comparing the Hungarian data with those from the United States and British Columbia studies, it is worth pointing out that the authors' choice of these two sets of data for comparisons were dictated by the following specific considerations: first, the United States data come from a prospective study and represent the results of a co-operative endeavour of 12 major medical centres (the so-called Collaborative Perinatal Project) which was designed from the outset to ensure "nearly complete ascertainment and accurate assessment of the malformations in the new-born" [M12]; consequently, these data were expected to provide a perspective of the situation if the ascertainment efficiency were close to 100%. Secondly, the British Columbia data with certain modifications now constitute a major basis for the evaluation of genetic radiation hazards in man; it is therefore instructive to inquire whether major differences between the

Hungarian and British Columbia data exist, particularly if the Hungarian data could be used as a basis for detriment calculations (see chapter VIII).

77. In the study from the United States, the analyses were based on data from about 56,000 pregnant women who had been followed up from the first few months of pregnancy, and 52,257 deliveries (24,153 whites, 25,126 blacks and 3,978 other ethnic groups) with the children having been followed up through one year of age. Myrianthopoulos and Chung did not use the scheme recommended in the Manual on International Classification of Diseases (hereafter to be referred to as ICD) [I5]. The anomalies were classified into major and minor and, within them, single and multiple. As Myrianthopoulos and Chung stated, ". . . the decision to assign a malformation to the major or minor group, though it followed certain guidelines, was in the last analysis, arbitrary and was based on expert advice as well as our experience and intuition, rather than any one criterion or set of criteria . . . Multiple malformations were defined as those . . . found in association with malformation of the same or any other system or type . . ."

78. The Hungarian data are more extensive and are based on a total of 1,992,773 births from 1970 to 1981. In Hungary, all deliveries take place in hospitals and the reporting of CAs diagnosed through the first year of life has been mandatory since 1962. Likewise, autopsies of all dead infants are also obligatory. The data derive from two principal sources: population-based epidemiological surveys for specific CAs and the Hungarian Congenital Malformation Registry (HCMR). The epidemiological studies were initiated in the late 1960s and used all possible sources of ascertainment. Data pertaining to about 30% of the conditions (i.e., ICD entries) to be discussed later (which correspond to about 80% of the case-load) come from this source. The completeness of ascertainment for these is close to 100%.

79. The HCMR has been operational since 1970 and has multiple sources of ascertainment. For obvious reasons, the data pertaining to the earlier years (particularly 1970) are likely to be underestimates. The five years between 1977 and 1981 represent those of most reliable birth prevalences, a result of increasing diagnostic expertise and consequently more complete reporting of cases to the HCMR. The general completeness of ascertainment for these five years is on the order of 80%, although there are significant differences in ascertainment efficiency, depending on the kinds of CAs. The HCMR is the source for about 70% of the conditions (i.e., ICD entries) accounting for about 20% of the cases, for which no epidemiological data are available. It is worth mentioning that both the epidemiological studies and the maintenance of the HCMR (and analysis of the data reported to it) are carried out by the Department of Human Genetics of the National Institute of Hygiene, Budapest, and thus they complement each other. Furthermore, the epidemiological studies provide a means of controlling the completeness of the reporting to the HCMR and of introducing appropriate corrections when necessary.

80. In the Hungarian work, all the CAs are registered using the ICD code numbers. In the WHO manual, the CAs are listed in Chapter XIV (entries 740-759), which includes chromosomal anomalies, but excludes congenital inguinal and umbilical hernias (ICD numbers 550 and 553) and congenital tumours (ICD numbers 227-228). Many teratologists, however, consider the latter three entities also as CAs. The CAs have been classified into two groups: isolated and multiple. Isolated CAs are those structural defects that can be traced back to one localized error in morphogenesis. In contrast, the multiple CAs represent the concurrence of two or more different (i.e., differently localized errors in morphogenesis) major CAs in the same individual. The Hungarian data presented in the paper of Czeizel and Sankaranarayanan refer mostly to the isolated group, although some multiple ones have also been included.

81. The British Columbia data derive from two sources: (a) the actual number of cases of congenitally malformed children born in British Columbia and recorded in the Registry for Handicapped Children and Adults; and (b) non-registered cases ascertained through a province-wide surveillance system of CAs. For this study period, there were 756,304 live births. The ICD system was used to classify the CAs.

82. Table 12 represents a comparison of birth prevalences recorded in the United States, Hungarian and British Columbia studies. The following general points should be made: (a) in the Hungarian and British Columbia studies, the prevalence figures are based on the number of affected individuals, whereas in the other study these figures refer to the number of CAs; (b) the prevalence figures for the United States are those extracted by Czeizel and Sankaranarayanan from the large appendix table of Myrianthopoulos and Chung, which in their view would correspond to those of their isolated CAs (the actual numbers of CAs—and thus not of affected individuals—on which the estimated prevalences given in column 3 are based, are given in parentheses); and (c) it was considered useful to separate congenital dislocation of the hip from the group of musculoskeletal and skeletal anomalies (ICD 754-756) and present totals including and excluding the above condition, the reason being that this condition has a very high birth prevalence in Hungary ($257.7/10^4$). In what follows, unless otherwise stated, the term prevalence will be used to denote births affected with CA (and not the number of CAs).

83. Considering first the overall prevalence figures (i.e., for conditions covered by ICD entries 740-759, 550, 553 and 227-228), it can be seen that the prevalence of $849.2/10^4$ total births for the United States is higher than that for Hungary ($735.9/10^4$ total births) by about 13%. Such a comparison between live birth prevalences in Hungary and British Columbia is not feasible since Trimble and Doughty's corrected figure of $428/10^4$ live births is only applicable to ICD entries 740-759.

84. If the comparisons are restricted to ICD entries 740-759 (and thus include the congenital dislocation of the hip), the estimated prevalences in the United

States range from $704.0/10^4$ to $846.1/10^4$ total births,[g] which is again higher than that for Hungary ($614.9/10^4$ total births). It can also be noted that the live birth prevalence of $597.4/10^4$ for Hungary is also higher than that for British Columbia ($428/10^4$ births).

85. The exclusion of the congenital dislocation of the hip (again limiting consideration to ICD entries 740-759) makes only a marginal difference to the total prevalence in the United States (the range is now from $632.1/10^4$ to $775.0/10^4$ total births[h]). However, the Hungarian figure is substantially reduced to $357.2/10^4$ total births. For British Columbia a comparable calculation cannot be reliably made; however, if the percentage contribution of this condition in the corrected estimate of $428/10^4$ is the same as that based on the actual observations during the period 1952-1972 (the latter is 6.3% or 1063/16,791), then the prevalence would be marginally reduced from $428/10^4$ to $401.8/10^4$ live births. For Hungary, the reduction is from 597.4 to $339.7/10^4$ live births.

86. A close inspection of columns 3 and 5 of Table 12 (United States versus Hungary comparisons; taking into account the fact that the United States figures refer to the number of CAs and those for Hungary to the number of affected births) shows that the prevalences are fairly similar for anencephaly and spina bifida, congenital cardiovascular malformations, anomalies of the urogenital system and for chromosomal anomalies (most of the cases of chromosomal anomalies in the above two studies, as well as that of British Columbia, were trisomy-21). The agreement is less good for other malformations, such as cleft lip with or without cleft palate, anomalies of the eye, ear, face and neck, anomalies of the respiratory system and anomalies of the digestive system, the figures from the United States being generally higher than those for Hungary. Particularly noteworthy is the finding that the prevalence of musculoskeletal and skeletal anomalies in the United States (even with the exclusion of the congenital dislocation of the hip) is about 6 times, and the prevalence of integumental anomalies more than 10 times, those in Hungary. Such a condition-by-condition comparison between the Hungarian and British Columbia figures is inappropriate, since the British Columbia data summarized in Table 12 for the different conditions refer to uncorrected estimates.

87. The principal conclusions that emerge from these comparisons are the following: (a) the total estimated

birth prevalences of CAs (ICD entries 740-759, 550, 553, 227-228) range from $849.2/10^4$ total births in the United States to $735.9/10^4$ total births in Hungary; with the exclusion of the hernias (ICD 550 and 553) and congenital tumours (ICD 227-228), the estimated figures range from $704.0/10^4$ to $846.1/10^4$ total births in the United States to $614.9/10^4$ total births in Hungary; (b) in live births, the CAs defined by the ICD entries 740-759 have a prevalence ranging from $428/10^4$ in British Columbia to $597.4/10^4$ in Hungary, but over 40% of this total for Hungary is due to congenital dislocation of the hip, a condition known to have a high prevalence in that country; and (c) in principle, it is possible to have similar or nearly similar total prevalences in different countries, but the relative contributions of the different CAs to the total could be different; this fact should be clearly borne in mind in attempting to arrive at average values applicable in a global context.

88. In this document, the Committee decided to use the Hungarian prevalence figure for CAs of $600/10^4$ live births for two principal reasons: (a) this figure per se does not seem to be an unrealistic average considering the three sets of data reviewed in the preceding paragraphs; and (b) only on the basis of the Hungarian data, it has been possible to arrive at estimates of detriment for CAs and this has been one of the principal aims of the Committee. The Committee is aware of the fact that congenital dislocation of the hip has a very high birth prevalence in Hungary; however, as discussed in chapter VIII, the contribution of this condition to real detriment (expressed as lost or actually impaired life) is so small that it does not distort the overall picture of detriment associated with CAs as a whole.

E. OTHER MULTIFACTORIAL DISORDERS (EXCLUDING CONGENITAL ANOMALIES)

89. On the basis of their data on the prevalence of Mendelian, chromosomal and other disorders in British Columbia, Canada, Trimble and Doughty [T9] estimated that the total prevalence of multifactorial disorders other than congenital anomalies was on the order of $470/10^4$ live births. As may be recalled, their estimate was based on a follow-up of individuals from birth to age 21. Since many of these multifactorial disorders are not scored at birth and have variable ages of onset with manifestation late in life, it is obvious that their estimate is applicable only to those that manifest themselves before age 21 and this underestimates their prevalence in the population as a whole.

90. The preliminary results of Czeizel et al. (unpublished, 1986) obtained from an extensive analysis of data in several epidemiological studies carried out in Hungary and in other parts of the world strongly support the thesis that the population prevalence of these multifactorial disorders is at least about $6000/10^4$. Some of the essential aspects of their data and analysis are briefly summarized below.

91. Since a compilation of an exhaustive list of these disorders with adequate and reliable information on

---

[g]The estimate of 704.0 is arrived at by assuming that the number of cases affected with hernias and congenital tumours is the same as the number of these CAs ($= 350$) and that $2051 - 350 = 1701$ cases had 2330 CAs or 1.37 CAs per affected case. Thus, $964.5/1.37 = 704.0$. The value of 846.1 is arrived at by assuming that 2051 affected births had 2330 CAs or roughly 1.14 per affected birth. Thus the number of affected births is $= 964.5/1.14 = 846.1$.

[h]The assumptions underlying these calculations are the same as those explained in footnote g. The estimate of 632.1 is arrived at by assuming that the number of births with congenital dislocation of the hip, hernias and congenital tumours is the same as the total number of these CAs (i.e., $177 + 350 = 527$) and that a total of $2051 - 527 = 1524$ births had 2153 CAs or roughly 1.41 CAs/affected birth. Thus, $891.2/1.41 = 632.1$. To arrive at the figure of 775.0, it is assumed that the affected births is $2051 - 177 = 1874$. These had 2153 CAs or 1.15/affected case. Thus, $891.2/1.15 = 775$.

prevalences, ages of onset, etc., would be a formidable task for several reasons, they excluded from consideration: (a) those disorders whose population prevalences are equal to or less than $1/10^4$; (b) pre-senile and senile dementias and other cerebral degenerative disorders (such as Pick, Creutzfeldt-Jacob and Alzheimer diseases with a high prevalence in the age group of 70 and above); (c) refractory errors of the eye (myopia, hypermetropia, astigmatism), strabismus, and tooth anomalies, although again, many of these disorders have a significant genetic component in their aetiology (the decision to exclude them stems from the fact that in spite of their high population prevalences, possibilities for visual or dental corrections exist in almost all countries and after such corrections, life impairment is minimal); (d) mental retardation, blindness and deaf-mutism, not only because these conditions are aetiologically or clinically quite heterogeneous, but also because they merit a separate and detailed analysis; (e) those disorders for which the evidence on the genetic contribution is either inadequate or equivocal (e.g., pernicious anaemia, migraine, Parkinson disease, neurosis, alcoholism); (f) those with too many different clinical end-points such as atherosclerosis, which is associated with myocardial infarction, senile dementia, cerebral haemorrhage, hypertension and obesity; (g) infectious diseases; and (h) all cancers, in spite of evidence suggesting that there is some genetic component in their aetiology (this exclusion was made because the subject is very complex and deserves to be treated in its own right).

92. The disorders included in their preliminary compilation together with estimates of their prevalences in Hungary and some of their important epidemiological features are summarized in Table 13. It should be stressed that the disorders included in this selected list are by no means homogeneous either clinically or aetiologically. Nevertheless, the compilation provides some idea of the kinds of disorders that fall under the category being considered in this section. It is worth mentioning that the figures were standardized for the study population. Thus, for instance, when only the data for the adult population (above age 14) were available, the prevalence figure was reduced by 21% since the population in the 0-14 age range represented 21% of the total population. The wide range of figures published in the literature for other countries no doubt reflects the scope, size and nature of the different studies, the age-groups included in the analysis and the variations in diagnosis, time, location and the degree of ascertainment.

93. It is obvious that: (a) the population prevalence of around $6000/10^4$ (considering the fact that several disorders have been excluded) is much higher than that reported in the British Columbia survey, which only included, however, those multifactorial disorders (other than congenital anomalies) that become manifest before the age of 21; (b) the Hungarian prevalence figures for individual conditions are not out of line with those published for other parts of the world; and (c) the actual frequency of affected individuals will be less than 60% because many of them will suffer from more than one of these disorders.

F. SUMMARY AND CONCLUSIONS

94. New data on the prevalence of certain Mendelian disorders in man that have become available since the publication of the 1982 UNSCEAR report do not warrant any revision of the Committee's earlier assessments in this regard. The earlier findings of Dubinin and Altukhov that the frequencies of rare electrophoretic variants (at over 20 genetic loci coding for the synthesis of enzyme proteins and erythrocyte antigens) are significantly higher in premature infants and in those with multiple congenital anomalies, could not be confirmed in an independent study of a similar nature carried out by Neel and Mohrenweiser.

95. A re-analysis of data on the contribution of chromosomal anomalies to spontaneous abortions and still births shows that about 40% of spontaneous abortions and 5.7% of still births are associated with chromosomal anomalies. The figure of 40% spontaneous abortions pertains to those that occur in weeks 5-28 of pregnancy (UNSCEAR's figure of 50% discussed in its earlier reports allows for developmental arrests that may occur before the fifth week of gestation). The currently available information suggests that about 5% of recognized conceptions are associated with chromosomal anomalies.

96. Studies on the parental origin of the extra chromosome in trisomies in spontaneous abortions show that, in most cases, the trisomies result from non-disjunction in maternal meiosis-I.

97. New data have been published on the effect of maternal age on chromosomally normal and abnormal spontaneous abortions. These show that the overall rate of spontaneous abortions is relatively constant from age 20 to 30, but, beginning in the mid-30s, there is a marked increase and, by 40 years of age, more than 25% of all registered pregnancies terminate in spontaneous abortions. In chromosomally abnormal spontaneous abortions, trisomies accounted for 20% of spontaneous abortions involving women under 25 years of age, but approximately 33% for those in the 30-35-year age group and no less that 67% in women aged 40 years or more.

98. The rates of numerical chromosomal anomalies in pre-natal (amniocentesis) cytogenetic studies have been determined and compared with maternal-age adjusted rates in live births. The results show that the frequencies of XXX and XXY conditions increase with maternal age while that for XYY shows a slight decrease with maternal age. The rates of trisomy-21 and for trisomy-18 in live births are about 20% and 70%, respectively, lower than the corresponding ones at amniocentesis. Another cytogenetic investigation showed that the prevalence of balanced structural rearrangements at amniocentesis is higher than in new-borns and that the mutation rate estimate (based on de novo balanced rearrangements) of $4.3 \ 10^{-4}/$ gamete/generation calculated on the basis of these data is higher than that of $1.88 \ 10^{-4}/$gamete/generation derived earlier on the basis of data from new-born surveys.

99. Recent results from new-born cytogenetic surveys using banding methods in Norway and in Denmark, despite the relatively small sample sizes involved, support the view that in the earlier surveys, which did not use chromosome banding methods, the frequencies of reciprocal translocations and inversions had been underestimated. These new data suggest that the total birth prevalence of chromosomal anomalies may be as high as 2%, but 30-50% of this frequency is made up of autosomal inversions, primarily of chromosome 9, that are regarded as variants rather than anomalies per se.

100. The prevalence of chromosomal anomalies in mentally retarded or otherwise handicapped individuals and in those with mental retardation and one or more congenital anomalies is higher (8 to 20%) than in new-borns. Similarly, in subfertile males the frequency of chromosomal anomalies is also higher, with XXY being the major contributor. Furthermore, there is a clear correlation between sex-chromosomal anomalies and azoospermia, the prevalence of these anomalies being much higher among azoospermic males than in new-borns (XXY, 100-fold higher; XX males, 160-fold higher).

101. The results of further studies on direct analysis of the chromosome constitution of human spermatozoa (after fertilization of hamster eggs in vitro) have been published. There is a high degree of inter-individual variation, the frequencies of chromosomal anomalies ranging from 0-28% in the different males studied. The anomalies detected include chromatid breaks, chromosome breaks, chromatid exchanges, acentric fragments, hypo-ploidy and hyper-ploidy. In cancer patients who underwent radiotherapy treatments, these frequencies were higher than before radiotherapy.

102. Considerable work has been carried out on fragile sites in human chromosomes during the last 2-3 years. The fragile sites are currently classified into two broad groups, the rare and the common or constitutive. Among the rare fragile sites are 16 folate-sensitive sites (the fragile site on the long arm of the X associated with mental retardation and macro-orchidism is included in this group), 2 distamycin-A-inducible sites, and 1 BrdU-requiring site. Among the common ones are: 6 aphidicolin-inducible sites, 2 azacytidine-inducible sites, and 3 BrdU-inducible ones. In addition to the sites that have been confirmed, at least 7 rare fragile sites and 17 common ones are grouped under the category of possible fragile sites needing further confirmation.

103. The fragile site on the X-chromosome that is associated with macro-orchidism and one form of X-linked mental retardation has now been localized to band Xq27.3.

104. Most fragile-X carrier females are not mentally retarded; there is an inverse relationship between the frequency of fragile-X expression in lymphocytes and IQ (e.g., mildly retarded females have higher frequencies of fragile-X expression than their intellectually normal counterparts). An inverse relationship between

fragile-X expression and IQ is also found in affected males, but it is less pronounced than in carrier females or not demonstrable at all.

105. There is also an inverse relationship between age and the frequency of fragile-X expression in mentally normal heterozygotes (older females have lower frequencies of fragile-X expression) and retarded carriers show higher frequencies at all ages.

106. The mentally retarded carrier females appear to have higher frequencies of early replicating fragile-X active X-chromosome than their mentally normal counterparts, but this relationship needs further study.

107. Analysis of the available data on the prevalence of non-specific, X-linked mental retardation in males suggests a rate of about $18.3/10^4$ males: about one-half of this is due to fragile-X, which makes the latter the second major contributor to mental retardation, after trisomy-21. A more recent estimate of the prevalence of fragile-X associated mental retardation is $4-5/10^4$ males. Genetic analysis of 110 fragile-X pedigrees allows a mutation rate estimate of about $2.4 \ 10^{-4}$/locus/generation (both sexes considered).

108. The results so far available from population cytogenetic studies show that the prevalence of fragile-X is very low in unselected neo-nates (in fact, no fragile-X positive case has been detected in 3558 neo-nates of both sexes screened) but higher in institutionalized retardates, in those attending special schools for the retarded and in hospital referral patients; the prevalence in these last groups ranges from 1.6 to 16.1%, obviously depending on the severity of the retarded individuals included in the different studies. Likewise, the limited data on autosomal folate-sensitive rare fragile sites suggest a low prevalence in unselected neo-nates (0.15%) and significantly higher ones in hospital referral patients, in children attending special schools and in institutionalized retardates (range from 0.38 to 1.6%). Data on other rare fragile sites (i.e., distamycin-inducible and BrdU-requiring sites) are less extensive.

109. There are reports in support of the working hypothesis that autism may be associated with the presence of the fragile-X chromosome. There are no conclusive data demonstrating that fragile sites (other than the Xq27) may be associated with adverse phenotypic effects such as congenital anomalies.

110. Data have been published that support the thesis that certain fragile sites may predispose the chromosomes carrying them to spontaneous breakage (visualized under specific lymphocyte culture conditions) or may be associated with the break-points in constitutional chromosome rearrangements (seen in spontaneous abortions, still births and in new-borns). There is also some evidence suggesting that non-random chromosomal changes associated with certain specific cancers may have break-points that coincide with, or are in proximity to, the fragile sites and that some of the latter may represent oncogenic sites. However, further data are needed to validate these findings.

111. The birth prevalence of isolated and multiple congenital anomalies in man has been re-assessed by comparing the estimates made in the British Columbia study with those of other studies in Hungary and the United States. The total estimated birth prevalence of these anomalies (included in chapter XIV of the International Classification of Diseases and conditions such as inguinal and umbilical hernias and congenital tumours not included in the above chapter) range from $849.2/10^4$ total births in the United States to $735.9/10^4$ total births in Hungary; with the exclusion of hernias and congenital tumours, the estimated figures range from $704.0/10^4$ to $846.1/10^4$ total births in the United States to $614.9/10^4$ total births in Hungary. In live births, the congenital anomalies included in chapter XIV of the Manual on the International Classification of Diseases alone have a prevalence ranging from $428/10^4$ in British Columbia to $597.4/10^4$ in the other series, while over 40% of the total for Hungary is due to congenital dislocation of the hip, a condition known to have a high prevalence in that country.

112. Considering the three sets of data, the Committee concluded the Hungarian prevalence figure for congenital anomalies of about $600/10^4$ live births is a reasonable average.

113. A similar, but preliminary re-assessment of the population prevalence of other multifactorial disorders in man has been made. In this work, only conditions that have a population prevalence of at least $1/10^4$ have been included. Excluded from consideration were those conditions with high prevalences in age groups of 70 and above, refractory errors of the eye, tooth anomalies, mental retardation, blindness and deaf-mutism, those conditions with a multiplicity of clinical end-points, disorders for which the evidence of genetic contribution is either inadequate or equivocal, infectious diseases and cancers. The overall prevalence (of about 25 entities) is on the order of $6000/10^4$ individuals for Hungary. This figure is within the range reported in the literature for other countries but is an order of magnitude higher than that estimated in British Columbia ($470/10^4$). It should be stressed, however, that in the latter study, only those multifactorial disorders that become manifest before the age of 21 were included.

II. THE APPLICATION OF RECOMBINANT DNA TECHNOLOGY TO THE ANALYSIS OF THE HUMAN GENOME AND GENETIC DISEASE

114. The latest update [M57] of McKusick's 1983 Compendium [M21] contains details of 1789 conditions, mostly diseases or pathological states determined at distinct gene loci, which are well documented as being inherited in a Mendelian manner. The breakdown is as follows: 1059 autosomal dominants, 610 autosomal recessives and 120 X-linked ones. In addition, a further 1886 conditions are included (971 autosomal dominants, 774 autosomal recessives and 141 X-linked ones) where the evidence of Mendelian inheritance is not complete. Apart from the fact that the total number of loci so far identified is a very small proportion of the total number of genes in man (variously estimated to be between 50,000 and 100,000; see [M21]), only about 450 have been mapped to specific chromosomes and the molecular basis for disease is known only in a small proportion of these conditions [M24].

115. The advent of recombinant DNA technology, one of molecular biology's most powerful tools, is now rapidly changing this situation. The application of these techniques to the human genome during the last few years is providing new opportunities for increasing the speed and precision of gene mapping, for defining the nature of the genetic lesions involved, for analysis of the action of specific genes in health and disease, including cancer, and for formulating new approaches in the management of heritable disorders. The potential, current achievements and future prospects of recombinant DNA technology have already been reviewed (e.g., [B16-B18, D15, E11, E18, J14, M58, R16, W17]). The present section is focused on some of the principal developments that have resulted from the use of recombinant DNA applications to human disease. The remarkable insights into oncogenic transformation that have emerged through the use of this technology are considered in a later chapter.

A. GENERAL PRINCIPLES

116. The British Genetic Manipulation Advisory Group (see [M58]) defined recombinant DNA technology as follows: "the formation of new combinations of heritable material by the insertion of nucleic acid molecules, produced by whatever means outside the cell, into any virus, bacterial plasmid or other vector system so as to allow their amplification and then incorporation into a host organism in which they do not naturally occur but in which they are capable of continued propagation". The major techniques and their biochemical and enzymological aspects have been extensively discussed in a number of publications (e.g., [D15, E11, R50, S39, W8-W10, W40]). The actual recombinant part of the technology, whereby new combinations of genetic material are generated, is relatively well defined and can be considered under four main headings: (a) the generation of DNA fragments using, for example, restriction endonucleases; (b) the incorporation of these fragments into a suitable vector; (c) the introduction of the vector into a particular host organism, which is then grown in culture to produce clones with multiple copies of an incorporated DNA fragment; and (d) the selection and harvesting of clones that contain a specific DNA fragment.

1. Production of DNA fragments: the use of restriction endonucleases

117. Although DNA can be reduced to fragments by mechanical shearing, the process is random because

there is no way of ensuring that a particular DNA sequence is isolated. The discovery in 1970, by Smith and Wilcox [S91] and Kelly and Smith [K38], of a group of enzymes that occur in microorganisms (referred to as class II restriction endonucleases) and that were found to cleave the DNA at sequence-specific sites, therefore, represented a major milestone in recombinant DNA technology (see also [M59]). In general, the target sequences are composed of particular tetra-, penta-, hexa-, or hepta-nucleotides. At present, well over 500 different restriction enzymes, with at least 100 different recognition specificities, are known [F10, K37, R17]. Each enzyme is designated according to the organism from which it is derived (for instance, EcoRI is an enzyme obtained from Escherichia coli strain R and was the first such enzyme isolated). Some enzymes may cleave the same site but are obtained from different organisms (e.g., HindIII and HsuI) or recognize the same sequence but cleave at different sites within the sequence (XmaI and SmaI). Table 14 provides some illustrative examples of the commonly used restriction enzymes and their specificities.

118. Because of the complementary base-pairing in the DNA [adenine (A) with thymine (T) and guanine (G) with cytosine (C)], restriction endonucleases produce double-strand breaks. For instance, the enzyme EcoRI specifically cleaves the DNA between the bases G and A in the sequence -GAATTC- producing staggered ends:

$$5' - G \overline{\underline{|A A T T}}\, C - 3'$$
$$3' - C\, T T A A\underline{|}\, G - 5'$$
$$\downarrow$$
$$-G \qquad AATTC-$$
$$-CTTA \qquad G-$$

The staggered ends with complementary bases are called sticky or cohesive ends. Other enzymes, however, produce "blunt-ended" fragments, e.g., SmaI.

$$5' - C C C\,|\,G G G - 3'$$
$$3' - G G G\,|\,C C C - 5'$$
$$\downarrow$$
$$-CCC \qquad GGG-$$
$$-GGG \qquad CCC-$$

The different types of ends produced by restriction enzymes have important implications in the strategy subsequently used to join two DNA molecules together.

2. Incorporation of the DNA fragments into a suitable vector

119. When a restriction enzyme produces sticky ends, as in the case of EcoRI, and is used on both the DNA to be incorporated into a vector (foreign DNA) as well as on the DNA of the vector itself, the cohesive ends will come together and be held by hydrogen bonding between the complementary bases. The two molecules can then be sealed (ligated) and stabilized by the joining enzyme, DNA ligase. There are several types of ligases and some (e.g., T4 DNA ligase) will actually link together DNA molecules with blunt ends. The choice of a particular restriction enzyme and

DNA joining strategy depends on a number of factors. In general, preference is given to an enzyme that has a single site on both the foreign and vector DNAs and that is readily available and relatively inexpensive.

120. The vectors used for cloning are of different types. Plasmids, bacteriophage lambda derivatives, bacteriophage M13 and cosmids are the most commonly used ones to clone fragments of foreign DNA and propagate them in E. coli. Despite differences in size and structure, these four types of vectors share the following properties: (a) they can replicate autonomously in E. coli, even when joined covalently to a foreign DNA fragment; (b) they can be easily separated from bacterial nucleic acids and purified; and (c) they contain regions of DNA that are not essential for propagation in bacteria; foreign DNA inserted into these regions is replicated and propagated as if it were a normal component of the vector [M32].

121. Plasmids. Plasmids are extrachromosomal genetic elements found in a variety of bacterial (and yeast) species. They are small circular molecules of double-stranded DNA that range in size from 1 kb (kilobase) to greater than 200 kb. They replicate as independent units as the host cell proliferates.[i] Plasmids often contain genes coding for enzymes that, under certain circumstances, are advantageous to the host bacterium. Among the phenotypes conferred by the different plasmids are: resistance to antibiotics, production of antibiotics and production of colicin. Under normal conditions, many plasmids are transmitted to new hosts by a process similar to bacterial conjugation. In the laboratory, they can be transferred to bacteria by an artificial process known as transformation (see next section).

122. Maniatis et al. [M32] list a number of properties that a plasmid must have to be useful as a cloning vector: (a) it should be relatively small and should replicate in a relaxed fashion (to ensure high copy numbers); (b) it should carry one or more selectable markers to allow identification of transformants and to maintain the plasmid in the bacterial population; and (c) it should contain a single restriction site for one or more restriction enzymes in regions that are not essential for plasmid replication; preferably, they should be located within genes coding for selectable markers so that insertion of a foreign fragment inactivates the gene. In terms of insert size, plasmid vectors can accommodate up to 5 to 6 kb of foreign DNA. The most widely used vector is pBR322, a plasmid under relaxed control that contains both ampicillin and tetracycline genes and a number of convenient restriction sites.

---

[i]In general, replication of plasmid DNA is carried out by the same set of enzymes involved in the replication of the bacterial chromosome. Some plasmids are under stringent control, i.e., their replication is coupled to that of the host so that only one or at most a few copies of the plasmid will be present in the bacterial cell [N19]. Plasmids under relaxed control, however, have copy numbers of 10-200; the copy number of the relaxed plasmids can be increased by several thousands per cell if host protein synthesis is arrested (e.g., by treatment with chloramphenicol [C33]). In the absence of protein synthesis, replication of relaxed plasmids continues whereas replication of chromosomal DNA and of stringent plasmids ceases [M32].

123. Bacteriophage lambda. Ever since the first demonstration of the feasibility of using bacteriophage lambda as a cloning vehicle [M33, R21, T21] a large variety of vectors have been constructed [W18]. Bacteriophage lambda is a double-stranded DNA virus with a genomic size of about 50 kb; only about 60% of its genome is necessary for lytic propagation of the phage, the middle one-third (the stuffer portion) being not essential. The maximum size of the insert tolerated by lambda derivatives is about 24 kb.

124. Cosmid. A cosmid [C34] is a type of artificially constructed small plasmid vector that can be packaged in vitro in lambda phage. Typically, it contains: (a) a drug resistance marker and a plasmid origin of replication; (b) one or more unique restriction sites for cloning; (c) a DNA fragment that contains the ligated cohesive (cos) end site of the phage. The cosmid is of small size, so that eukaryotic DNA fragments up to 50 kb in length can be accommodated.

125. M13 phage. M13 is a single-stranded DNA bacteriophage with its circular DNA genome being about 6500 nucleotides in length [D28]. The primary advantage of M13 as a cloning vehicle derives from the fact that the phage particles released from the bacterial cell contain single-stranded DNA that is homologous to only one of the strands of the cloned DNA fragment and can therefore be used as a template for DNA sequencing. M13 vectors and specific primer DNAs have been developed to allow sequencing of up to 350 bases from a single clone.

3. Cloning and the production of multiple copies of the inserted DNA fragment

126. After a fragment of foreign DNA is inserted into a suitable vector (plasmid, lambda phage, cosmid, etc.), the next step is to introduce the vector into a host organism. Host organisms that have been used in recombinant DNA technology include E. coli, strain K-12 (the most favoured), Bacillus subtilis and the yeast Saccharomyces cerevisiae. In the case of plasmid vectors, in order to generate recombinant plasmids, the plasmids are first isolated from a bacterial host by disruption and centrifugation and the bacterial DNA and debris are discarded. The plasmid DNA and foreign DNA are then exposed to an appropriate restriction enzyme, mixed together and treated with ligase. To reduce the likelihood of the plasmid recircularizing without incorporating the foreign DNA, the former is treated with the enzyme alkaline phosphatase. The recombinant plasmid DNA is then introduced into a bacterial cell (by treating the latter with calcium chloride, which renders its cell membrane permeable to the plasmid DNA), a process referred to as transformation. The transformed bacteria are then grown on nutrient agar in petri dishes. Each colony of cells represents the progeny of a single cell and therefore all the cells in a colony have the same genetic constitution and all the cells in a clone will contain the same inserted segment of foreign DNA. Individual colonies can be subsequently sub-cloned to generate multiple copies of a particular recombinant DNA sequence.

127. Cloning in lambda vectors involves the following steps: (a) the vector DNA is digested to completion with the appropriate restriction enzyme, and in the case of replacement vectors,[j] the left and right arms are separated from the central stuffer fragments by velocity gradient centrifugation or gel electrophoresis; (b) the two arms are then ligated in the presence of fragments of foreign DNA having termini compatible with those of the arms; and (c) the resulting recombinant DNAs are packaged in vitro into viable phage particles that form plaques on the appropriate hosts. The strategies used with other vectors are basically similar.

4. Selection and characterization of recombinant clones

128. If a clone has become transformed by a plasmid carrying resistance to a particular antibiotic, then this could be detected by the ability of this clone to grow in the presence of the antibiotic; in the case of the phage, this will be revealed by the formation of plaques. The next step is to determine whether the vector has acquired foreign DNA. In the case of a plasmid, this can be recognized by an altered antibiotic resistance, using replica plating techniques. For instance, in the case of the plasmid pBR322, if foreign DNA has been incorporated at the PstI site (thus destroying the ampicillin resistance gene), colonies will not grow in the presence of ampicillin (though they will remain resistant to tetracycline) and can therefore be identified, picked off and cultured separately. In the case of phage vectors, advantage is taken of the fact that certain strains normally produce blue plaques when plated in the presence of a particular chromogenic substance (Xgal), but if foreign DNA is successfully inserted in the gene responsible for this colour change, then they form colourless plaques.

129. A number of ingenious techniques have been developed to characterize the recombinants that contain a specific DNA sequence (genetic, hybridization with an appropriate probe, hybrid-arrested protein translation,[k] electron microscopy, etc.). A probe is a segment of single-stranded DNA or RNA that has been labeled either radioactively (e.g., ^{32}P) or with some biochemical marker such as biotin [L25]. A gene-specific probe may be produced in several ways from its constituent nucleotides, either because these are already known or can be inferred from the aminoacid composition of the gene product, or by first isolating mRNA from a relevant tissue and, using this as a template, and with reverse transcriptase, synthesizing the complementary copy of the DNA (cDNA). The important point here is that a probe will search out and detect (hybridize with) complementary sequences in the presence of a large amount of noncomplementary DNA. Hybridization of DNA extracted

---

[j]Lambda derivatives having a single target site at which foreign DNA is inserted are known as insertion vectors and those having a pair of sites spanning a segment that can be removed and replaced by foreign DNA are known as replacement or substitution vectors.

[k]Hybrid-arrested translation (HART) is a technique used to identify DNA sequences by hybridization with RNA and then study the products of in vitro protein synthesis [P32].

from a clone can also be carried out on an electrophoresis gel using the method introduced by Southern and therefore referred to as a Southern blot [S42].

130. In the Southern blotting method, the DNA extracted from a clone is first exposed to an appropriate restriction enzyme and the resultant DNA fragments subjected to electrophoresis on agarose gels and separated according to size. The DNA is then denatured with alkali (to render it capable of hybridization with the complementary sequences of the probe) and transferred to a nitrocellulose filter (Southern blotting). The DNA or RNA probe is labelled with ^{32}P and hybridized to the filter bound DNA. The sequence complementary to the probe used would appear as bands on autoradiographs. When the sequences analysed are less than 1 kb, polyacrylamide gels may be used [M34] for their separation, as used for sequencing DNA [M35, M36]. The DNA fragments in this case may be transferred from the gel to the filter electrically.

131. The Southern blotting method cannot, however, be applied to RNA fragments separated by gel electrophoresis because RNA does not bind to nitrocellulose. A modification of the procedure, called the Northern blotting method, has therefore been developed for use with RNA [A7].

B. CONSTRUCTION OF LIBRARIES

132. Through the use of techniques briefly discussed in the preceding paragraphs, it has been possible to make libraries of cloned DNA fragments [W11]. The advances in this area have been so rapid and phenomenal that, currently, gene libraries, some chromosome-specific libraries and genomic libraries are available (see [D15] for details). A cDNA (copy DNA or complementary DNA) library is constructed by synthesizing a double-stranded copy of the mRNA population (using RNA-dependent DNA polymerase or reverse transcriptase) and integrating these cDNA molecules into a restriction site in a plasmid [W11]. The cDNA library is representative of mRNA sequences expressed in the particular cell type from which it is derived and is useful for studying tissue- or stage-specific gene expression. It contains fewer repetitive DNA sequences than a genomic library and is a source of the coding sequences of the genome. A genomic library contains all the coding and non-coding sequences [M22, F11], including single copy sequences and repetitive sequences. It has also been possible to construct libraries of clones of at least some individual human chromosomes (chromosome-specific libraries), mostly from hybrid cell lines, following various enrichment procedures, such as chromosome sorting [D15].

C. RESTRICTION FRAGMENT LENGTH POLYMORPHISMS (RFLPs)

133. As mentioned earlier, the DNA restriction enzymes recognize specific sequences in the DNA and cleave them, yielding fragments of definite lengths.

These fragments can be separated according to molecular size by electrophoresis on agarose gels. Differences among individuals in the length of a particular restriction fragment (RFLP) can be due to several kinds of genotypic differences: differences in one or more nucleotide bases (resulting in loss of a cleavage site or formation of a new one) or insertion or deletion of a stretch of DNA within a fragment (resulting in an alteration of fragment size). These changes, which seem to occur approximately every 100-200 base pairs in the normal population, are apparently without any phenotypic effects, are inherited in a Mendelian co-dominant manner and thus can be used in family linkage studies to localize specific genes of interest [B19, D16-D18, H18, H19, K12, M23, O6, S40, S41, W12]. Cooper and Schmidtke [C35] have published a list of DNA polymorphisms found in the human genome by restriction enzyme analysis.

D. RECOMBINANT DNA TECHNOLOGY IN HUMAN GENETICS AND MEDICINE

134. Over the last six years or so, recombinant DNA technology has revolutionized the study of the human genome. It has led to the successful cloning of cDNA for a large number (well over a hundred) of human structural genes, among which are several proto-oncogenes, genes with known functions, as well as unique sequences whose functions will ultimately become known [B45, D19, E18, S40, S43, S44]. It has permitted greater insights to be made into the fine structural organization of genes, the nature of molecular defects that lead to disease states, gene regulation and gene expression and has helped in the pre-natal diagnosis of certain heritable disorders. It has provided a powerful tool for gene mapping and for delineating linkage relationships. Table 15 is taken from the paper of Cooper and Schmidtke [C35] and provides a useful summary of these advances (see also [J14]). Some illustrative examples are discussed below.

1. Direct analysis of genes

135. Globin gene clusters. The genetic analysis of human globin genes and mutations that affect their structure and synthesis of haemoglobin (and thus lead to diseased states, the haemoglobinopathies) has frequently set the pace and established precedents for studies in the area of normal gene structure and function, as well as mechanisms of abnormal gene expression leading to specific diseases [B46, W17, W42]. There are at least two reasons for this: (a) on a global scale, the haemoglobinopathies cause far more illness than Mendelian conditions, since about a quarter of a million severely affected individuals are born every year with one or more of these disorders [W17]; and (b) the study of haemoglobinopathies has been made easier by the fact that cells in which gene expression is limited to the synthesis of globin chains of haemoglobin can be obtained relatively easily (peripheral blood reticulocytes).

136. Haemoglobin is a tetramer consisting of two alpha-like and two beta-like globin subunits. These

subunits are encoded by two clusters of globin genes, the alpha and beta gene clusters, the former located on the short arm of chromosome 16 and the latter on the short arm of chromosome 11. The alpha gene cluster consists of two active alpha genes and a zeta gene. The beta gene cluster consists of an epsilon gene, two different gamma genes, a delta gene and a beta gene. The zeta and epsilon genes are only active in the embryo, the gamma genes normally only in the fetus and the beta and delta genes only in the adult.

137. The advances in understanding of the structure and organization of these genes, which have resulted from the application of recombinant DNA methods have been reviewed in a number of publications (e.g., [A18, F12, M61, O7, O14]. Among the important results are: (a) the delineation of linkage relationships between the alpha [E19, L26, O15] and between the beta genes [B47, F31, F32, L27, L28, M62, P33, R51, T32]; (b) the identification of non-expressed globin pseudogenes[l] within the globin gene clusters [F33, J21, P34]; (c) the discovery of intervening sequences (introns) which separate the coding regions [F38], similar to those already known from studies of rabbit and mouse globin genes [J22, T33]; (d) the identification of repetitive sequence elements within globin gene clusters [F33, M61]; (e) the detection of DNA polymorphisms in the globin gene clusters and their characterization (reviewed in [A18, O14]) with their applications for pre-natal detection of haemoglobinopathies; and (f) the establishment of phylogenetic relationships among mammalian and human globin genes [E20].

138. Haemoglobinopathies. These belong to two major groups: the first group includes those in which there is a structural alteration in one of the globin peptide chains; the second includes those in which the basic abnormality is a defect in globin chain synthesis, rather than a structural abnormality in the globin chain itself. The classical example for the first group is sickle cell anaemia and for the second, the thalassaemias. Sickle cell anaemia is a consequence of a point mutation (transversion) at the sixth codon from the 5' end of the beta globin gene, which results in the replacement of glutamic acid by valine [M25]:

(glutamic acid)

$$\beta^A.....CCT\ \ GAG\ \ GAG....$$
$$\downarrow$$
$$\beta^S.....CCT\ \ GTG\ \ GAG....$$

(valine)

139. It is now possible to detect directly the above mutation by restriction enzyme analysis. The $A \rightarrow T$ substitution in codon 6 alters the recognition site for restriction enzymes MnlI, DdeI and MstII [C21, G19, K14, W15]. For strictly practical reasons, only the last is useful when standard Southern blot analysis is performed. Loss of the cleavage site at codon 6 produces a 1.3 kb beta-gene fragment, compared with a 1.1 kb normal fragment. This method has been

[l]These are DNA sequences which share sequence homology with the well-established globin loci (in this case) but do not correspond to known globin polypeptide chains. Globin pseudogenes have also been identified in other animal species such as rabbit, mouse, goat and sheep [F12].

successfully used in pre-natal detection studies [C21, K14, O14].

140. Another approach that has been used for direct detection of the β^S-mutation (and also of several different beta thalassaemia defects) is the use of synthetic oligonucleotides as probes. Under appropriate experimental conditions, short synthetic DNA fragments (oligonucleotides, oligomers) can hybridize to their homologous sequences but not to heterologous sequences, i.e., those with any degree of mismatch. A probe 19-nucleotide long (19-mers) directed to the normal beta globin sequence in the region of the β^S-mutation can hybridize efficiently with the normal gene, but not with DNA containing the β^S-mutation. Conversely, a 19-mers probe strictly homologous to the altered sequence will hybridize only with the β^S-containing DNA [C38].

141. With respect to thalassaemias, the whole array of recombinant DNA techniques has been used, including the screening of genomic libraries with cDNA probes, the isolation, characterization and sequencing of globin genes, and in vitro translation and protein synthesis. As a result of these studies, it is now known that the molecular defects in β^o-thalassaemia (complete absence of beta globin synthesis) include nonsense mutations due to base substitutions, nonsense mutations due to base deletions or insertions causing frameshift, base substitutions at junctions between introns and exons totally preventing normal precursor mRNA processing and partial beta globin gene deletion. Likewise, in β^+-thalassaemia (where beta globin synthesis is present but markedly reduced), the lesions include base substitutions in introns causing defects in precursor mRNA processing and base substitutions in the 5'-flanking DNA that cause reduced transcription of the beta globin gene. The majority of beta globin defects, however, are the result of point mutations (reviewed in [F12, M61, O7, O14]; see also [O10 and P51] for the use of synthetic oligonucleotides for the direct detection of β^+-thalassaemia and β^o-thalassaemia in pre-natal diagnosis).

142. Other examples. Alpha-1-antitrypsin deficiency (an autosomal recessive syndrome) predisposes the individuals to the development of pulmonary emphysema and, for reasons still not clear, such a deficiency may also present as infantile liver cirrhosis. The alpha-1-antitrypsin cDNA clone has been constructed [K15] and nucleotide sequence analysis has shown that the deficiency is due to a point mutation involving a G to A transition, which leads to a single aminoacid substitution from glutamic acid to lysine at residue 342 [W14], a situation analogous to the sickle cell haemoglobin. Since this point mutation does not create or destroy a restriction enzyme recognition site, probes of oligonucleotides complementary to the normal and mutant genes were synthesized and employed to identify homozygous recessive individuals. The probe specific for the normal gene sequence yielded significant hybridization signals only with the chromosomal DNAs of normal individuals. Since only the recessive homozygotes will manifest the disease, this methodology will permit the identification of fetuses lacking the normal gene sequence and allow for pre-natal diagnosis of the deficiency syndrome.

143. Studies with the arginosuccinate synthetase locus (deficiency of this enzyme causes the disease citrullinaemia characterized by ammonia intoxication, mental retardation and early death) have now shown that this locus involves an expressed gene on chromosome 9 and a family of related pseudogenes dispersed to at least nine other chromosomes, including 6, X and Y. Analysis of the genomic DNA suggests that the expressed gene is larger ($>$ 50 kb) with at least nine introns and the presumptive pseudogenes are smaller ($<$ 6 kb). Analysis of cultured fibroblasts from citrullinaemia patients demonstrated the presence of hybridizable mRNA which was shown to be defective [B20].

144. Hypoxanthine-guanine phosphoribosyl transferase (HPRT) which functions in the metabolic salvage pathway of purines, is encoded by an X-linked gene in man. Partial HPRT deficiencies are associated with gouty arthritis, while the absence of activity results in Lesch-Nyhan syndrome. Although a complete characterization of the human HPRT gene has not yet been achieved, the complete structure of the mouse HPRT gene has been determined by restriction mapping of lambda recombinants and selective DNA sequencing; the gene was shown to be 33 kb long and to be split into 9 exons [M37]. From this study, the human gene appears to be of similar length. This estimate is in agreement with that of Jolly et al. [J15] based on analysis of HPRT-deficient mouse cell transformants that carried a functional human HPRT gene. The coding regions of the mouse, hamster and human HPRT genes share a substantial ($>$ 95%) homology, with a divergence in the 3' and 5' untranslated regions [F13, N15, N16]. The mature mRNA for the human HPRT is only about 1.6 kb in length [B29, J15, L13]; thus the functional mRNA is only about 5% of the genomic DNA that codes for HPRT and this discrepancy in length is explained in part by the presence of long non-coding introns that interrupt the coding exons [W20]. There is evidence for the existence of four autosomal cross-hybridizing sequences in the human genome [N16], located on chromosomes 3 (one), 5 (one) and 11 (two) [P22]. The hybridization of specific cDNA fragments to the autosomal sequences, as well as partial sequence analysis, suggest that these HPRT-like sequences represent processed or intronless pseudogenes.

145. A characterization of mutant genes of 28 Lesch-Nyhan patients using recombinant DNA techniques showed that, in 23 of them, the Southern blot patterns were identical to that found among normal controls, while five showed patterns suggestive of major gene alterations: one of them showed a total deletion of the HPRT gene (exons 1-9), one a partial deletion (exons 4-9), one a smaller partial deletion (exons 7-9), one a partial duplication (in the region starting with the 5' end and extending to exon 4) and, finally, one an altered pattern (exons 4-6), which could not be delineated [P22, Y9]. A similar conclusion, namely, that the nature of the alterations was different in different individuals, was reached by Wilson [W20] from studies of 5 unrelated patients, first by comparative mapping of tryptic peptides with the use of high pressure liquid chromatography and more recently by restriction enzyme analysis.

146. Rees et al. [R62] have obtained evidence that, in a patient with a severe form of haemophilia B, the only significant difference from the normal factor IX gene (the clotting factor gene) is a point mutation within the donor splice junction (one that is essential for the normal splicing of pre-mRNA to mRNA), which changes the obligatory (and highly conserved) GT to TT. In addition, the authors used oligonucleotide probes specific for this mutation to demonstrate the feasibility of carrier detection and pre-natal diagnosis for relatives of the patient.

2. Indirect analysis of genetic disease using gene probes to detect linked polymorphisms

147. The techniques of restriction endonuclease analysis of DNA have allowed the identification of a number of polymorphisms (RFLPs), which in turn have been found to have a number of applications in clinical practice and human genetics. In general, if an RFLP is closely linked to a locus for a serious genetic disease, this can be used for pre-natal diagnosis, for the detection of dominant disorders before symptoms appear or for the detection of female carriers of X-linked diseases. Thus, for instance, Kan and Dozy [K13] detected a HpaI site polymorphism located at the 3' flanking segment of the beta globin gene that was adjacent to the gene for sickle cell anaemia. This has enabled its use in pre-natal diagnosis. As has been mentioned earlier, direct detection of the β^S gene has now become possible using the endonucleases MstII and DdeI [C21, G19, K14, O8, W15].

148. There is general agreement that several different genes are probably involved in rendering an individual susceptible to atherosclerosis and coronary artery disease, additional important environmental factors being cigarette smoking and overeating. The genetic control of lipoproteins is clearly important since there is an association of atherosclerosis with raised plasma levels of low-density lipoproteins (LDL) and reduced plasma levels of high-density lipoproteins (HDL). It seems that while LDL may predispose the individual to atherosclerosis, HDL affords protection against the disease. Apolipoprotein A-1 (apoA-1) is the major protein constituent of HDL. The normal gene for apoA-1 has now been isolated, cloned and characterized, the coding region of the mature apoA-1 mRNA consisting of 804 nucleotides [K39]. It has been found using apoA-1 probes that, at least in some individuals, premature atherosclerosis is associated with a variant apoA-1 gene with an insertion in the coding region [K20, K21].

149. Using a cDNA clone for human phenylalanine hydroxylase (PH), which is responsible for phenylketonuria (PKU), Woo et al. [W21] demonstrated that the PH gene is present in the cellular DNA of PKU patients, suggesting that the classical PKU is not caused by a deletion of the entire PH gene. Since PH is a hepatic enzyme not readily detectable in pre-natal diagnosis, the detection of 8 distinct polymorphisms at this locus allows for pre-natal diagnosis of classical PKU and identification of carriers of the trait [W21]. Likewise, discoveries of multiple restriction site polymorphisms detected within the 60 kb of DNA of the

beta globin gene cluster have permitted the detection of about 85% of the pregnancies at risk for β-thalassaemia, using amniocytes alone [A6, D22, J6, K14, T13].

150. Some progress has been made in understanding the genetic basis of susceptibility to diabetes mellitus [type I or insulin-dependent diabetes mellitus (IDDM) or juvenile onset diabetes mellitus]. The human insulin gene is located at 11p15 about 14 cM from the β-globin gene [L29] and has been isolated, cloned and sequenced [B48]. It is 1430 bp (base pair) in length with two introns. About 360 bp upstream from the starting point of transcription is a region with a very high frequency of DNA length polymorphisms, referred to as a hypervariable region. Taking advantage of this polymorphism and the availability of cDNA insulin probes, attempts have been made to determine the susceptibility to IDDM diabetes by studying the frequency of DNA polymorphisms in this region in affected individuals. Depending on the fragment sizes generated by restriction enzymes, Bell and Karam [B49] found three classes of alleles defined by their different lengths due to the numbers and arrangements of tandem repeats at the polymorphic locus. Class 1 and class 3 alleles are the most frequent, while class 2 alleles are rare, at least in Caucasians. In Caucasians it appears that class 1 alleles occur significantly more frequently in those with IDDM than in healthy controls [B50].

3. Indirect analysis of genetic disease using cloned DNA segments to detect linked DNA polymorphisms

151. Since RFLPs can be used simply as genetic markers, any disorder caused by a major locus and segregating in pedigree can be mapped. The advantage of such a procedure is that it does not require knowledge of the biochemical basis of the disorder in question or the isolation of a specific gene [B17, D15, W44]. Disorders that fall into this category include, among others, Huntington disease (HD) (autosomal dominant), myotonic dystrophy (autosomal dominant) and the X-linked Duchenne and Becker muscular dystrophies. It should be realized, however, that the chance of detecting a linkage between a randomly selected probe and a particular RFLP is very small. The statistical aspects of the problem—how many markers are needed, how polymorphic each marker must be, how many informative families are needed, etc.—have been dealt with, among others, by Botstein [B17], Bishop and Skolnik [B19], Southern [S46], Skolnik and White [S41] and Lange and Boehnke [L8].

152. The location of the gene for Huntington disease was unknown until recently. Gusella et al. [G27] have now discovered a polymorphic region in close linkage to the gene. The probe used in this case, termed G8, maps to chromosome 4; its close linkage to HD indicates that the locus (or one of the loci) for this degenerative disorder lies on chromosome 4. A promising aspect of G8 is that it is likely to make possible the identification of the HD gene itself and thus clarify the mechanism of this neurological disease.

153. Myotonic dystrophy is another autosomal disorder for which the age of onset and the degree of severity are highly variable; this can make it very difficult to determine whether an individual at risk is carrying the gene [H45]. The biochemical basis of this disorder is not understood, but the gene is known to be on chromosome 19 [E21, W43] and shows close linkage to a very infrequent peptidase D protein polymorphism [O16] as well as loose linkage to the complement [C3], secretor and Lutheran loci [D16, E21]. Apolipoprotein CII is one of a group of genes coding for apolipoproteins, which has also been mapped to chromosome 19, and the cDNA probe for this gene detects an RFLP due to a variable TaqI site about 2 kb downstream of the gene itself [M63]. In a recent study, Shaw et al. [S92] examined the possibility of linkage of this polymorphism to the myotonic dystrophy locus in families and found that the two loci are in fact closely linked (only one recombination between the disease and marker loci in a total of 53 informative meioses) but pointed out that further family studies are required to increase the precision of their estimate of genetic distance.

154. Duchenne muscular dystrophy (DMD) is a severe X-linked disorder normally affecting only males and leading to their early death; its biochemical basis is also unknown at present [M64]. The disease has also been found in a few girls so far, and in some instances, an X-autosome translocation is present in which the exchange point in the X is in band Xp21 near the middle of the short arm (see [D44] for citations of the relevant literature). The concurrence of the repeated translocation breakpoint with DMD phenotype suggests that band Xp21 may be the site of the DMD gene. This map location is consistent with family studies that have shown linkage of the DMD locus to two RFLPs (recognized by probes L1.28 and RC8), flanking the Xp21 region [D17, D18, H19, M23]. In order to achieve a more refined localization of the DMD gene, De Martinville et al. [D44] analysed panels of somatic cells of hybrid lines carrying various structural rearrangements of the human X-chromosome short arm with 21 X-chromosome-specific cloned DNA fragments. The finding of interest was that the ornithine transcarbamylase gene and four anonymous DNA sequences mapped within band Xp21, flanking the presumed DMD locus.

155. In a detailed study on the isolation of probes detecting RFLPs from X-chromosome-specific libraries, Hofker et al. [H46] found that two of the isolated probes detected a high frequency of RFLP. One, No. 754, maps between Xp11.3 and Xp21 and the other, termed 782, maps between Xp22.2 and Xp22.3. In a pilot study of families at risk for DMD, the authors found that the recombination fraction between DMD and 754 is less than 3 cM (between DMD and 782, it is 17 cM). These results suggest that probe 754 is probably the most powerful probe currently available for linkage studies with DMD. This suggestion has received support from the work of Francke et al. [F34]. In a male patient who manifested four different disorders (DMD, retinitis pigmentosa (RP), chronic granulomatous disease and McLeod phenotype), these investigators found a subtle interstitial deletion of part

of band Xp21. Not only were they able to confirm the deletion by somatic cell and molecular studies, but they also showed that the probe 754 recognizes an RFLP of high frequency; their linkage data suggest a genetic distance of about 3 cM between the DMD locus and 754, with 95% confidence limits of 1-12 cM. (For a similar attempt to map DNA sequences in a human Xp interstitial deletion that extends across the region of the DMD locus, see Ingle et al. [I10].)

156. In other studies, linkage between L1.28 and a non-lethal form of X-linked muscular dystrophy, the Becker muscular dystrophy (BMD) (which had long been thought to be a different clinical entity), was demonstrated. On the basis of data from analysis of 10 X-linked DNA polymorphisms (5 mapping on the short arm and five on the long arm), Roncuzzi et al. [R52] confirmed linkage of the Becker gene to L1.28 and also showed that the locus is located between L1.28 and B24. It has been surmised that the locus for Becker muscular dystrophy and that for DMD may be the same [K12, K22]. Brown et al. [B69] used the p754 probe to study 14 DMD and 8 BMD kindreds; their linkage data suggest that both the disease loci are in p21 (short arm of the X) at a distance of about 15-20 cM from the 754 locus. Data from families informative for both the p754 and L1.28 polymorphisms suggest that p754 is closer than L1.28 to the disease loci.

157. The X-linked variety of retinitis pigmentosa (RP) found in 14-22% of RP families in the United Kingdom, is one of the most severe clinical forms of RP with onset in males in the first decade and progressive blindness by the third or fourth decade. Female carriers are difficult to identify because of only partial manifestation due to random X-inactivation. Bhattacharya et al. [B28] have reported close genetic linkage between this X-linked disorder and a RFLP identified by L1.28. This probe is potentially useful for carrier detection and early diagnosis, though only approximately 40% of the cases (heterozygotes) appear informative for this probe, provided genetic heterogeneity can be excluded by further family studies.

4. Other applications of recombinant DNA technology

158. Molecular studies on Down syndrome. Some progress towards understanding of the molecular biology of Down syndrome has been made in recent years. The gene locus for superoxide dismutase (SOD-1) is located on 21q22 which is very near, at least, to the region of chromosome 21 involved in Down syndrome, since trisomy for this small segment is sufficient to cause Down syndrome (e.g., [H47, N27, P35, S93, W45]). The gene for SOD-1 has been cloned [L30, L31] and may well contain the DNA sequences involved in the pathogenesis of Down syndrome, or at least provide a convenient starting point for chromosome analysis. Work currently under way on regional mapping of DNA sequences in chromosome 21, construction of a linkage map of this chromosome, etc., has recently been presented [E22].

159. Through the use of a recombinant clone containing a sequence that occurs only in human chromosome 21, Davies et al. [D29] were able to find a two-allele RFLP showing Mendelian inheritance. Studies of DNA from Down syndrome patients and from their parents enabled the confirmation of trisomy-21 by dosage hybridization to Southern blots and the determination of the origin of the extra chromosome 21.

160. In a recent paper, Antonarakis et al. [A19] tested the hypothesis that there is a genetic predisposition to non-disjunction and trisomy-21 associated with DNA sequences on chromosome 21. They used DNA polymorphism haplotypes for chromosome 21 to examine the distribution of different chromosomes 21 in Down syndrome and control families from the same ethnic group in Greece. Four common polymorphic sites adjacent to two closely linked single-copy DNA sequences (namely pW228C and pW236B), which map on the proximal long arm of chromosome 21, were found. One particular haplotype was much more commonly associated with chromosomes 21 that underwent non-disjunction in the Down syndrome families, suggesting that an increased tendency for non-disjunction may be due to DNA sequences associated with a subset of chromosome 21 bearing this haplotype.

161. Fetal sexing. In X-linked disorders, which cannot as yet be diagnosed pre-natally, selective abortion of any male fetus may be acceptable to a mother at risk of having an affected son. In such circumstances, fetal sexing is usually carried out by karyotyping cultured amniotic fluid cells, or more recently, chorionic tissue. However, probes are now being developed that contain DNA sequences specific for the human Y chromosome, which can also be used for fetal sexing [B51, G40].

162. The immune system. Recombinant DNA techniques have provided detailed information on the genetic organization of the major histocompatibility complex (MHC) or the HLA system. While the association of specific serologically detectable alleles at these loci to a number of diseases (reviewed in [D20, R18]) has long been known, the availability of molecular clones for the different genes of the HLA system is enabling the detection of a variety of polymorphisms that distinguish allelic forms of the various segments of MHC and may prove useful in studies correlating MHC haplotypes to propensity to certain diseases [D21, E12, P14]. Likewise, the application of DNA methods to the study of genes controlling the synthesis of immunoglobulins has been extremely useful in understanding how antibody diversity is generated [E18, L32, L33, R53, T35, Z5] and is likely to provide insights into the nature of defects that may underlie the generation of specific antibodies known in certain inherited sensitivities (atopies).

163. Diagnosis and typing of tumours and lymphomas. Recombinant DNA techniques have potential in providing additional information for diagnosis and typing of tumours and lymphomas. Thus, for instance,

Cleary et al. [C39] recently described the use of the Southern blot hybridization technique to diagnose B-cell lymphoma by detecting clonal immunoglobulin gene rearrangements in lymphnodes and other biopsy tissues. The analysis of immunoglobulin gene re-arrangements, which characterize B-cell lymphoma, offers several advantages over conventional diagnostic methods.

164.   Biosynthesis of valuable hormones and proteins. One of the major applications of recombinant DNA technology is in the synthesis of medically important drugs. In 1977, Itakura and colleagues [I11] reported the first successful synthesis of somatostatin, a peptide inhibiting the growth hormone, used in the treatment of children with excessive growth. Since then, a number of other valuable hormones and proteins have been synthesized (insulin [G41], growth hormone [G42], F-interferon [T34], L-interferon [N28, G43]).

165.   Radiation genetics and genetic risk assessments. In the 1972 UNSCEAR report [U3], the Committee stated "... the past decade has witnessed an almost explosive growth of molecular biology ... impressive as these developments are, molecular biology has not yet provided information on the relationship between the damage from ionizing radiation at the DNA level and mutational events to explain or to predict the array of mutational responses observed with different dose-rates, cell stages, etc., in mammals". As will be evident from the preceding discussions, the situation is rapidly changing. Molecular methods have been greatly refined and applied to the study of gene structure, organization and function and the nature of spon-taneously arising mutations. Applied to human genetic disorders, these studies have exposed considerable genetic heterogeneity in many of these disorders at the molecular level. This unmasking of genetic hetero-geneity may have implications in the context of estimating the additional burden of these disorders due to radiation exposures. Furthermore, molecular methods are currently being extended to investigate the molecular basis of induced mutations (see chapter VI) and to examine differences in the spectra of mutations (including radiations of different quality). These advances are bound to add more precision, both in formulating questions and obtaining answers that are relevant for genetic risk assessment.

E.   SUMMARY AND CONCLUSIONS

166.   Recombinant DNA technology has provided a formidable array of new opportunities to study the human genome; it has increased the speed and precision of gene mapping and has helped to define the nature of genetic lesions and to analyse the action of specific genes in health and disease. The methods consist of generating DNA fragments in vitro by restriction endonucleases, incorporating these frag-ments into a suitable vector, introducing the vector into a host organism, producing multiple copies of the incorporated fragments and, finally, selecting, harvest-ing and characterizing the cellular clones containing the fragments of interest.

167.   Restriction endonucleases—of which over 500 are currently known—are DNAses that recognize specific oligonucleotide sequences in the DNA and break the DNA within or near the sequences, generat-ing DNA fragments of defined length and sequence. Some of the fragments generated have free protruding 5′ or 3′ ends (cohesive or sticky ends) while others have blunt ends. The vectors used for cloning in E. coli are plasmids, bacteriophage lambda derivatives, cosmids and bacteriophage M13. In terms of insert size, plasmids can accommodate up to 5-6 kb, bacterio-phage lambda derivatives up to 15 kb and cosmids up to 50 kb of foreign DNA.

168.   The use of recombinant DNA techniques has permitted the establishment of gene-specific, chromo-some-specific and genomic libraries. A cDNA library is constructed by synthesizing double-stranded copy of the mRNA population using reverse transcriptase and integrating these cDNA molecules into a restriction site of a plasmid; it is a source of the coding sequences of the genome. A genomic library consists of all coding and non-coding sequences. The chromosome-specific library, as the term implies, is specific for individual chromosomes.

169.   The DNA fragments generated by restriction endonucleases differ in length among individuals (restriction fragment length polymorphism or RFLP); these differences are apparently without any pheno-typic effects, are inherited in a Mendelian co-dominant manner and thus can be used in family linkage studies to localize specific genes of interest.

170.   The Southern blotting method is a very impor-tant technique for locating specific DNA fragments on electrophoresis gels; the analysis of defects in the processing of RNA molecules is possible by Northern blotting.

171.   The major advances achieved during the past few years using recombinant DNA techniques in the study of gene structure and organization and muta-tional alterations leading to disease states in man can be broadly grouped under three headings: (a) direct analysis of the normal and mutant genes using gene probes or synthetic oligonucleotides (e.g., globin gene clusters, thalassaemias, sickle cell anaemia, HLA gene system, diabetes, haemophilia B, HPRT, antithrombin III deficiency, alpha antitrypsin deficiency); (b) indirect analysis of genetic disease (i.e., mutant states) using gene probes to detect closely linked polymorphisms (sickle cell anaemia, atherosclerosis, hypertriglyceri-daemia, phenylketonuria, osteogenesis imperfecta, etc.); and (c) indirect analysis of genetic disease using cloned DNA fragments to detect linked polymorphisms (fragile-X, Huntington disease, muscular dystrophies, myotonic dystrophy, retinitis pigmentosa, etc.). Several findings emerging from these studies have applications in pre-natal diagnosis and in the diagnosis and typing of tumours and lymphomas. At the level of disease management, recombinant DNA methods are proving to be very useful in the synthesis of medically important drugs.

172. It is hoped that the application of the recombinant DNA methods to radiation- and chemically-induced mutations will help to unravel differences in mutational spectra and to gain more precise insights into repair processes, dose-rate and dose-fractionation effects in experimental systems, aspects that are pertinent to the evaluation of genetic radiation hazards in man.

III. GENES, CHROMOSOMES AND CANCER

173. In the 1982 UNSCEAR report, several Mendelian disorders with predisposition to neoplasia and a number of specific chromosomal defects associated with cancer in man were considered in some detail (see also reviews by Neri [N20], Radman et al. [R25] and Sasaki [S62]). During the last few years, some major breakthroughs in this area have been reported and these have significantly advanced knowledge about the genetic basis of cancer. Paradoxically, these advances have come about from studies of tumour viruses (although most naturally occurring tumours, particularly in man, do not appear to be caused by viruses) and through the convergence of thought and techniques from viral oncology, cell genetics and molecular biology. These advances have been reviewed in several publications [B1, B3, B13, B52, C3, C40, C61, D11, D45, H48, K3, K23, K40, L15, R12, S71, V13, W4, W25, W30, Y4] and thus only some of the salient aspects are briefly summarized below.

A. THE ONCOGENES OF RETROVIRUSES
(v-oncs)

174. The fact that certain viruses can cause rare malignant tumours in chicken, mice, rats, cats and a variety of other species has been known for a long time. Studies with retroviruses[m] and particularly with some members of this group, the acute transforming viruses,[n] showed that their genomes contain specific genes (viral oncogenes or v-oncs) responsible for oncogenicity as well as unrelated sequences required for viral replication. Currently, about 20 different onc-specific sequences have been identified in retroviruses [B13, C5, D11, D12, V13, W4]. Table 16 lists most of these oncogenes and the viral prototypes in which they were first diagnosed, with a brief description of their oncogenic properties. Some of these genes regularly cause multiple types of tumours (e.g., the onc gene of MC29 causes myelocytomatosis, carcinoma and sarcoma) while other genes like src of the Rous sarcoma virus or the onc gene of the avian myeloblastosis virus AMV cause one predominant type of tumour.

---

[m]Retroviruses are a family of RNA viruses that replicate by way of a DNA provirus integrated in cellular DNA.

[n]The acute transforming viruses are highly oncogenic; they efficiently transform cells in culture and induce neoplastic disease with short latent periods in infected animals. Approximately 20 viruses of this type isolated from chickens, mice, cats, rats and monkeys have been characterized.

175. The product of at least 8 of these oncogenes is a protein kinase, a phosphorylating enzyme. Six of these kinases have so far been shown to phosphorylate the aminoacid tyrosine and at least five of the kinases bind to the plasma membrane [B1, B13, H48]; the pp60^{v-src} of the Rous sarcoma virus and the p20 of the Abelson leukemia virus are among the best known examples of the protein products of these genes.

B. PROTO-ONCOGENES (proto oncs) OR CELLULAR ONCOGENES (c-oncs)

176. The biochemical definition of several v-oncs was subsequently followed by the development of cDNA probes made from the RNAs of Kirsten and Harvey sarcoma viruses [S29, S30, T10], Rous sarcoma virus [S31] and Maloney sarcoma virus [F8] and their hybridization (in molecular hybridization experiments) to cellular DNA. The data that emerged from these and other studies [A13, C14, C15, F9, S32, W5, W29, Z4] led to the discovery that avian and mammalian genomes contain nucleotide sequences related to retroviral oncogenes. Homologues of over a dozen other viral onc genes have since been found in normal cells of vertebrates [W4]. In addition, nucleotide sequences similar to the oncs of Rous sarcoma virus, MC29, Abelson and feline sarcoma viruses have even been found in Drosophila [L6, S33]. Likewise, sequences similar to the Harvey and Kirsten sarcoma viruses have been found in the yeast Saccharomyces cerevisiae [D46, G44].

177. These and other findings lend support to the view that some of these sequences emerged quite early and have been conserved over extensive periods in the course of evolution. It therefore seems unlikely that the vertebrate sequences in question represent genes of endogenous retroviruses. The use of restriction endonucleases and molecular cloning have given substance to this view. The cellular prototypes of most known viral oncs have since been cloned and compared with viral counterparts by heteroduplex analysis, endonucleases site mapping, fingerprinting and complete sequence analysis. Such comparisons have revealed that: (a) those parts of viral oncs that are unrelated to essential genes of retroviruses have closely related counterparts in normal cells; and (b) these counterparts, which are not linked to any of the genes essential to retroviruses, display minor structural polymorphisms of the sort found in recognized cellular genes and have (at least several of them) intervening sequences (introns) that interrupt the coding sequences (exons) [B1, B13, D11]. Consequently, it has been suggested that retroviral transforming genes are present in normal cells in a latent form. Recent structural analyses have indicated that the viral oncs and cellular genes, which share specific sequences, are not isogenic and that they differ from each other in scattered point mutations and in unique coding regions [D11].

178. A variety of experimental results support the view that the cellular homologues of retrovirus oncogenes constitute a group of normal genes. The latter have been designated by the generic name proto-oncogenes. The wealth of data currently available

suggests that these cellular genes have oncogenic potential and thus can be referred to as cellular oncogenes or c-oncs. The function of proto-oncogenes is unknown. However, they are commonly expressed in most or all tissues and sometimes regulated in temporal or lineage-specific fashion [B13], implying that they might play a central role in growth and development, processes that seem particularly likely to be altered during neoplasia. The latter idea has received confirmation by the findings that c-sis appears to encode the platelet-derived growth factor [D33, W28] and c-erbB, the epidermal growth factor receptor [D60].

C. CELLULAR GENE ONCOGENESIS

179. Studies on the potential oncogenic activity of cellular genes are dependent on an assay for determination of the biological activity of purified cellular DNA. In this assay (termed transfection), recipient cell cultures are exposed to donor DNA in the form of a calcium phosphate precipitate [G2]. The efficiency of transformation obtained varies with the cells used as recipients. The established mouse cell line (fibroblasts) NIH/3T3 is most commonly used as a source for recipient cells.

180. The potential of normal cellular genes in inducing transformation has been investigated in a number of studies. High molecular weight DNAs (> 30 kilobases, kb) from normal cells (chicken embryonic fibroblasts, non-transformed mouse cell lines and normal human embryonic lung fibroblasts) were found to be ineffective in inducing transformation in transfection assays. However, after fragmentation to sizes of 0.5-5 kb, normal cell DNAs induced transformation with efficiencies (0.003 transformant per microgram of DNA) that were similar to subgenomic src-containing fragments of DNA of RSV-transformed cells [C5]. DNAs of cells transformed by normal cell DNA fragments induced transformation with high efficiencies (0.1-1.0 transformant per microgram of DNA) in secondary transfection assays, indicating that these transformed cells contained activated transforming genes that could be efficiently transmitted by transfection [C5].

181. If carcinogenesis involves dominant genetic changes (either by mutations or by gene rearrangements) affecting the structure or regulation of such potential transforming genes, it is possible that the DNAs of some neoplasms contain activated transforming genes and therefore induce transformation with high efficiencies upon infection. Several groups have reported that the DNAs of a variety of tumours are indeed able to induce transformation of NIH/3T3 mouse fibroblasts. In a number of cases, the transforming activities have been shown to be localized to discrete DNA segments present in the tumour cell genome and several of these have been isolated using molecular cloning techniques (Table 17); a high proportion of those have proved to be mutant members of the ras gene family. It was found that the DNA of normal cells contains sequences closely related to those of the isolated tumour oncogenes; this

suggests that the latter are probably derived from normal cellular sequences, presumably by a process of somatic mutation or rearrangement occurring in the target tissue during carcinogenesis [G17, P11, S34, V13, W6].

182. DNAs of approximately 80-90% of chemically induced and spontaneously arising tumours, however, do not induce efficient transformation on transfection [V13]. Carcinogenesis in these neoplasms may involve epigenetic changes or recessive genetic alterations that would not be detectable by transfection of tumour DNAs. Alternatively, these neoplasms may contain dominant transforming genes, which do not induce transformation of the NIH/3T3 cells used as recipients in transfection assays.

D. RELATIONSHIPS BETWEEN CELLULAR ONCOGENES DETECTED IN TRANSFECTION ASSAYS AND THE TRANSFORMING GENES OF ACUTE TRANSFORMING RETROVIRUSES

183. As discussed above, cellular transforming genes have been defined either by their affiliation with retroviruses or by transfection of DNAs of tumours that were not, in large part, induced by viruses. The relationships between different cellular transforming genes detected by transfection of NIH/3T3 cells have been clarified by the discoveries (Table 17) that many of these genes represent cellular homologues of the oncogene v-Ha-ras of the Harvey murine sarcoma virus or the oncogene v-Ki-ras of the Kirsten murine sarcoma virus [D4, P1, S7, S35]. For example, the transforming activity associated with the T24(EJ) human bladder carcinoma line [D4, P1, S7] and several chemically induced mouse squamous cell carcinomas [B14] corresponds to an activated version of the cellular homologue c-Ha-ras1 of v-Ha-ras. Transforming genes corresponding to the cellular homologue c-Ki-ras2 of v-Ki-ras are found in human cell lines established from bladder, lung, colon and gall bladder carcinomas, as well as biopsy tissue from lung, pancreas and colon carcinomas and a rhabdomyosarcoma [P2, D4, S35, M13]. Other cases of homology between ras genes and transfected tumour genes are coming to light [W6]. The most obvious consequence of these newly discovered homologies is a realization that at least some of the cellular sequences can become activated via one of two routes: by recombination with a retroviral sequence or by non-viral somatic mutational events.

E. OTHER TRANSFORMING GENES

184. Shimizu et al. [S64] first described a new transforming gene termed N-ras in a human neuroblastoma cell line, which was only weakly homologous to v-Ha-ras and v-Ki-ras. Subsequently, transforming genes of the N-ras type were also found in a number of other cell lines (Table 17). No retroviral oncogene corresponding to N-ras has been described. By transfection of chicken B lymphoma DNA into NIH/3T3 cells, Goubrin et al. [G18] detected a new transforming gene unrelated to known oncogenes of acute

transforming viruses. Subsequently, Diamond et al. [D13] showed that the same type of transforming gene could be isolated from six Burkitt lymphoma cell lines. Thus it was called B-lym-1. Human B-lym-1, like the chicken B-lym-1, was not found to be homologous to molecular clones of any retroviral transforming genes tested. Cooper et al. [C43] reported on the molecular cloning of a new transforming gene from a chemically transformed human osteosarcoma-derived cell line and showed that this is unrelated to known oncogenes (chromosomal location: 7p11.4-7qter). Eva and Aaronson [E23] published the first report of another new transforming gene associated with a human diffuse B-cell lymphoma and have designated it as dbl.

F. HOW MANY ONCOGENES?

185. Currently, at least 17 distinct retrovirus onco-genes are known (Table 16), each with a corresponding cellular c-onc. Transfection with tumour DNA has also uncovered 6-7 new oncogenes. The number of new oncogenes will increase with continued efforts in this direction. However, it appears that the number of cellular oncogenes may not be very large. The fact that most of the oncogenes first found in retroviruses have been identified more than once in the same host species, that several have turned up in more than one species and that some of the oncogenes isolated from tumour DNA had already been encountered in the study of retroviruses, all suggest that the majority of cellular oncogenes may already be in view. Bishop [B13] has ventured the guess that there may be no more than 50-100 oncogenes. Some of the 20 or so currently recognized oncogenes are assignable to at least two distinct gene families: the ras family, with at least four distinct oncogenes, and the src-yes-mos family, with another three [W6].

G. MECHANISMS OF ACTIVATION OF PROTO-ONCOGENES

186. Proto-oncogenes do not transform NIH/3T3 cells. In contrast, 10-20% of DNAs from different tumour cells lead to neoplastic transformation of NIH/3T3 cells after transfection. Cellular transforming genes are derived from proto-oncogenes by activation steps leading to qualitative or quantitative changes in the corresponding gene product. There are several possible mechanisms for activation of proto-oncogenes (see [W25, V13] and [G32] for reviews); some of these have been shown to occur in human tumours and others have been found in model systems.

1. Point mutations in proto-oncogenes

187. Nucleotide substitutions and concomitant amino-acid change in members of the ras gene family is the genetic alteration that most commonly explains the transforming activity of tumour cell DNA. Table 18 presents a summary of the available data and shows that changes affecting the same codons (12 and 61)

have been encountered in multiple mutant alleles of c-Ha-ras1, c-Ki-ras2 and N-ras. The question of whether repeated lesions at the same site imply a hot spot for mutations or selection for random mutations that confer transforming activity upon a proto-oncogene has not yet been resolved. There are, however, different lines of evidence from in vitro studies, suggesting that positions 12, 59 and 61 are functionally important in $p21^{c-Ha-ras}$ and that it is probable that random mutations at these sites are selectable (see [V13] for details). Of particular importance in this context is the work of Fasano et al. [F35] who used sodium bisulphite to produce C to T transitions at many positions in c-Ha-ras1 gene and then tested cloned mutants for their ability to transform NIH/3T3 cells. Oncogenic mutants occurred only at a restricted number of sites, including codons 12, 13, 59, 61 and 63. Three of these sites (12, 59 and 61) conform precisely to the positions of mutations encountered in spontaneous tumours and in viral ras oncogenes (Table 18) and all are close to such sites. The change observed at position 59, ala to thr, is particularly interesting because it is one of three differences in amino acid sequence between c-Ha-ras1 and v-Ha-ras, implying that the viral oncogene has acquired two alterations independently sufficient to induce cellular transformation.

188. Further evidence for non-random nucleotide substitutions at a specific site come from the work of Bos et al. [B53]. These authors tested DNAs from 4 patients with acute myeloid leukaemia (AML) by an in vivo selection assay in nude mice using transfected mouse NIH/3T3 cells; in addition, the DNA from one other AML patient was tested in the focus-forming assay. All five were found to contain an activated N-ras oncogene. With synthetic oligonucleotide probes, it was possible to demonstrate that, in all of them, the activation was due to a point mutation at codon 13, resulting in a replacement of gly to either val or asp; there was no evidence for the activation of any other ras oncogenes. The question of why N-ras should be preferentially activated in these leukaemias has not been answered and the authors have speculated that N-ras, rather than other ras genes, may be critically involved in the control of proliferation and differentiation of cells in the haematopoietic lineage.

189. There are now several papers (e.g., [B14, E23, G45, S94, Z6]) documenting the thesis that specific oncogenes are activated by exposure of experimental mammals to carcinogens in vivo. For instance, in mice, Guerrero et al. [G45] induced thymomas with methylnitrosourea [MNU] (i.p. injection, 30 mg/kg body weight, once a week for five consecutive weeks) or gamma irradiation (4 weekly doses of 1.5 Gy each) and used the DNA from the tumours to transfect NIH/3T3 cells. A high percentage of the tumours transformed the recipient cells and the oncogenic phenotype was found to be due to the activation of N-ras oncogene (MNU experiment) or the K-ras onco-gene (gamma-ray experiment). Although the authors did not clone the genes in question, they found that there was no evidence for any rearrangements in the Southern blot analysis. They therefore concluded that the presumed changes were point mutations.

190. Sukumar et al. [S94] used MNU (single i.p. injection, 30 μg/g body weight) to induce mammary carcinomas in Buf/N female rats and examined the transforming activity of the DNA from these carcinomas in transfection experiments with NIH/3T3 cells. Each of the nine mammary carcinoma DNA tested induced the appearance of foci of morphologically transformed cells. Upon analysis of whether the transforming activity was related to the altered rat ras sequences, it was found that, in all cases, transformed H-ras1 oncogenes were present. Molecular characterization of these revealed a nucleotide change at the 12th codon (GGA to GAA) of the normal gene with the result that there was an aminoacid change from glycine to glutamic acid. As was mentioned earlier, codon number 12 is one of the most important sites at which mutations lead to activation of the proto-oncogene. These studies were subsequently extended [Z6] using restriction enzyme analysis and it was shown that in 48 out of 58 DNA samples from MNU-induced carcinomas studied, the Ha-ras1 had been activated by the same G to A transition, the type of mutations preferentially induced by MNU.

2. Attachment of strong promotors/enhancers to proto-oncogenes

191. Another mechanism of proto-oncogene activation has been studied in two other experimental systems. Blair et al. [B30] covalently linked the molecularly cloned long terminal repeat sequence (LTR) of Moloney murine sarcoma provirus DNA (Mo-MSV) to mouse c-mos, the proto-oncogene homologous to v-mos. These constructs transformed NIH/3T3 cells as efficiently as cloned subgenomic Mo-MSV fragments containing both v-mos and LTR. This is explained by transcriptional activation of c-mos caused by promotor and/or enhancer elements in the LTR DNA sequence. The resulting overproduction of the c-mos gene product is apparently sufficient for malignant transformation of NIH/3T3 cells. The above observation was confirmed in a related experimental system by Chang et al. [C41]. In this work, viral LTR sequences were ligated to the human c-Has-ras gene. After transfection of the constructs into NIH/3T3 cells, the recipient cells became highly tumorigenic and expressed high levels of the p21 gene product. (For other examples, see [D45].)

192. It is worth noting here that, unlike the mouse c-mos gene, the human c-mos gene could not be activated by insertion of Mo-MSV elements at the 5' end of the coding sequence [W26]. Duesberg [D11] points out that promotor-activated c-mos and c-ras genes have not been found in naturally occurring murine tumours, although leukaemia viruses that could provide LTR sequences are ubiquitous in mice. Thus, increased expression of proto-oncogenes due to promotor attachment or insertion may not be sufficient to transform normal mammalian cells in vivo, although established cell lines like NIH/3T3 can be transformed in this way by promotor-activated mouse c-mos and human c-Ha-ras.

3. Promotor (enhancer) insertion near proto-oncogenes

193. This mechanism may be similar or identical to that discussed above. In contrast to the transformation of NIH/3T3 cells by hybrid LTR-oncogene constructs, however, activation of proto-oncogenes can also be achieved by insertion of a slow transforming virus into DNA flanking the proto-oncogene, but not immediately adjacent to it. Hayward et al. [H33] reported that avian leucosis virus (ALV, a slow transforming retrovirus lacking a known oncogene), which causes B-cell lymphomas in the chicken after a latent period of more than 6 months, was found to be integrated near (within 5 kb) the c-myc gene in the cells of some but not all B lymphomas. Fung et al. [F21] found that ALV-LTR had integrated at least 0.5 kb upstream of c-erb-B gene locus in the genome of chicken erythroblastosis cells. Since it is now known that enhancers of transcription act over longer distances than promotors [K24], it is possible that the observed effects are due to enhancer activity of retroviral LTR sequences. Although the possibility envisaged above may sometimes contribute to the tumorigenicity of slow transforming viruses, arguments can be advanced against the generalization of this hypothesis [D11]: (a) promotor (enhancer) insertion and elevated expression of c-myc are not found in all chicken B lymphomas; and (b) the insertion hypothesis would call for a more rapid induction of tumours than is reflected by the long latency period actually observed for the appearance of B-lymphoma or erythroblastosis in ALV-infected chicken. (See also [V13].)

4. Amplification of proto-oncogenes

194. Amplification of proto-myc DNA sequences (up to 20-fold) has been found in human myeloid leukaemia cell line HL60 [C42, D30] and in the human colon cancer cell line Colo 320 [A11]. The Ki-ras proto-oncogene was amplified 30- to 60-fold in cells of the mouse adrenocortical tumour cell line Y1 [S66]. The amplified Ki-ras proto-oncogene was localized in double minute chromosomes in homogeneously staining regions (HSR), i.e., in cytological structures characteristic of amplified genes in cultured cells. In none of these cases has it been shown that amplification of the corresponding oncogene is an obligatory event in tumorigenesis, although it is tempting to speculate that such amplification may be involved at some stage of the multi-step process of malignant transformation of normal diploid cells ([L34, B54]; see also [P37, S96, V13]).

5. DNA transposition and rearrangements

195. Rechavi et al. [R13] have reported on the first case of proto-oncogene activation in a non-virally induced tumour by a process of DNA transposition. The oncogene studied was the c-mos, the progenitor of the transforming information in the Moloney murine sarcoma virus [F8, C18]. Previously, it had been shown that the molecularly cloned 14-kb c-mos gene was inactive when assayed for its ability to

transform NIH/3T3 cells in transfection experiments. To demonstrate the biological activity of this gene, it was necessary to ligate a viral long terminal repeat (LTR) upstream from the 5' end of the gene [O4]. In screening the DNAs of several BALB/c mouse myelomas by Southern blot analysis, Rechavi et al. detected an additional hybridization band, XRPC24, in one of the tumours. Further studies revealed that the c-mos gene in this case has undergone DNA rearrangement at the 5' end of the gene including the insertion of a 159 bp DNA fragment having the structure of an insertion element (IS). This gene, designated as rc-mos (rearranged c-mos) was active in transfection assays with NIH/3T3 cells.

196. Other instances of proto-oncogene activation as a result of DNA rearrangements stemming from chromosomal rearrangements, as well as those involving joint action of cellular transforming genes, are considered in the next section.

H.   HUMAN ONCOGENE LOCALIZATIONS AND THE ACTIVATION OF C-ONCOGENES THROUGH CHROMOSOMAL ABERRATIONS

197.   During the past few years, a number of cellular homologues (c-oncs) of retroviral oncogenes have been localized to specific chromosomes or chromosomal regions of the human complement (Table 19). Although karyotypic abnormalities have been known to exist in human tumours for quite some time [M15, U1, Y4], the remarkable similarity between the chromosomal location of some of the c-oncs and the breakpoints involved in some specific chromosomal aberrations are noteworthy [C61, F2, G29, R12, R55, Y4].

198.   The best example studied is c-myc (an oncogene originally found in B-cell avian myeloblastoma), which is now assigned to 8q24. The translocation common in Burkitt's lymphoma (between the long arms of chromosomes 8 and 14) involves a break in chromosome 8 (at the 5' site of the c-myc gene) and a break in chromosome 14 (at band q32) within the locus for the immunoglobulin heavy chain, which is active in these lymphoma cells [K11]; the break in chromosome 14 seems to occur in different nucleotide sequences in different Burkitt lymphoma lines. Dalla Favera et al. [D14] reported that the break is in the variable region, but Taub et al. [T12] assigned it to the switch region of the gene. In either case, the net result is translocation of the c-myc gene from its normal position on chromosome 8 to a new location adjacent to the immunoglobulin heavy chain locus on chromosome 14. The c-myc transcription has been found to be increased (up to 20 times) over the normal level in some patients, while there is no clear increased transcription in others, but rather an altered gene product [B15, D14, M18, S37, T12]. It is not without significance that the other chromosomes involved with chromosome 8 in translocation events in Burkitt lymphoma (chromosomes 2 and 22) contain the sites of the immunoglobulin kappa and lambda chains, respectively: the lymphomas express the kappa chain

in the case of t(8;2) and the lambda chain in the case of t(8;22) [C19, K3, K11, M19].

199.   Recently, Rabbits et al [R27] have provided evidence suggesting that c-myc oncogene activation in Burkitt lymphoma occurs by disruption of a normal control mechanism in which the c-myc protein itself is involved. A translocation similar to that in Burkitt's lymphoma occurs in mouse and rat plasmocytomas [K3]. In the mouse, the terminal segment of chromosome 15, carrying the c-myc gene, rearranges with chromosome 12 at the switch region of the heavy chain constant-region gene [C20, D14, S37, T12].

200.   Another interesting correlation is between c-abl and the translocation of chromosomes 9 and 22 in chronic myeloid leukaemia (CML). The chromosomal regions involved are 9q34 and 22q11. The oncogene c-abl has been localized to 9q34, and it was possible to demonstrate that, in CML cases with the Philadelphia Ph¹ chromosome, the c-abl sequences have been translocated from chromosome 9 to chromosome 22 at a position distal to AK1 (adenylate kinase-1) locus on chromosome 9, resulting in the activation of c-abl expression [D5].

201.   Mapping of the break-points on chromosome 9 indicated variable distances 5' (upstream) of the first known exon of c-abl: in one individual, the break-point was 14 kb 5' of the oncogene; and in others it occurred further upstream and has not yet been accurately mapped [H49]. The situation on chromosome 22 is different: the break-points in different CMLs occurred in a restricted region of about 5.8 kb; this region was termed break-point cluster region or bcr [G46, H50] and its consistent rearrangement in CML patients strongly implicates it in the pathogenesis of CML.

202.   Shtivelman et al. [S97] recently cloned and characterized complementary DNA of the normal and CML-specific c-abl RNA and showed that the latter is a hybrid molecule, a fused transcript of bcr and c-abl sequences. Nucleotide sequence analysis indicated that the protein translated from this 8-kb long fused RNA has bcr information at its amino terminus and that it retains most but not all of the normal c-abl protein. The authors were able to show that the sequence at the RNA function point is derived from the 3' end of a 78-bp bcr exon and the 5' end of the 174-bp abl exon II. Therefore, the normal splice signals of the two genes are used to form the hybrid transcript.

203.   Although the information summarized above shows good correlation between the break-points associated with consistent translocations or deletions and the bands containing the oncogenes, no generalizations are as yet possible. For instance, c-fes, which maps at 15q24-25, has been correlated with the break-point in chromosome 15 which is involved in the translocation t(15;17) associated with ANLL-M3. However, recent evidence [R12, Y4] indicates that the break-point in chromosome 15, is at q22, i.e., at some distance away from c-fes (a single chromosome band may contain 2000-3000 kb); furthermore, Sheer et al.

[S38, cited in R12] have shown that the 15q⁺ chromosome does not contain c-fes, which presumably has been translocated to chromosome 17.

204. Likewise, the assignment of c-Ha-ras1 to 11p11 → p15 raised the possibility that this oncogene might be involved in the predisposition to nephroblastoma (Wilms' tumour, WT) seen in the aniridia-WT association (AWTA) that is frequently caused by an interstitial deletion of band 11p13. However, the results reported by Martinville and Francke [M20] and Huerre et al. [H17] appeared to rule out such a possibility and also showed that the c-Ha-ras1 is located at 11p11.12 or 11p14.2 [M20] or 11p15.1 → 11p15.5 [H17], in any case outside the region deleted in these patients (see also [F23]).

205. Evidence is accumulating to suggest that the mechanism(s) of tumorigenesis in Wilms' tumour may be heterogeneous, as was demonstrated for retinoblastoma, another childhood tumour. In the latter, the locus has been assigned to chromosome 13 (13q14). Although the hereditary pattern in familial retinoblastoma is that of an autosomal dominant mutation, there is evidence that the defect is recessive at the cellular level [B31, C37]. At least four mechanisms for the development of homozygosity of recessive alleles in the region of 13q14 have been documented in retinoblastoma cells in culture: loss of an entire chromosome [B31, C37], loss of one chromosome 13 homologue, with the reduplication of the remaining chromosome 13 homologue [C37], somatic recombination with subsequent segregation resulting in homozygosity at all loci distal to the recombination site [C37, D32], and deletion of a segment of chromosome 13 including 13q14 [B31]. Data consistent with these mechanisms have also been reported for Wilms' tumour [F24, K25, O12, R28].

206. More recent results of Reeve et al. [R28], based on DNA analysis of tumour DNA from patients with sporadic Wilms' tumour, show that, in both cases studied, one of the two c-Ha-ras1 allele was absent. One tumour had a reciprocal translocation between the short arm of chromosome 11 (at 11p13) and the long arm of chromosome 12, with no visible loss of chromosome material. The other tumour had two cell types: one showing marked hypo-diploidy with very contracted chromosomes (so that no deletions could be detected) and the other with apparently normal karyotype. The authors point out that: (a) their demonstration of the loss of the c-Ha-ras1 allele may reflect events affecting the Wilms' tumour locus and the quite distinct distally placed c-Ha-ras1 gene; and (b) although the consensus of a gene mapping meeting placed c-Ha-ras1 at 11p15 [G30], the localization of c-Ha-ras1 by Jhanwar et al. [J17] at 11p14.1 (using in situ hybridization studies with meiotic chromosomes) places the above locus immediately adjacent to the translocation break-point (11p13) in one of the two tumours they studied. In their view, until the chromosome location of c-Ha-ras1 has been determined with certainty, one cannot exclude the possible functional involvement of c-Ha-ras1 in Wilms' tumour development. (See also [M65].)

I. ONCOGENIC TRANSFORMATION OF CELLS IN VITRO (IN TRANSFECTION EXPERIMENTS) VERSUS ONCOGENIC ACTIVATION AND PATHOGENESIS OF NEOPLASMS IN VIVO

207. As discussed earlier, the established mouse fibroblast cell line NIH/3T3 has been used with remarkable success over the past few years, as a principal in vitro transformation assay to demonstrate the presence of transfectable transforming genes in the DNA of certain human and rodent tumour cell lines. However, as is well known, carcinogenesis in vivo is a multi-stage process and it was thought, therefore, that the NIH/3T3 cells—chosen because of their particular competence in taking up and expressing exogenous DNAs—which are well adapted to grow indefinitely in monolayer cultures, probably deviate substantially from normal target cells for oncogenesis in vivo. In other words, the NIH/3T3 cells may already have acquired several alterations usually developed by a cell during its tumorigenic progression that make them susceptible to tumorigenic conversion by a single-hit event. The problem has been addressed by three groups of investigators, in three different kinds of study [L7, N13, R15].

208. Newbold and Overall [N13] found that Syrian hamster dermal fibroblasts immortalized by treatment with chemical carcinogens (benzopyrene, dimethyl sulphate and others) can be transformed to anchorage-independent growth by the human bladder carcinoma EJ-c-Ha-ras1 transforming gene and that the transforming activity was elicited only in newly immortalized cells. From these and other results, the authors concluded that fibroblast immortality is a prerequisite for transformation by the EJ-c-Ha-ras1 gene.

209. Land et al. [L7] reported that the EJ-c-Ha-ras1 gene transformed rat embryo fibroblasts only to limited proliferation in semi-solid agar medium. However, in combination with the v-myc gene, or a gene construct consisting of an early simian virus-40 transcriptional promotor attached to c-myc, or certain genes from DNA tumour viruses (middle and large T antigen gene from polyoma virus[o] isolated as separate molecular clones used either alone or in combination with one another, or the EIA gene[p] from adenovirus), the EJ-c-Ha-ras1 gene transformed rat embryo fibroblasts to tumorigenicity. Furthermore, Land et al. found that EJ-c-Ha-ras1, together with the large T polyoma antigen gene, or the EIA gene led to unlimited tumour growth, whereas, EJ-c-Ha-ras1 in combination with the v-myc gene transfected into diploid rat fibroblasts produced tumours of a limited size in the nude mice. The authors concluded that the myc gene greatly enhanced the transformed phenotype created by the EJ-c-Ha-ras1 but did not lead to fully transformed cells after co-transfection with the genes of DNA tumour viruses.

[o]The middle-T antigen induces morphological alteration and anchorage independence while the large-T antigen affects serum dependency and cell immortalization.

[p]The adenovirus early region IA is responsible for establishment function, i.e., the ability of cells to grow idefinitely in culture.

210. The work of Ruley et al. [R15] involved the use of primary baby rat kidney cells as recipients for transfection with EJ-c-Ha-ras1, the polyoma virus middle-T antigen and the adenovirus EIA gene. It showed that the polyoma virus middle-T and EJ-c-Ha-ras1 genes are individually unable to transform the rat kidney cells. However, the adenovirus EIA provides the functions required by these genes to transform such cells following DNA-mediated gene transfer. These results, like those of Newbold and Overall [N13] and of Land et al. [L7] mentioned above, strongly support the notion that carcinogenesis is at least a two-step process to which different transforming genes must contribute and that separate establishment and transforming functions are required for oncogenic transformation of primary cells in culture [C45, L2].

211. Further evidence that many neoplasms involve activation of at least two distinct oncogenes, suggesting that different oncogenes may function at different stages of neoplasm development have been summarized by Cooper [C40].

J. GROWTH FACTORS: MECHANISM OF ACTION AND RELATION TO ONCOGENES

212. The proliferation of normal diploid cells in culture is under the control of exogenous growth factors. In the absence of the proper mitogens, cells leave the cell cycle and become reversibly arrested in the G_1/G_0 phase. Transformed cells, on the other hand, have relaxed cell cycle control and may go through the cell cycle in the absence of growth factors. The lack of growth factor requirement thus seems to be an important feature of transformed cells which contribute to their defective growth control. The view that has gained increasing currency in recent years is that proto-oncogenes are involved in cell cycle regulation and that any regulatory component in the chain of events linked to normal growth, if inappropriately expressed or activated, may have oncogenic properties. The subject has been extensively reviewed by Heldin and Westmark [H32] and therefore only a few essential aspects are pointed out below.

213. In addition to nerve growth factor [Y12] there are three well-characterized families of growth factors: platelet-derived growth factor family (PDGF), epidermal growth factor family (EGF) and insulin-like growth factor family (IGF) (see [C46, S67, W27 and Z3] for reviews). Evidence that a viral oncogene may code for a growth factor comes from a number of recent studies. For example, the sis oncogene of the simian sarcoma virus displays striking homology to the PDGF [D33, W28], a small polypeptide that stimulates growth of connective tissue cells [S67]. A portion of the sequence of the receptor for EGF is virtually identical to another oncogene (erb-B) carried by avian erythroblastosis virus [D34]. Moreover, several growth factor receptors, including those for PDGF [C47, E15, N22], EGF [H34, U7] and insulin [K26, P24] as well as 10 different oncogene protein products [B13] share functional homology in that they are all associated with tyrosine kinase activity (see Table 16).

214. Information on growth factors and their receptors has been obtained in studies in which BALB/c3T3 fibroblasts, arrested in their growth by serum starvation, have been allowed to undergo synchronous progression through the cell cycle, by the addition of serum. In the absence of serum, 3T3 cells enter G_0 in which cell division and growth stop and many metabolic processes are arrested. The addition of serum initiates a complex series of events (G_1), which culminates 14-20 h later in DNA synthesis. The PDGF is the serum component that renders 3T3 cells competent to undergo DNA synthesis [A12, D35, H35], although additional components such as EGF and the somatomedins (progression factors) seem to be necessary to maintain cell viability [P25, S68-S70, V7].

215. The availability of cloned DNA probes for a variety of cellular genes has made it possible to undertake studies on transcriptional events resulting from growth factor stimulation [C48, G31, K27]. For instance, Kelly et al. [K27] showed that PDGF (fibroblast mitogen), lipopolysaccharide (B-cell lymphocyte mitogen) and concanavalin-A (T-cell lymphocyte mitogen) stimulate the expression of c-myc (whose abnormal expression is implicated in a wide variety of naturally occurring tumours) in those cells that normally respond to them; within 1-3 hours after the addition of these mitogens to the appropriate cells, c-myc mRNA concentration was increased between 10- and 40-fold with a return to baseline levels well before the onset of DNA synthesis. The activation of c-myc by PDGF is particularly noteworthy in the light of the very close relationship between the sequence of one chain of PDGF and that of the product of the c-sis oncogene [D33, W28].

216. Greenberg and Ziff [G31] measured the effect of a mitogenic signal on the transcription of a range of different c-onc genes using isolated nuclei from BALB/c3T3 cells. Within 15 minutes of serum stimulation, there was a striking (15-fold) increase in the transcription of c-fos (the normal cellular homologue of the transforming gene of FBJ-osteosacroma virus), which returned to its initial levels within 30 minutes. No further changes in c-fos transcription were observed as the cells progressed from G_1 to S. The authors also observed a small but reproducible increase in c-myc transcription after serum stimulation, which peaked approximately 2 hours after stimulation and decreased significantly within 4 hours. Under similar conditions, many other c-oncs displayed barely detectable levels of transcription at all times after serum stimulation.

217. Campisi et al. [C48] measured c-myc expression during growth and quiescence in three cell lines: the non-tumorigenic mouse fibroblast line A31 and two tumorigenic derivatives, BPA31 and DA31, both transformed by chemical carcinogens. The growth of all these lines can be arrested by starvation (though the tumorigenic cells are slower to respond). While arrested A31 cells cease to express c-myc, the transformed cells continue to express c-myc at the same level after arrest. It would thus seem that c-myc expression, and thus growth competence, is no longer subject to regulation by serum growth factors after transformation. The authors point out that these

observations are consistent with the existing evidence that the activation of c-myc depends on the disruption of the genetic control of its expression and not with mutations affecting the function of the product (as seems to be the case with respect to c-oncs of the ras family).

218. These and other results support the view that the proto-oncogenes play an active role in the regulation and control of cellular proliferation and that growth factor independence and autonomous growth of transformed cells might be due to the constitutive expression of any of the controlling elements along the normal mitogenic pathway. The constitutively expressed factors, which function as transforming proteins in the malignant cell, may be encoded by oncogenes, or, alternatively, their expression may be under the control of oncogenes.

K. SUMMARY AND CONCLUSIONS

219. This section contains a discussion of the exciting advances that have been made during the last few years in the study of the genetic basis of cancer; these advances have come about from convergent research on retroviruses, DNA-mediated gene transfer, application of recombinant DNA methods and cell genetics.

220. The genomes of retroviruses contain specific genes (viral oncogenes or v-oncs) responsible for the production of tumours in a number of avian and mammalian species. The discovery that mammalian and other genomes contain nucleotide sequences related to v-oncs and that these cellular proto-oncogenes have oncogenic potential, and the identification of the activated forms of the proto-oncogenes (transforming genes) in tumour cells, have helped to catalyse and accelerate research in this area, bringing the understanding of the genetic basis of cancer a step closer.

221. The potential transforming activity of cellular genes has been studied in transfection assays. In these experiments, normal cellular DNA fragmented to sizes of about 0.5-5 kb and transfected to NIH/3T3 cells (recipients) induced transformation with relatively low efficiencies. However, DNAs of cells transformed by normal cellular DNA fragments induced transformation with high efficiencies in secondary transfection assays. The transforming activities were found to be localized to discrete DNA segments present in the tumour cell genome. Several of these have been isolated using molecular cloning techniques.

222. The relationships between different cellular transforming genes detected in transfection assays have been clarified by the discovery that many of these represent cellular homologues of the oncogene c-Ha-ras of the Harvey murine sarcoma virus or the oncogene v-Ki-ras of the Kirsten murine sarcoma virus. A number of new transforming genes not belonging to the ras family have also come to light. Currently, we know of at least 17 distinct cellular oncogenes, each with a corresponding retroviral oncogene. The most obvious consequence of these newly discovered homologies is the realization that at least some of the cellular sequences can become activated through certain mechanisms, leading to qualitative and quantitative changes in the corresponding gene product.

223. The discovery that the genetic lesion leading to the activation of the c-Ha-ras1 proto-oncogene in human bladder carcinoma is a point mutation resulting in the replacement of glycine by valine at the 12th aminoacid in the protein product of the gene, led to other discoveries: the c-Ki-ras2 and its activated version in certain lung and colon carcinomas differ by the same $G \rightarrow A$ transversion at the 12th codon; in certain other cell lines derived from other tumours, mutations at position 61 were responsible for the transforming activity elicited in NIH/3T3 cells. It would thus appear that codons 12 and 61 are the major hot spots for activation of proto-oncogenes (members of the ras family) studied so far.

224. The first case of proto-oncogene activation in a non-virally induced tumour by a process of DNA transposition has been reported. There are now a number of instances in which proto-oncogene activation seems to be mediated through chromosomal rearrangements. In these the remarkable concordances between the chromosomal localization of the cellular oncogenes and the break-points involved in some specific chromosomal aberrations are noteworthy (Burkitt's lymphoma, chronic myeloid leukaemia, acute lymphoblastic leukaemia, etc.). These findings do not necessarily mean that all non-random chromosomal changes involved in several kinds of tumours are associated with events in which the activation of proto-oncogenes occurs through chromosomal changes involving the proto-oncogenes.

225. Other possible mechanisms for proto-oncogene activation have been explored in experimental systems, which include: attaching of strong promotors/enhancers to proto-oncogenes, inserting promotors/enhancers near proto-oncogenes and then using these constructs to study transformation in NIH/3T3 cells. The evidence that there is amplification of proto-oncogenes in certain tumour cell lines has led to speculation that such amplification may be involved at some stage in carcinogenesis.

226. The apparent conceptual conflict between cellular transformation as studied in transfection assays and the multi-step nature of carcinogenesis in vivo has been the subject of research in a number of laboratories. It is clear that fibroblast immortality is a prerequisite for transformation in vitro and that while NIH/3T3 cells are a useful tool, they deviate from normal cells in their ability to grow indefinitely in monolayer cultures and thus probably contain already several alterations that make them susceptible to tumorigenic conversion in vitro. Furthermore, evidence is emerging to suggest that different transforming genes must contribute to the carcinogenic process and that they function in different stages of neoplastic development.

227. The question of the normal cellular functions of proto-oncogenes has been investigated in a number of

studies. The findings that several protein products of viral oncogenes share homologies with growth factors and/or receptors support the view that proto-oncogenes are actively involved in the regulation and control of cellular proliferation and that growth factor independence and autonomous growth of transformed cells probably result from the inappropriate expression or activation of these controlling elements.

IV. MOVABLE GENETIC ELEMENTS AND SPONTANEOUS MUTATION RATES

228. The conceptual framework for one of the most active areas of current genetic research—the one dealing with movable genetic elements—was established by McClintock over three decades ago [M3-M7]. Meticulous analysis of the results of crosses between certain genetically marked maize plants led her to postulate the existence of what she called controlling elements, which had the capacity to move from one chromosomal location to another. When a controlling element was inserted next to a gene, it inhibited that gene's activity and, conversely, when the element moved away from a gene, the activity of that gene reappeared. However, the realization that the phenomenon observed by McClintock and the effects generated as a consequence (induction of novel variation at particular loci, localized high mutability, localized chromosome breakage) are not genetic oddities but represent events of a more general nature, had to await confirmation in other organisms and the availability of means to explore the problem more fully.

229. Movable genetic elements have now been discovered in a number of species including bacteria, blue green algae, yeast and Drosophila. The possibility exists that they will eventually be discovered in man. Some of these movable genetic elements have been characterized at the molecular level and there is evidence for some similarities between these and the integrated proviruses of some vertebrate retroviruses. The current state of the art with respect to movable genetic elements has been the subject of a recent symposium [C6] and a book edited by Shapiro [S72]. Some salient aspects of these elements are briefly discussed below, focusing on bacteria, yeast, Drosophila and the mouse and on some speculations concerning their possible presence in man.

A. BACTERIA

230. Some of the first major insights into movable genetic elements came from bacterial genetics in the late 1960s and early 1970s with the discovery of small, transposable DNA sequences that can insert themselves into bacterial chromosomes or into DNA of temperate bacteriophages or plasmids [F3, J2, S130]. Some of these DNA sequences are devoid of a recognizable phenotype, and contain no detectable genes unrelated to insertion functions [C49, C50]. These are called insertional sequences (IS). Other insertions carry additional detectable gene(s), unrelated to insertion functions and are called transposons (Tn). The properties of these elements have been extensively reviewed [B4, C62, H36, I8, K4, K28, K29, S9, S10].

231. Insertional sequence elements were first detected as a cause of spontaneous mutations in E. coli (reviewed in [S9]). Insertion of discrete segments 0.8-1.5 kb long led to interruption of structural genes or strong polar effects. Reversion to the original phenotype was observed. Occasionally, insertion of an IS element in front of a gene resulted in an activation of gene expression.

232. Recent developments in rapid DNA sequencing techniques have allowed the elucidation of the structure of several IS elements. The IS elements range from 0.8 to about 1.5 kb in size. The termini of these carry perfect or near perfect inverted repeats of about 10-40 base pairs; they are believed to serve as recognition sequences for the transposition enzymes in their role of fusing the ends of the IS elements with the target DNA. The number of IS elements varies from 1 to 40 and on the basis of the copy number of the known IS elements (over 10 have been well characterized in E. coli), it is possible to calculate that at least 1-2% of the E. coli K12 chromosome consists of various IS elements [I8].

233. Integration of the IS elements shows a certain site specificity and the degree of specificity varies for the different insertion elements. Their insertion into a gene abolishes its functions, leading to a mutation. Most of these mutations revert to wild type, indicating the exact integration and excision of the IS element. Reversion cannot be enhanced by mutagens. Both integration and excision are independent of RecA [J3, J4]. In addition to exact excision, secondary chromosomal aberrations (deletions, duplications) are often detected in the vicinity of IS elements. The presence of an inserted segment of DNA can be demonstrated by a number of biophysical techniques.

234. Insertion of an IS element is accompanied by a short duplication of target DNA such that the transposed element is flanked by direct repeats of target DNA. The length of the duplication, but not its nucleotide sequence, is usually specific for the particular IS element. Different IS elements transpose at different rates, depending on the genotype and the physiological state of the host organism, as well as on the particular structures of the donor and target sequences. Rates varying between 10^{-3} (or perhaps more usually 10^{-5}) and 10^{-9} per cell division per IS element, have been reported.

235. Many of the notions and concepts about the properties of IS elements are those extrapolated from the results of transposons (Tns), which contain one or more genes in addition to those involved in insertion functions, rendering them more amenable to study. Among the transposons, the properties of the members of the Tn3 family and Tn10 have been extensively investigated [H36, K28]. About 20 transposons belonging to

the Tn3 family have been isolated from at least 50 different bacterial genera. Most of these genera are gram-negative bacteria but Tn551 (encoding erythromycin resistance) was isolated from Staphylococcus aureus [K41]. Other members of the Tn3 family encode tetracycline resistance, and several others encode multiple antibiotic resistance.

236.   Tn3 and its immediate relatives Tn1 and Tn2, carry the most common penicillinase gene found in gram-negative bacteria. These transposons are found in plasmids from antibiotic-resistant bacteria, but may transpose to bacteriophages and to the chromosomes of E. coli and many other bacteria. The Tn3-like elements have a similar structure and are transposed by a common mechanism. Tn3 is 4957 kb long and has a short inverted sequence of 38-bp at its end. The presence of such short repeated sequences is a characteristic feature of the members of the Tn3 family, other common features including the following: (a) they encode a related high molecular weight protein that is essential for transposition; (b) they are transposed by a two-step mechanism (in the first step, the donor and recipient DNA molecules become fused via a duplication of the transposon (co-integrate), and in the second, the duplicated copies undergo recombination to yield a precise transposition); (c) most insertions are clustered in narrow regions of the target DNA, which are A + T rich [H36]; (d) they exhibit a phenomenon known as transposition immunity, which limits multiple insertions of the same transposon into a plasmid [R29]; and (e) there is evidence that host functions are required for transposition.

237.   The ampicillin transposon Tn1 transposes from plasmid RP4 into E. coli chromosome with a frequency of about (1-3) 10^{-4}/cell. Treatment of the bacteria with UV light, mitomycin-C or nitrosoguanidine leads to an increase in the frequency of transposition. Mutation in lexA and RecA genes blocks the induction of transposition; chloramphenicol (protein synthesis inhibitor) and rifampicin (inhibitor of transcription) decrease the effect of UV-induced transposition [K42, S98]. Mutants that lead to high efficiency of transpositions (het mutants) have been isolated [I12]. (See also [G47].)

238.   The intact Tn10 transposon is 9300-bp long and has 1400-bp inverted repeats at its ends. The 6500-bp of non-repeated material include the 2500-bp tetracycline-resistance determinant and (probably) other determinants the functions of which are not known [J23, K43]. The 1400-bp repeats at the ends are closely related but non-identical IS elements, IS10-right and IS10-left, that encode the sites and functions responsible for Tn10 transposition and that co-operate with one another to mediate transposition of the intervening tetracycline determinant [F36]. Of these two ISs (right and left), the IS10-right is the functional transposition module in Tn10. Insertion of a transposon into a gene causes a mutation in that gene and inexact excision leads to deletions adjacent to the transposon. For details of these and other effects, as well as molecular models that have been proposed, see [H36] and [K28].

B.   YEAST

239.   The Ty (transposon yeast) elements were first described by Cameron et al. [C15], who characterized a Ty sequence (the Ty1) present at the yeast SUP4 locus (tyrosine-inserting suppressor locus; one of the eight yeast tyrosine transfer RNA genes). In this study, the evidence for the transposability of Ty1 was obtained both from the observation of the location of Ty1 in different isolates and from the observation of such changes during growth of a single isolate S288c of Saccharomyces cerevisiae. The Tys are a family of dispersed repetitive DNA sequences [R30]. Each member consists of a central region of about 5.6 kb pairs of DNA flanked by direct repeats of approximately 330 bp sequence called delta; there are 30-35 Ty elements per haploid yeast genome. In addition to the delta elements associated with Ty sequences, the yeast genome contains at least 100 solo delta sequences. The presence of terminally repeated sequences indicates structural similarities to the prokaryotic transposons. The Ty elements show considerable sequence divergence and differ from each other by simple base pair changes and also by insertion, deletion and substitution mutations. Likewise, the delta sequences associated with the Ty elements show considerable sequence heterogeneity.

240.   Mutants that arose as a result of transposition of Tys have been isolated at the histidine-4 locus, alcohol dehydrogenase locus and cytochrome-c locus [E6, R31, R32, W31]. Cloning of these genes, restriction mapping and sequence analysis indicated that these mutations resulted from the insertion of an intact Ty element into the 5′-non-coding region of the affected gene. Insertions into structural genes appear to be rare, but more data are needed before generalizations can be made [R30, S99].

241.   As in the case of bacterial transposons, Ty transposition results in a duplication of the target DNA at the site of transposition. In addition to the ability of Tys to transpose, they have been implicated in a variety of genomic rearrangements, including deletions, tandem duplications, inversions and chromosome translocations [R30]. These various rearrangements appear to be the result of general recombination between different homologous Ty elements and not the result of the transpositional activities associated with Tys.

C.   DROSOPHILA

242.   Presumptive evidence for the occurrence of movable genetic elements in the Drosophila genome first came from genetic studies of mutable or unstable genes ([G8-G10]; reviewed in [G3, G4 and G7]). Such mutations were found to revert to wild type at high rates and generate chromosomal rearrangements. By analogy with what is known about the genetic properties of IS-mediated mutations in bacteria, the above observations were interpreted on the assumption of involvement of IS elements of unknown origin.

1. MR-chromosomes

243. In 1971, Hiraizumi [H6] reported low but significant levels of spontaneous recombination in certain types of hybrid males whose second chromosomes were derived from flies captured in nature. Such chromosomes were designated as MR (for male recombination). It soon became clear that MR chromosomes are present in all the natural populations of Drosophila studied in this respect, sometimes at high frequencies (reviewed in [T6]). In studies of Drosophila populations caught at a number of widely separated sites in the Soviet Union, Berg [B6] found that: (a) males with the recessive singed bristles (sn) occurred relatively frequently in collection of wild flies; and (b) an inordinately high frequency of sn mutants occurred among the descendants of wild-caught males when bred in the laboratory. A subsequent detailed analysis of the sn mutants derived from wild-caught males showed them to be mutationally unstable: they reverted to wild type frequently and/or generated deletions at the sn locus. It was hypothesized that the sn mutants were the product of MR action. The test of this hypothesis [G6, G7] demonstrated its validity: MR chromosomes of diverse geographical origins generate unstable sn mutants at very high frequencies (100-200 mutants/10^5 chromosomes). Concurrent tests of MR chromosome on several X-linked loci demonstrated that three of them (ras, raspberry eye colour; y, yellow body colour; and cm, carmine eye colour) were also susceptible to MR action. The ras and y mutants, as with the sn mutants, proved to be mutationally unstable, whereas a few of the cm mutants tested were stable (see also [E3]).

244. There is evidence that MR element(s) may themselves transpose [M8, S12, Y1]. Transposition of the MR element implies that, generally, the element can be mapped to a specific chromosomal location. For the second chromosome, a major MR element exhibiting both male recombination-inducing and mutator capacities has been mapped to the left arm of this chromosome [M8, S13, S14]. The analysis of the nature and distribution of MR-induced mutations [E26] showed that: (a) most of these mutations (10 out of 13 tested) are due to the insertion of a particular mobile element (P-element); and (b) the distribution of these mutations [E26] is not identical with that reported for mutations [L58].

245. In experiments on the effects of MR on radiation-induced genetic damage in males, Sobels and Eeken [S15] found that the frequencies of autosomal translocations in the MR-containing males were not significantly different from those in males that did not contain the MR; however, the frequencies of sex-linked recessive lethals were higher in the MR than in the non-MR males. A more specific interaction of x rays and the mobile element P was observed when recessive lethals were induced by x irradiation in a chromosome that carried P-elements at known sites. The cytological analysis, using polytene chromosomes, showed that among these lethals, there were specific breakage events at the site of the inserted P-elements [E31].

246. In other studies, Eeken and Sobels [E4] focused attention on the reversion of a specific insertion mutation (sn^{MR}, which was originally induced by MR and which reverts spontaneously to sn^+ under the influence of MR) by two chemical mutagens, ethyl nitrosourea (ENU) and methyl methanesulphonate (MMS). Since MR acts primarily in gonia, the two chemicals were fed to first instar larvae. With ENU (1 mM and 3 mM), the reversion of sn to sn^+ was either unaffected (1 mM) or increased by a factor of 2 (3 mM), suggesting a possible threshold. With MMS, however, there were no demonstrable increases in reversion frequencies in the MR + MMS group relative to the MR group.

247. Eeken and Sobels [E5] also examined the extent to which excision and incorporation of DNA sequences by MR is affected by enzymatic pathways involved in DNA repair. MR chromosomes were introduced into males deficient for excision repair (mei-9 mutant) or post-replication repair (mei-41 mutant) or into males carrying both repair-deficient mutations. MR activity was recorded using the induction of sn and ras mutants as indicators. The interesting finding was that, in the double mutant with MR, there was a striking enhancement (by a factor of 5-10) of the frequencies of these mutational events, relative to the double mutant without the MR. With the single mutants mei-9 or mei-41, there was also an enhancement of the frequencies of sn and ras mutants in the presence of MR, but this effect was of borderline significance. In another study [E6], repair deficiency (again, mei-9, mei-41 or both) reduced the reversion of sn to sn^+ by more than 50%, suggesting that DNA repair defects do interfere with the action of MR.

2. The P-M system of hybrid dysgenesis

248. In the mid-1970s, Kidwell and Kidwell [K44], Kidwell et al. [K5] and Sved [S100] advanced a unifying general hypothesis to account for the variety of unusual phenomena that have been reported in the literature on Drosophila, such as those associated with the MR chromosomes, and introduced the term hybrid dysgenesis. This was defined as "a syndrome of correlated genetic traits that is spontaneously induced in hybrids between certain mutually interacting strains, usually in one direction only" [K5, K44]. These include such phenomena as male recombination, male and female sterility, transmission ratio distortion, chromosomal aberration and high mutability, which occur only in certain classes of outcrossed flies (and thus never within homogeneous strains). By examining the F_1 hybrids from a series of inter-strain crosses, Kidwell et al. [K5] found that each strain could be unambiguously classified as either P (paternally contributing) or M (maternally contributing). The traits were most pronounced in the progeny of crosses between M females and P males, greatly reduced in the reciprocal cross and virtually absent in the progeny of all P × P or M × M crosses. In most cases, the P strains were those recently derived from wild populations and the M strains were long established (10 years or longer) laboratory stocks. The traits themselves showed common features, such as pre-

ferential occurrence in the germline. The subject of hybrid dysgenesis has recently been reviewed [B5, B56, E25].

249. Further investigations into the inheritance of these traits revealed that the causative factors could be mapped to multiple locations in the genome of P strains [E24, S100]. The number and genomic locations of these factors varied among the different P strains and not in the M strains. Such elements operationally defined by their dysgenic traits were designated as P factors. Considerable heterogeneity among P factors was implied by the observation that the relative magnitude of each dysgenic trait was a function of the particular P strain involved. In its simplest form, the hypothesis of hybrid dysgenesis states that P factors are present in P strains where their transposition is repressed and are absent from M strains. When chromosomes carrying P factors are placed in the M cytotype, these elements become derepressed and transpose at high rates. Among other effects, P factors would then induce mutations by inserting into and disrupting genetic loci. Such dysgenesis-induced mutations would be expected to be stable in the P cytotype, where P factor transposition is repressed, but unstable in the M cytotype, where they could revert by excision of the P factor. Biochemical evidence for this hypothesis has now been obtained. Using molecularly cloned P-elements from hybrid dysgenesis-induced mutations at the w (white) locus, Rubin et al. [R56] and Bingham et al. [B55] were able to show that such mutations are due to insertions of P-elements; these elements bore homology to one another in sequence, although heterogeneous in size (0.5-1.4 kb in length). They were present in about 50 dispersed copies in P strains (as seen by in situ hybridization of labelled P element sequences to polytene chromosomes) and, as would be expected, absent in M strains.

250. O'Hare and Rubin [O17] have now sequenced the DNA of what they consider the primary P-element. It is 2907 bp long with precise inverted repeats of 31 bp at the termini; unlike many other transposable elements, it has no long direct repeats. In addition to the 2.9 kb element, there are many smaller elements, and sequence studies have revealed that they can all be derived from the major one by internal deletions that always leave the 31 bp repeats intact. The size of the deletions range from a few hundred bp to more than 2000.

251. A mutation caused by the presence of a P-element can be considered an insertion mutation if the parental chromosome is known to lack the element at that locus. Such is the case for four independent mutations at the w locus [R56, S101]. In addition, eight independent mutations at the singed (sn) locus and one at the yellow (y) locus were examined by in situ hybridization techniques and each had a P site at the expected cytological position that was not present in the parental chromosome [E25]. Examination of the structures of the wild-type phenotypic revertants of four different P-element insertion mutations in white (w) indicated that phenotypic reversion was accompanied by excision of the P-element [R56]; the

excision appeared to be precise within the limits of resolution of the analysis, which was estimated to be less than about 50 bp. There is evidence for a variety of partial excisions at the y locus (for details see [E25] and [R33]). Three of the P-element insertions at the w locus were found to occur at tightly clustered or identical sites within the w locus, suggesting some insertional site specificity. Site preference for insertion of P-elements could account for the observed differences in the frequencies at which mutations arise at various genetic loci in dysgenic individuals.

3. The I-R system

252. Another independent system of interacting strains is that denoted by I-R (for inducer and reactive) described by Picard [P5] and discovered through its effect on female sterility. The interaction postulated here is between chromosomally located inducer factors (I) and a cytoplasmic state called reactive (R). The combination in a female fly of a strong I factor, which can be linked to any of the four chromosomes, and an R cytoplasm leads to female sterility. In females heterozygous for the I factor, a phenomenon called chromosomal contamination occurs. In such females, homologous or non-homologous chromosomes lacking I acquire it. Genetic evidence favours the interpretation that chromosomal contamination involves the transposition of I from one chromosome to another [B5, P5]. One other feature of the I-R system is its mutator activity. After the transiently sterile females recover fertility, sex-linked recessive lethal and visible mutations occur among their progeny at very high frequencies; the recessive lethals do not map randomly and, among the visibles, some occur in clusters and some are unstable, reverting at high rates [P5]. The mutator effects parallel those observed for MR and suggest that the unstable mutants are probably insertions.

4. Interrelationships between the MR, P-M and I-R systems

253. The designations of the three mutator systems discussed above reflect the mode of origin of the mutator. Thus, MR reflects the increased frequency of mitotic crossing-over occurring in males carrying particular second chromosomes isolated from wild flies [H6]; hybrid dysgenesis refers to the high frequency of occurrence of dysgenic traits among the progeny of wild type (natural populations) males crossed to laboratory strains of females; and the I-R refers to a type of transitory sterility observed among females obtained by crossing particular laboratory strains (all these in Drosophila). All these mutator systems are of interest, not only because they generate high frequencies of mutations at various loci (mutants which to a large extent appear to be insertion events) but also because they produce all types of chromosomal aberrations. It is worth noting that both the MR and P-M systems involve chromosomes derived from wild flies.

254. The question of whether there exists some inter-relationships between these mutator systems, or whether they are all different, has been raised (see Green [G48] for a recent review). As may be recalled, I-R as a mutator functions only in females, in contrast to MR and P-M where mutator activity occurs in males and females. Thus it is reasonable to conclude that I-R represents a discrete mutator system, distinct from MR and P-M. The MR and P-M systems share a number of features including the following: (a) mutator activity is manifest only when the chromosomes (MR) or chromosomes (P-M) are patroclinously inherited; (b) there is an inordinately high frequency of unstable mutants induced at the X-chromosome locus, sn; and (c) there are elevated frequencies of male mitotic crossing-over. However, comparison of results of studies with MR and P-M system show that mutator action is not a predictor of hybrid dysgenesis [G48].

255. Biochemical evidence substantiating the thesis that, in the P-M system, the P-elements are involved has already been discussed. It was also shown, in experiments of two kinds, that MR activity is associated with the P-elements. In one experiment [G48], Southern blot analysis for the presence of 1.2 and 3 kb P-elements in DNA extracted from larvae of MR strains was carried out. In the other [E26], sex-linked recessive lethals isolated using an MR chromosome were mapped genetically and further examined in hybridization experiments in situ using a cloned P-element, described as p6.1 by Rubin et al. [R56]. In the first study, all the six strains examined carried the P-elements; in the second, in 10 out of 13 cases, hybridization was observed over the region where the lethals were genetically localized. It thus seems clear that the MR and P-M systems are "part and parcel of the same mutator system" [G48]. The absence of gonadal dysgenesis in the MR system needs further study.

5. Mobile genetic elements inferred from biochemical studies

256. The existence of the mobile genetic elements discussed so far was inferred from genetic studies, although molecular methods were subsequently used to identify them. Quite independently of these studies, students of Drosophila molecular genetics have identified the presence, in Drosophila DNA, of several dispersed moderately repetitive DNA sequences[q] [R5, R33, S102]. In fact, such repeated gene families compose nearly one-sixth of the Drosophila chromosomal DNA and most of the fly's middle repetitive DNA. The genes that characterize these families are designated as 412, copia and 197 among others [A4, F4, I3, R5].

257. The first biochemical evidence that elements of these repeated gene families transpose came from observations of polymorphisms in the number and positions of several dispersed, moderately repetitive DNA sequences between different stocks of Drosophila [I3, S103], between cell lines and their parental fly stocks [P38] and between Drosophila melanogaster and its sibling species, Drosophila simulans [L35]. These observations were soon extended to include a large number of other moderately repetitive DNA sequences [D48, M66, P39, Y2, Y3]. The biochemical and genetic properties of these have been recently reviewed [G49, R33] and only a few important points are mentioned below.

258. On the basis primarily of internal structures, the dispersed moderately repetitive sequences have been classified by Rubin [R33] into: (a) copia-like elements, including copia, 412, 297, mdg1 (mobile dispersed genetic elements) (the fragments described in earlier publications as Dm 225 and Dm 234 are part of the complete mdg1 element [B104]), gypsy and a number of others not yet well-characterized; (b) fold-back (FB) elements; (c) P-elements; and (d) other dispersed repetitive families.

259. The copia-like elements range in size from 5 to 8.5 kb, carry long direct terminal repeats (169-571 bp) and occur at approximately 10-100 copies in widely scattered locations in the chromosome arms as well as the centric heterochromatin. There is now direct evidence that several Drosophila mutations (e.g., white-apricot (w^a), bithorax (bx)) result from the insertion of copia-like elements [B57, G11, G50, L36]. Rubin et al. [R56] obtained evidence for the trans-position of a copia element into the w locus, following a cross between two strains known to produce hybrid dysgenesis. It is possible that hybrid dysgenesis, in addition to the dramatic increase it produces in the transposition rate of P-elements, also increases the rate of transposition of copia-like elements.

260. The FB elements described by Potter and colleagues [P40] comprise a family of heterogeneous, but cross-homologous sequences ranging in size from a few hundred base pairs to several kilobases. Each FB element carries long terminal inverted repeats; in some cases, the entire element consists of these inverted repeats and in other cases, a central sequence is located between these inverted repeats. The genetic properties of mutations caused by the insertions of FB elements are revealed by the behaviour of two such mutations, w^c (white-crimson) and w^{DZL} (white domi-nant zeste-like) [K45, L37]. A large transposable element of the X-chromosome called the TE, which usually carries w and an adjacent gene (roughest), has FB elements flanking it [G50] contrary to the original hypothesis of Gehring and Paro [G11] that the copia transposable element is present at both ends of TE.

261. The properties of P-elements have already been described. Other dispersed repetitive families include insertions ranging from 0.5 to 5 kb in length found in ribosomal genes, as well as what are referred to as "scrambled clustered arrays of moderately repetitive DNA sequences", which are 0.3-1 kb in length. Their properties have been reviewed [R33].

---

[q]Eukaryotic DNAs contain different sequence classes whose constituent members can be broadly classified as: (a) unique (approximately one copy per haploid genome); (b) moderately repetitive (~ 10^6 copies per haploid genome); and (c) highly repetitive [B60].

6. Similarities between Drosophila transposable elements and those in other systems

262. The possibility that the transpositions of discrete elements are analogous phenomena in prokaryotes and eukaryotes such as Drosophila or yeast has been discussed. For the element copia in Drosophila, this analogy holds at the molecular level [R6]. Rubin et al. [R6] have listed the following common features between copia and bacterial transposons: (a) the elements are inserted within many different target sequences that share no obvious homology to each other or to the ends of the transposable elements; (b) upon insertion, the elements generate a duplication, in direct orientation, of a few base pairs of the target sequence found immediately adjacent to the ends of the element; (c) an element has the same terminal sequence when inserted at different chromosomal locations; and (d) the element contains a terminal repetition binding the main body of the element. These features are also shared by the Ty1 element in the yeast Saccharomyces cerevisiae [F5, G12] and the Dm 297 in Drosophila. The integrated proviruses of the avian retrovirus SNV (Spleen Necrosis Virus, an avian reticuloendotheliosis virus) [S17] and the Moloney murine sarcoma provirus (M-MuSV) [D6, M9] also share the structural features mentioned above, although they are not known to transpose. Although at present their significance is not clear, the structural analogies are striking.

263. There is now evidence that among eukaryotes, the transposition of copia-like elements in Drosophila and of Ty1 in yeast may involve reverse transcription, i.e., their transposition is mediated through an RNA intermediate ([B58, S104], also reviewed in [B59] and [G49]). Such transposable elements dependent on reverse transcriptase have been termed retroposons [R57] or retrotransposons [B59].

D. MOUSE

264. The fact that the chromosomal DNA of inbred and wild-type mice contains one or more copies of endogenous murine leukaemia virus[r] (MuLV) sequences and that the MuLV expression follows Mendelian segregation in many strains, has been known for some time (see Chan et al. [C22] and Chattopadhyay et al. [C23] and references cited therein). Several high leukaemic strains such as AKR, C58, C3H/Fg, etc., carry multiple copies (3-5 per haploid genome) of ecotropic viral DNA sequences, whereas many low leukaemic strains such as DBA, BALB/c and C3H/He contain a single copy per haploid genome. The structure of most ecotropic MuLV genomes in high and low leukaemic strains is similar to the prototype Gross-AKR MuLV, but the endogenous ecotropic MuLVs are integrated at multiple sites in mouse chromosomes in different strains, though possibly at a constant site within a strain.

---

[r]Endogenous MuLVs have been divided into three related classes on the basis of their host ranges which are determined by the viral envelope glycoprotein: ecotropic, which infect only murine cells, xenotropic which infect primarily heterologous cells and amphotropic which replicate efficiently in cells of both types.

265. Jenkins et al [J7] studied the chromosomal location of the DBA/2J ecotropic provirus Emv-3 by Southern blotting and hybridization with an ecotropic-specific DNA probe in a number of inbred and specially constructed hybrid mouse strains. It was found that the Emv locus was near the d (dilute coat colour) locus on chromosome 9 and that it co-segregated with the d allele, suggesting close linkage. Analysis of DNAs prepared from inbred strains and substrains that carried the wild-type allele of d, showed that they did not carry the proviral sequence. Furthermore, a spontaneous revertant (d → d⁺) in the DBA/2J strain, was associated with the concurrent loss of most of the proviral sequence.

266. Further work [C76] demonstrated that, at least for two germline revertants of d to d⁺, reversion was accompanied by excision of the Emv provirus, by a process of homologous recombination between the proviral LTRs. Furthermore, this recombination process left behind exactly one LTR at the integration site [H64] in d⁺ revertants. Thus, the proviral insertion itself probably induced the d mutation by integrating into non-coding regions in or around d. These observations have been interpreted by the authors as providing evidence for the thesis that the d locus mutation in the DBA/2J mice is associated with the integration of the provirus. The authors have evidence for a close association between a unique MuLV sequence and another coat colour mutation (the A^y locus). The question of whether the relatively high spontaneous reversion rates associated with the a and d loci (reversion rates about 3 times the forward mutation rate) recorded in the earlier work of Schlager and Dickie [S47] is in any way related to the integration and excision of MuLV sequences is still unclear, but, at least for d, proviral excision due to homologous recombination may be responsible for the increase in reversion rate.

267. The possibility of inactivation of cellular genes through insertion of retroviral sequences in chromosomal DNA in vivo was investigated in the mouse by Jaenisch et al. [J8]. Mouse embryos were exposed to Moloney murine leukaemia virus [M-MuLV] and 13 substrains were obtained in which the virus was stably integrated into the germ line chromosomal DNA, but at different locations or integration sites (the Mov loci). Twelve of these sub-strains were generated in experiments involving infection of pre-implantation embryos and one was from infection of post-implantation embryos. The substrains were maintained by mating normal females with males heterozygous for a given Mov locus. The virus-carrying offspring were identified by testing for viraemia or for the presence of virus-specific sequences in DNA from liver biopsies. Each of the substrains carried one copy of the virus and the pattern of inheritance followed Mendelian rules. For instance, in crosses involving heterozygotes for a given Mov gene, the expected number of Mov/Mov homozygous embryos at term were observed. However, in one substrain that carried the Mov-13 gene (this strain was the one derived from infection of post-implantation stages), homozygosity was lethal. Examination of pregnant females (the cross: +/Mov 13 × +/Mov 13) revealed that about

25% of the embryos were degenerated. DNA extracted from these embryos invariably revealed homozygosity at the Mov 13 locus. Schniecke et al. [S133] have shown that the Mov 13 provirus integrates into the α1(I) collagen gene and embryos homozygous for this mutation begin to die at approximately day 12 when α1(I) collagen transcription normally becomes predominant in wild type.

268. There is one group of stable inserted elements in the mouse, the intra-cisternal A-particle genes (IAPs). The IAPs are retroviral-like elements, but appear to have no infectious or recognized extracellular phase; they are similar to the virus-like copia RNA particle in Drosophila and are present in about 1000 copies per genome. Recently, Kuff et al. [K30] have shown that these particles are responsible, by insertion, for mutations involving the kappa immunoglobulin light chain gene in mouse hybridoma cells and emphasize that the family of IAP-related genes may be considered as potential movable elements and a source of insertional mutations in the mouse.

269. Suggestions exist that other dispersed repeats (human Alu-type, see below) in the mouse—the B1 and B2 sequences—may also be candidates for transposable genetic elements, since they usually are flanked by short direct repeats, specific for each copy of the repeat. For details, see [G49, J9, K46, K47].

E. MAN

270. The human genome contains between 300,000 and 500,000 copies of a 300 bp repeat sequence that act as substrate for the Alu restriction enzyme[s] and are referred to as Alu repeats [J9, J24, S73]. Since the genome contains 3×10^9 bp, these repeats must be one of the most predominant groups of repetitive sequences in the human genome and account for approximately 4% of the total DNA. The Alu repeats are present in all mammalian genomes and a 40 bp sequence appears to have been conserved throughout mammalian evolution. Of particular interest is that most Alu elements are flanked by direct repeats of sequences of some 7-20 nucleotides long [G33, H37], a feature in common with movable genetic elements; they are therefore considered prime candidates for mobile genetic elements within the genome.

271. There is the possibility that pairs of Alu sequences might be able to act as pairs of insertion sequences in transferring intervening DNA segments, inter-Alu DNA around the genome, in other words, acting the same way as bacterial transposons. Recently, Calabretta et al. [C24] have found that both chromosomal and extra-chromosomal forms of inter-Alu DNA in normal and human neoplastic tissues show considerable inter-tissue and inter-individual variation (polymorphisms). From these and other results, the authors have suggested that such chromosomal and extra-chromosomal segments of inter-Alu DNA reflect

the presence of transposable elements, that they may be involved in genetic rearrangements, and that the interspersion of Alu repeats may arise from sequential excision of the Alu sequence and their subsequent reinsertion elsewhere in the genome.

F. RELEVANCE IN THE CONTEXT OF RISK EVALUATION

272. The findings that transposable genetic elements so far studied in various species are capable of causing appreciable alterations in spontaneous mutation frequencies have documented the concept that, far from being interesting curiosities in a background of genomic stability, the transposable genetic elements are important factors in the genetic control of mutation phenomena in general. The question of whether their mobility can also be substantially altered by mutagenic agents such as x rays has not yet been resolved since the currently available data are very limited and do not lend themselves to generalizations.

273. The possible relevance of mobile-genetic-element-mediated spontaneous mutations in the context of risk evaluations using the doubling dose method has recently been discussed by Sankaranarayanan [S132] and can be best illustrated by the following assumptions (which are not exhaustive) and the consequences of these assumptions:

(1)   All spontaneous mutations arise through mechanisms that have been envisaged before the advent of the "mobile genetic element era" and represent rare errors made during DNA replication and/or repair (mechanism A). The contribution of transposable-genetic-element-mediated spontaneous mutations (originating by mechanism B) to the total is zero. There are no qualitative differences between spontaneous mutations and those induced by irradiation and radiation merely increases the frequency and types of events that lead to spontaneous mutations. If these assumptions are valid, then it is safe to use the doubling dose method for risk estimation.

(2)   Spontaneous mutations are of two kinds, namely, those that arise by mechanism A and those by mechanism B mentioned above (i.e., those independent of mobile genetic elements and those that are dependent on these). The frequencies of both kinds of mutations can be enhanced by irradiation. If these assumptions are true, the consequences would be indistinguishable from those obtained for situation (1).

(3)   This is the same as situation (2), except here it is assumed that only the frequencies of mutations that arise by mechanism A (i.e., those that are independent of movable genetic elements) can be enhanced by radiation exposure while those that arise by mechanism B are not. If these assumptions are true, it is proper to estimate the doubling dose only for mutations that arise by mechanism A. If one lets the proportion of spontaneous mutations that arise by mechanism A vary from 1 to zero (and thus

---

[s]The name Alu derives from the fact that these sequences have been identified using restriction endonuclease AluI (from Arthrobacter luteus) which recognizes A G C T sequences in the DNA and cleaves them between G and C.

the B-type mutations from zero to 1), and since the induction rate one estimates is applicable only to A-type mutations, it is easy to see that, as the proportion of A-type mutations decreases, the doubling dose will decrease, i.e., the relative mutation risk will increase. When all spontaneous mutations are caused by mechanism B, it is not correct to estimate the doubling dose as a ratio of the average spontaneous and induction rates of mutations, since the numerator will be zero.

274. The prediction for situation (3) can be illustrated by the following example. In this, P_A is the spontaneous prevalence of autosomal dominant and X-linked disorders that have arisen by mechanism A (expressed as the number of cases per 10^6 live births); P_B is the same for the disorders that arise by mechanism B; m_1 is the average spontaneous rate of A-type mutations; m_2 is the average rate of induction per unit dose; c is the doubling dose in Gy; 1/c is the relative mutation risk; and E, the expected increase in the number of cases (per 10^6) at equilibrium following irradiation at a rate of 1 Gy per generation. The results of calculations summarized below show that: (a) as the proportion of spontaneous mutations arising by mechanism A decreases, the estimate of the doubling dose also decreases (since the induction rate measured is assumed to be applicable only to those mutations that arise by mechanism A and therefore held constant); and (b) from the standpoint of the population, the total number of induced mutations will remain the same (the E values given below).

P_A	P_B	m_1	m_2	c	1/c	E
10,000	0	10^{-5}	10^{-5}	1	1	10,000
7,500	2,500	$0.75 \, 10^{-5}$	10^{-5}	0.75	1/0.75	10,000
5,000	5,000	$0.50 \, 10^{-5}$	10^{-5}	0.50	1/0.50	10,000
2,500	7,500	$0.25 \, 10^{-5}$	10^{-5}	0.25	1/0.25	10,000

It is worth reiterating that there is as yet no hard evidence as to whether the transposition rate of the transposable elements is increased under conditions of radiation exposure and there is no evidence on the proportion of spontaneous mutations in man that could reliably be attributed to the transposable elements. Consequently, it is fruitless to make further speculations at the present time.

G. SUMMARY AND CONCLUSIONS

275. The classical studies of transposable controlling elements in maize were the first to indicate the presence of chromosomally located mobile and transmissible elements in the genome that induce chromosome breaks, duplications, a variety of other structural changes, as well as changes in gene expression at many loci. These observations were made before the first demonstration of mobile DNAs in bacteria in the form of plasmids and bacterial viruses (bacteriophage), which could insert themselves into the genome, but also detach themselves completely and replicate independently in the cell.

276. Movable genetic elements have now been discovered in a number of other species studied in this respect (bacteria, blue-green algae, yeast and Drosophila) and there are indications that they may be present in mammals including man, although they have not yet been demonstrated to transpose.

277. Bacterial transposable elements are of two kinds: IS (insertion sequences; these contain only genes related to insertion functions) and Tns (containing other detectable genes unrelated to insertion functions). The IS range in size from 0.8 to 1.5 kb and carry perfect or near-perfect repeats of about 10-40 base pairs at their termini. It has been estimated that at least 1-2% of the genome of E. coli K12 consists of various insertion elements. Integration of the IS elements shows a certain specificity of sites. Their transposition into a gene abolishes its functions, leading to a mutation. Insertion of an IS element is accompanied by a short duplication of target DNA. Different IS elements transpose at different rates.

278. Among the bacterial transposons, those belonging to the Tn3 family and Tn10 have been extensively studied. Transposons are generally somewhat longer than IS elements although their properties are basically similar.

279. There is evidence for the thesis that treatment of bacteria with UV, mitomycin-C, or nitrosoguanidine may increase the rate of transposition of at least one transposon (Tn1).

280. The transposable elements in yeast (the Tys) are a family of dispersed repetitive sequences consisting of a central region of about 5.6 kb of DNA flanked by direct repeats of approximately 330 bp sequences called delta. There are about 30-35 Tys per haploid genome. The evidence that Tys are transposable comes from the the analysis of mutations at a number of genetic loci. Most of the Ty insertion mutations studied so far have occurred in the regulatory and not in the structural genes.

281. The first evidence for mobile DNA elements in Drosophila was provided by the behaviour of a small number of unstable mutations. These mutations display genetic properties analogous in many respects to those of mutations caused by the insertion of transposable elements in maize and prokaryotes. Such unstable mutations revert to wild type at unusually high rates and generate deletions and other chromosomal rearrangements. Three mutator systems that generate unstable mutations, the MR, the P-M and the I-R, have been the subject of a number of genetic studies.

282. In experiments in which the effect of MR on radiation-induced genetic damage in males was studied, it was found that the frequencies of autosomal translocations in MR-containing males were not significantly different from those in non-MR males; the frequencies of sex-linked recessive lethals were about 50% higher in the MR-bearing males. There is some evidence that DNA repair defects may interfere with the action of MR. In one case there appears to be direct interaction between a P-element and x rays, resulting in site-specific chromosome breakage events.

283. The occurrence of hybrid dysgenesis, "a syndrome of correlated genetic traits that is spontaneously induced in hybrids between certain mutually interacting strains, usually in one direction only" and that includes phenomena such as male and female sterility, high mutability, chromosomal aberrations and male recombination, has been extensively documented in Drosophila. In the so-called P-M system, the strains could be classified as either P (paternally contributing) or M (maternally contributing). The traits mentioned above occur in crosses between P strain males and M strain females, are much less pronounced in the reciprocal cross and are absent in P × P or M × M crosses. The hypothesis that the occurrence of hybrid dysgenesis in the P-M system is due to the insertion of P-elements (insertion sequences) has been tested biochemically and found to be correct. These P-elements are present in about 50 dispersed copies in P strains and, as expected, absent in M strains.

284. The question of whether the P-elements in the P-M system and the MR factors discussed earlier are similar has been examined in a few studies, using genetic and molecular techniques. It has become clear that both systems are integral parts of the same mutator system, although they were originally identified by different experimental approaches.

285. Another independent system of interacting strains in Drosophila is that designated as I-R (for inducer and reactive), discovered originally through its effect on female sterility. Genetic evidence favours the interpretation that the mutator effects observed in this system are also due to DNA insertions.

286. In addition to the transposable elements in Drosophila, which were originally identified in genetic studies (with a molecular follow-up), there is extensive evidence for the presence of several moderately repetitive DNA sequences that are capable of transposition from one chromosome location to another. These include the copia-like elements, fold-back elements, P-elements (already described) and several other dispersed repetitive families as yet not fully characterized. Their insertion into genes results in mutations and a number of such insertion mutations have been described.

287. In the mouse, there is evidence for unique MuLV (murine leukaemic virus) sequences being closely associated with two coat colour loci, called a and d; in the case of the d locus, a spontaneous revertant from d to d⁺ was associated with the concurrent loss of the proviral sequence. Exposure of mouse embryos to exogenous Moloney leukaemic virus results in the stable incorporation of the virus into the germ line chromosomal DNA, but at different locations or integration sites (the Mov loci); homozygosity for one such locus seems to disrupt a gene function essential for normal development and consequently to produce lethality of the homozygotes.

288. One group of stable inserted elements in the mouse is constituted by the intra-cisternal-A-particle genes (IAPs), which are retroviral-like elements. They are responsible, by insertion, for mutations involving the kappa immunoglobulin light chain in mouse hybridoma cells. Furthermore, dispersed repeats such as the B1 and B2 sequences may be potential candidates for movable genetic elements in the mouse.

289. The human genome contains between 300,000 and 500,000 copies of a 300 base-pair repeat sequence that act as substrate for the Alu restriction enzyme (the Alu repeats); these repeat sequences constitute about 4% of the human DNA. They are flanked by direct repeats of sequences of some 7-20 nucleotides long, a feature they share with movable genetic elements studied in other species. There is evidence that the Alu repeat sequences may be transposable within the human genome.

290. The finding that a sizeable proportion of spontaneous mutations in experimental organisms studied in this respect can be caused by transposable genetic elements may have implications for the evaluation of genetic radiation hazards in man using the doubling dose method. Such implications have been outlined.

V. EXPERIMENTAL DATA ON THE MECHANISMS INVOLVED IN THE PRODUCTION OF CHROMOSOMAL ABERRATIONS IN CELLS IN VITRO

291. The 1982 UNSCEAR report reviewed the progress in studies on the relationship between DNA repair processes and chromosomal aberration phenomena in mammalian cell systems. Among the aspects covered were: (a) the molecular mechanisms involved in the production of chromosomal aberrations; (b) the isolation of mammalian cell lines hyper- or hyposensitive to DNA damaging agents; and (c) the delineation of complementation groups for repair-deficient syndromes in man. New data that have become available since then shed further light on the molecular mechanisms, particularly on the nature of primary lesions in the DNA that lead to chromosomal aberrations and on the role of DNA repair processes. The aim of this chapter is to summarize some of the principal findings. For recent reviews, see Collins et al. [C52], Miwa et al. [M38] and Ishihara et al. [I9].

A. NATURE OF THE PRIMARY DNA LESIONS INVOLVED IN THE FORMATION OF CHROMOSOMAL ABERRATIONS

292. Among the wide variety of lesions that are induced in cellular DNA by x rays and other mutagens (single-strand breaks (SSBs), double-strand breaks (DSBs), base damage, mis-matches, DNA-DNA cross-links, DNA-protein cross-links, etc.), DSBs seem to be the principal ones involved in the production of chromosomal aberrations. Direct evidence for this was provided by Natarajan and colleagues [N3, N4, N23, O2] and this was reviewed in the 1982 UNSCEAR report. Briefly, these authors treated x-irradiated CHO cells with an enzyme—Neurospora

endonuclease (NE)—that recognizes SSBs in the DNA and converts them into DSBs. The prediction was that, should the DSBs be the principal lesions involved in the formation of chromosomal aberrations, then the frequencies of aberrations should be increased in the x rays + NE group relative to the x rays alone group. This increase was in fact observed. Biochemical evidence for the conversion of SSBs to DSBs by NE was subsequently provided [N3]. However, when cells are irradiated with neutrons—a treatment that produced predominantly DSBs—no potentiating effect of NE would be expected; this possibility was also tested and found to be true [O2].

293. Another possible way to inquire into the nature of the lesions responsible for the formation of chromosomal aberrations is to choose agents that will induce only one class of specific lesions in cellular DNA and then study their efficiency in inducing chromosomal aberrations. Restriction endonucleases (discussed in chapter II) represent such a class of agents; they produce either blunt-ended or cohesive-ended DSBs in the DNA. This approach was utilized in independent studies by Bryant [B32], Natarajan and Obe [N24] and Obe et al. [O21].

294. In the work of Bryant, two restriction enzymes, PuvII and BamHI, which generate blunt-ended and cohesive-ended DSBs, respectively, were used to treat permeabilized V-79 Chinese hamster cells. Under the conditions of their experiments, PuvII induced blunt-ended DSBs resulted in both chromosome- and chromatid-type aberrations (exchanges and deletions) including a high frequency of triradials (the latter were assumed to arise from exchanges between isochromatid and chromatid breaks). The total frequency of aberrations was proportional to the amount of enzyme used up to 100 units per treatment flask (at the highest enzyme concentration, the aberration frequency was 10 times the control frequency). Further increases in enzyme concentration produced no further increase in aberration frequencies. In contrast with these results, BamHI (even at concentrations higher than the highest used in the PuvII experiments) did not induce aberrations above the spontaneous level. The ineffectiveness of DSBs with cohesive ends in causing aberrations has been explained as being due to the stabilizing influence of the hydrogen bonding, and consequent ease with which restitution can occur. Because of a lack of such stabilization, DSBs induced by PuvII may behave as true DSBs and are probably more easily brought out of alignment and rendered irreparable or have a higher chance of interacting illegitimately with other DNA strands, leading to chromosome exchanges.

295. In the experiments of Natarajan and Obe [N24] three restriction enzymes that produce blunt-ended breaks (EcoRV, PuvII and SmaI) and three that produce cohesive-ended breaks (BamHI, AsuIII and NunIII) were used to treat CHO cells or PG-19 mouse fibroblasts. The results showed that both kinds of endonucleases induced chromosome-type (the most frequent class) and chromatid-type aberrations; however, the endonucleases that produce blunt-ended DSBs were clearly more efficient than those that

produce cohesive-ended DSBs. Though there was some indication for an increase in frequencies with increasing concentration of the enzymes, no clear-cut dose-response relationships could be demonstrated. In experiments on the cell-cycle stage dependence of aberrations induction, it was found that cells in G_1 and G_2 are relatively resistant to treatment and S phase cells are more sensitive. In several respects, the pattern of aberrations induced was similar to that induced by ionizing radiation, namely, sub-chromatid and chromatid-type aberrations in G_2, chromatid-type in S, chromosome and chromatid-type in late G_1 and early S and chromosome-type in G_1.

296. In independent experiments, Winegar and Preston [W53] reported linear dose-response relationships for aberrations induced by AluI, RsaI and MspI. In addition, they found that for RsaI (blunt-end) and MspI (cohesive-end) the frequency of aberrations was the same for equivalent restriction enzyme doses. The calculated frequency of cutting in CHO cells was the same for these two enzymes. The authors suggested that an improved cell permeabilization technique, which they used, could account for the differences between their results and those of other authors.

297. In those experiments in which treatment with ara-C (cytosine arabinoside, a specific inhibitor of DNA polymerase alpha) or caffeine (an inhibitor of DNA repair and one that is known to abolish the block in G_2 stage induced by different mutagens) was used in addition to PuvII, there was a doubling of the breakage rate (except that, with caffeine, this was only evident at low induction rates). Though ara-C is a specific inhibitor of DNA polymerase alpha, it is known to inhibit excision repair; the ultimate effect of ara-C on excision repair is deduced to be the inhibition of the ligation step. The finding that the presence of ara-C during treatment with endonucleases leads to an increase in the frequency of aberrations strongly suggested that ara-C affects ligation of DNA double-strand breaks.

298. Further data on the induction of chromosomal aberrations in CHO cells by restriction endonucleases have been presented by Obe et al. [O21]. The authors found that the G_1 stage of the cell cycle is particularly sensitive in this regard. The differential yields of aberrations recorded with different restriction endonucleases appeared to be correlated with the number of recognition sites in the genome.

299. From entirely different kinds of experiments, but all involving ara-C treatment, Preston [P7, P26] has favoured the involvement of DNA base damage in the origin of chromosomal aberrations induced by x irradiation. The premiss and the approach were the following: (a) ara-C has been shown to inhibit the repair of DNA damage induced by a variety of agents; (b) ara-C inhibits repair replication, leaving a single-strand gap in the DNA; and (c) this effect of ara-C can be reversed by the addition of deoxycytidine. The general approach has been to treat human lymphocytes in various stages of the cell cycle with x rays or chemical mutagens and to incubate the cells for different periods of time with ara-C. In this way,

single-strand gaps can be accumulated by the inhibition of repair replication. If these accumulated gaps can be converted to aberrations on reversing the ara-C inhibition with deoxycytidine, then increased aberration frequencies will result, compared with those in cells given no ara-C treatment.

300. When human lymphocytes were x irradiated in G_0 and then incubated with ara-C for 1, 2, or 3 hours, the yields of dicentrics, rings and acentric fragments were all increased, compared with cells that received only x irradiation [P7]. There was an approximately linear increase in aberration frequency as a function of ara-C incubation time. The dependence of the increase in aberration yield with the duration of ara-C post-treatment suggested to Preston that misrepair of base damage was most likely to be involved in the induction of aberrations since most of the DNA strand breaks would be rapidly repaired.

301. Natarajan [N25] pointed out that there are at least three arguments that are not in support of this line of reasoning: (a) Bender and Preston [B9] found that the maximum increase in aberration frequencies (80%) occurred during the first one hour of ara-C post-treatment of x-irradiated (G_0) lymphocytes, a period when most of the strand breaks are repaired; (b) when irradiated G_0 lymphocytes are challenged with ara-C after one hour of incubation in normal medium, the potentiating effect of ara-C is greatly reduced [N25]; and (c) while there is a profound oxygen effect for x-ray- or gamma-ray-induced chromosomal aberrations and DNA strand breaks, the oxygen effect is minimal for base damage [P27]. The finding in the more recent studies of Natarajan and Obe [N24] with restriction endonucleases (ara-C post-treatment of restriction endonuclease-treated cells leads to an increase in aberration frequency and this effect is most likely a consequence of ara-C-mediated inhibition of ligation of DSBs) provides one additional argument against the hypothesis of Preston. These different points of view need to be resolved by further experiments.

B. THE ROLE OF DNA REPAIR PROCESSES IN THE FORMATION OF CHROMOSOMAL ABERRATIONS INDUCED BY IONIZING RADIATION

302. The approach of treating mutagenized cells with selective inhibitors of DNA repair/replication to gain insights into the different stages of the repair pathways has been gaining increasing momentum. Among the studies in this area that have been made over the past few years, several are focused primarily on the biochemistry of repair processes, while some have attempted to elucidate the role of such repair processes in the formation of chromosomal aberrations induced by ionizing radiation. Only the latter kind of study is considered in the present section (see [N2-N5, N25 and K6] for recent reviews).

303. The inhibitors that are commonly used can arbitrarily be divided into those that inhibit DNA synthesis (e.g., 5-fluorodeoxyuridine, FdUrd; 2'-de-

oxyadenosine, 2'Ado; hydroxyurea, HU; aphidicolin, APC) and those that inhibit DNA repair (e.g., ara-C; 3-aminobenzamide, 3-AB; benzamide, B). This distinction, however, is not an absolute one since compounds such as HU, ara-C and aphidicolin can all inhibit both replication and repair [D7], and APC was first discovered as a specific inhibitor of DNA polymerase alpha (and thus of DNA synthesis) and subsequently found to inhibit DNA repair as well [K6].

1. Inhibitors of DNA synthesis

(a) Effects at the molecular level

304. The three inhibitors to be discussed here are FdUrd, 2'Ado and HU. A common property of these inhibitors is that they act at a late stage in the synthesis of the immediate precursors of DNA. Their action leads to a disturbance of the balance within the DNA precursor pool and a consequent reduction in DNA synthesis. After phosphorylation to 5-fluoro-deoxyuridilic acid, FdUrd is a powerful and specific inhibitor of the enzyme thymidylate synthetase, which catalyses the synthesis of thymidylic acid from deoxyuridilic acid [C7, H7]. The inhibition is irreversible. Both HU and the triphosphate of 2'Ado are inhibitors of the enzyme ribonucleotide reductase, which catalyses the reduction of ribonucleoside diphosphates to the corresponding deoxyribonucleoside diphosphates. The inhibition is reversible (see [K6] for a listing of the relevant references).

(b) Production of chromosome aberrations

305. All three substances, FdUrd, 2'Ado and HU, are capable of producing chromosomal aberrations themselves in both plant and cultured animal cells. In cells treated in early interphase, exchange aberrations predominate, whereas those treated in late interphase show mainly breaks and large gaps. It is believed that these compounds produce aberrations by disturbing the normal semi-conservative DNA synthesis in the S phase.

306. Similarly, all three inhibitors significantly enhance the chromosomal damage produced by agents such as x rays; this is true for Vicia faba root tips, Chinese hamster cells and human lymphocytes. For instance, in Chinese hamster cells and human lymphocytes, post-treatments with HU or 2'Ado during G_2 have a strong potentiating effect on the chromosomal damage produced by S-independent agents in S or G_2 and by S-dependent agents in G_0, G_1 or S [H8, H9, K7, N5].[1] The types of aberrations increased by

---

[1]Ionizing radiation produces aberrations in all stages of the cell cycle; these can be recovered at the first mitosis following irradiation (i.e., their formation is S-(DNA synthesis)-independent). Antibiotics belonging to the bleomycin group also act via S-independent mechanisms. However, for UV and most chemical mutagens, which are capable of inducing lesions in chromosomes in all stages of the cell cycle, the lesions require DNA and chromosome replications (i.e., they are S-dependent) to be transformed into aberrations that are always of the chromatid type, irrespective of the stage of cell cycle treated.

HU post-treatments are gaps and breaks, whereas exchange-type aberrations are unaltered or even decreased. In human lymphocytes, the most marked potentiation of x-ray-induced chromosomal damage is obtained when HU is given 2 hours before harvesting [K6].

307. It has been assumed that the enhancement of the frequencies of chromosomal aberrations is a consequence of the suppression of some form of DNA synthesis that takes place late in G_2 when chromosomal DNA is damaged by mutagenic agents. Presumably, the DNA synthesis affected by the inhibitors is required for the repair of the induced chromosomal damage.

2. Inhibitors of DNA repair

(a) Inhibitors of DNA polymerases

308. There are several inhibitors that are relatively specific to the activity of alpha, beta and gamma DNA polymerases. This specificity, however, seems to depend on the cell type and the state of the cell during treatment (stationary versus exponentially growing cells). Of these inhibitors, APC, which is absolutely specific for polymerase alpha, and ara-C, which preferentially inhibits polymerase alpha, have been used in experiments to study their influence on spontaneous and induced chromosomal aberrations [K6].

309. Ara-C inhibits DNA replication as well as repair replication in cells following treatment with a variety of mutagenic agents. The probable mechanisms by which ara-C inhibits DNA repair have been discussed by Fram and Kufe [F25]. There is evidence for the incorporation of ara-C into DNA rather than RNA and this incorporation is both concentration and time dependent. Furthermore, the degree of inhibition of DNA synthesis is correlated with the extent of its incorporation into DNA [F25]. While the mechanisms underlying the effect of ara-C on DNA repair are not known, both the competitive inhibition of DNA polymerase alpha and the incorporation of ara-C into DNA segments may play a role in drug action.

(b) Effects on chromosomal aberrations

310. Ara-C is capable of inducing chromosomal aberrations not only in the DNA synthetic (S) phase of the cell cycle but also in cells in the pre- (G_0 or G_1) and in the post-DNA synthetic phases of the cell cycle [B7-B9, K8, N5, P7]. The experiments of Preston [P7] on post-treatment effects of ara-C (following x irradiation of human lymphocytes) were discussed earlier. In another study, Preston and Gooch [P8] treated G_1 lymphocytes with 4-nitroquinoline-N-oxide (4-NQO) and, as would be expected of an S-dependent agent, there was no increase in aberration frequency compared with untreated controls. However, if 4-NQO-treated cells were incubated with ara-C for 6 hours, aberrations were observed, but they were of the chromosome type. The conclusions were that: (a) chromosome-type aberrations can be induced in G_1 by

chemicals that normally do not induce them, if repair is inhibited by ara-C; and (b) in order to produce a significant frequency of aberrations, rather long (at least relative to x rays) ara-C incubation times are required. The latter conclusion suggests that the repair of the 4-NQO damage that is converted into aberrations is rather slow, compared with the repair of the x-ray damage involved in aberration production. This leads to the general conclusion that the frequency of aberrations, and in many instances the spectrum of aberration types, is determined by the rate of repair of the DNA damage responsible for aberration production.

311. In a more recent paper, Heartlein and Preston [H51] advanced and tested the hypothesis that ara-C-inhibitable DNA damage provides a measure of inter-specific difference in the sensitivities of lymphocytes to the induction of chromosomal aberrations by x rays. Human, rabbit, marmoset and pig lymphocytes were irradiated in G_0 (0.5-3.0 Gy), incubated with ara-C for 0-4 h and processed for cytogenetic analysis. In all four species, the frequencies of dicentrics increased with incubation time (up to 3-4 hours), but the rates of increase were different and approximately proportional to the ratios of x-ray-induced aberrations observed in the absence of ara-C. Thus, for example, human lymphocytes are about twice as sensitive as rabbit lymphocytes to the induction of dicentrics by x rays and the rate of increase of aberrations in the presence of ara-C was about twice as great in human relative to rabbit lymphocytes. The authors suggest that these findings are consistent with the existence of possible inter-specific differences in excision or resynthesis associated with the repair of damaged bases and that this approach may be useful in explaining differences in sensitivity to aberration induction (by x rays) among species or cell types and differences of dose-response curves.

312. The experiments of Natarajan et al. [N29] were aimed at a further clarification of the effects of ara-C on the repair of x-ray-induced lesions in human G_0 lymphocytes. Attention was focused on the following aspects: (a) inhibition of repair by ara-C during 15 to 60 min following x irradiation and its effects on chromosome aberration yields; (b) the effect of delayed ara-C treatment on aberration yields; (c) estimation of the rate of strand-break repair following x irradiation in the presence of ara-C, by nucleoid sedimentation technique; and (d) the effects of ara-C during the first 30 min following x irradiation, using the technique of prematurely condensed chromosomes.

313. The results showed that treatment with ara-C for a time as short as 15 min following x irradiation increased the yields of chromosomal aberrations in a very striking manner; longer durations (up to 2 hours) also led to further increases in aberration yields, but these were quite small, relative to the increase observed with a 15 min treatment. These data thus suggest that ara-C may inhibit, predominantly, the repair of short-lived x-ray-induced lesions. If this interpretation were correct, with ara-C administered 1 hour after x irradiation, the potentiating effect of ara-C would be expected to be greatly reduced and this was in fact

what was observed. Biochemical studies (nucleoid sedimentation) revealed that ara-C prevented rejoining of breaks very effectively and this inhibition was maximal already with a 30 min ara-C treatment; with delayed ara-C treatment (given 1 hour after x irradiation), the effect on repair of strand breaks was negligible, as would be expected. On the basis of these results and their earlier data with restriction endonucleases, those of Iliakis and Bryant [I13] and of Holmberg and Gumauskas [H52], Natarajan et al. [N29] concluded that ara-C can inhibit the repair of directly induced single- and double-strand DNA breaks and this accounts for the increased yields of chromosomal aberrations. The results obtained with the premature chromosome condensation technique (discussed in the next section) are in line with this interpretation.

314. Aphidicolin (APC), another inhibitor of DNA polymerase alpha, does not induce chromosomal aberrations in human lymphocytes when treated in G_0 [N5]. The chromatid-type aberrations observed by Bender and Preston [B9] after treatment of G_0 lymphocytes with APC are probably the result of residual APC present in the medium [Z1]. APC, however, induces chromatid breaks and gaps when human lymphocytes or CHO cells are treated in G_2 [B9, N5], indicating the occurrence of a residual DNA synthesis during the G_2 stage.

315. The frequencies of chromosome-type aberrations are potentiated when x-irradiated G_0 lymphocytes are post-treated with APC [B9]; both breaks and exchange-type aberrations increase with the duration of post-treatment. However, the finding that APC induces lesions in G_0 which synergistically interact with x-ray-induced lesions to produce an increase in chromatid-type aberrations [B9] appears to be due to residual APC in the medium [Z1]. When G_0 lymphocytes are x-irradiated and post-treated with APC, there is a 2- to 3-fold increase in the frequencies of chromatid breaks but either no increase or a slight decrease in the frequencies of exchanges, indicating an inhibitory effect of APC on the rejoining of DNA strand breaks. With CHO cells in G_1, however, post-treatment with APC after x irradiation produces only a slight potentiation of the chromosome damage. This may be due to the possibility that the inhibition of repair of damaged DNA by APC depends on the metabolic state of the cells, inhibition being more effective in stationary than in proliferating cells [N5, Z1].

(c) Inhibitors of ADP-ribosyl transferase (ADPRT)

316. ADP-ribosyl transferase (ADPRT), which is also known as poly-(ADP-ribose) polymerase or synthetase, is a DNA-dependent nuclear enzyme on which a considerable amount of work has been done during the last few years. This enzyme covalently attaches ADP-ribose moieties derived from NAD to proteins to form mono- or poly-ADP-ribosyl derivatives [H11, S21]. ADPRT activity is strongly stimulated by breaks in DNA [B10] and the enzyme is required for efficient DNA repair [C8, D8]. The evidence so far available indicates that, in most cases, the ADPRT activity is

not required for the incision, excision or repair synthesis steps, but is required for the strand-rejoining step, particularly that mediated by DNA ligase-II [S21, S76].

317. Exposure of cells to alkylating agents or to radiation results in an inhibition of glycolysis, due to a drastic fall in cellular NAD levels. This drop in cellular NAD induced by DNA damaging agents, in particular by streptozotocin, a derivative of MNU, methyl nitrosourea, is due to activation of ADPRT and not to inhibition of NAD biosynthesis or to activation of NAD glycohydrolase [W32]. Furthermore, cytotoxic agents that do not directly affect the integrity of DNA, such as colchicine or FdUrd, do not have this effect on cellular NAD [S21]. In addition to the clear evidence suggesting that ADPRT is required for efficient DNA repair, there is also evidence that ADPRT activity is required for certain types of cell differentiation [F6, J5].

318. Inhibitors of ADPRT activity such as 3-aminobenzamide (3-AB) and benzamide (B) prevent the depletion of cellular NAD that is caused by DNA-damaging agents. These inhibitors also retard DNA strand rejoining in some cell types after certain kinds of DNA damage, such as simple alkylating agents in permanent cell lines like L1210 lymphoid cells, in cell strains such as human skin fibroblasts and in protozoa [S21]. There is a small retardation of DNA strand rejoining after ionizing radiation, but no evident effect of ADPRT inhibitors after ultraviolet radiation [S21, C9].

319. A number of investigators have studied the effects of inhibitors of ADPRT activity on the spontaneously arising and mutagen-induced chromosomal aberrations, sister chromatid exchanges (SCEs) and point mutations [N2, N5, N6, H12, O3]. Under normal culture conditions (F10 medium with 15% fetal calf serum) when human lymphocytes or CHO cells are incubated in the presence of 3-AB or B even at high concentrations (10 mM), there is no evidence for an increase in the frequency of chromosomal aberrations [N5, N6]. However, if CHO cells are grown in Eagle's MEM or in a medium deficient in nicotinamide and in the presence of 10 mM of BrdUrd, 3-AB induces chromatid aberrations, especially of the exchange type [H12], suggesting that the metabolic condition of the cells is an important factor for the manifestation of the effects of 3-AB. Fibroblasts derived from human chromosome instability syndromes such as ataxia telangiectasia or Fanconi's anemia (which have low but significant levels of spontaneously arising chromosomal aberrations) respond to 3-AB with increased frequencies of aberrations in a dose-dependent manner [N2]. These observations have been interpreted as an interference of 3-AB on the repair of spontaneously arising DNA breaks in these cells.

320. When human lymphocytes are x-irradiated in G_0 and incubated in a medium containing 3-AB for 6 hours prior to mitogenic stimulation, or during the entire period of 48 hours of culture, the frequencies of chromosomal aberrations increase 2- to 3-fold [N6].

The increase due to 3-AB post-treatment is similar, irrespective of the duration of post-treatment, indicating that most of the aberrations induced by x rays are fixed immediately after irradiation. The observed increases in aberration yields are interpreted as due to the slowing down or partial prevention of restitution of DSBs in DNA by this inhibitor, thus allowing for an increased possibility for the formation of exchanges.

321. Treatment of CHO cells in G_2 with 3-AB following x irradiation also increases the frequencies of induced aberrations (breaks and exchanges) by a factor of 2-3. As will be recalled, the other inhibitors of DNA repair such as APC and HU which act by different mechanisms when given immediately after x irradiation of G_2 cells increase only chromatid breaks and not exchanges [K7, N6, Z1]. Thus, 3-AB is different in its mode of action in that it does not completely inhibit the rejoining of breaks but only causes a delay in the repair of breaks.

322. The results obtained with short-wave UV show, however, that 3-AB post-treatment does not affect the yields of induced chromosomal aberrations [N6], unlike ara-C, HU and APC, which have marked effects (enhancement of the yields of chromosomal aberrations).

323. It is now established that several inhibitors of ADPRT induce SCEs [N6, O3]. Interestingly, under conditions in which very high frequencies of SCEs were obtained, there was no increase in the spontaneous frequencies of chromosomal aberrations. From detailed studies on the mechanism of induction of SCE induction by 3-AB, Natarajan et al. [N2] have concluded that the replication using BU-containing strand as template is responsible for the increased frequencies of SCEs in cells grown in a medium containing 3-AB. The rationale was that BU-containing DNA is fragile and during replication is susceptible to spontaneous breaks. The repair of such breaks is slowed down by 3-AB, thus allowing the possibility to form SCEs. Shiraishi et al. [S48, S49] reported similar results with Bloom's syndrome [BS] cells. They demonstrated that, in BS cells (which, as is well known, are characterized by a high spontaneous frequency of SCEs), most of the SCEs occur during the second cell cycle when BU-containing DNA is used as a template for replication.

324. When cells are treated with a mutagen in the presence of 3-AB or B, the response to the induction of SCEs varies, depending on the mutagen and the inhibitor used. Thus, in experiments with CHO cells, there is no, or only very weak, potentiation of SCE induction by short-wave UV or mitomycin-C; with EMS (ethyl methanesulphonate) and MMS (methyl methanesulphonate), there is strong potentiation and with ENU (ethyl nitrosourea), there is again only weak potentiation [N2].

325. Neither 3-AB nor B induce mutations at the HPRT locus in CHO cells, either when treated alone or in the presence of BrdUrd for two cell cycles, a condition that induces about a 10-fold increase in the frequency of SCEs [N6]. Post-treatment with 3-AB

after EMS, ENU and short-wave UV treatment of cells had no effect on the frequencies of HPRT mutations. Yet, as mentioned in the preceding paragraph, for SCEs there is strong potentiation effect for EMS.

C. PREMATURELY CONDENSED CHROMOSOMES: A MODEL SYSTEM FOR VISUALIZING EFFECTS OF DNA DAMAGE, REPAIR AND INHIBITION OF REPAIR AT THE LEVEL OF CHROMOSOME STRUCTURE

326. In most in vitro cytogenetic studies on the effects of mutagens, the cells treated at a given stage in the cell cycle are allowed to proceed to mitosis to evaluate chromosomal damage. In 1970, Johnson and Rao [J18] described a phenomenon whereby if mitotic and interphase cells were fused, factors from the mitotic component would cause nuclear membrane breakdown and premature condensation of the interphase chromatin. The resulting chromosome units were called prematurely condensed chromosomes (PCC). Thus, one can visualize the interphase chromosomes as discrete units. Their morphology reflects the stage of the cell in the cell cycle at the time of fusion. Cells from G_1 phase yield PCC with a single chromatid per chromosome, S cells show a fragmented appearance and G_2 cells give rise to PCC with two closely aligned chromatids per chromosome. The number of PCCs per cell equals the number of chromosomes observed at mitosis and G_1 and G_2 PCCs approximate mitotic chromosomes in size and location of the centromere.

327. The formation of PCCs occurs very quickly after fusion of mitotic and interphase cells and can take place across species barriers (e.g., mitotic CHO cells can induce PCC in fish or human cells). The fact that this technique allows the visualization of interphase chromosome means that structural damage can be assessed directly in interphase cells. Waldren and Johnson [W33] found that chromosome damage after x irradiation could be immediately assayed in G_1 cells by counting the number of fragments of G_1 PCC. Since the number of G_1 PCCs prior to treatment equals the number of chromosomes in the cell, a chromosome break would result in the formation of an additional chromosome piece. Using this technique, Waldren and Johnson observed a linear dose-response curve for G_1 HeLa cells after x irradiation. Similarly, Hittelman and Rao found that chromosome damage could be immediately visualized in the G_2 PCCs of CHO cells after gamma irradiation, bleomycin and adriamycin treatment [H38-H40].

328. During the past few years, the potential of this technique has been exploited to study the induction of chromosomal aberration in mammalian cells and probe into the molecular mechanisms operating during DNA and chromatin repair. The use of DNA repair inhibitors in these studies have been particularly helpful in unravelling the consequences of repair inhibition at the chromosomal level. These and other themes have recently been reviewed by Hittelman [H41].

329. In the experiments of Natarajan et al. [N29] mentioned earlier, the effects of inhibition of repair by ara-C was studied in irradiated (2.0 Gy) human G_0 lymphocytes using the PCC technique. Irradiated lymphocytes, after appropriate post-treatments with ara-C were fused with mitotic CHO cells and subsequently processed for chromosome analysis. It was found that: (a) the yield of fragments in cells irradiated and fused immediately was similar to that in irradiated cells treated with ara-C for 30 min before fusion; and (b) irradiated cells treated with ara-C 30 min after irradiation responded with somewhat lower frequencies of fragments. These observations have been interpreted by the authors as indicating the inhibitory effect of ara-C on x-ray-induced short-lived lesions. Since, in these studies, only fragments were scored, the question of whether the changes in the numbers of fragments reflect corresponding changes in the frequencies of exchange aberrations and/or simple fragments as such could not be answered.

330. Pantelias and Wolff [P41] examined the effects of ara-C treatment on irradiated and unirradiated G_0 human lymphocytes using the PCC technique and showed that, with long treatment durations (up to 8.5 hours), ara-C alone induced a significant increase in the frequencies of fragments per cell, but during the first hour, there was no increase. X rays alone induced chromosome fragments, which decreased during the first hour in the presence of ara-C; then, however, the number of fragments increased, so that by the end of the 8.5 hours treatment period, the yield was increased by about 30% over the starting period of time zero. In the absence of ara-C, the yield of fragments did not increase, but continued to decrease for about 5 hours. The total yield of fragments in the ara-C + x-ray group was simply the sum of yields induced by ara-C and x rays individually. The use of very long treatment durations with ara-C, the finding that the clastogenic activity of ara-C was expressed in only about 50% of cells and the fact that it is not possible to discriminate between ara-C effects on x-ray-induced exchange aberrations or fragments, make comparisons with other data obtained through metaphase analysis difficult.

D. SUMMARY AND CONCLUSIONS

331. A number of recent studies have shed further light on the nature of the lesions in DNA that lead to chromosomal aberrations in somatic cells in vitro and the processes of DNA repair associated with the formation of these aberrations. Particularly interesting are the new data obtained with the use of DNA-restriction enzymes, which provide further direct evidence for the thesis that double-strand breaks in DNA are the principal lesions involved in aberration formation.

332. The role of the DNA repair processes in chromosome aberration formation has been extensively studied during the past few years using specific inhibitors of replication and/or repair. All these inhibitors have in common the property of enhancing the frequencies of chromosomal aberrations induced by

physical or chemical agents, although the mechanisms and the magnitude of the potentiation effect varies, depending on the metabolic state of the treated cells, the mutagen and the specific inhibitors used.

333. One of the principal repair enzymes that is activated in mutagenized cells is ADP-ribosyl transferase; this is a nuclear enzyme that is sensitive to DNA breaks and it may modulate the rate of their rejoining, possibly by regulating the activity of DNA ligase II. Inhibition of the activity of this enzyme by inhibitors such as 3-aminobenzamide leads to an enhancement in the frequency of radiation-induced chromosomal aberrations. Fibroblasts derived from carriers of human chromosome instability syndromes such as ataxia telangiectasia or Fanconi's anaemia (which have low but significant levels of spontaneous chromosomal aberrations) respond to inhibitors such as 3-aminobenzamide with increased frequencies of aberrations.

334. It is clear that several inhibitors of ADP-ribosyl transferase induce sister chromatid exchanges (SCEs). Under conditions in which high frequencies of SCEs are obtained, there is no increase in the frequencies of chromosomal aberrations. An examination of the function of bromodeoxyuridine used in the technique for detecting SCEs has provided evidence showing that these inhibitors are more effective at enhancing SCEs when the template DNA strand during S phase contains bromodeoxyuridine.

335. The potential of the technique of premature chromosome condensation by artificial fusion of mitotic and interphase cells is being exploited to study the induction of chromosomal aberrations and the associated molecular mechanisms.

VI. OTHER RELEVANT DATA

A. STUDIES IN EXPERIMENTAL MAMMALS INCLUDING PRIMATE SPECIES

1. Production of heritable tumours in mice and rats following irradiation and/or chemical treatment

336. The earlier work of Nomura [N9] demonstrating that congenital anomalies and tumours could be detected in the progeny of irradiated ICR mice was discussed in the 1982 UNSCEAR report. In a subsequent paper, Nomura presented the detailed results of this and other work with urethane [N7]. Of particular interest is the finding that both x-irradiated and urethane-treated male or female mice produced progeny with a much increased tumour incidence, with a clear dose-response relationship for treated post-meiotic stages in males and less clear-cut results for spermatogonial treatment; oocytes at late follicular stages were resistant to x rays in the range of 0.36-1.08 Gy, but very sensitive to higher doses. At the highest dose of 5.04 Gy, the tumour incidence in the offspring was around 30% following irradiation of

spermatids in the male or oocytes in the female, a frequency that is 6 times that in the controls. The spectrum of tumours in controls and in offspring of treated parents was similar, with about 90% being papillary adenomas of the lung and the remainder various malignant tumours of other organs. Matings continued down to the F_3 generation clearly demonstrated heritability of the induced high tumour incidence and the pattern of inheritance resembled that of a dominant trait with 40% penetrance, on average. Although x irradiation of males resulted in dominant lethals and cytologically demonstrable translocations, no such effects were observed in animals treated with urethane. Nomura has argued that the mutations that result in excess tumours are probably not gross chromosomal rearrangements.

337. In further studies, Nomura [N30] extended these results to LT and N5 strains of mice. In these experiments, adult males were exposed to 0.504 Gy of x irradiation, mated to unirradiated females and the F_1 progeny scored for tumours. Since the LT mice were very sensitive to x irradiation and fertility was never recovered, only the progeny derived from irradiated post-meiotic germ cells were available for scoring. The data showed that the frequencies of tumour-bearing progeny as well as of tumours were higher following irradiation. In the LT mice, these frequencies were the following: tumour-bearing progeny, 21.3% (16/75) in the x-ray group versus 9.0% (37/411) in the controls; and frequency of lung tumours, 16% (12/75) in the x-ray group, and 5.4% (22/411) in controls. In addition, 5.3% of the progeny in the x-ray group had leukaemia, whereas this frequency was only 1% in the controls. In the N5 strain, following spermatogonial irradiation, the frequencies of tumour-bearing progeny and of tumours were likewise higher than in controls: tumour-bearing progeny, 33.2% (76/229) in the x-ray group and 23.0% (56/244) in the controls; lung tumours, 21.0% (48/229) in the x-ray group and 14.3% (35/224) in the controls. In experiments with N5 mice, 3.9% of the progeny had leukaemia (relative to 0.4% in controls) and, among the female progeny, 28 out of 123 (22.8%) in the x-ray group had ovarian tumours compared to 18/116 (15.5%) in the controls. It was noted that the frequencies of lung and other tumours in these experiments were in the same general range as those in the ICR strain. Nomura's results with the N5 strain also indicated that induced lung tumours showed a dominant pattern of inheritance with an average penetrance of about 40%.

338. In the same paper, Nomura [N30] presented results of studies aimed at examining whether the induced tumours were benign or malignant through transplantability of induced tumours. Among 26 induced tumours in the N5 strain (11 lung tumours, 2 fibrosarcomas, 3 undifferentiated tumours, 2 hepatomas, etc.) only 3 (1 lung tumour and 2 hepatomas) were not transplantable, suggesting that most of the induced tumours were malignant.

339. In other experiments, Nomura [N8] focused on the problem of whether or not the manifestation of such presumed tumour mutations could be enhanced.

The rationale was the following: if germ-line mutations lead to heritable tumours, then all the cells comprising the organ in question (in this case the lung) must carry the mutations and have the potential to develop tumours. However, most often, not more than one tumour nodule was present in the lung of the tumour-bearing progeny (experiments discussed above) and, as already mentioned, the average penetrance of the presumed tumour mutations is only about 40%. Consequently, if the progeny of irradiated parents (some of which must carry the tumour-inducing mutations) are given an exposure to a carcinogen such as urethane, whose mode of action, at least under certain conditions, is promotion of carcinogenesis [B12, N10], then it should be possible to increase the level of expression of tumours (i.e., both the number of tumour-bearing animals and the number of tumours per animal).

340. As in earlier experiments, mice of the ICR strain were used. In some experiments, mature (60-65 day old) male or female mice were irradiated with 2.16 Gy of x rays and mated to unirradiated animals of the other sex to produce F_1 progeny. In others, pregnant females were irradiated on day 9 or 15 after the appearance of the vaginal plug. The F_1 progeny were divided into two groups: one group was killed eight months after birth; the other group received a single subcutaneous injection of 5μmol/g body weight of urethane at 21 days of age and was killed 5 months later. Offspring of non-irradiated parents were similarly treated with urethane. The numbers of tumour nodules in the lungs were counted.

341. The main results were the following: (a) x irradiation significantly increased the incidence of lung tumours in the progeny, regardless of which sex was irradiated and 88 out of the 93 tumour-bearing offspring developed only one tumour nodule in the lung while the remainder developed two nodules; (b) in the group treated with x rays and urethane (x irradiation of parental post-meiotic stages or late follicular stages), the number of progeny developing large clusters of tumour nodules was strikingly enhanced; (c) in the group treated with urethane alone, 2 out of 71 animals developed clusters of tumour nodules; (d) with in utero irradiation, there was a slight non-significant increase in tumour frequency, but additional treatment with urethane similarly enhanced the incidence of animals with large clusters; (e) when all the data were considered together, the proportion of affected progeny with large clusters of tumour nodules was 18% (34/1889) in the group treated with x rays and urethane; when corrected for the control incidence (2.8%, in the group treated with urethane alone), this figure became 15.6%, which is more than twice the frequency (6.3%) in the group treated with x ray alone. It is instructive to note that in the experiments of Russell [R58] no specific locus mutations were recovered in 13,315 F_1 offspring derived from urethane-treated (1750 mg/kg body weight) spermatogonia. Neither did Nomura [N9] observe the induction of mutations causing tumours after spermatogonial treatment with urethane, although a large increase in somatic mutations was observed in melanocytes [N41].

342. In rats, Strel'tsova et al. [S106] found that x irradiation (1 Gy) 5 days before mating led to increased incidence of breast tumours in the female progeny, irradiation of females being more effective in this regard. Following ^{90}Sr injection (14.8 kBq g^{-1}) to female rats, there was a higher incidence of sarcomas in the progeny, than in controls [N31]. Likewise, injection of a single intraperitoneal dose of ^{238}Pu (185 kBq kg^{-1}) to female rats 5 days before mating, led to a significantly higher incidence of tumours in the progeny conceived 300 days after injection; the experimental progeny exhibited certain malignancies (osteosarcoma, liver tumours) not observed in controls [L39]. The same dose of ^{238}Pu injected into male rats also produced tumours in the progeny, but the frequencies were lower [L39].

2. Radiation-induced congenital anomalies in mice

343. In its 1982 report, UNSCEAR discussed the information available at that time [K16, N9] on the induction of congenital anomalies in the progeny of irradiated mice. Kirk and Lyon [K17] have now obtained further data from two experiments. In the first, male mice were exposed to x-ray doses of 1.08, 2.16, 3.60 and 5.04 Gy and mated to unirradiated female mice at various intervals (1-7, 8-14, 15-21 and 64-80 days post-irradiation) so as to sample both post-meiotic stages and spermatogonial stem cells. In the second, only spermatogonial stem cells were sampled following a single x-ray exposure to 5.0 Gy and a fractionated exposure to 10 Gy (5 Gy + 5 Gy, 24 hours interval between the fractions). Contemporaneous controls were maintained. Pregnant mice were killed on day 19 following the appearance of vaginal plug and the uterine contents examined for the presence of congenitally abnormal fetuses.

344. The results showed that: (a) in the first experiment, while the frequencies of congenital anomalies in the irradiated series were higher than in controls, there were no statistically demonstrable differences, either between the effects of different doses or between different intervals, except in week 3 (treated spermatids), at which sampling interval the frequencies increased with increasing dose (from 1% to 5%); (b) the overall frequency of congenital anomalies was $2.0 \pm 0.3\%$ (40 abnormal fetuses among 1950 examined) in the irradiated series (summed over all doses and the first three sampling intervals), which is significantly higher than that in contemporaneous controls $(0.24 \pm 0.17\%, 2/831)$, the lowest frequency found in the authors' various experiments); (c) the data on the induction of congenital anomalies following spermatogonial irradiation in experiment 1 were equivocal, as the frequencies varied from 1.1 to 2.0% between the different doses, and were not significantly different from that observed in the corresponding controls (2.1%); (d) in the second experiment (spermatogonial irradiation), however, the frequencies recorded $(2.2 \pm 0.5\%$ after 5 Gy and $3.1 \pm 0.6\%$ after 5 + 5 Gy) were not significantly different from each other, but higher than the control frequency of $0.7 \pm 0.3\%$; in any case, the enhancing effect of dose fractionation (expected on the basis of results with specific locus

mutations and reciprocal translocations) was not observed; and (e) dwarfism (i.e., less than 75% of the average body weight of the rest of the litter) and exencephaly were the most commonly observed malformations in all series.

345. In studies aimed at testing whether irradiation of post-implantation maternal environment would have any effect on the induction of congenital anomalies by irradiation, West et al. [W46] transferred pre-implantation embryos surgically between females that had been irradiated (3.6 Gy, x rays) before conception or left unirradiated. The results were equivocal: in the group in which the embryos (3.5 days post-coitum) were transferred from untreated donors to irradiated recipients (group D), the frequency of congenital anomalies was not significantly different from that in which the transfer was from untreated donors to untreated recipients (group E, negative control) and that in which the females were irradiated prior to conception and no embryo transfer was made (group A, positive control). In the group in which the embryo transfer was from irradiated donors to untreated recipients (group C), the frequency was not significantly lower than in group A, although the frequency in group C was higher than in group E. The embryo transfer experiments also showed that irradiation of the uterus had no significant effect on the frequency of subsequent post-implantation mortality or mean fetal weight.

346. In further experiments, West et al. [W47] showed that when mouse ovaries were surgically exteriorized and selectively irradiated or shielded in a specially constructed apparatus, and the abdomen (and uterus) irradiated (3.7 Gy of x rays) 15-21 days prior to conception, there was no significant effect on either post-implantation mortality or congenital anomalies attributable to irradiation of the abdomen (and uterus) alone. Exposure of the ovaries to 3.27 Gy of x irradiation, however, during the same period increased the frequency of both post-implantation mortality and congenital anomalies.

3. Further data on spontaneous and radiation-induced non-disjunction and chromosome loss in mice

347. The subject of non-disjunction and chromosome loss in experimental mammals has been reviewed in the earlier reports of the Committee, including the 1982 UNSCEAR report. Recent reviews have been provided by de Boer and Tates [D36], Lyon [L16] and Russell [R36]. The fact that maternal age plays an important role in the aetiology of human aneuploidy is well established. In the mouse also, there is evidence for an increase in the frequency of aneuploid embryos in aged females of some strains [G34, F26, T17]. Several hypotheses have been put forward to explain this age effect. For instance, Polani et al. [P28] suggested that, in human females, the failure of dissolution of the nucleolus in aged oocytes may be a possible mechanism leading to non-disjunction of the D and G group acrocentric pairs. Henderson and Edwards [H42] proposed the so-called production line hypothesis according to which: (a) developmental and

nutritional gradients may occur in the fetal ovary; (b) these gradients could give rise to a reduction in chiasma frequency in the late-formed, relative to the early-formed, oocytes in the meiotic sequence; (c) the first-formed oocytes with high chiasma frequencies are the first that are ovulated in the adult female; those formed later with lower chiasma frequencies and perhaps some achiasmatic chromosome pairs would be ovulated later in life; and (d) the loss of chiasmata may affect the small chromosome pairs more than the large and, as univalents, they may subsequently undergo irregular segregation at anaphase I, leading to aneuploidy.

(a) Cytogenetic methods

348. Speed and Chandley [S77] tested the production line hypothesis using the random-bred Swiss albino and the inbred CBA/Ca mouse strains. In the first set of experiments, surface-spread oocyte preparations were made from fetal ovaries by the method of Speed [S78]. Examination under the light microscope was carried out on oocyte preparations from day 15 of gestation and day 1 post-partum (day 20). A total of 1150 oocytes from 71 ovaries were analysed in the Swiss strain and 676 oocytes from 50 ovaries in the CBA strain.

349. The results showed that in neither of the two strains was there any evidence of gradients in oocyte development or production line; errors in synapsis were rare and oocytes containing univalents were even rarer. When such abnormalities occurred, they were evenly distributed over several gestational days, being no more common in the late than in the early stages of oocyte maturation. Furthermore, there was no evidence that nucleolar material interfered in any way with prophase pairing. One observation of some significance was that of a premature desynapsis of the smallest chromosome pair (19) in late pachytene oocytes; this was observed in about 6% of CBA oocytes analysed over days 17-19 and in about 8% of the Swiss strain oocytes analysed over the same period. The authors believe that the premature desynapsis of bivalent 19 is a normal feature of late oocyte development in the mouse.

350. In another set of experiments, Brook et al. [B33] obtained further data that were inconsistent with the production line hypothesis but that supported the notion that biological and not chronological age of the female is an important factor in the genesis of aneuploidy. In these experiments, inbred CBA/Ca mice 6-8 weeks old were allocated at random to two groups: one group was unilaterally ovariectomized (uni-ovx) and the other sham operated. They were mated to males of known fertility at different ages (63-91 days, 154-182 days, 245-280 days, and 308-350 days) and the pregnant females were killed on day 4 for counts of corpora lutea and uterine analysis of pre-implantation embryos to determine the incidence of aneuploidy. In addition, the oestrous cycle of 20 uni-ovx and sham-operated mice was determined between 60 and 390 days. A further group of about 60 females was used to study the rate of utilization of primordial follicles.

351. The results were the following: (a) the uni-ovx mice had fewer subsequent oestrous cycles (a mean of 15.3 over the period between 90 and 390 days versus 20.4 in the sham-operated mice) and an earlier onset of acyclicity (at 330 days of age versus some 40 days later in the sham-operated ones); (b) the mean number of embryos obtained per animal was higher in sham-operated animals at all ages, though the difference was most marked among the oldest groups; (c) trisomic embryos were not found in either sub-group at ages 63-91 days, whereas monosomics were present in both sub-groups (11.9% and 6.1%, in uni-ovx and sham-operated groups, respectively); in the intermediate age group (154-182 days), the proportion of monosomic embryos was virtually unchanged but three trisomic embryos (4.0%) were found in the uni-ovx group (the overall incidence of monosomic and trisomic together was 17.3% in the uni-ovx group relative to 4.3% in the sham-operated one); (d) the highest incidence of aneuploidy was found in the uni-ovx animals at 245-280 days (22.0% versus 12.1%, but the numbers are small); and (e) quantitative histological studies showed that the rate of primordial follicle utilization was not increased by unilateral ovariectomy, but the rate of their depletion was comparable with that in the sham-operated animals.

352. The authors pointed out that their observations are not amenable to interpretation on the basis of an earlier utilization of the last remaining oocytes which, according to the production line hypothesis, are most likely to be defective; neither can they be explained by any factor that is determined strictly by the chronological age of the female. Rather, they seem to suggest that abnormal meiotic chromosome segregation is an epiphenomenon of the process of physiological ageing of the reproductive system. They further suggest that their results may have implications for human aneuploidy and Down syndrome in particular; they imply that unilateral ovariectomy may be an additional risk factor for Down syndrome. Furthermore, any factor that depletes the oocyte population could advance the maternal age effect for aneuploidy.

353. Tease [T17] investigated the x-ray induction of non-disjunction in young and old mice. Females 10-14 week or 43-54 weeks old were super-ovulated with 5 i.u. of pregnant mare's serum gonadotrophin, followed 45 hours later by 5 i.u. of human chorionic gonadotrophin. Three hours after the latter treatment, they were irradiated with 0.10, 0.25 or 0.50 Gy of high-dose-rate x rays. They were mated overnight to males and fertilized eggs were recovered the following day. The eggs were cultured in vitro to metaphase of the first cleavage division. Under this regimen, maternal and paternal pronuclei remain separate and can be distinguished through differences in chromosome staining and contraction. Only the numbers of hyper-haploid pronuclei were used as measures of chromosome non-disjunction. The results showed that: (a) spontaneous non-disjunction occurred more frequently in oocytes of old females (1.54%) compared to young females (0.19%); (b) after x irradiation, both young and old females displayed significant linear increases in hyperhaploidy with absorbed dose, but the slopes of the regressions did not differ significantly;

(c) the numbers of structural aberrations in maternal pronuclei showed significant linear relationships to absorbed dose in young and old females, but there were no significant differences between young and old females in this respect; and (d) there was no evidence for an increase in sensitivity to radiation induction of either numerical or structural aberrations as a function of maternal age.

354. In a subsequent study, Tease [T38] used higher x-ray doses (1-6 Gy) to various dictyate oocyte stages (sampled at 3.5, 9.5, 16.5 and 23.5 days after irradiation of females 10-14 weeks old) and studied the induction of hyperhaploidy using the same techniques as described in the preceding paragraph. Significant increases were found in the irradiated groups relative to the controls; the frequencies of hyperhaploidy increased with dose and the latter was consistent with either a dose-squared or a quadratic dose-effect relationship. Furthermore, oocytes sampled 3.5 days after irradiation were less responsive than the others, the order of increase in sensitivity being 3.5 days, 9.5 days, 23.5 days and 16.5 days. Structural chromosomal anomalies also increased with dose and could be described either by a dose-squared or a quadratic relationship; the general order of increase in sensitivity for the induction of structural anomalies was roughly similar to that for hyperhaploidy.

355. In other experiments, Tease [T18] examined whether the use of gonadotrophic hormones to induce ovulation altered the radiosensitivity of the oocytes to the induction of structural or numerical aberrations. Young mice were stimulated to ovulate with either low or high doses of hormones and then irradiated (0.5 Gy of x rays) followed by analysis of the first cleavage embryos, as in earlier work [T17]. There was no evidence for a hormonal dose-related difference in spontaneous or radiation-induced chromosome non-disjunction. Radiation-induced chromosome fragments were observed at a higher frequency in maternal pronuclei of 1-cell embryos from females treated with large amounts of hormones; this increase, however, was not statistically significant.

356. Tease and Fisher [T42] have now investigated the extent to which radiation-induced non-disjunction may be related to the clastogenic properties of x rays. Acute x-ray doses between 0.1 and 1.0 Gy were given to preovulatory oocytes (with the same regime as that given in [T17]) and chromosomal aberrations were scored at metaphase I. The yield was markedly higher than after irradiation of dictyate oocytes, but the dose-response was similar, with best fit to a quadratic curve. By comparing these results with those for non-disjunction frequencies after the same doses to the same oocyte stage, Tease and Fisher concluded that: (a) visible damage to the centromere is not the principal mechanism of radiation-induced non-disjunction; and (b) the involvement of induced multivalents as the principal mechanism is quite likely, in view of their high frequency and of the fact that they may generate tertiary trisomic embryos.[u] However,

[u] The model of chromatid-interchange-mediated non-disjunction was proposed more than 15 years ago from the results observed on radiation-induced non-disjunction in Drosophila immature oocytes (see [P52] for a review).

the relative proportions of primary and tertiary trisomic embryos following x-ray-induced non-disjunction have yet to be determined.

(b) Genetic methods

357. The numerical sex-chromosome-anomaly (NSA) method was employed by Russell [R34] in an experiment designed to test whether advancing age increases the incidence of either spontaneous or radiation-induced non-disjunction or chromosome loss in female mice. The NSA method [R35, R36] permits detection of maternal or paternal non-disjunction or chromosome loss by way of genetic markers that affect external phenotype. Irradiated (200 R, x rays) or control Ta/+ females of various ages were mated to Ie/Y males (Ta and Ie are X-linked markers). A number of abnormal sex-chromosome genotypes can theoretically result from maternal or paternal non-disjunction (each occurring in first or second division), maternal or paternal chromosome loss, mosaics involving any of these, or certain sex-linked translocations. Some of these are unequivocally diagnosable by phenotype. Others require genetic and/or cytological verification.

358. Old females (11.5-12 months at irradiation), divided into virgins (1289 offspring) and pluripara (1103 offspring), were compared with young females (2.5-3 months at irradiation, 2451 offspring) irradiated concurrently. There were 6 groups of contemporary controls, aged up to 15 months at time of mating, with the 11.5-12 month group divided into virgins and pluripara, as was the case for the irradiated females. Altogether, 15,986 offspring were observed. Among these were 115 possible exceptionals, of which 45 were tested genetically, 4 cytologically, and 38 both genetically and cytologically. These tests yielded only 2 exceptional sons, one Ta/Ie/Y (due to paternal non-disjunction) and one Ta/+/Y///+/Y (i.e., mosaic resulting from maternal non-disjunction). There were 41 certain and 13 questionable exceptionals among daughters, with most of them being due to paternal non-disjunction of sex chromosomes and thus not obviously resulting from the variable parameters of the experiment. Neither maternal non-disjunction nor maternal chromosome loss was increased by advancing age of female in either the treated or untreated group. At any one age, radiation did not increase the incidence of maternal events. The $X^M X^M Y$ male, albeit a mosaic, is the first proven case of maternal sex-chromosome non-disjunction on record for the mouse.

359. Searle and Beechey [S105] have discussed the various genetic approaches to studying autosomal non-disjunction in mice through the use of Robertsonian translocations, including the one devised by Lyon et al. [L38]. Cattanach et al. [C53] described two conceptually similar genetic methods involving the use of marker genes and Robertsonian translocations, the latter present only in tester parents, to detect events in chromosomally normal mice. In the first, designated as the Rb method, normal mice are mated to tested stock animals that are heterozygous for one or more

Robertsonian translocations with appropriate markers on the chromosomes to enable detection of non-disjunction or loss of the autosomes under study. In the second method, termed the MBH method, normal mice are again mated to tester stock animals doubly heterozygous for two different Robertsonian translocations that share a common arm (monobrachial homology or MBH) and with appropriate markers.

360. In their experiments using the Rb method, Cattanach et al. chose the Rb 1 Robertsonian translocation (a translocation between chromosomes 1 and 3) and in those using the MBH method, the Robertsonian translocations were those involving chromosomes 1 and 3 and 1 and 15. The chromosome 1 markers were ln (leaden) and fz (fuzzy). The Rb method was used to study: (a) loss of chromosome 1 in female mice attributable to either non-disjunction or other mechanisms following absorbed x-ray doses of 0, 1, 2, 3 and 4 Gy; (b) chromosome 1 gain attributable to non-disjunction in female mice following a single absorbed x-ray dose of 4 Gy; and (c) maternal chromosome 1 loss following x irradiation (1 Gy) of 1-cell zygotes. The MBH method was used to study chromosome loss following x irradiation of spermatozoa and spermatids (3.0 Gy), and for determining non-disjunction of chromosome 1 after irradiation (0.75 and 1 Gy) of spermatocytes. Appropriate cytological analysis and breeding tests were carried out on the exceptional animals.

361. The results were the following: (a) with the Rb method, the frequencies of chromosome 1 losses showed an approximately linear increase with increasing dose (mature oocytes, slope of $(6.44 \pm 1.94) \ 10^{-4} Gy^{-1}$); (b) at the dose of 4 Gy, there was a single non-disjunctional case among 3353 progeny (mature oocytes); and (c) the frequency of maternal chromosome loss following irradiation of zygotes was 0.69% at 1 Gy.

362. In the MBH experiments (irradiation of post-meiotic male germ cells), 9 exceptional (loss of chromosome 1) progeny were found among a total of 2586 (0.35%), which was significantly higher than in the controls (2/4150 or 0.05%). No exceptional progeny were recovered following irradiation of spermatocytes. The authors pointed out that: (a) the two new tester methods have potential for screening for chromosome loss and non-disjunction; (b) the one non-disjunctional exception found after irradiation of mature oocytes does not establish that this was induced by x rays, but provides the first definitive genetic evidence of autosomal non-disjunction; (c) while the NSA method only detects chromosome loss among female progeny, with the Rb method both sexes of progeny are informative regarding non-disjunction; the estimated frequency of x-ray-induced chromosome 1 loss is about 16 times higher than that of X-chromosome loss at near equivalent doses (mature oocytes, zygotes); and (d) with the MBH method, the spontaneous and x-ray-induced frequencies of loss of paternal chromosome 1 are similar to corresponding frequencies of sex chromosome loss, as scored by the NSA method.

363. All the various genetic methods used for the detection of non-disjunction with the aid of Robertsonian translocations depend on successful complementation of a gamete with an extra chromosome from one parent and a gamete with corresponding loss of a chromosome from the other. Searle and Beechey [S134] pointed out that, for certain mouse chromosomes, there is defective complementation, with lethality of the expected complementation product. This is especially true of complementation where there is maternal chromosome duplication combined with paternal deficiency and is known to involve at least mouse chromosome numbers 2, 6, 7 and 8. Cattanach and Kirk [C77] described a similar phenomenon in mouse chromosome 11, in which maternal duplication and paternal deficiency led to offspring that were only half the normal size at birth, while the reciprocal cross led to abnormally large offspring. Thus, for the affected chromosomes, genetic tests for non-disjunction may give misleading results, by suggesting absence of non-disjunction where there is really absence of normal complementation.

4. Further data on the induction of reciprocal translocations in mouse spermatogonia

364. The 1977 UNSCEAR report [U2] considered the data available then [G15] on the induction of heritable reciprocal translocations following spermatogonial irradiation in mice. It was found that: (a) the frequency of F_1 males heterozygous for reciprocal translocations (genetic tests) increased with exposure up to 600 R (although the difference between the yields after 150 R (0.6%) and 300 R (0.88%) was not significant); (b) at exposure levels of 300 R and above, the ratio of translocations was roughly 1/8 of that found earlier by Ford et al. [F7]; and (c) at the lower exposure of 150 R, this ratio was 1/4 (although not significantly different from 1/8 in view of the small number of F_1 males tested).

365. Generoso et al. [G16] have now obtained more extensive data (summarized in Table 20) from which it can be seen that, at all radiation exposures, the frequencies are higher than in the controls. The shape of the exposure-frequency curve is humped and the ascending portion of the curve is consistent with linearity. The coefficients per R per gamete at 150 R, 300 R and 600 R are very close to one another; the average coefficient (weighted by the reciprocal of the variances, on the basis of data collected after acute as well as fractionated exposures) can be estimated as $(3.89 \pm 0.25) \ 10^{-5}/R/gamete$. A comparison of the absolute frequencies at the different exposure levels with the frequencies expected on the basis of cytological results (last column, the latter were calculated using the same assumptions as those employed by Ford et al. [F7]) shows that these are in agreement at 150 R; at higher exposures, the observed frequencies are lower than expected.

366. The finding of Ford et al. [F7] that, after spermatogonial x irradiation (600 + 600 R, 8-week interval) of male mice, the frequency of semi-sterile males in the F_1 was only one-half of that expected on the basis of multivalent configurations diagnosed cytogenetically in spermatocytes (descended from irradiated

spermatogonia) of the irradiated males themselves was discussed in the 1972 report. Ford et al. [F7] suggested that this differential transmission to the F_1: (a) may be due to selection acting against translocation-carrying cells after metaphase I; and (b) that such a selection could be related to the occurrence of male sterility in heterozygotes for translocations that cause spermatogenic arrest both before and after metaphase I (see also [C63] and [S107]). If the disparity between the yields of translocations in cytogenetic and genetic experiments is due to the latter cause, then one would expect a progressive reduction in frequency through male meiosis both before and after meiosis. However, if it were due to the possibility that spermatocytes carrying translocations tend to take longer to pass through metaphase I (see for instance [N32]), then the frequency of translocations estimated on the basis of metaphase analysis would represent an overestimate of the true frequency. Crocker [C64] conducted experiments to test these possibilities.

367.   In these experiments, male mice homozygous for certain Robertsonian translocations (the MC and RIB stocks) and normal mice carrying only acrocentric chromosomes were exposed to 500 R of x rays. From 12 to 16 weeks later, the animals were killed and testes preparations made for spermatocyte analysis by two methods: (a) scoring of the proportion of translocations that involved metacentrics (for comparison with the proportion expected to be induced in spermatogonia on the assumption of random exchange between metacentrics and acrocentrics); and (b) scoring of the number and sizes of clones of acrocentric and metacentric translocations from individual tubules (since each clone represents a single induction event, factors such as meiotic delay or selection acting after induction should affect clone size, but not the number of clones). It was found that, with both these methods, the frequency of metacentric translocations was enhanced at metaphase I. Furthermore, the clone size of the metacentric translocations, was higher relative to that of clones from acrocentric translocations but the number of clones of metacentric translocations was as expected. These observations therefore suggest that the enhancement was due to events occurring after induction. Since selection would be expected to produce the opposite effect, Crocker concluded that his results provide evidence in favour of the delay hypothesis. He further suggested that, if delay is capable of enhancing the frequency of metacentric over acrocentric translocations, it is possible that a similar difference in retardation between normal cells and those carrying acrocentric translocations could account for the differential transmission to the F_1.

368.   In an earlier cytogenetic study involving unequally fractionated x-ray exposures to mouse spermatogonia, van Buul and Léonard [V8] obtained some indications for a possible threshold effect for spermatogonial sensitization between 75 and 100 R. In this work, discussed in the 1982 UNSCEAR report, a total exposure of 1000 R was administered in two unequal fractions (separated by 24 hours) of 100 + 900 R, 75 + 925 R, 50 + 950 R and 25 + 975 R. Appropriate single exposure controls were run concurrently. It was found that, when the conditioning exposure was below

100 R, there was no enhancement of the translocation frequencies in the fractionation experiments relative to the single-exposure controls.

369.   According to the authors [V8], the results supported the idea that depletion of the stem cell population is the important cause in triggering survivors into the more active cycle (as has been postulated by Cattanach and Crocker [C54]) because at exposures below 100 R, stem cell depletion would be relatively slight though there would be major killing effects upon differentiating spermatogonia. Van Buul and Léonard [V9] conducted another set of experiments using BALB/c and Swiss random-bred mice, with conditioning exposures as low as 12.5 R (the total exposure was always 1000 R). However, contrary to earlier results, the present ones showed considerable variation between experiments, in spite of the same or very similar fractionation regimes and mouse strains (in one experiment there was no enhancement effect of the 100 + 900 R regime, whereas this showed a striking increase in the earlier study) so that the earlier assumption of a threshold for spermatogonial sensitization could not be upheld. These and other data have recently been reviewed by van Buul [V10].

370.   Pomerantseva et al. [P42] compared the cytogenetic effects of chronic versus acute ^{137}Cs gamma irradiation on the induction of reciprocal translocations in mouse spermatogonia. Doses of 1.5-4.5 Gy were delivered at four different rates (i.e., 2.7 10^{-6}, 5.8 10^{-6}, 9.4 10^{-6} and 4.5 Gy per min). The results showed that the frequencies of translocations at the dose rate of 9.4 10^{-6} Gy/min were, on the average, only about one-tenth of those at the highest dose rate, in conformity with earlier results from their laboratory and other laboratories. Further reduction in dose rate did not lead to a concomitant reduction in yields. However, at a dose of 3 Gy, delivered at 2.7 10^{-6} Gy/min, the yield is about twice if the results from one mouse with a high frequency of translocations (15/79 or 19%) are excluded; if not, the yield is about 4 times higher than that at dose rates of 5.8 10^{-6} and 9.4 10^{-6} Gy/min (1.18 ± 0.29% versus 0.56 ± 0.16% and 0.42 ± 0.13%; the numbers of analysed cells were, respectively, 1679 or 1600, 2514 and 2400).

5.   Elimination of x-ray-induced chromosomal aberrations induced in pre-ovulatory mouse oocytes by early embryonic death

371.   Reichert et al. [R37] re-examined the question of the elimination of chromosomal damage induced by x irradiation of pre-ovulatory oocytes in vivo, through cytogenetic analysis of MII oocytes or embryos at the 2-cell stage. In one set of experiments, NMRI female mice 10-12 weeks old were superovulated (treated with pregnant mare's serum and human chorionic gonadotrophin), irradiated with x rays (0.2-6 Gy) and the oocytes were prepared for MII analysis; in another experiment, pre-implantation embryos (mainly 2-cell stages) were examined after an x-ray dose of 2 Gy; and in a third experiment,

treatment was identical to the second, but the animals were killed 13.5 days after appearance of the vaginal plug for intra-uterine analysis and chromosomal preparation from the liver of the embryos. About 87% of the MII oocytes showed structural chromosomal aberrations after irradiation with 2 Gy; in contrast, among the 2-cell stages, only 69% carried aberrations. The 13.5-day-old fetuses were practically aberration free. These results suggest an almost complete elimination of chromosomally damaged oocytes and zygotes already before birth. The structural aberrations included breaks, translocations and deletion and numerical aberrations were mostly hypoploidies.

6. Aneuploidy and structural aberrations (spontaneous and radiation-induced) in the germ cells of rodents

372. Mikamo and colleagues carried out a number of studies using the Chinese hamster (in some, using rats) to examine the primary incidence of spontaneous chromosomal anomalies in oocytes and zygotes, their mechanisms of production and radiosensitivity profiles. Some of these data were discussed in the 1982 UNSCEAR report. Illustrative recent results are briefly considered below.

(a) Effect of pre-ovulatory overripeness of rat primary oocytes on the incidence of chromosomal anomalies

373. The artificial arrest of the normal sequence of oogenesis is known to exert a deleterious effect on the ovum when the delay exceeds a certain time limit (see Mikamo and Hamaguchi [M39] and the references cited therein). Since Mikamo [M40] first described a teratogenic effect of pre-ovulatory overripeness of the primary oocytes on the embryos of Xenopus, it has been recognized that overripeness causes developmental and chromosomal anomalies [M67]. In the work of Kamiguchi et al. [K31], sexually mature female rats with consistent 4-day oestrous cycles were intraperitoneally injected with sodium pentobarbital on two successive days (once on the day of proestrous and twice on the second day) to delay ovulation. On the third day, the treated females were mated to males and 2-cell embryos were collected from oviducts 52 hours after fertilization for scoring of morphological abnormalities. Chromosome analysis was carried out on morphologically normal embryos (a great majority of the morphologically abnormal ones did not reach metaphase of the second cleavage).

374. It was found in the treated group that: (a) the frequency of developmental abnormalities was increased by a factor of over 2 (15.1% versus 6.4%) and the frequency of unfertilized eggs was also higher (13.5% versus 1.6%); and (b) there was a striking increase in the frequency of aneuploid and mosaic embryos (10.1% versus 4.0%), suggesting that delayed ovulation induced non-disjunction and anaphase lag of chromosomes during both the meiotic and first cleavage divisions. There was also a significant increase of polyploidy, a consequence of polyspermy in the treated group.

(b) Incidence of spontaneous chromosomal anomalies in Chinese hamster and mouse oocytes and early zygotes

375. Using an improved cytogenetic technique [K32, M41] Mikamo and Kamiguchi [M42] examined the spontaneous incidence of chromosomal anomalies in Chinese hamster oocytes and early zygotes. Secondary oocytes were collected from the ampullary region of oviducts of female hamsters 5-8 months old and used for chromosome preparations. To arrest mitosis of 1-cell and 2-cell zygotes, colchicine was injected into copulated females and the zygotes were subsequently collected by flushing of the oviducts. In secondary oocytes, 1.6% (31/1970) were aneuploid (0.6% hyper- and 1% hypo-haploidy); 0.4% were diploid (giant diploid oocytes twice the normal size) and there were no diploid oocytes caused by a suppression of the first polar body. A further 1.8% carried structural aberrations.

376. In 1-cell embryos, 3.2% (37/1146) were aneuploid with approximately equal numbers in the hyper- and hypo-haploidy groups, 1.5% of the embryos were triploid (0.9% of diandry, 0.3% of digyny and 0.3% of uncertain cases), and 2.8% carried structural anomalies. In 2-cell embryos, the incidence of triploidy (1.6%) and haploidy (0.4%) were similar to those in 1-cell zygotes. However, the incidence of aneuploidy was lower (2.0%), suggesting selective death of some aneuploids. The frequencies of structural anomalies were higher in the embryos (2.8%, in 1-cell zygotes and 3.7% in 2-cell zygotes) relative to those in oocytes. The authors found that: (a) the incidence of aneuploidy in 1-cell zygotes of maternal origin (2.1%) was 3 times that of paternal origin; (b) first-division meiotic errors were also 3 times higher than second-division errors (1.6% versus 0.5%); and (c) the incidence of female-derived structural aberrations was the same as that of the male-derived ones (1.3% and 1.4%, respectively).

377. In another study, Sugawara and Mikamo [S79] analysed the effect of maternal aging on the configuration of chiasmata, formation of univalents and segregation of first meiotic chromosomes in young (5-8 months) and old (16-19 months) Chinese hamsters. Primary oocytes were collected from mature follicles approximately 10 hours before ovulation and secondary oocytes were obtained from the oviducts 5 hours after spontaneous ovulation. It was found that the average number of chiasmata per oocyte was significantly lower in the old hamsters than in the young ones, but terminal chiasmata were more frequent in the old animals, results reminiscent of those of Henderson and Edwards [H42]. Since the 11 meiotic chromosomes could be divided into four morphologically distinguishable sub-groups, it was possible to determine whether the same bivalent forming univalents at MI actually underwent non-disjunction in the following meiotic division. The incidence of both MI oocytes with a univalent pair (2.0% versus 9.1%) and aneuploid MII oocytes (1.5% versus 3.6%) due to first meiotic non-disjunction was significantly higher in the aged group than in the young group; however, univalents occurred almost exclusively in the small metacentric chromosomes (96%) whereas non-disjunction took place nearly equally in each chromosomal

sub-group. These results demonstrate no correlation between the univalents seen at MI and non-disjunction during the first meiotic division and this is true of both young and old hamsters.

378. In a further study, Sugawara and Mikamo [S80] adduced evidence for a striking induction of non-disjunction in Chinese hamster primary oocytes by intraperitoneal colchicine injection (3 μg/g body weight) at the onset of formation of the first meiotic spindle in oocytes of females with a normal oestrous cycle. The incidence of aneuploid MII oocytes was 25.9% in the experimental group, while it was 2.0% in the controls. Their results support the notion that maternal age-effects known for aneuploidy may in part be associated with incomplete formation of spindle microtubules, which in turn can lead to increased incidence of meiotic chromosome non-disjunction in oocytes of aged females.

379. Tease and Fisher [T43] used lower doses of colchicine (0.25 and 0.5 μg/g) in similar work with female mice and obtained only a 10% increase over controls in hyperhaploidy and a 20% increase in hypohaploidy. However, they found a marked age effect of colchicine in that old (50-56 weeks) female mice had a higher sensitivity to metaphase I arrest at the smaller dose, as compared with young (9-12 weeks) females, but a lower sensitivity at the higher dose. The authors consider that the maternal age effect on non-disjunction may be related to a difference in spindle behaviour in young and old females.

(c)   X-ray induction of structural chromosome aberrations in Chinese hamster and mouse oocytes

380. The earlier data of Mikamo et al. [M43] on stage-dependent changes in chromosomal radiosensitivity of primary oocytes in Chinese hamster were discussed in the 1982 UNSCEAR report. These results demonstrated that early diakinesis was the most radiosensitive phase, the incidence of metaphase II oocytes with structural aberration being about 15 times that after treatment of early dictyotene stages of dioestrus (43% versus about 3%) (see also Mikamo [M44]). Irradiation of subsequent stages, (i.e., late MI-anaphase I, telophase I, polar body emission), however, yielded fewer chromosomal aberrations, and more dominant lethals and might be related to the occurrence of unrepaired lesions and a reduction in DNA repair capacity, for which there is some evidence from mouse studies [M68] after UV irradiation.

381. In subsequent experiments, Kamiguchi and Mikamo [K33] determined the dose-frequency relationship for structural chromosome aberrations in early diakinesis (over a range of x-ray doses from 0.1 to 4.0 Gy). The types of aberrations found were breaks, deletions, fragments and exchanges and the metaphase II aberrations were mainly of the chromatid type. The frequencies were found to increase with dose (from 0.0033/cell after 0.1 Gy to 0.814 in the 2.0 Gy group) the data being consistent with a quadratic model. A comparison of these results with those published by Reichert et al. [R38] for the mouse (in both studies,

the meiotic stage of the oocytes and chromosome analysis were similar) shows that the rate of induction in the hamster is only about one-half of that in the mouse. This is in contrast with earlier results where the spermatogonia and lymphocytes of both these species were found to have similar radiosensitivities [B34, B35].

382. Tease and Fisher [T42] obtained much higher aberration yields than Reichert et al. [R37] after similar radiation regimes with mouse oocytes, but the aberrations were scored at metaphase I rather than at metaphase II. They considered that these differences most probably reflect the greater accuracy of the metaphase I method for assessing chromosomal damage. Similarly to Reichert et al., however, they reported that the data on chromatid interchanges best fitted a quadratic model.

383. Tease [T44] also investigated whether dictyate oocytes of old (42-52 weeks) female mice were more radiosensitive than those of young (10-15 weeks) ones when metaphase I chromosome preparations were made from superovulated females 3.5 or 12.5 days after 0.5 Gy or 2.0 Gy acute x irradiation. Very few aberrations were found after 0.5 Gy, but, as expected from previous work, after 2.0 Gy the aberration frequencies were significantly higher at 12.5 days than at 3.5 days of sampling. At this latter dose level, there were more chromosomal aberrations in metaphase I cells from old females than from young ones, but the differences were not significant.

384. Searle and Beechey [S135] also compared chromosome aberration yields in young (8-12 weeks) and old (about 48 weeks) female mice after the same x-ray doses of 0.5 Gy and 2.0 Gy, but with a slightly longer interval of 2-3 weeks between irradiation and metaphase I chromosome preparations. Although the interchange frequencies were not significantly higher in the old females, the overall frequencies of the aberrations scored (interchanges + fragments) were significantly higher after 2.0 Gy in oocytes of old females (35.5%) than of the young ones (12.5%). Thus, there is some evidence that maturing oocytes of older females are more sensitive to aberration induction, although data are limited and more work is needed.

(d)   Synaptonemal complexes as indicators of induced structural change in chromosomes of Syrian hamster spermatogonia and of post-meiotic germ cells in the mouse

385. The conventional cytogenetic method of studying induction of chromosomal damage in spermatogonia of experimental mammals involves the analysis of spermatocytes (descended from treated spermatogonia) at diakinesis/metaphase I. The translocations give rise to multivalent configurations, which, given good cytological preparations, are relatively simple to detect at diakinesis/metaphase I. This technique has been very successfully used over the years in quantitative radiation cytogenetic studies, particularly those aimed at ascertaining the frequencies of reciprocal

translocations. However, for multivalent associations to persist until diakinesis/metaphase I, homologous segments must synapse and there must be chiasma formation in at least one of the translocated segments, as well as in the non-translocated segment. As Evans [E17] pointed out, this requirement for chiasma formation may mean that rearrangements of small segments may be missed unless pachytene cells are analysed.

386. Cawood and Breckon [C55] compared the efficiency of the conventional method mentioned above with that involving the analysis of pachytene cells using synaptonemal complexes as visible markers (the SC method) and Syrian hamsters as experimental material. Following testicular irradiation with 2.6 Gy, the animals were kept for 5-15 weeks before they were killed. One testis from each of 7 animals was used for making cytological preparations with the conventional and the SC methods. The results showed that, despite variation in the frequencies of abnormal cells (i.e., those carrying multivalent configurations) between animals, the overall frequencies with the SC method were about twice as high as those with the conventional methods (8.6% versus 4.6%). The authors considered that the analysis of diakinesis/metaphase I cells alone may lead to a serious underestimation of the amount of structural change induced in spermatogonia after irradiation and that the SC method can provide information not obtainable by any other method. Kalikinskaya et al. [K55] reached similar conclusions in their experiments. They also pointed out that the SC method could be useful in the analysis of the causes of sterility of F_1 males descended from irradiated P_1 males.

7. Induction of reciprocal translocations in spermatogonia of non-human primate species

387. Cytogenetic data on the induction of reciprocal translocations in stem cell spermatogonia of non-human primates and in those of man were reviewed in the 1977 and 1982 UNSCEAR reports. The overall conclusions were that: (a) the sensitivity of the spermatogonia of the marmoset Saguinus fuscicollis is higher than that of the rhesus monkey, Macaca mulatta; (b) at the dose levels studied, the yields of translocations from irradiated human spermatogonia are roughly comparable to those in the marmoset species mentioned above; (c) following acute x irradiation, the dose-effect relationship in all the three species is humped with a maximum around 1 Gy; and (d) the dose-effect relationship up to the dose of peak yield is consistent with linearity. Some additional data have now become available from studies with the rhesus monkey at low dose rates and after fractionated exposures [V14, V15] and with two new primate species, namely, the marmoset Callithrix jacchus [V5, V11] and the crab-eating monkey, Macaca fascicularis [M27, M69, T45]. All the currently available primate data are summarized in Table 21 (see also Figure I).

388. Van Buul [V14] and Van Buul et al. [V15] found (Table 21) that, when an x-ray dose of 1 Gy is delivered to rhesus monkey spermatogonia at a dose

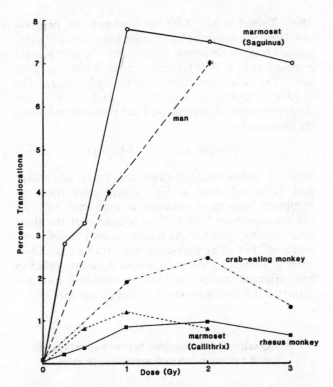

Figure I. Dose-response relationships for the induction of reciprocal translocations in stem-cell spermatogonia of some primate species by high dose-rate x or gamma irradiation.

rate of 0.002 Gy/min, the yield of translocation is about one-half of that at the same x-ray dose delivered at 0.3 Gy/min. A gamma-ray dose of 1 Gy delivered at either 0.14 or 0.0002 Gy/min gave similar yields, however, and these were about the same as that obtained at an x-ray dose of 1 Gy delivered at 0.002 Gy/min. When an x-ray dose of 4 Gy was delivered into two equal fractions separated by an interval of 24 hours, the yield was higher relative to that after a single dose of 4 Gy, and less than one-half of that expected on the basis of additivity of yields; the latter observation is in contrast with that obtained in mouse experiments [L57, M80] in which, with similar fractionation regimes, the yields continued to increase linearly with dose.

389. The data for Callithrix jacchus suggest that the sensitivity of this species to the induction of translocations by acute x or gamma irradiation may be similar to that of the rhesus monkey, but clearly lower than that of Saguinus fuscicollis studied by Brewen et al. [B61]. However, Macaca fascicularis responds with frequencies that are intermediate between those observed in the rhesus monkey on the one hand and Saguinus fuscicollis on the other [M27, M26]. The possible basis for these differences is discussed below (chapter VI, section C). Comparing their data for Macaca fascicularis with those for different rodent species published in the literature, Matsuda et al. [M69] noted that, over the dose range below 1 Gy, the sensitivity of Macaca fascicularis (slope of $1.79 \ 10^{-2} \ Gy^{-1}$) is similar to that of the mouse, the Chinese hamster and the rabbit (slopes per Gy: mouse, $(1.39-2.56) \ 10^{-2}$; Chinese hamster, $2.15 \ 10^{-2}$; rabbit, $1.39 \ 10^{-2}$). The values for the guinea pig are different in two different studies: $0.98 \ 10^{-2}$ [L41] and $2.75 \ 10^{-2}$ [B62]; consequently, it is difficult to make rigorous comparisons.

390. Tobari et al. [T45] have a study in progress involving the induction of translocations in spermatogonia of the crab-eating monkey by chronic gamma irradiation (1.8 10^{-5} Gy/min; about 0.024 Gy/22 h/day). The total doses are: 1.0, 1.5 and 2.0 Gy. The results available so far (at 1.0 and 1.5 Gy) are consistent with a linear dose-effect relationship defined by the equation

$$Y = 0.91 \ 10^{-3} + 0.16 \ 10^{-2} \ D$$

where Y is the yield of translocations in percentage and D is the dose in Gy. When these data are compared with those obtained at high dose rates by the same authors (Table 21) it is clear that the slope after chronic gamma irradiation is only about one-tenth of that after high-dose-rate irradiation. Thus, there is evidence for a pronounced dose-rate effect in this primate species, in contrast with the situation recorded for the rhesus monkey (see paragraph 388).

8. Qualitative comparison between spontaneous and radiation-induced mutations in mice

391. Detailed genetic analysis of mutations recovered from irradiated and control parents in mouse specific-locus experiments indicates that the mechanisms by which spontaneous mutations arise may differ from those involved in the radiation induction of mutations [R39]. The frequency of fractional (mosaic) mutants at all 7 of the marked loci was roughly similar in offspring of irradiated and control mice [R40], and the same was true in a large sample in which the study was restricted to the c locus [R41]. Thus, radiation does not induce fractionals, and the observed fractional mutants in irradiated as well as control groups are presumably of spontaneous origin. At the c locus, the large majority of spontaneous mutations were fractionals, and, at d, almost one-half were also fractionals. (Fractionals would probably be non-detectable at se and more poorly detectable at d than at c.) Analysis of segregation ratios derived from 16 c-locus fractionals [R71] led to the conclusion that the mutations had occurred in one strand of the gamete DNA, or in a daughter chromosome derived from pronuclear DNA synthesis of the zygote, or in one of the first two blastomeres prior to replication.

392. Another mechanism implicated in the production of certain spontaneous mutations is the so-called double non-disjunction, whereby the offspring receives two copies of the marked chromosome and no copies of the wild-type chromosome. Several spontaneous d se mutants [R42] as well as an Hbb^d c$^+$ mutant are apparently of this type.[v] The event is detectable only where two or more markers are present on the chromosome involved. When only one marker is present, the result is indistinguishable from a repeat mutation to the marker allele. Since there is no

evidence that either mosaic or double non-disjunction mutants are induced by radiation exposure of the germ cells, Russell [R39] has proposed that the population of spontaneous mutants might have a strong admixture of types not present in the population of induced mutants and has, therefore, raised questions on the appropriateness of the doubling-dose approach in the calculation of genetic risk.

393. It is possible to make a rough calculation of the maximum extent to which the spontaneous mutation frequency, and therefore the doubling dose, would be changed if all double non-disjunctional events were excluded in specific locus data in males. In all, the spectrum and viability of 32 specific locus mutations recovered from unirradiated male mice have been reported [E33, S136]. There were no simultaneous c^{ch}p mutations among these, but one out of 2 d se mutations was homozygous viable and therefore probably the result of double non-disjunction. There were no mutations at the a locus while only one out of 9 at the s locus might have been viable in the homozygote. The 9 mutations at the b locus included a cluster of 2, which seems much more likely to be the result of a spontaneous mutation early in gametogenesis than a double occurrence of double non-disjunction. All but one of the others which could be fully tested seem viable repeats of b. Thus, between 1 and 8 out of the 32 mutations or 3-25% might have been the result of double non-disjunction and therefore should be excluded from doubling dose calculations.

394. Since, in all, 60 specific locus mutations in 1,005,363 offspring of control males have been reported [E33, R69a, R70], i.e., a mutation frequency per locus of 8.5 10^{-6}, the exclusion of possible non-disjunctional events would lead to a corrected control frequency within the range of 8.2 10^{-6} and 6.4 10^{-6} per locus. Russell and Kelly [R70] derived a regression coefficient of 7.34 10^{-6} per Gy from all the specific locus spermatogonial data for chronic gamma-ray exposure of male mice. Use of the corrected control rate range and the induction rate mentioned above gives a corrected doubling dose estimate of between 1.12 Gy and 0.87 Gy. Clearly, the currently used doubling dose estimate for chronic gamma-ray exposures of 1 Gy would remain appropriate.

9. Molecular analysis of mouse specific locus mutations

395. The original spontaneous d (dilute) mutation and the closely linked se (short ear) are used among the seven markers in mouse specific-locus mutation-rate studies. Mutations involving the wild-type allele of these markers can lead to altered melanocyte morphology, abnormal cartilage development, central nervous system disorders, or embryonic death. A large number of radiation-induced mutations involving d, se, or both loci were genetically analysed by complementation and deficiency mapping [R43]. These analyses resulted in the characterization of at least 16 complementation groups and the identification of 6 pre-natally lethal and 2 neo-natally lethal loci between and around d and se. Since the original d mutation was caused by the integration of MuLV

---

[v]However, the results of translocation intercrosses involving chromosome 7 (on which the c and Hbb loci are located), as well as the lack of simultaneous c^{ch}p mutant offspring in specific locus experiments, indicate non-complementation of gametes with gains and losses of chromosomes [S134]. It seems probable, therefore, that the Hbb mutant arose by a different mechanism.

into chromosome 9 (see chapter IV), this provirus can be used as a marker to gain molecular access to the d-se region. Cellular DNA sequences flanking the provirus have been cloned and used to probe genomic DNA from several of the genetically characterized mutants in this region [R44]. Specific DNA fragments have been correlated with specific deletions, and a physical map of one deletion break-point has been constructed [R71]. The molecular analysis also provides physical proof that many of the mutations are deletions, confirming what had earlier been surmised on the basis of genetic evidence.

10. Genetic and cytogenetic effects of incorporated radioactive isotopes in mice

396. Data on genetic and cytogenetic effects of incorporated radioactive isotopes were reviewed in the earlier reports of the Committee and more recently by Searle [S81]. This section focuses on data that became available since the publication of Searle's review.

397. Balonov and Kudritskaya [B36] compared the effects of tritium, administered as tritiated water (^{3}HOH), and chronic gamma irradiation on the induction of dominant lethality in post-meiotic and meiotic male germ cell stages. Spermatids were found to be more radiosensitive than either spermatocytes or spermatozoa. The effect did not depend on the dose rate in the range from $1 \ 10^{-3}$ to 1.7 Gy/min (total doses from 0.5 to 3.7 Gy). The RBE of tritium (relative to chronic gamma irradiation) increased with decreasing dose, reaching a value of about 2.5 at doses less than 0.1 Gy. These studies were subsequently extended to include the induction of reciprocal translocations in spermatogonia [P43]; they showed that the RBE of tritium increased from 1 at a dose of 1 Gy to 2 at a dose of 2 Gy.

398. In another study, Pomerantseva et al. [P29] examined the effects of incorporated ^{14}C after single, long-term (33 days) and chronic (6 and 12 months) treatment of male mice ((CBA × C57BL) F$_1$) with ^{14}C-glucose. The frequencies of dominant lethals in post- and pre-meiotic germ cells, of translocations in spermatogonia (analysis of spermatocytes) and of sperm abnormalities were determined. The estimated absorbed gonadal doses were the following: 0.22, 0.50 and 1.01 Gy (single-exposure experiments), 0.74 and 1.47 Gy (long-term exposures), 0.006 and 0.031 Gy (chronic exposures for 6 months), 0.031 and 0.066 Gy (12-month chronic exposure).

399. In the single-exposure groups, the frequencies of dominant lethals (expressed as the ratio of live embryos per female in the experimental group to that in the control group) increased approximately linearly with increasing dose in post-meiotic cells; in pre-meiotic cells, there was no induction. In the long-term exposure group, the frequencies were somewhat lower than in the single-exposure groups (post-meiotic as well as pre-meiotic cells). In the 6-month chronic group, the frequencies were again low and there was no measurable induction in the 12-months chronic group. The frequencies of translocations induced in

spermatogonia were low (0.34-0.84% in single-exposure groups; 0.20-0.60% in the long-term group; and 0.06-0.10% in the chronic groups) and only in the single-exposure and long-term-exposure groups were the frequencies higher than in controls. Sperm abnormalities were about 1% in all the groups, except in the 13-month exposure group where they were between 3.4 and 4.6% (control, 1.8%). On the basis of their earlier results with external chronic gamma irradiation, the authors concluded that ^{14}C is no more effective than chronic gamma rays.

400. Balonov et al. [B63] showed that tritiated glucose (3.3 MBq/g, corresponding approximately to an absorbed dose of 1 Gy) administered to male mice induced dominant lethals (in post-meiotic cells) and reciprocal translocations (in spermatogonia) with a pattern similar to that of tritiated water. In other studies, Pomerantseva and Ramaiya [P44] found that intraperitoneal injection of ^{238}Pu-nitrate ($18.5 \ 10^5$-$0.28 \ 10^5$ Bq/g) with estimated doses of between 0.06 and 0.47 Gy induced dominant lethals in post-meiotic cells and translocations in spermatogonia. Relative to chronic gamma irradiation, the absorbed dose from ^{238}Pu (alpha irradiation) was about 20 times more effective, confirming earlier results [U2].

401. In the experiments by Generoso et al. [G55], a ^{239}Pu-citrate solution (about 379 kBq/kg body weight) was injected into the tail vein of male mice ($101 \times$ C3H/F$_1$), which were then mated to T stock females. Two series of experiments were carried out. In the first series, the intervals from treatment to mid-points of mating periods were 23.5 and 52.5 weeks (with estimated spermatogonial stem cell doses of 0.54-1.07 Gy for the first mating period and 1.42-2.85 Gy for the second). In the second series, these intervals were 29 and 56.5 weeks (with estimated spermatogonial stem-cell doses of 0.70-1.41 Gy and 1.55-3.09 Gy). The male progeny were screened for the presence of translocations in genetic tests and those that were found to be sterile or partially sterile were examined cytologically.

402. In the first series, the frequencies of translocations were 0.20% (2/987, first interval) and 0.39% (6/1560, second interval). In the second series, the corresponding frequencies were 0.23% (6/2633) and 0.56% (14/2505). Thus, there was an increase in frequency with time (i.e., accumulated dose). With correction for control frequency (from another study carried out with a different strain; 3/8095 or $3.7 \ 10^{-4}$), the rate of induction per Gy has been estimated to be between 1.45 and $2.91 \ 10^{-3}$. The effectiveness of alpha irradiation does not appear to be markedly different from that of acute x rays (rates of $3.89 \ 10^{-2}$ per Gy [G16] and $3.42 \ 10^{-3}$ per Gy [L50]). (Since there are no genetic data on translocation induction after chronic gamma rays, the effectiveness at low dose rates could not be calculated.)

11. Sensitivity of the mouse, Chinese hamster and primate oocytes to the killing effects of radiation

403. Data on the radiosensitivity changes between oocytes in different stages of development and in

different mammalian species were discussed in the earlier UNSCEAR reports and more recently by Dobson and Felton [D37] and Dobson et al. [D49]. The new data on the radiosensitivity of mouse primordial oocytes have raised some questions on the validity of extrapolation of mouse radiation mutagenesis results to human females. Primordial oocytes of two primate species studied show also striking differences and oocytes of neo-natal Chinese hamsters show some important differences relative to the situation in the mouse and rats. This section is devoted to a discussion of these results.

(a) The mouse

404. The fact that primordial mouse oocytes are very sensitive to the killing effects of x or gamma radiation is well known. For instance, if a young female mouse is exposed to a gamma-ray dose of 0.4 Gy and the ovaries are examined a few days later, the remarkable finding is that no immature primordial oocytes (which constitute about 90% of the oocyte population) are present; only growing and maturing oocytes (which are about 10% of the oocyte population) remain [D52, O13]. The LD_{50} is of the order of 0.06 Gy. Similar results were obtained following single intra-peritoneal injections of ^3HOH, reflecting the generally very high radiosensitivity of mouse oocytes to radiation-induced killing [D39, D51, D52]. When the animals are chronically exposed to low levels of ^3HOH in body water during early life (from conception to 14 days after birth), there is a dose-dependent germ cell destruction at all tritium levels examined in a more than 100-fold range of concentrations, from 0.4 MBq/ml to 31 kBq/ml, without any evidence of a threshold (exponential decrease in oocyte survival with an LD_{50} of about 74 kBq/ml). When these results are compared with those obtained after similar chronic low-level exposure to gamma rays, the RBE of tritium increases from about 1.5 (at about 0.035 Gy/day; dose 0.5-0.6 Gy) to nearly 3 at low dose rates and low doses (less than 0.005 Gy/day and an effective dose of less than 0.05 Gy) ([D39, D40]; see Figure II). The increase of RBE with decreasing dose is not due to any increased effectiveness of tritium, but to a decreased effectiveness of gamma rays at low doses.

405. The exceptionally high sensitivity of mouse oocytes to the killing effects of ^3HOH and gamma rays, together with the finding that ^3H-TdR incorporated in the chromosomes is much less effective in this regard [B64], have prompted the suggestion that the target for killing effects in these cells is not in the nucleus but at some distance away from it. The realization that the target most likely involves cytoplasmic structures, adjacent follicle cells or the plasma membrane prompted studies with neutrons for information on target cross section. These studies [S82] indicated that the target area, assumed to be circular, had a diameter larger than the nucleus but smaller than any combination of oocyte plus follicle cells. Together with an estimated target volume (determined from gamma-ray data) of about $4 \mu m^3$, these results suggest that the plasma membrane or something similar to it in geometry and location is the likely target.

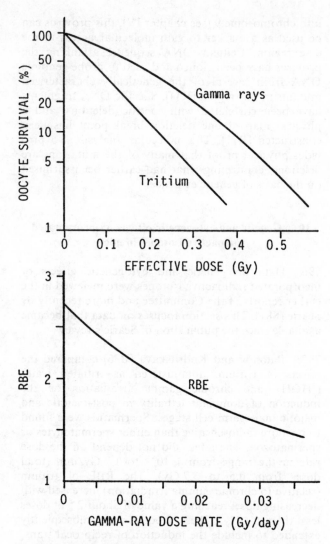

Figure II. Survival of primordial oocytes (as a function of dose and dose rate) in mice chronically exposed from conception to 14 days of age to tritiated water or to cobalt-60 gamma rays, and the RBE of tritium compared with gamma radiation.
[D40]

406. Assuming that the membrane is the target, the data for tritium, neutrons and gamma rays can be reconciled, and in each case the D_{37} dose corresponds to a deposition in the plasma membrane of about 500 to 1000 eV. Monte-Carlo calculations show that for an x-ray exposure of 50 R to female mice, the predicted oocyte survival (cells with mean plasma membrane dose not exceeding D_{37}) was about 1%, which is in agreement with observations [D41]. The authors state that in the experiments with exposure of 50 R done by Russell, the nuclear dose to the surviving oocytes could be much less, too low "to give scorable yields of mutations". They argue that this could explain the negative findings, and that this has implications for the estimation of genetic risk.

407. The possibility that the nuclear dose to surviving oocytes might be less than the exposure given was first suggested by Russell in 1965 [R72] as one of the three possible explanations for the absence of mutations induced in early oocytes by fission neutrons. He stated

that "the mechanism could conceivably be the survival of only those oocytes that escaped having a proton track pass through their genetic material". However, he went on to argue that, if this were the explanation, "the effect would not be seen with x or gamma rays". In a large experiment with 50 R of x rays, the effect was seen, namely, a very low or zero induced mutation rate in early oocytes [R73]. Russell's argument that a reduced dose to the nucleus could not be invoked to account for this was based on the view that the distribution of ionizations in the cell with x rays would be so diffuse that the dose to the large nucleus could not differ appreciably from the exposure of 50 R administered. Current concepts of microdosimetry still agree with this view.

(b) Chinese hamsters

408. Tateno and Mikamo [T25] studied the response of the neo-natal Chinese hamster ovaries (ovaries exposed to 1 Gy on days 0, 2, 5, 6, 8, 10, 12 and 14 after birth) to the killing effects of x irradiation. The ovaries were excised 48 hours after irradiation, examined histologically and the results compared with those obtained with unirradiated controls. The important findings are the following: (a) the Chinese hamster oocytes are highly resistant to radiation during the pachytene stage (at birth all ooctyes are at pachytene) and become extremely susceptible to the killing effects of x rays when the oocyte maturation advances further, especially during diplotene and the very early dictyate phases (on day 4 the majority are at diplotene and by day 6 nearly all oocytes reach the diplotene or dictyate phase); there is an almost complete killing by 1 Gy at these stages; (b) with the onset of the resting phase (day 10 onwards) the oocytes become increasingly resistant, reaching levels similar to pachytene; these observations are in contrast with those in rats where the increase in resistance is more gradual and the pachytene levels are never reached [M45]. Furthermore, whereas high sensitivity is restricted in the Chinese hamster to days 4-8 (diplotene-dictyate), after which the oocytes become progessively more resistant, high sensitivity persists in the mouse for a longer period (neo-nates from 8 to 26 days old). (See [T25] for a discussion.)

(c) Primate species

409. Pregnant squirrel monkeys (Saimiri sciureus) were exposed continuously to ^{3}H in drinking water from conception to birth of the young (153 days) and the ovaries of the offspring were examined at birth [D37, D50, D52]. Concentrations of ^{3}HOH in maternal drinking water ranged from 204 down to 2.6 kBq/ml and corresponding body-water levels were measured at 116 down to 1.9 kBq/ml, delivering doses of about 6.8-0.1 mGy/day. The surprising finding was that there was a massive oocyte loss which increased exponentially with dose. The LD_{50} level was 18.5 kBq/ml (giving 1 mGy/day), which is about one-fourth of that found in mice. With other primates (the rhesus monkey, Macaca mulatta, and the bonnet monkey, Macaca radiata), and with similar treatment schedules

(from the time of proof of pregnancy, day 25, to parturition, day 164; ^{3}HOH in maternal drinking water at 185 kBq/ml; ^{3}H body-water concentrations level by day 60 at 144 kBq/ml; dose rate of 8.6 mGy/day during the second and third trimesters), the ovaries of the new-born showed about a 20% loss of oocytes (and thus much less than in squirrel monkeys). By 6 months, however, more fully expressed losses were striking: 59% in the rhesus monkey and 95% in bonnet monkeys.

410. Dobson [D50] suggests that, judging from these data, early germ-cell losses exceeding 50% may lead to premature menopause in women. Since effective oocyte LD_{50} values for pre-natal rhesus monkey, bonnet monkey and squirrel monkey were about 600, 200 and 100 mGy, respectively, and if such doses were accumulated over the second half of human gestation (160 days), doses of 3.8, 1.2 or even 0.6 mGy/d may already suffice to produce early menopause.

12. Summary and conclusions

411. Further data have become available on the radiation induction of heritable tumours in mice. Spermatids in males and maturing oocytes in females seem to be the most sensitive stages for the induction of genetic changes leading to tumours in the progeny. The spectrum of tumours in controls and in the offspring of irradiated parents is similar, with about 90% being papillary adenomas of the lung. The pattern of transmission of these tumours is consistent with a dominant mode of inheritance and a penetrance of about 40%. These data, originally obtained with the ICR strain, have now been extended to include two others (the LT and N5 strains). Furthermore, evidence showing that most of the tumours were malignant has been obtained.

412. Treatment of the F_1 progeny descended from irradiated parents (or in utero irradiation of pregnant mice with the known carcinogen urethane) led to an enhancement of tumour incidence relative to those in the progeny that were not treated with urethane, suggesting that urethane may promote carcinogenesis.

413. X irradiation of rats or treatment with radioactive isotopes (^{90}Sr, ^{238}Pu) increased the frequency of tumours in the progeny.

414. Further data on the radiation induction of congenital anomalies in the offspring of irradiated mice have been obtained. In these experiments, males were irradiated and mated to unirradiated female mice and the progeny screened, by intra-uterine examinations, for the presence of congenital anomalies. The overall frequencies of these anomalies (ignoring the different radiation doses of between 1 and about 5 Gy) were significantly higher following irradiation of post-meiotic germ cells. The results of spermatogonial irradiation were variable: some experiments showed significant increases over controls, while others did not show such differences. Dwarfism and exencephaly were the most commonly observed malformations.

415. The question of whether irradiation of post-implantation maternal environment would have any effect on the induction of congenital anomalies was studied in experiments involving embryo transfers and in others where the ovaries were surgically exteriorized and the abdomen selectively irradiated. No significant effects were found.

416. A number of recent studies on spontaneous and radiation-induced non-disjunction and chromosome loss in mice have been reviewed. The so-called production line hypothesis advanced to explain the effect of maternal age on spontaneous non-disjunction was tested using two different approaches. These data showed that the hypothesis could not be confirmed and that abnormal meiotic chromosome segregation is associated with the process of physiological aging of the reproductive system. A comparison of the frequencies of chromosomal aberrations and of non-disjunction after irradiation of pre-ovulatory oocytes suggested the possibility that the induction of chromosomal exchanges might be the principal mechanism of radiation-induced non-disjunction. This would be in line with previous findings in Drosophila.

417. New cytogenetic (examination of the fertilized oocytes in vitro at the first cleavage divisions) and genetic (use of the numerical sex-chromosomal anomaly method) data have been reported concerning the effects of maternal irradiation on the incidence of non-disjunction. In the cytogenetic experiments, in controls, the frequency of hyper-haploid female pro-nuclei was higher in the oocytes of old, as compared with young, females; but after irradiation, the increases that were found did not show a relationship to age. In the genetic experiments, however, neither maternal non-disjunction nor maternal chromosome loss was increased by advancing age of the females in either the irradiated or the unirradiated group.

418. Two new methods have been designed to study autosomal non-disjunction and chromosome loss in normal mice, making use of tester stocks containing Robertsonian translocations and appropriate genetic markers. While the evidence for radiation-induced chromosomal loss was strong, confirming earlier results for sex chromosomes, that for induced non-disjunction was, at best, weak.

419. Further data on the radiation induction of heritable reciprocal translocations in male mice (following spermatogonial irradiation) have been presented. These show that up to 600 R, there is an exposure-dependent increase in frequency, the slope being $(3.89 \pm 0.25)\ 10^{-5}$ per R. A comparison of the absolute frequencies at the different exposures obtained in this study with those from cytogenetic studies at the same exposure levels shows that the frequencies after 150 R are consistent with expectations (i.e., one-quarter of the frequencies observed in spermatocytes); at higher exposures, the observed frequencies of heritable translocations are only one-half of the expected ones. Data have been obtained from cytogenetic studies suggesting that these discrepancies may be due to spermatocytes carrying translocations taking longer to pass through metaphase I.

420. Cytogenetic studies designed to examine the loss of radiation-induced chromosomal aberrations in pre-ovulatory oocytes, 2-cell embryos and fetuses show that most of the structural aberrations induced in the oocytes are efficiently eliminated by cell death before development proceeds to a fetal age of 13.5 days. Most of the elimination already occurs by the 2-cell embryonic stage.

421. In rats, there is now evidence that pre-ovulatory overripeness of primary oocytes (prevention of ripening through the use of pentobarbital) leads to a striking increase in the frequency of aneuploid embryos derived from them.

422. The frequencies of spontaneously occurring chromosomal anomalies in Chinese hamster oocytes and early zygotes have been determined using an improved chromosome preparation technique. The data support the notion that the incidence of aneuploidy of maternal origin (2.1%) is three times higher than that of paternal origin and first division meiotic errors are about three times more frequent than second division errors. In experiments in which the effect of maternal age on chiasma configuration, formation of univalents and segregational errors at meiosis I of Chinese hamster oocytes were studied, there was no evidence for any correlation between univalents seen in metaphase I and non-disjunction during the first meiotic division.

423. There is evidence to suggest that, in Chinese hamster females, the early diakinesis stage is most sensitive to the induction of structural aberrations of chromosomes. A comparison of the radiation data available for this stage in Chinese hamsters and mice shows that the former species is only one-half as sensitive as the latter.

424. New data using a technique for the analysis of pachytene cells and the associated synaptonemal complexes for the study of radiation-induced translocations in spermatogonia of Syrian hamsters have provided evidence for the thesis that the conventional method of analysing diakinesis/metaphase I cells underestimates the frequency by a factor of 2.

425. Further cytogenetic data on the induction of reciprocal translocations by x or gamma rays in some primate species have now been published (acute high-dose-rate exposures). The marmoset Callithrix jacchus has been found to have a sensitivity similar to that of the rhesus monkey; both these species are much less sensitive than the other marmoset species, Saguinus fuscicollis. The crab-eating monkey, Macaca fascicularis, however, is more sensitive than the rhesus monkey and Callithrix jacchus but less sensitive than Saguinus fuscicollis in this regard. Furthermore, there is a pronounced dose-rate effect after chronic gamma irradiation of the crab-eating monkey (spermatogonial exposure), the yield being about one-tenth of that obtained at high dose rates.

426. The finding that the frequencies of fractional mutations recovered at the specific loci studied in mouse experiments are similar in control and after irradiation suggests that fractionals are not induced by irradiation. Furthermore, there is some evidence that spontaneous mutations, but not radiation-induced mutations, may arise via double non-disjunction. Since the population of spontaneous mutations may thus represent an admixture of types not occurring in radiation experiments, it has been suggested that the validity of using the doubling dose method for risk evaluations may become questionable; however, the influence of the doubling dose estimate is likely to be small.

427. The recent demonstration that, in the mouse, spontaneous d locus mutations are associated with the integration of murine leukaemic virus and the cloning of cellular DNA sequences flanking the provirus, has now opened up the possibility of molecular dissection of genetically characterized mutants at this locus.

428. The most recent data on the genetic and cytogenetic effects of incorporated radioactive isotopes in mammals relate to the effects of ^{3}H (given as tritiated water to male mice) on the induction of dominant lethals (post-meiotic germ cell sampling) and to those of ^{14}C (given as ^{14}C-labelled glucose to male mice) on the induction of dominant lethals (post-meiotic and pre-meiotic cells) and of reciprocal translocations in spermatogonia. The ^{3}H results suggest that the RBE (relative to chronic gamma rays) increases with decreasing dose reaching a value of about 2.5 at doses of gamma rays lower than 0.1 Gy. The ^{14}C results show that radiocarbon and chronic gamma rays are nearly equal in producing the effects mentioned. The effects of tritiated glucose are similar to those of tritiated water. The cytogenetic data obtained with ^{238}Pu are confirmatory of those reviewed in the 1977 UNSCEAR report. The genetic data on reciprocal translocations show that alpha-ray doses from ^{239}Pu are no more effective than from acute x rays.

429. A detailed study on the radiosensitivity of oocytes of neo-natal Chinese hamsters has been carried out. The results show that oocytes in the pachytene stage (most of the oocytes present at birth) are very resistant; this resistance abruptly decreases at diplotene or early dictyotene, remains at the same level until day 8 (nearly all the oocytes reach diplotene or dictyate phase) followed by a steep rise thereafter. These changes in radiosensitivity profile in the Chinese hamster are more marked than in the mouse or rat.

430. The three primate species studied from the standpoint of the sensitivity of their primordial oocytes to the killing effects of ^{3}H show that the squirrel monkey is even more sensitive than the mouse. The other two, the rhesus monkey and the bonnet monkey, do not manifest this unusually high sensitivity.

B.   STUDIES WITH IN VITRO SYSTEMS

1.   Spontaneous and radiation-induced thioguanine resistant cells in human lymphocytes

431. In the 1982 UNSCEAR report, the data of Albertini [A6] and Strauss and Albertini [S23] on spontaneous 6-thioguanine resistant (6-TG^R) variants in peripheral blood lymphocytes were presented. As may be recalled, these authors made use of the cytotoxicity of 6-TG to human lymphocytes possessing normal HPRT levels to distinguish, and select for, viable 6-TG^R variants. In autoradiographic studies, such variants were shown to undergo DNA synthesis (incorporation of ^{3}H-labelled thymidine) and survive in the presence of normally toxic levels of 6-TG following PHA stimulation.

432. These studies have now been extended by Vijayalaxmi et al. [V2, V16] to lymphocytes from Bloom syndrome (BS) and Fanconi anaemia (FA) patients. In the 7 BS patients, the corrected (i.e., corrected for cycling S-phase cells) variant frequencies were in the range 8.5-24.9 10^{-4} with a mean of 17.3 10^{-4}. In the age- and sex-matched controls, the range was 1.6-2.8 10^{-4} (mean, 2.1 10^{-4}), indicating that, in BS patients, the variant frequencies are clearly higher (by about 8 times) than in controls. Likewise, in the 2 FA patients studied [V15], the corrected variant frequencies were 11.4 10^{-4} and 17.7 10^{-4}, which are higher than in controls (1.5 10^{-4} and 1.8 10^{-4}). It is instructive to note that even the control frequencies determined by the autoradiographic method are higher than those recorded in fibroblast work (around 1.0 10^{-5}) [C69, D62].

433. The autoradiographic technique has the disadvantage that the 6-TG^R cells are killed during the procedure and the evidence that they are mutants is therefore circumstantial. Recently, it has become possible to clone human lymphocytes from peripheral blood [M46, M47] and the high efficiency of this method has made it possible to detect [A14] and enumerate [M48] 6-TG^R lymphocyte clones. The frequency of 6-TG^R lymphocyte clones that could be detected by this technique is 10^{-6} to 10^{-5} in healthy young adults, and the frequency increases with age [T26]. Following expansion of the clones, it has been shown that they are unable to incorporate hypoxanthine and direct measurements show little or no HPRT activity [A14, M48].

434. In a recent paper, Albertini [A20] reviewed the autoradiographic and cloning assays from the selection of 6-TG^R mutants in human lymphocytes. The TG^R mutant frequencies determined by the clonal assays were found to be in the range from 10^{-6} to 10^{-5} for normal adults; autoradiographically determined variant frequencies were also in the same range for normal adults, when the lymphocytes were cryopreserved before study to remove phenocopies. Thus, the generally higher frequencies recorded with the autoradiographic method without the use of cryopreservation, as was done in earlier studies (see also [V15]), is due to the presence of phenocopies in the mutant samples.

435. Vijayalaxmi and Evans [V4] used the T-cell cloning technique to select and clone 6-TG^R cells present in human peripheral lymphocytes in vivo. It was found that the incidence of such cells ranged from $0.83 \ 10^{-5}$ to $2.53 \ 10^{-5}$ (mean: $1.48 \ 10^{-5}$) in healthy individuals aged between 19 and 79 years. There were no sex differences. However, the frequencies increased with age at a rate of 2.4 cells/10^7 lymphocytes/year. Exposure of G_0 lymphocytes in vitro to x-ray doses of up to 2 Gy resulted in a dose-dependent increase in the TG^R cell frequencies; the rate of increase was approximately proportional to the square of the dose although statistically a linear dose-effect relationship could not be excluded. With the latter model, the estimated rate of increase was $1.95 \ 10^{-5}$/cell/Gy. Both the spontaneous and induced rates were similar to those recorded for fibroblasts in a number of earlier studies and were from 10- to 20-fold lower than those observed with the autoradiographic method.

436. A similar but independent study has been carried out by Sanderson et al. [S83]. Mutation induction to 6-TG^R resistance was studied in freshly isolated lymphocytes from healthy individuals, using x rays and UV irradiation. In 8 of the 11 individuals whose G_0 lymphocytes were studied using x irradiation, proliferating lymphocytes on day 3 of culture were also studied in the x-ray experiments. In addition to studying mutation induction, data on survival and expression time were also collected. The results showed that: (a) the expression time was between 3 and 7 days; (b) with both kinds of radiation, there was a dose-dependent increase in mutation frequency, measured on day 10 after irradiation. For the G_0 lymphocytes, for instance, the frequencies were $2.3 \ 10^{-5}$ after 2 Gy and $9.2 \ 10^{-5}$ after 4 Gy; lymphocytes irradiated on day 3, i.e., proliferating ones, showed a lower mutation induction and a higher mortality relative to G_0 lymphocytes. The frequency at 2 Gy is quite similar to that recorded in the work of Vijayalaxmi and Evans [V4] in whose studies a 48 hours expression time was used.

437. In the study of Vijayalaxmi et al. [V16] mentioned earlier, the T-cell cloning technique was also used to determine the spontaneous frequencies of TG^R mutants in 5 FA patients, 5 FA heterozygotes and their age- and sex-matched controls. In the FA patients, the frequencies were in the range 0.41-$1.54 \ 10^{-5}$ (mean, $0.98 \ 10^{-5}$) compared to frequencies for controls, which were in the range 0.34-$0.44 \ 10^{-5}$ (mean, $0.40 \ 10^{-5}$). Two of the FA patients had frequencies similar to controls, whereas in the other three there was a 3-fold elevation. There were no significant differences between FA heterozygotes and controls, in all of whom the range was 1.2-$1.9 \ 10^{-5}$, which is similar to that observed in an earlier study of 24 healthy controls [V4]. It is instructive to note that the controls for FA patients had lower spontaneous frequencies than those for FA heterozygotes. This is interpreted by the authors as a reflection of the difference in their ages (controls for FA patients ranged between 8 and 17 years old and controls for FA heterozygotes from 36 to 51 years old) and is in line with the earlier observation [V4] that the incidence of TG^R lymphocytes increases with increasing age.

438. Messing and Bradley [M73] also used the T-cell cloning technique to study the frequency of TG^R mutants in lymphocytes of 12 breast cancer patients before and after radiotherapy (gamma rays) and in patients with heart disease unexposed to radiation. In the normal controls (n = 12, mean age 35 years), the average mutant frequency was $1.1 \ 10^{-6}$, which is well within the range found by Morley et al. [M48]. The frequency of mutants in the heart patients (n = 12, mean age 52.4) was $2.4 \ 10^{-6}$, which is not significantly different from the above. In the cancer patients before radiotherapy, however, the mutant frequency was higher, being on average $8.6 \ 10^{-6}$ (range, 0.1-$54.7 \ 10^{-6}$). Although the radiotherapy patients were older than the controls, the authors point out that it is unlikely that age alone accounts for the difference, since the older heart patients had a frequency close to that of the controls. After exposure of cancer patients to 50 Gy (2 Gy per working day for 5 weeks to the chest wall and surrounding lymph nodes; the treatment began 1-2 months after surgery), or an estimated 5 Gy received by lymphocytes, the average frequency was $36.8 \ 10^{-6}$ (range, 7.6-$102.2 \ 10^{-6}$). It was also found that sampling after 6 Gy revealed no effect on the average mutant frequency, since blood was usually drawn from these patients 3 days after the start of the treatment, a period insufficient to permit phenotypic expression [S83].

2. Induction of mutations and chromosome aberrations in mammalian (including human) somatic cells at low doses and dose rates

439. Making use of a special line of Chinese hamster fibroblasts (V79S) capable of exponential growth in suspension culture, Crompton et al. [C27] examined the mutational response of the cells to low-dose-rate ^{60}Co gamma radiation (0.032-0.04 Gy/hour), administered over a period of 2-3 weeks in continuous (chemostat) cultures. At periodic intervals, cells were removed, tested for viability and allowed to multiply. Following an expression period of 6-10 days, the cells were again tested for viability and for the induction of 6-TG^R mutants. In addition, the mutational responses of cells to acute x irradiation (1.9 Gy/min) following growth in unirradiated continuous culture for 3-6 days were also determined. The results showed a clear-cut increase in mutation frequencies under conditions of long-term exposure to low-level irradiation and there was no indication of a reduced effectiveness of chronic exposures. The authors suggested several possible explanations for their findings, including the following: (a) differences in the distribution of cell cycle phases in continuously irradiated cultures relative to normal ones; (b) differences in doubling times between irradiated and unirradiated cultures; (c) induction of error-prone repair processes; and (d) build-up of mutagenic intermediates in cultures during the extensive irradiation periods.

440. Pohl-Rüling et al. [P16] have now published the results of a co-ordinated research programme of the International Atomic Energy Agency in which the in vitro responses of human peripheral blood lymphocytes to low doses of x irradiation (0.004, 0.01, 0.02,

0.03, 0.05, 0.1 and 0.3 Gy) were studied. Blood from 2 donors was used to conduct one master experiment and the culture time was 48 hours. The coded slides were scored by investigators from 10 participating laboratories. The main findings, based on over 60,000 cells scored were the following: (a) the frequencies of all types of chromosomal aberrations at 0.004 Gy were, according to the authors' analysis, significantly lower than the control values; (b) there was no increase in the frequencies of dicentrics up to 0.02 Gy and in those of terminal deletions up to 0.05 Gy; (c) the mean frequencies of all aberrations considered together were not significantly different from one another at 0.01, 0.02, and 0.03 Gy; and (d) over the entire dose range the dose-effect relationship is clearly non-linear. A fit of these data to a linear-quadratic model showed that the observed total aberration frequencies at doses of 0.01, 0.02, 0.03, 0.04 and 0.05 Gy were below the curve defined by the model. The authors explained these observations on the basis of possible altered kinetics of aberration induction at very low doses, probably due to DNA repair mechanisms operating in these cells.

3. Molecular approaches to the study of mutations and DNA repair in mammalian somatic cells

441. The molecular approaches that are currently being used to study mutations and DNA repair in mammalian somatic cells, the results so far obtained and the prospects for the future have recently been reviewed by Lehmann [L17] and Thacker [T28]. Some illustrative examples are discussed below.

442. Thacker et al. [T15] introduced the E. coli XGPRT gene[w] into HPRT deficient V79 Chinese hamster cells by transfection (those expressing XGPRT activity were selected by their resistance to the purine synthesis inhibitor azaserine). Two sublines designated as XGPRT+6 and XGPRT+10, which showed no tendency to lose their resistance to azaserine despite over 40 generations in non-selective conditions, were selected for further analysis. Restriction enzyme and Southern blot analyses revealed that the XGPRT gene has been incorporated in each subline as a single copy. Since bacterial XGPRT will also use 6-thioguanine (6-TG) as a substrate, the authors carried out experiments in which XGPRT+10 cells were x-irradiated and mutants deficient in XGPRT activity (XGPRT−) were selected using 6-TG resistance as a marker. The results showed a linear increase of mutant frequencies with x-ray dose, and higher spontaneous and induced frequencies of these mutants over the corresponding frequencies for HPRT deficiency in the parental V79 line. In other experiments in which the hamster HGPRT gene was introduced into HG-PRT− cells, x irradiation also led to the recovery of high frequencies of mutants. All these data thus suggest that this high mutability is a property of the chromosome sites at which the transferred DNA integrates. Of particular interest is the finding that the majority of 6-TG

---

[w]XGPRT: the bacterial gene coding for xanthine-guanine phosphoribosyl transferase, which has now been cloned. The bacterial XGPRT enzyme has functional similarity to the mammalian HPRT, but XGPRT can utilize xanthine as a substrate, while HPRT (and mammalian cells in general) cannot.

resistant mutants of XGPRT+10 show deletions of the introduced gene (as defined in hybridization experiments).

443. In a similar study, Tindall et al. [T27] introduced the E. coli XGPRT gene into a CHO line deficient in HPRT activity and used the transformant cell line in x-ray and UV mutagenesis studies. The results showed a dose-dependent induction of TG[R] mutants with maximal recovery of UV-induced mutants after 7-9 days of expression time. While this cell line (designated as gpt+) showed a cell-killing response comparable to the normal CHO-HPRT+ cell line following irradiation, there is a 10-25-fold increase in mutation induction at the gpt+ locus versus the HPRT locus for a given dose of radiation. Two TG[R] clones (one spontaneous and one x-ray induced) so far analysed by Southern blot hybridization were found to contain deletions involving at least a portion of the gpt+ gene.

444. **Thompson and colleagues [T29, T39] have** isolated a number of UV-sensitive CHO cells deficient in excision repair; these lines fell into five complementation groups. Two of these lines were sensitive to both UV and mitomycin-C. Using human DNA as donor and these cell lines as recipients in DNA transfer experiments, Rubin et al. [R47] obtained a number of transfectants that were no longer sensitive to UV and mitomycin-C. Molecular analysis suggested that the transfected human sequences contained the wild-type alleles of the defective gene. UV-resistant transfectants were also obtained by MacInnes et al. [M49] by transferring wild-type hamster DNA into a different repair-deficient recipient.

445. Using another repair-deficient CHO cell line (complementation group 2) as recipient for human DNA, Westerveld et al. [W34] obtained evidence for the correction of the repair defect in the CHO cells; these authors subsequently cloned (in a cosmid vector) the complete human gene, which corrects the defect in the hamster mutant. This gene, designated as ERCC-1, is about 17 kb long. This work represents the first successful attempt at cloning a human repair gene and is likely to be of use in studies devoted to the nature, control and function of the ERCC-1 gene product in excision repair.

446. In contrast with the relative ease of correcting repair defects in Chinese hamster cell lines, studies using human cells (xeroderma pigmentosum (XP), ataxia telangiectasia (AT)) as recipients have had only limited success (see [L17]). However, indications have been obtained that at least one AT cell line may have a defect in the cellular equilibrium between ligation and exonuclease digestion of DSBs in DNA [C56] and that, despite the postulated DNA repair defect in AT, these cells are competent recipients in DNA transfer experiments [D42].

447. Meuth and colleagues [G35, M50, N26] analysed mutations induced in the hamster adenine phosphoribosyltransferase (APRT) gene using the cloned APRT gene probe [L18]. It was found that most EMS-induced mutations in Chinese hamster cells resulted from changes below the level of detection and could be single base-pair changes or deletions of less than

50 base pairs; most of the spontaneous mutations were also point mutations. Mutations induced under conditions of deoxynucleotide pool imbalances were also predominantly point mutations. Two of the nine gamma-ray-induced mutations at the dihydrofolate reductase locus (studied with the aid of a cDNA probe) contained altered restriction patterns consistent with their being deletions, insertions or rearrangements [G36].

448. Spontaneous and UV-induced mutations at the HPRT locus in Chinese hamster cells have been analysed using HPRT gene probes. One out of 10 spontaneous mutations and one out of 9 UV-induced ones had large deletions in the HPRT gene [F27]. Fenwick at al. [F28] studied a HPRT mutant of Chinese hamster cells and its wild-type revertants. There was no evidence for an altered restriction pattern in the mutant cell line, suggesting that it contained a point mutation. Some of the spontaneous revertants produced a much stronger hybridization signal, suggesting that the gene had been amplified up to 20 times, with a corresponding overproduction of mRNA.

449. Vrieling et al. [V17] examined 19 x-ray-induced (600 R) HPRT-deficient mutants in V79 Chinese hamster cells with Southern blotting using a mouse cDNA probe. Twelve of the mutants had large deletions (> 10 kb) of the HPRT DNA sequences. Cytological studies of chromosome preparations of these 12 showed that, in at least 3 of them, part of the long arm of the X-chromosome was lost. The authors estimate that at least 70-80% of x-ray-induced mutants at this exposure are caused by large deletions. In the work of Thacker [T40] 43 gamma-ray-induced (5 Gy) and 15 alpha-particle-induced (1.2 Gy) HPRT deficient mutants in V79 Chinese hamster cells were studied with Southern blotting using a full length hamster HPRT cDNA. Twenty of the 43 gamma-ray-induced mutants were found to lack the functional HPRT gene and another 10 showed various partial gene deletions and/or rearrangements; the remaining 13 showed no detectable changes. In the alpha series, 6 out of the 15 were total gene deletions, 5 had partial deletions and/or rearrangements and 4 had no detectable changes. Thus, it would appear that about 70% or more of radiation-induced HPRT deficient mutants arise through large changes in the HPRT gene, especially deletion.

450. Albertini et al. [A21] reported that 3 out of 11 TG^R-lymphocytes derived from a single normal individual (by a T-cell cloning technique) showed definite changes by Southern blot analyses with a 947-bp full length HPRT cDNA clone, 4 showed uncertain changes and in the remaining 4, there were no detectable changes in the genomic DNA after digestion with 5 restriction endonucleases. These results provide unequivocal evidence that the 6-TG^R mutants are in fact mutants. Similar results were reported by Turner et al. [T41]. Twelve of the 21 mutant clones (57%) had alterations not evident cytogenetically; these involved major changes including deletions, exon amplification and novel, sometimes amplified, bands on Southern analysis.

4. Use of somatic cell hybrids to identify repair genes and their chromosome locations in human cells

451. Mouse cells repair UV-induced DNA damage with about 5-10% of the efficiency of human cells. Lin and Ruddle [L9] reported that somatic cell hybrids between primary mouse cells and SV-40-transformed XP cells (complementation group A) exhibited wild-type (human) levels of DNA repair capacity, as judged by the levels of unscheduled DNA synthesis; they also demonstrated that mouse chromosome 4 was involved in compensating the DNA repair defect in XP cells. Lalley et al. [L10] isolated human x mouse somatic cell hybrid clones, employing human cells normal for UV repair, UV-irradiated them and examined their repair profiles using the BrdUrd photolysis assay. It was found that some of the hybrid clones had a pattern of repair similar to that of human cells, some had a pattern similar to that of mouse and some fell in between. Since the numbers of dimers per 10^8 dalton were the same in mouse, human and hybrid cells, they examined hybrid clones for the presence or absence of individual human chromosomes. A strong correlation between the presence or absence of human chromosome 3 and the presence or absence of UV repair was found. In these three clones, there was also a correlation between human chromosome 14 and excision repair capacity, although there was one clone that was positive for chromosome 14 but negative for repair.

452. Lalley et al. [L10] also examined whether mouse cells could contribute one or more steps required for excision repair of UV damage in XP cells. Fusion experiments were carried out between cells from 5 of the XP complementation groups (A-E) and mouse cells. The resultant hybrid clones segregated human chromosomes. When the XP x mouse hybrid cells were analysed for repair ability, it was found that mouse cells reduced the level of defective repair of XP cells in complementation groups A-D but not in E. When the XP x mouse hybrids lost certain human chromosomes (the chromosomes not specified), they lost the ability to be complemented by the mouse genome, suggesting that these hybrids had lost the gene(s) coding for the repair step that is rate-limiting in the mouse.

453. An essentially similar approach has been used by Hori et al. [H21] to study repair in mouse cells. These authors examined somatic cell hybrids produced by fusion between the UV-sensitive, excision-repair-deficient Q31TG3 cell line (derived from mouse lymphoma L5178Y cells) and PHA-stimulated human lymphocytes for their UV sensitivity and unscheduled DNA synthesis (UDS). From the initial two hybrid clones, subclones were isolated at various intervals and segregation of UV-sensitive clones was tested. Most of the UV-resistant clones exhibited nearly the same resistance as the parental L5178Y cells, whereas most of the UV-sensitive clones showed UV hypersensitivity similar to that of the Q31 mutant; the UDS capacity of the UV-resistant clones was similar to that of human lymphocytes. Analysis of the distribution of specific human chromosomes in each subclone showed a positive correlation between UV sensitivity and the presence or absence of human chromosome 13.

5. Inducible (SOS-like) responses to DNA damage and adaptive responses in mammalian cells

(a) Inducible SOS-like responses

454. The fact that E. coli and other bacteria respond to various adverse conditions by inducing SOS responses[x] is well established [K48, L42, R59, W48]. These observations and indications that inducible functions may be associated with the tolerance of DNA damage in living cells catalyzed a search for analogous phenomena in eukaryotic cells. Although there are data suggesting that mammalian cells respond to physiological perturbations (which in E. coli act as inducing signals for SOS responses), there is as yet no unequivocal evidence for the de-repression of previously repressed genetic functions and no indication that eukaryotic cells respond to inducing signals by expressing a battery of genes under the control of a common regulatory system, as is true in E. coli [F37]. Thus the evidence for SOS-like responses in mammalian cells is largely phenomenological. It has been recently reviewed [H53, F37] and only a few illustrative examples are discussed here.

455. Viruses have been widely used as probes to study a variety of cell functions since they offer the possibility to separate the effects of cell treatment from those resulting from the treatment of the viruses. Table 22 taken from the paper of Herrlich et al. [H53] provides a summary of results obtained using viruses. In these studies, the virus is UV-irradiated and allowed to infect UV-irradiated or chemically treated host cells (or unirradiated or untreated host cells). Evidence for an enhanced reactivation (ER: survival of irradiated virus on treated host/survival of irradiated virus on non-treated host) and enhanced mutagenesis (EM: mutation frequency of the irradiated virus in treated host/mutation frequency of the irradiated virus in non-treated host) was sought. As can be seen in Table 22, UV-irradiated virus such as Herpes, SV40 or adenovirus or transfected viral DNA survived better in host cells that had been pre-treated with mutagen than in control cells. The ER factor increases as the time interval between cell treatment and infection increases, until a maximum is reached after which the expression of ER decreases. The ER factors are in most cases on the order of between 1 and 5 and certainly less than those observed with lambda phage after infection of E. coli. The kinetics suggests that inducible repair processes might be involved in ER. The UV reactivation of HSV (herpes simplex virus) and of Kilham virus (a single-stranded parvovirus) is inhibited in the presence of cycloheximide [L46], suggesting a requirement for active protein synthesis. Cycloheximide does not block protein synthesis selectively in mammalian cells, however, and DNA synthesis is also arrested. In general, ER is associated with treatments that cause breaks or gaps in cellular DNA or that inhibit DNA synthesis [B68]. Its expression in human cells appears to be independent of excision repair, since the phenomenon can also be shown in XP cells that are excision-repair deficient [L48].

456. With respect to EM (enhanced mutagenesis), the process presumed to be activated or induced appears to be mutagenic, or partly mutagenic [D54, S109, S110]. The rate of reversion to the wild type of UV-irradiated SV-40 temperature-sensitive mutants grown in UV-irradiated monkey kidney cells is increased relative to that in unirradiated cells [G52, S110]. Sequence analysis in one case suggested that the reversion occurred at a site opposite to a possible thymine dimer, indicating that the mutation was probably targeted[y] [S110, S111]. The same conclusion of targeted mutagenesis can be deduced from the fact that the degree of mutagenesis depended largely on irradiating the virus prior to infection [C65, C66].

457. Some laboratories have reported increased mutagenesis of non-treated virus in mutagen pre-treated cells [C65, D54], but others [D55, S109, S110] have failed to see such an increase. In cases where untargeted mutagenesis has been recorded, this could be the result of an error-prone damage tolerance mechanism that is activated by host-cell DNA damage, an observation that is in line with untargeted mutagenesis recorded in phage-bacterial systems.

458. Integrated DNA from DNA or RNA viruses can be activated to produce viral particles by treatment of cells with a variety of DNA-damaging agents (reviewed in [F37]). This process bears at least a superficial resemblance to prophage induction in lysogenic bacteria. An interesting parallelism in dose-response curves has been found for UV induction of SV-40 provirus and enhanced reactivation of irradiated HSV [Z7], and for the induction of SV-40 provirus and the formation of SCEs following exposure to ethylmethanesulphonate or mitomycin-C [K49]. But it remains to be established whether these correlations signify a common regulation of the expression of the three functions.

459. Another approach that has been used to study induction of repair in mammalian cells is the use of split-dose protocols, in which a first relatively small dose is given (and is presumed to be the inducing stimulus), followed by a large DNA damaging dose. When CHO cells are exposed to a small UV dose several hours prior to a larger dose, and are subsequently pulse labelled and analysed in alkaline sucrose gradients, the DNA synthesized after exposure to the second dose is smaller than that observed for DNA from cells that did not receive the first small dose. However, the DNA increases in size when the cells are subsequently incubated in unlabelled medium;

---

[x]The term SOS responses in bacteria denotes the initiation of a regulatory signal causing a simultaneous de-repression of a number of genes. The products of some or all such genes enhance the survival of the bacterium or of its normal resident phages, prophage induction, phage mutagenesis, cell filamentation, cellular responses to DNA damage (including excision repair and DNA damage tolerance) and genetic recombination [F37].

[y]A mutation is targeted if it occurs at the site of the original mutagenic interaction, e.g., UV-induced pyrimidine dimer. In contrast, the term untargeted mutation occurs in an unirradiated phage when SOS proficient host cells are previously induced. These could be divided into mutations opposite spontaneous depurinations and into truly untargeted replication errors. These cannot be distinguished at present [M70].

this apparent enhanced rate of chain elongation is not observed in cells incubated with cycloheximide between the two UV treatments, suggesting the need for de novo protein synthesis. These results have been interpreted in terms of a possible mechanism for enhanced DNA synthesis that facilitates replication past dimers [D57].

460. Studies of the overall rate of DNA synthesis through autoradiography of cells labelled with ^{3}H-thymidine also show enhancement in split-dose protocols [M71]. However, in mutation experiments with CHO cells, in which they were first irradiated with x rays at times 0 and 17 hours before being irradiated with UV, there was no evidence for an enhanced recovery of ouabain-resistant or 6-TG^R mutations (x rays in these experiments is a putative inducer of error-prone cellular replicative response, since it is known that they do not induce ouabain-resistant mutations) [C67].

461. Cornelis et al. [C66] studied the problem of whether the expression of inducible error-prone repair processes could be correlated with an increased sensitivity to oncogenic transformation. In these experiments, the authors determined the transformation frequency in unirradiated and UV-irradiated human VH12 cells, using a deletion mutant of SV40 lacking the origin of DNA replication. The results showed that UV-irradiated cells were transformed more efficiently than unirradiated cells. This enhanced transforming activity (defined as the ratio of the efficiency of transformation per cell in UV-irradiated cultures to that in unirradiated cultures) increased as the interval between cell irradiation and transfection with viral DNA increased. Susceptibility to transformation decreased again after a maximum was reached when the cells were infected three days after irradiation. Since transformation with SV40 is thought to be due to the insertion of the virus genome into host sequences by a process involving recombination, this observation provides evidence for the existence in human cells of a UV-inducible recombination process.

462. The data discussed in the foregoing paragraphs (and others discussed in [F37] and [H53]) strengthen the possibility that SOS-like responses are inducible in mammalian cells, all following DNA damage or arrest of replication. Formal proof, however, requires knowledge of the type of reactions involved or of the genes coding for repair enzymes involved in this pathway, both of which are not available at present.

(b) Adaptive responses

463. The SOS-like responses in mammalian cells discussed so far result in increased survival as well as increased yields of mutations. In 1977, Samson and Cairns [S112] reported that chronic exposure of E. coli cells to very low non-toxic levels of the simple alkylating agent N-methyl-N'-nitro-nitrosoguanidine (MNNG) results in the de novo induction of an adaptive DNA repair pathway. Once induced, this pathway affords the cells considerable protection against both the killing and the mutagenic effects of alkylating agents, i.e., it is antimutagenic and thus is different from SOS-like responses. Adaptation is specific for alkylation damage; it can be induced by, and provide protection against, all the simple alkylating agents that have been so far tested (methyl-nitrosourea, methyl-methanesulphonate, ethyl-methanesulphonate, N-ethyl-N'-nitrosoguanidine). Adaptation cannot be induced by, nor protect against, UV light or 4-nitro-quinoline-1-oxide damage [J27, S113].

464. Since the resistance of MNNG did not develop when protein synthesis was inhibited by chloramphenicol, it was proposed that a protein was responsible for the (error-free) repair of mutagenic lesions induced by the exposure to a low level of MNNG. Subsequent work confirmed that such an explanation was indeed correct. Of the several adducts formed in the DNA upon exposure to alkylating agents, 0^6-alkylguanine is implicated as premutagenic [G53, L47] and precarcinogenic [G54]; if left unrepaired, 0^6-alkylguanine is recognized as adenine during DNA replication and so causes GC AT transitions. Schendel et al. [S114] and Robins and Cairns [R61] demonstrated that, in the MNNG experiments, the adapted E. coli cells are exceedingly efficient at removing 0^6-methylguanine from their DNA. This removal is extraordinarily rapid [C68] and achieved by a hitherto undescribed DNA repair mechanism, which is now termed as the adaptive response mechanism. Surprisingly, the 0^6-methylguanine is not eliminated by nucleotide excision repair but rather by a direct transfer of the methyl group from the 0^6 position of guanine to a cysteine residue, which is probably the adaptive enzyme itself (DNA methyltransferase). The enzyme has been recently purified [D58]. It became clear that the adaptive enzyme can act only once, and is therefore consumed during the DNA methyltransferase reaction [L48, R61]. The mutagenic protection provided by the adaptive response therefore shows an unusual and characteristic saturation at very high doses of the alkylating agent [S114, S115].

465. Studies have been carried out to examine whether adaptive responses could be demonstrated with mammalian cells; they represent a logical extension of those in bacteria. Most of these studies, carried out with alkylating agents, have been recently reviewed by Samson and Schwartz [S113] and Frosina and Abbondandolo [F38] and are beyond the scope of the present section. There is, however, one study with radiation in which presumptive evidence for an adaptive response has been obtained and this is considered below.

466. Olivieri et al. [O18] cultured human peripheral blood lymphocytes in ^{3}H-thymidine-containing medium (^{3}H-thymidine was added 4-6 hours after culture initiation and was the source of low-level chronic radiation) and irradiated them with 1.5 Gy of x rays at 7, 9 or 11 hours before fixation. Appropriate controls were maintained. It was found that in the

^{3}H-thymidine + x-ray group, the yield of chromatid aberrations (chromatid and iso-chromatid deletions and chromatid interchanges) was less than the sum of the yields of aberrations induced by ^{3}H-thymidine and x rays separately. At the same fixation times, non-radioactive thymidine did not affect the yield of x-ray-induced aberrations. In another experiment, the effects of continuous treatment with ^{3}H-thymidine on the frequency of chromatid aberrations treated with 0.4 Gy of x rays 50 hours after stimulation (and fixed 3 hours later) were studied. The findings were similar. The authors suggest that these responses are analogous to the adaptive response to alkylating agents, whereby prior treatment with small doses for a long period of time reduces the damage occurring after larger doses of similar agents given for a short time.

6. Summary and conclusions

467. New data on the incidence of spontaneous 6-thioguanine resistant variants (studied with the autoradiographic method) in human lymphocytes from Bloom syndrome and Fanconi anaemia patients have been published; they show that these are about eight times higher than in controls. The frequencies determined by the autoradiographic methods are generally higher than those known for mutants studied at the same locus with the same selective agent in human fibroblasts. However, if the lymphocytes are cryopreserved before study to eliminate phenocopies, the frequencies become lower and comparable to those recorded in fibroblast work and in T-cell cloning work (see below).

468. The newly developed T-cell cloning technique has been successfully used in studies on the determination of spontaneous as well as radiation-induced 6-thioguanine resistant mutations in human peripheral blood T-lymphocytes. The spontaneous frequencies are in the range between 10^{-6} and 10^{-5} in healthy young adults and the frequency increases with age. With x irradiation, there is a dose-dependent increase in mutation frequency. Both the spontaneous and induced frequencies are comparable with those known from work on fibroblasts and from autoradiographic work on lymphocytes in which the lymphocytes are first cryopreserved before study.

469. The spontaneous frequencies of 6-thioguanine resistant mutations determined by the T-cell cloning technique, show that, in Fanconi anaemia patients, they are about 2-3 times higher than in controls. With Fanconi anaemia heterozygotes, there is no such difference.

470. Breast cancer patients who have undergone radiotherapy show elevated levels of 6-thioguanine resistant mutants in their lymphocytes (T-cell cloning method) and these are higher than those in the same patients before therapy, in controls and in heart patients.

471. New data on the induction of 6-thioguanine resistant mutations by chronic gamma irradiation of Chinese hamster fibroblasts (over a period of 2-3 weeks in chemostat culture) suggest that there is no reduced effectiveness of chronic versus acute irradiation.

472. Recent results of a collaborative study on the x-ray induction of chromosomal aberrations (over the range from 0.004 to 0.3 Gy) in human peripheral lymphocytes in vitro (G_0 irradiation) show no increase in aberration yields up to 0.05 Gy, beyond which the increase is linear with dose.

473. Molecular approaches are being used to study mutation and DNA repair in mammalian cells. Among the possibilities explored are: (a) introduction of the E. coli XGPRT gene (by transfection) into HPRT$^-$ Chinese hamster fibroblasts and their use in radiation mutagenesis experiments; (b) correction of excision repair deficiency of certain excision repair Chinese hamster cell lines through introduction of wild-type human DNA; (c) cloning of the first human repair gene; (d) similar attempts to correct repair defects in human cells (xeroderma pigmentosum, ataxia telangiectasia) through trasfection of suitable donor DNA; and (e) molecular characterization of spontaneous and radiation-induced mutations using appropriate cDNA probes. The currently available data suggest that a majority of radiation-induced 6-thioguanine resistant mutants in Chinese hamster cells are large deletions.

474. Somatic cell hybrids (mouse × human) have also been used to identify repair genes and their chromosomal locations in human cells. Indications that human chromosomes 13 and 14 may carry genes involved in the correction of excision repair deficiency in XP cells have been obtained.

475. A number of studies have been carried out to examine whether inducible SOS-like repair processes (known from earlier work with bacteria) could be demonstrated in mammalian cells following DNA damage. Most of these data have been collected in experiments using viruses as probes. They provide evidence for the occurrence of such repair processes. However, there is as yet no unequivocal evidence for the de-repression of previously repressed genetic functions and no indication that eukaryotic cells respond to inducing signals by expressing a battery of genes under the control of a common regulatory system, as is the case in E. coli.

476. Most of the studies that bear on the problem of adaptive responses—cellular responses to mutagenic treatments that result in higher survival and lower yield of mutations—carried out in mammalian cells have used chemical mutagens and carcinogens. In one study with human lymphocytes, in which low-level ^{3}H-irradiation was used to stimulate the putative repair process involved in adaptive response before giving doses of 0.4 or 1.5 Gy of x radiation, evidence for a possible adaptive response was obtained: the yield of chromosomal aberrations is lower in the ^{3}H + x-ray group than in the group given x rays alone.

C. INTERSPECIFIC COMPARISONS OF KARYOTYPES AMONG PRIMATE SPECIES: RELEVANCE FOR THE CHOICE OF PRIMATE SPECIES CLOSE TO MAN FOR RADIATION CYTOGENETIC STUDIES

477. The work of Dutrillaux et al. [D59] on the chromosomal evolution in primates was discussed in the 1982 UNSCEAR report. From this work, the authors concluded that: (a) the pattern of chromosomal evolution is not the same in the different branches of the evolutionary tree, i.e., the types of rearrangements that have occurred vary from one group to another (suborder, family, genus); (b) there is a very close similarity between the chromosome banding patterns of the simians studied and man; and (c) all the quantitative and some of the qualitative variations detected involve the heterochromatin. From the standpoint of comparisons of chromosomal sensitivity of radiation (or other mutagens) to the induction of different kinds of aberrations, two principal questions remained unresolved: firstly, can the evolutionary tree provide any clue with respect to the inducibility of a given kind of chromosomal aberration in different species and in man and the pathological consequences that may derive from such induced aberrations; and, secondly, can quantitative and qualitative comparisons based on the induction of one kind of aberration in different species provide a proper perspective and a basis for predicting the relative radiosensitivity of human chromosomes to damage that is relevant in the context of induced pathological states?

478. Dutrillaux and colleagues have now devised a scheme [D60] for comparing the karyotypes of different primate species that is potentially capable of providing some answers to the above questions. In this scheme, the karyotype of each species is transformed into two histograms, one on the basis of distribution of distances to telomeres (or more precisely, the half-length of the chromosomes) and the other, on the basis of distances to centromeres (= arm length). To draw the first histogram, the individual chromosomes are ordered in terms of decreasing length (in R-banded preparations) and the relative half-lengths are expressed as a percentage of the total length of the genome. Each chromosome is assigned a constant width of 2 units so that the relative half-length and width define an area for each chromosome and the total area for each genome is 100 units. The second histogram makes use of distance to the centromeres (arm length), ordered as above in terms of decreasing length (i.e., relative length of the chromosome arms), which, together with a constant width of 1 unit, likewise define a relative area for each chromosome arm. Here too, the total area for all the chromosome arms is 100 units. The heterochromatin at the telomeric regions and in the short arms of acrocentrics is considered separately from the euchromatin and the centromeric heterochromatin. The amount of each of these is arbitrarily counted as 0.25% of the haploid karyotypes.

479. The karyotypes of the different species characterized as above (each as two histograms) were used to discern similarities and differences between them. Furthermore, since the histograms represent the distribution of all the chromosome segments of the karyotype, they can be used as a basis to predict the relative sensitivities of chromosomes of the different species to a given clastogenic agent. For instance, if the chromosome breaks (involved in the different kinds of rearrangements) are randomly distributed among the different chromosomes and the chromosome arms (i.e., show a proportionality to the chromosome lengths and arm lengths), the breakpoint distribution profiles should be superimposable on the above histograms. However, if breaks are not located at random (e.g., excessive number of breaks in centromeric or telomeric regions or preferential involvement of short or long arms), the break-point profile will not be superimposable on the histograms representing the species karyotype.

480. Among the eight primate species (including man) characterized as indicated above, the orangutan (Pongo pygmaeus) and the marmoset (Callithrix jacchus) have karyotypes most similar to man, followed by the gorilla (Gorilla gorilla), chimpanzee (Pan troglodytes), the crab-eating monkey (Macaca fascicularis) and the squirrel monkey (Saimiri sciureus). The profile of the African green monkey (Cercopithecus aethiops) is clearly different from all the rest and, finally, the chimpanzee and gorilla have karyotypes most similar to each other. When the comparisons are restricted to the distributions of the relative lengths of the chromosomes only, the marmoset is clearly the closest to man, followed by the gorilla and chimpanzee. If, however, only the distributions of the relative lengths of the chromosome arms are considered, the orangutan is the species closest to man, followed by the crab-eating monkey (if acrocentric short arms of human chromosomes are neglected) and the gorilla. If the heterochromatin distributions are taken into account, the karyotype of orangutan appears closest to that of man.

481. In order to test their model with respect to break-point distributions after irradiation, Muleris et al. [M72] and Paravatou-Petsota et al. [P45] performed experiments in which peripheral blood lymphocytes of the crab-eating monkey and of the chimpanzee were gamma-irradiated in vitro (2 and 3 Gy). The break-points involved in the different rearrangements were carefully mapped and the profiles so obtained compared with those expected on the basis of a random distribution of break-points. In the work with the crab-eating monkey, from the sample of 319 rearrangements, a total of 603 break-points could be accurately mapped. The results were the following: (a) the overall distribution of break-points showed a significant excess in smaller chromosomes, as had been found earlier in work with human lymphocytes and fibroblasts [D9, D10]; (b) in the case of reciprocal translocations, smaller chromosomes were more frequently involved than expected on a random basis; the break-points showed a slight but non-significant tendency to be located near the telomeres and the overall pattern of break-point distribution could be characterized as random; (c) for dicentrics, there was a significant excess of breaks in the juxta-telomeric regions, but no

significant excess near the centromeres; (d) for pericentric inversions, there was a significant deficit of juxta-telomeric breaks, an excess of breaks far from telomeres (i.e., near to centromeres) and a greater involvement of longer chromosomes; and (e) for paracentric inversions, there was a slight non-significant excess of juxta-telomeric breaks and of breaks near the centromeres and a non-random involvement of longer chromosomes and longer chromosome arms.

482. In the work on chimpanzees [P45], the situation was different. From a sample of 460 cell karyotypes after R-banding, 1047 rearrangements were detected and the break-points mapped. It is important to note that the chimpanzee has terminal heterochromatin in many of its chromosome arms. A comparison of the number of breaks in the euchromatin (1008) and in heterochromatin (138) in relation to their relative sizes (100 units and 7 units, respectively) showed a large excess of breaks in the heterochromatin, and these were located both in the terminal heterochromatin as well as in the short arms of the acrocentrics. In the case of reciprocal translocations, again, there was a significant excess of breaks in the juxta-telomeric regions and in the short arms of the acrocentrics. For dicentrics, there was a significant excess of breaks, again, in heterochromatin and a significant lack of breaks in the euchromatin, except in the distal regions; the terminal Q-bands were even more affected than the short arms of acrocentrics. In the case of pericentric inversions, there was a tendency for chromosomes with relatively small arms to be preferentially involved. (In fact, chromosomes 9, 22 and 16, which are relatively small metacentrics, were among the most frequently affected chromosomes in relation to size.) Finally, for paracentric inversions, almost all the breaks were in the euchromatin (29/30) and no such inversions were detected in the short arms of the acrocentrics.

483. Paravatou-Petsota et al. [P45] have pointed out that the high sensitivity of chimpanzee lymphocytes to the x-ray induction of dicentrics (2.2-fold higher than with human lymphocytes at a dose of 2 Gy) recorded in the work of Léonard et al. [L49] may in fact be related to the presence of terminal heterochromatin in about half of the chromosome arms. Among the primates, the only other species that has terminal heterochromatin is the gorilla and its lymphocytes would be expected to be more sensitive than those of man to the induction of dicentrics: this in fact had been found to be the case ([D61, L49]; 1.6 times more sensitive than human lymphocytes). From all these findings, the authors concluded that: (a) there are real differences in break-point distribution, between different rearrangements in the same species and between different species; (b) the presence of juxta-telomeric heterochromatin may be an important factor in the sensitivity of the lymphocytes of the different species to dicentric induction; and (c) the differences in break-point distributions and differential involvement of chromosomes in the various types of rearrangement suggest that dicentrics may not be representative of the sensitivity of induction for other rearrangements and, therefore, dicentrics may not be the appropriate cytological end-points in inter-specific comparisons of radiosensitivity.

VII. RE-EXAMINATION OF AND FURTHER APPROACHES TO RISK ASSESSMENTS

A. MUTATIONAL DAMAGE

1. Consistency of the genetic findings in Hiroshima and Nagasaki studies with those expected from radiation genetic studies with mice

484. As may be recalled, in its 1977 [U2] and 1982 [U1] UNSCEAR reports, the Committee extrapolated from the data on the induction of dominant skeletal and dominant cataract mutations in mice to risks from the induction of mutations having dominant effects in the first generation progeny. Furthermore, in the 1982 report the results of continuing genetic studies [S128] on the progeny of the survivors of the Hiroshima and Nagasaki bombings were discussed. In these studies, Schull et al. [S128] used four indicators of genetic effects, namely, untoward pregnancy outcomes (i.e., still birth, major congenital defects and death during the first post-natal week), occurrence of death in live-born during the first 17 years of life, frequency of children with sex-chromosomal aneuploidy and frequency of children with mutations resulting in electrophoretic variants. As Schull et al. stated, "... in no instance is there a statistically significant effect of parental exposure ... but for all indicators, the observed effect is in the direction suggested by the hypothesis that genetic damage resulted from the radiation exposure ...".

485. Ehling [E29, E30] examined the question of whether the above conclusion is consistent with expectations based on mouse results with dominant cataract and dominant skeletal mutations. He used the estimate of the genetically significant dose (sustained by the survivors of Hiroshima and Nagasaki) of $1.1 \ 10^4$ man Sv arrived at by WHO in its report [W52] on the "Effects of nuclear war on health and health services". The expected increases in the frequencies of dominant mutations in 19,000 children were derived as follows:

		Cataracts	Skeletal mutations
(1)	Mutations/gamete/Sv	$0.45\text{-}0.55 \ 10^{-4}$	$10.1 \ 10^{-4}$
(2)	Genetically significant dose (man-Sv)	$1.1 \ 10^4$	$1.1 \ 10^4$
(3)	Expected number of cases of cataracts/skeletal mutations [= (1) × (2)]	0.5-0.6	11
(4)	Multiplication factors for the overall dominant mutation rate	41	5
(5)	Total number of expected dominant mutations on the basis of the cataract/skeletal mutation data [= (3) × (4)]	20-25	56

486. It is clear that, in the sample of 19,000 children born to Hiroshima and Nagasaki survivors, less than 1 cataract mutation and about 11 dominant skeletal

mutations would be expected; the total number of expected dominant mutations will be in the range 20-25 (on the basis of the cataract data) or about 56 (on the basis of the skeletal mutation data). Ehling argues that with the kinds of end-points used in the Hiroshima and Nagasaki studies: (a) it is not surprising that no clear-cut positive evidence for the induction of genetic damage could be demonstrated; and (b) the Hiroshima and Nagasaki results are not inconsistent with the expectations based on the cataract and dominant skeletal mutation data.

487. Abrahamson [A24] and the report of the United States Nuclear Regulatory Commission [E32] arrived at similar conclusions. In their analysis of the Japanese data, they used: (a) the paper of Schull et al. [S131] (specifically Table 7 of this paper in which mortality up to age 17 for 16,713 children of exposed parents is given according to the distribution of parental doses) as a basis; (b) the linear-quadratic equation for the induction of gene mutations and of chromosomal aberrations developed independently of the Japanese data on the basis of experimental results (with the mouse for mutations and with the marmoset Saguinus fuscicollis for translocations); and (c) average doses for each exposure group (parents), i.e., 0.05 Gy (0.01-0.09 Gy group), 0.295 Gy (0.10-0.49 Gy group), 0.745 Gy (0.50-0.99 Gy group) and 200 Gy (> 1.00 Gy group). These values were introduced into the equations to project the number of cases of each genetic event relative to the child sample size in each of the 32 sectors of exposure in the matrix by Schull et al.

488. As summarized in the United States Nuclear Regulatory Commission report ". . . among the 16,713 children born to parents, one or both of whom were exposed, we conclude that there should have been about 50 total cases of genetic defects distributed as follows: 24 dominant, 5 X-linked, 4 aneuploid and 15 unbalanced translocations (early deaths) plus 55 cases of balanced translocation (detectable in otherwise normal individuals). In addition, the lower limit prediction is about 8 additional cases of genetic defects plus 6 individuals with balanced translocations and the upper limit prediction is approximately 170 additional cases of genetic defects plus 137 individuals with balanced translocations. It should be obvious that the central estimate prediction of cases should lead to a statistically insignificant, that is, undetectable increase in genetic disorders among the 16,713 progeny of irradiated parents. For example, there were 1040 deaths in this group of 16,713 progeny up to the age of 17 (6.22%). In the unexposed groups, there were 2,191 deaths of 33,976 progeny produced (6.45%) and the two frequencies are not significantly different, nor would they have been even if 50 additional cases were added to the exposed group."

2. Risks from the induction of recessive mutations

489. In the 1977 and 1982 UNSCEAR reports, the risk from the induction by radiation of recessive mutations was considered negligible and no attempt was made to quantify this risk. Instead, attention was focused on the induction of mutations having harm-ful dominant effects, and the risk from the induction of recessives having heterozygous effects was considered as one component of the risks (see also [B79, B80, O22]). Searle and Edwards [S126] have now provided a numerical estimate of risks for recessive disorders, the principal considerations being that: firstly, harmful recessive mutations presumably can arise at all loci coding for essential proteins (perhaps at least 10,000), and mutations to dominant alleles may be a property of relatively few loci; and, secondly, while many recessives doubtless remain to be discovered, those known at present tend to have earlier and more severe effects than dominants. Induced recessive mutations can cause harm by: (a) partnership with a defective allele already established in the population; (b) partnership with another recessive mutation induced at the same locus; (c) the formation of homozygous descendants, i.e., identity by descent; and (d) heterozygous effects.

490. Searle and Edwards based their calculations on a combination of data from observations on human populations and from mouse experiments and found that: (a) a genetically significant dose of 0.01 Gy of x or gamma radiation received by each parent once in a stable population with a million live-born would induce up to 1200 extra recessive mutations; (b) from partnership effects, about 1 extra case of recessive disease would be expected in the following ten generations; (c) homozygosity resulting from identity by descent would not normally occur until the fourth generation after exposure, but, under certain assumptions, about 10 extra cases of recessive diseases would be expected from this cause by the tenth generation; and (d) in the same period, about 250 recessive alleles would be eliminated in heterozygotes, on the assumption of a 2.5% heterozygous disadvantage. Searle and Edwards have argued that these deleterious heterozygous effects should not be combined with those of dominants. However, this would only apply to slightly deleterious effects; more serious ones would probably be included in the dominant category.

3. First-generation litter size reduction following irradiation of spermatogonial stem cells in male mice: a measure of deleterious effects of induced mutations (including deletions) and translocations

491. Selby and Russell [S127] used the data on litter size reductions routinely obtained in the course of specific locus experiments of Russell and colleagues between 1950 and 1961 to study the effects of irradiation of spermatogonial germ cells for this endpoint of genetic damage. The data come from 14 experiments (carried out at different x-ray and gamma-ray exposures, both at high and low dose rates) and involve a total of 158,490 litters. Litter sizes were compared between experimental and control groups at about three weeks after birth. In order to reduce variability, comparisons were made only with concurrent controls and between groups of litters having mothers of approximately the same age.

492. The main results were the following: (a) at the high exposure rate of 90 R/min, litter size reduction

(LSR) at weaning showed a humped exposure-frequency curve (similar to those recorded earlier for the induction of specific locus mutations and of translocations), being significantly lower after 1000 R than after 300 R or 600 R; (b) there was a pronounced effect of exposure rate, the responses being much less at rates of 0.009 R/min and 0.001 R/min, and, at 300 R, the exposure-rate reduction factor could be estimated as about 6.7; and (c) for the nine chronic gamma-irradiation experiments, the slope (defining the induction of LSR per R) was $(0.00194 \pm 0.00076)\%$. On the basis of these results, it can be estimated that if male mice were exposed to 1 R of low-LET, low-dose-rate irradiation, the total number of induced deaths between conception and weaning age (i.e., 3 weeks), would be about 19 out of every million F_1 mice that would have lived to three weeks of age in the absence of irradiation. The authors suggested that about half of these deaths would be the consequence of induced reciprocal translocations and the other half due to gene mutations and small deficiencies.

493. In his population studies in which a testicular x-ray exposure (high exposure rate) of 276 R was administered to male mice in every generation, Lüning [L59] demonstrated that the net productivity (i.e., the number of weaned young per female) in the irradiated population was reduced by about the same amount from the first to the 18th generation, i.e., there was no evidence for an accumulation of genetic damage having adverse effects on productivity. His data and analysis pertain to a total of 5034 litters and 30,995 progeny at birth in the irradiated population and 5693 litters and 36,430 progeny at birth in the control. The total numbers of young at weaning were, respectively, 25,766 and 30,484. Litters with no weaned offspring were excluded from the analysis. The results showed that: (a) the ratio of litter sizes at birth between the irradiated and the control population was 0.9629 (average value based on tests in generations 7-10, 11-14 and 15-18), indicating a 3.71% reduction in litter size at birth in the irradiated, relative to the control, population; and (b) the ratios of the number of weaned offspring to total births in the irradiated and control populations were, respectively, 0.8368 (again an average value based on tests in the generations mentioned above); the ratio of these two figures (i.e., irradiated/control) is 0.9934, indicating a 0.66% induced death between birth and weaning in the irradiated population. Thus, the total amount of induced death between conception and weaning can be calculated as 4.37% at 276 R (it should be noted that 85% of this induced death occurs before birth and the remainder between birth and weaning).

494. On the basis of these data and on the assumption of linearity, the rate of induction of genetic changes causing death between conception and weaning can be estimated as 0.01583% per R. If the exposure-rate reduction factor of 6.7 (estimated by Selby and Russell at an exposure of 300 R) is used to correct the above figure for effects expected at low dose rates, then the rate becomes 0.002363% per R, corresponding to 24 cases of death between conception and weaning per R per million. This figure is in close agreement with the 19 cases per R per million estimated by Selby

and Russell. Furthermore, if the relative proportions of deaths between conception and birth and between birth and weaning estimated for high-dose-rate irradiation (i.e., 0.85 and 0.15, respectively) are applicable, then about 20 of the 24 induced deaths will occur before birth and 4 between birth and weaning.

495. At the request of the Committee, Searle and Papworth [S137] have now carried out an analysis of litter sizes at birth and at weaning in 48,165 offspring of male mice exposed over 12 weeks to fission neutrons or gamma rays. In the analysis, litters in which no young was weaned were excluded. Mean litter sizes at birth were 2.3% lower after paternal (stem-cell spermatogonial) exposure to 2.14 Gy fission neutrons + 0.93 Gy gamma rays, as compared with 6.06 Gy gamma rays + 0.025 Gy fission neutrons, the difference reaching a significant level in male offspring. Moreover, the proportion of offspring which survived to weaning fell significantly by 1.9% in the neutron series. On the assumption of a Q value of 20 for neutrons for the induction of these genetic changes having dominant sub-lethal effects (on the basis of results for dominant visible mutations, see [B81]) the authors estimated that the extra pre- and post-natal mortality was induced by an extra dose equivalent of 37.17 Sv. This is equivalent to 6 extra pre-natal and 5 extra post-natal deaths per million offspring induced by a dose equivalent of 0.01 Sv, i.e., a total of 11 extra deaths in all. Thus, in this experiment, 55% of the induced extra lethality acted at or before birth and 45% after birth (versus 85% and 15%, respectively, in Lüning's experiments).

496. It is thus clear that three entirely different sets of experiments lead to similar conclusions, namely, that low-LET irradiation of male mice at low doses and low dose rates would be expected to result in extra deaths in F_1 between conception and weaning, totalling 19 per million per R in the experiments of Selby and Russell, 24 per million per R in those of Lüning and about 11 per million per 0.01 Sv in the analysis of Searle and Papworth. The relative proportions of post-natal mortalities in the studies of Lüning and of Searle and Papworth are, respectively, 0.15 and 0.45, i.e., 3 and 5 cases per million per R (or per 0.01 Sv); if these relative proportions are applied to the data of Selby and Russell, then the corresponding estimates are about 3 or 9 per million per R. The Committee favours the use of a range between 5 and 10 per million per R to avoid the impression of too much precision in these estimates.

497. Considering now the relevance of these data in the context of risk assessment, it is important to note that, in the past, the methods used by the Committee for estimating dominant genetic damage have relied on data collected in mouse experiments in which the events were scored at weaning or in adult mice; consequently the question remained open as to whether induction of genetic changes having dominant sub-lethal effects had been overlooked. If the results obtained in the mouse and discussed above are considered applicable in the human context, it can be concluded that the risk of induction of genetic changes with dominant sub-lethal effects is relatively small.

While it is not possible to be precise as to when the extra post-natal mortality (observed in the mouse) will become manifest in the human beings, it would probably occur sometime in early life after birth.

B. CHROMOSOMAL DAMAGE

1. An estimate of the percentage of conceptions with an unbalanced reciprocal translocation that survive birth

498. In the 1972 report, in the context of estimating risks from the induction of reciprocal translocations in man, UNSCEAR estimated that about 6% of all human conceptions with a structurally unbalanced chromosome complement may result in live births with congenital anomalies. This figure was also used in the 1977 and 1982 UNSCEAR reports and was estimated on the basis of limited data on the incidence of unbalanced structural rearrangements in cytogenetic surveys of new-born children (0.03%; 7/21,996) and on that in spontaneous abortions (1.07%; 8/747) then available and on the view expressed by Carr [C73] that about 45% of all conceptions spontaneously terminate before birth. The proportion of conceptions that have an unbalanced chromosome complement and that survive to live birth should therefore be

$$\frac{p_1 \, a_1}{(p_2 \, a_2) + (p_1 \, a_1)}$$

where p_1 is the proportion of conceptions that result in live birth (0.55); a_1 is the frequency of unbalanced structural rearrangements in live-born (0.0003); p_2 is the proportion of conceptions that result in abortions (0.45); and a_2 is the frequency of unbalanced structural rearrangements in abortions. However, an arithmetic error was made in the calculations, resulting in the estimate of 6%, as has recently been pointed out by Russell [R69]. The correct estimate of conceptions with unbalanced structural rearrangements among all conceptions with unbalanced structural rearrangements, with the data then used, is 3.5%. As Russell pointed out, the estimate of 6% instead of 3.5% can hardly be regarded as serious in view of the size of the sampling errors of the human data.

499. Leaving aside the arithmetic error that led to an estimate of 6%, it is instructive to inquire whether a new estimate can be derived that will be consistent with current knowledge. Important in this exercise are the following considerations: (a) more extensive data on the frequencies of chromosomal anomalies in spontaneous abortions and in new-borns have become available since the publication of the 1972 report; and (b) in the 1972 report, the frequencies of all unbalanced structural rearrangements were taken into consideration, whereas in fact the calculations should be restricted to the presumed unbalanced products of reciprocal translocations only, since radiation does not appear to induce Robertsonian translocations.

500. In discussing the review of Hook [H1] on the contribution of chromosomal anomalies to spontaneous abortions (and still birth) in relation to gestational age (see I.B), it was pointed out that an estimated 15% of all conceptions recognized by 5 weeks of gestation onwards terminate in spontaneous abortions. This figure does not include early pre-implantation losses occurring prior to the clinical recognition of pregnancy or the early post-implantation losses, both of which probably occur [H60]. Tests are now available that allow the detection of pregnancies within a week of implantation; the results of one study [M78] of early pregnancy loss suggest that 33% of pregnant women abort spontaneously. However, there are as yet no data on the incidence of chromosomal anomalies in these early pregnancy losses. It is therefore preferable to use the commonly accepted figure of 15% for spontaneous abortions in the human species, since this estimate is backed by extensive data.

501. From an analysis of cytogenetic data from published surveys of spontaneous abortions (n = 5726) and new-born (n = 59,454), Jacobs [J10] estimated that the total frequency of unbalanced structural rearrangements was 1.54% in the abortus material and 0.050% in new-born. The frequencies of stable structurally abnormal chromosomes (i.e., monocentric chromosomes that have missing and/or additional material, equivalent to unbalanced products of reciprocal translocations) alone were 0.681% in the abortus material and 0.012% in new-born (for the latter, the estimate based on 67,014 babies summarized in the 1982 UNSCEAR report is 0.01% which is almost identical to Jacobs' estimate).

502. With these data, it is possible to make a new estimate of the proportion of conceptions with an unbalanced structural rearrangement (or with an unbalanced product of reciprocal translocations) that will result in live birth, relative to all conceptions that have an unbalanced structural rearrangement (or an unbalanced product of a reciprocal translocation). For making the overall estimate, the values to be used are: $p_1 = 0.85$, $p_2 = 0.15$, $a_1 = 0.0005$, and $a_2 = 0.0154$. With these, the estimated value is 15.5%. If only the unbalanced products of reciprocal translocations are considered, the figures to be used in the equation are: $p_1 = 0.85$, $p_2 = 0.15$, $a_1 = 0.00012$, and $a_2 = 0.00681$ and the estimated figure is 9.1%. In other words, 15.5% of all conceptions with unbalanced structural rearrangements will survive birth, and 9.1% of all conceptions with an unbalanced product of reciprocal translocation will survive birth. The Committee believes that it is preferable to use a round figure of 9% for the percentage of unbalanced products of reciprocal translocations that will survive to birth, in the context of risk estimations.

2. Model radiation studies with human peripheral blood lymphocytes and fibroblasts to estimate the proportion of balanced reciprocal translocations, which if induced in germ cells may generate viable imbalances after meiosis

503. Genetic theory dictates that a carrier of a balanced reciprocal translocation will, after meiosis, produce three kinds of gametes with respect to their chromosomal constitution: normal (i.e., not carrying the translocation), translocation carrying, and un-

balanced (i.e., with various deletions and duplications for defined chromosome segments). While usually no adverse viability or phenotypic effects are expected to be associated with the zygotes (and the progeny), with the normal chromosome complement or with the balanced reciprocal translocation-carrying complement, the majority of the zygotes with the unbalanced complements will not be viable and will be eliminated through early embryonic losses or abortions. A small proportion of them, however, may be viable despite the chromosomal imbalance and may thus result in children with one or another kind of birth defect. In general, the extent of imbalance that is likely to be generated and its effects on viability depend, among other things, on the location of the break-points in the chromosomes involved in the translocation, the lengths of the chromosome segments translocated, the genic content of these segments and the segregational properties of the translocations in meiosis. Segregation and fertility analyses of familial reciprocal translocations (ascertained through balanced or unbalanced probands) [A5, D66, D67, I14, V19] provide some clues about the nature, variety and the extent of imbalances compatible with live birth, but there are no data on the proportion of balanced reciprocal translocations induced in human germ cells that may generate chromosome imbalances that are viable. This information is an essential prerequisite for the realistic appraisal of the risks stemming from the induction of translocations by radiation.

504. In order to provide at least a partial answer to this question, Dutrillaux and colleagues carried out model experiments with human peripheral blood lymphocytes [D9] and fibroblasts [D10]. In the lymphocyte study, G_0 lymphocytes were irradiated in vitro with gamma-ray doses of 1 and 3 Gy, cultured for 48-96 hours, and processed for the scoring of translocations. All the mitoses were analysed in photographs after R-banding. A total of 247 translocations, each resulting from two chromosome breaks, were scored. The break-points of the translocations were accurately determined and the segments involved in the translocations were quantified by using the band-length unit defined in earlier work [A5].[z]

505. In the fibroblast work, the cells were derived from skin biopsies from individuals who underwent cosmetic surgery or from growing cells from other biopsies. These were irradiated with doses of 1, 3 or 6 Gy. A total of 124 independent translocations were ascertained. In addition, 90 other translocations were detected in cultures developed from the skin of a young boy acutely irradiated in an accident with an iridium-92 source [M10]. The break-points, lengths of segments involved, etc., were defined in R-banded preparations for all the 214 translocations, as in the case of those derived from lymphocytes.

506. The authors used the information obtained from the analysis of these translocations: (a) to inquire into the minimum possible imbalance that each of these translocations will generate, should they occur in

germ cells, by considering the different types of segregation; and (b) to compare these estimates with those available from studies of cases of partial monosomies and trisomies reported in the literature and that are known to be compatible with live births.

507. The main conclusions are the following: with the lymphocyte-derived translocations, 116 out of the 247 (47%) are capable of generating viable imbalances, should they occur in germ cells; 25 of the 247 (10%) may give rise to imbalances regarded as possibly not viable; and with the remaining 106 (43%), the imbalances would be of such a magnitude as to be incompatible with survival. The amounts of imbalance expressed in units of band length are 4.5, 5.5 and 10.2, respectively, for the viable, possibly not viable and not viable categories. If the last two categories are combined, the imbalance is 9.3 units. In 43 families where the translocations had been ascertained through abnormal probands (i.e., individuals who carried the unbalanced forms of the translocations and who were viable), calculations showed that the mean amount of imbalance was 4.1 units, an imbalance that is close to the 4.3 units classified as viable in the radiation experiment. In families where the translocations had been ascertained through balanced probands (24 families) and where the unbalanced products were known to have led to spontaneous abortions, sterility, etc., the mean imbalance was 8.0 units, again not strikingly different from 9.3 units mentioned above for the possibly not viable and not viable categories. The authors believe that the proportion of translocations (116/247) giving rise to viable imbalances in the lymphocyte-derived translocations may be a slight overestimate and that about 2/5 may be more reasonable.

508. The conclusions were essentially the same for the fibroblast-derived translocations, the breakdown among the categories of viable, possibly not viable and not viable being 83 out of 214 (39%), 24 out of 214 (11.5%) and 107 out of 214 (50%), respectively. This remarkable similarity in the distributions of translocations despite the differences in the tissue of origin suggest that it is possible to extrapolate from one tissue to another at least qualitively (i.e., to infer the nature of the translocations and their segregational consequences). It also indicates that the mean length of the exchanged segments is probably very similar in the two tissues and that it is unlikely that the response of the germ cells will be any different.

509. The authors stress that what they have attempted to establish is the proportion of translocations that may give rise to viable chromosome imbalances in the progeny, should they be induced in germ cells. Their finding that about 2/5 of the translocations may give rise to viable imbalances is only a first step, not sufficient in itself to allow estimation of the risk of chromosomal imbalance in terms of abnormal progeny. For the former, it should be pointed out that reciprocal translocations are known to be induced in mitotically dividing germ cells (namely, spermatogonia) as well as in meiotic and post-meiotic ones. For the latter, information is particularly needed on: (a) the probability that a translocation-carrying germ cell that

---

[z]Total length of the autosomes is 280 band-length units; one unit is thus 1/280 of the total length [A5].

may give rise to viable imbalance will actually produce a gamete of this particular karyotype; and (b) the probability that a zygote derived from such a gamete will actually survive to birth rather than leading to an early embryonic loss or an abortion.

510. In the mouse, about one-half of the gametes from male germ cells carrying a reciprocal translocation are chromosomally unbalanced; the two common types of imbalance involve duplication of one of the segments exchanged combined with the deletion of the other, while in some translocations tertiary trisomy for a small translocation product may also be relatively common. On the basis of these results, Searle [S129] suggested that if about one-half of the unbalanced gametes from a viable imbalance type of translocation led to zygotes that may survive to birth, then one-half of 40% (or 20%) of unbalanced gametes might lead to malformations at birth. He cautioned that, in view of the great variation in expression of these chromosomal anomalies, it is difficult to be certain how many of the zygotes would actually survive to birth. Furthermore, extrapolation from mouse results to man is fraught with uncertainty and probably incorrect with respect to the risk of producing unbalanced progeny, for the following reasons: (a) the mouse has only acrocentric chromosomes whereas most human chromosomes are non-acrocentric; (b) translocations with two distal breakpoints (i.e., close to telomeres) are those most likely to be viable; and (c) a karyotype with n acrocentrics has only half as many such regions as a karyotype with n non-acrocentric chromosomes. This means that $(1/2)^2 = 1/4$ of the number of exchanges between telomeric regions will occur in the first type of karyotype compared with the second. Therefore, the risk of producing viable imbalances (from balanced reciprocal translocations) may be much higher in man than in the mouse.

C. SUMMARY AND CONCLUSIONS

511. Ehling examined the principal conclusion of the continuing genetic studies on the children of survivors of the atomic bombs in Hiroshima and Nagasaki, namely, that there are no statistically significant effects of parental exposure. In doing this, he took into account the sample sizes involved, the genetically significant dose estimated to have been received by the parents, the sensitivity of the end-points (untoward pregnancy outcomes, sex-chromosomal anomalies, survival through the first 17 years of life and the frequency of biochemical variants) and calculated what would be expected on the basis of mouse data. He concluded that the absence of significant genetic effects in the Hiroshima and Nagasaki studies is not inconsistent with expectations based on the mouse data. Similar conclusions were reached by Abrahamson and by the United States Nuclear Regulatory Commission.

512. Basing their calculations on a combination of human and mouse data, Searle and Edwards attempted to estimate the risk from the induction of recessive mutations in man, in terms of recessive diseases. According to them, if a genetically significant dose of 0.01 Gy of x or gamma radiation is received by each parent once in a stable population with a million live-born, there will be about one extra case of recessive disease in the following ten generations, i.e., only a minority of the recessive mutations actually induced would become manifest as recessive diseases within ten generations.

513. Three sets of data on litter size reduction in mice in the first generation following spermatogonial irradiation of parental males were analysed and compared with respect to the amount of pre-natal (between conception and birth) and post-natal (between birth and weaning) mortality induced by irradiation. All these data sets are consistent with each other in that they provide evidence for the induction of genetic changes that lead to pre- and post-natal mortality. The rate for the latter has been estimated to be about 5-10 cases per million births per R of low-LET, low-dose-rate irradiation of males. If it is assumed that the situation would be similar following irradiation of human males, then such death would presumably occur some time in early life after birth.

514. The question of whether the estimate of 6% used in the 1972 and subsequent UNSCEAR reports for the percentage of human conceptions with an unbalanced reciprocal translocation that survive birth needs revision was re-examined in the light of new data. It was concluded that these data permit an estimate of 9% to be made, and that this figure can now be used in the context of estimating risks stemming from the unbalanced products of induced reciprocal translocations.

515. Model radiation studies with human peripheral blood lymphocytes and fibroblasts were conducted to ascertain the proportion of balanced reciprocal translocations (should they be induced in human germ cells) that may generate viable chromosome imbalances. It was concluded that roughly 40% of the induced translocations may do so, but this figure in itself is not sufficient to allow estimation of risks of chromosomal imbalance in terms of abnormal progeny.

VIII.   CURRENT RISK ASSESSMENTS

516. As will be evident from the data reviewed in the preceding chapters (see also [S138]) human genetics and experimental radiation genetics are now passing through a period of rapid growth and development. Several advances in mammalian radiation genetics throw light on the magnitude of genetic risks and allow some gaps in our knowledge to be filled, at least partially. The data concerned are discussed below.

517. *Induction of genetic changes having dominant sub-lethal effects in the first generation.* In the 1982 UNSCEAR report, the risk of induction of dominant deleterious mutations was assessed mainly from data on the induction of dominant mutations causing hereditary cataracts or skeletal abnormalities in mice, combined with information on known dominant

diseases in man. In the experiments, the mutations were scored at weaning (cataract mutations) or in adult progeny (skeletal mutations) and the question remained open, therefore, as to whether the induction of genetic changes having dominant sub-lethal effects had been overlooked. Analysis of three extensive sets of data on litter size reduction in mice (generated in experiments involving spermatogonial irradiation of the parental males; see paragraphs 491-497) lend credence to the view that such risks are small, as recapitulated below.

518. The data of Selby and Russell [S127] allow an estimate of $19 \ 10^{-6}$ per R for the rate of induction of dominant genetic changes (acting between conception and weaning) that lead to reduction in litter size. The rate of $24 \ 10^{-6}$ per R that could be obtained from Lüning's [L59] data (see paragraph 492) is quite comparable to that of Selby and Russell. Lüning's data, however, permit a partitioning of the total mortality rate into that occurring before birth (about $20 \ 10^{-6}$ per R) and that occurring between birth and weaning ($4 \ 10^{-6}$ per R). From a comparison of litter sizes at birth and of survival between birth and weaning in experiments involving chronic gamma-ray (6.06 Gy + 0.025 Gy neutrons) and fission-neutron (2.14 Gy + 0.93 Gy gamma-ray) exposures, Searle and Papworth [S137] found that the extra mortality observed in the neutron series could be attributed to an extra dose equivalent of 37.17 Sv (on the assumption of a Q value of 20 for chronic neutrons relative to chronic gamma rays). Their estimated rates are $6 \ 10^{-6}$ per 0.01 Sv for pre-natal mortality and $5 \ 10^{-6}$ per 0.01 Sv, for mortality between birth and weaning. Although the results of Selby and Russell do not permit the partitioning of the total mortality occurring before and after birth, by applying the relative proportions for these estimated in the other two studies (Lüning: $0.85 : 0.15$ and Searle and Papworth: $0.55 : 0.45$) it may be inferred that the rate of post-natal mortality in the work of Selby and Russell would be about 3-9 cases per 10^6 births per 0.01 Gy. Thus, when all the results are considered together, the induction rate of dominant genetic changes causing death between birth and weaning, can be estimated to be about 5-10 cases per 10^6 births per 0.01 Gy. If these results can be considered applicable to man, they would point to about 5-10 cases of death some time between birth and early life per 10^6 live births per 0.01 Gy of low-LET, low-dose-rate irradiation of males in the parental generation.

519. *Induction of hereditary tumours.* Recent work by Nomura ([N8, N30], paragraphs 338-342) has revealed that radiation can induce heritable pulmonary and other tumours (average of 40% penetrance) in the F_1 generation. Thus, in principle, this effect should also be included among those for the estimation of dominant genetic risks. However, these tumours show a very mild expressivity. As it is not yet known whether any serious health effects may be associated with these tumours, they have not been included in the present risk estimates.

520. *Induction of recessive genetic diseases.* It is now possible to provide new quantitative estimates of risk of recessive disease, stemming from the induction of recessive mutations (paragraphs 489-490). These estimates show that a one-time exposure to 0.01 Gy of low-LET, low-dose-rate irradiation of the parental generation is not associated with any appreciable risk of induced genetic disease in the first generation (the same conclusion was reached in the 1982 UNSCEAR report); however, this exposure could result in one extra case per million live-born by the tenth generation. The most serious detrimental effects of recessive mutations in heterozygous condition would probably be included in the dominant category of risk estimates by the direct method (Table 23).

521. *Fragile-X-linked genetic disease.* It has become clear that the heritable fragile site on the human X-chromosome is a major case of X-linked mental retardation, next only to Down syndrome (paragraphs 47-62). The prevalence of this condition is currently estimated as $400 \ 10^{-6}$. This means that the prevalence of X-linked disorders in man may need to be revised upwards from about $1000 \ 10^{-6}$ to $1400 \ 10^{-6}$. However, since it is not yet known whether the fragile site on the X-chromosome is inducible by radiation, it remains difficult to include this condition into the risk estimates.

522. *Risk from the induction of reciprocal trans-locations.* Data are available on the induction of reciprocal translocations by chronic gamma irradiation of spermatogonia of both the rhesus and the crab-eating monkeys ([V15, T45], paragraphs 387-390, and Table 21). In the former species, the observed frequency of 0.43% (in spermatocytes descended from irradiated spermatogonia after 1 Gy of gamma irradiation at 0.0002 Gy/min) after correction for controls (0.08%) allows an induction rate estimate of $0.35 \ 10^{-4}$ per 0.01 Gy. From this, the rate of balanced reciprocal translocations in the F_1 progeny could be estimated as $0.09 \ 10^{-4}$ per 0.01 Gy and that of unbalanced products, $0.18 \ 10^{-4}$ per 0.01 Gy (on the assumption of no reduction in transmission). If, as indicated earlier (paragraph 502), 9% of the unbalanced zygotes result in children with congenital malformations, then the risk for the latter can be estimated as $1.62 \ 10^{-6}$ per 0.01 Gy.

523. In the cytogenetic work with the crab-eating monkey, the dose-effect relationship after chronic gamma irradiation was consistent with linearity, the coefficient of induction being $0.16 \ 10^{-4}$ per 0.01 Gy. The same calculation as that for the rhesus monkey data leads to an estimate of $0.72 \ 10^{-6}$ surviving offspring per 0.01 Gy, reasonably close to the estimate of $1.62 \ 10^{-6}$ per 0.01 Gy made for the rhesus monkey data. It would therefore seem that a combined estimate of $1 \ 10^{-6}$ per 0.01 Gy can be used as the lower limit of risk (instead of $0.3 \ 10^{-6}$ per 0.01 Gy used in the 1982 UNSCEAR report) of malformed progeny, associated with the induction of reciprocal translocations in human males. Since, at present, it is unknown which of the non-human primate species may be the best model for man, the Committee prefers to retain the earlier estimate (made in 1977 and 1982, on the basis of the limited cytogenetic data in man and in the marmoset species Saguinus fuscicollis) to define a possible upper limit of risk, but with an appropriate correction introduced to take into account the newly estimated proportion of unbalanced zygotes (i.e., 9%) that will survive and result in congenitally

malformed children. This revised upper limit estimate of risk is $15 \cdot 10^{-6}$ per 0.01 Gy. Thus, the risk from the induction of translocations, expressed as congenitally malformed children in the F_1, is now estimated to lie in the range of 1-15 cases per million live births per 0.01 Gy.

524. *Induction of congenital anomalies in the progeny of irradiated parents.* Kirk and Lyon [K17] and Nomura [N9] have demonstrated the induction of congenital anomalies (scored shortly before birth) following spermatogonial irradiation of mice (paragraphs 343-344). However, neither the true nature of the dose-effect relationship nor the extent to which mice with these anomalies would survive to birth and thus overlap with other categories of genetic damage is yet clear. Therefore, these data have not been used in the present risk estimates.

525. *Summary of risk estimates obtained using the direct method.* These are given in Table 23. It can be seen that: (a) the estimates of the risk of induction of mutations leading to dominant genetic disease (based on the skeletal and cataract mutation data in mice) are the same as those arrived at in the 1982 UNSCEAR report (i.e., about 10-20 cases of affected individuals per 10^6 live births per 0.01 Gy of parental irradiation and about 0-9 cases of affected individuals per 10^6 live births per 0.01 Gy of maternal irradiation); (b) the risk estimate from the induction of genetic changes with dominant sub-lethal effects (based on the data on litter size reduction in mice) is given in footnote b of Table 23, since there is uncertainty about the extent to which such data can be extrapolated to the human situation (namely, the comparability of death between birth and weaning in mice with death in early extra-uterine human life); and (c) the risk associated with the induction of reciprocal translocations is now revised (relative to that given in the 1982 UNSCEAR report) to encompass a range of 1-15 cases of affected individuals per 10^6 live births per 0.01 Gy of low-LET paternal irradiation (and about 0-5 cases per 10^6 live births per 0.01 Gy under the same conditions for irradiation of females). This change was dictated by the new data obtained in the rhesus and crab-eating monkeys and the new analysis on the percentage of conceptions with unbalanced genomes that may result in children with congenital anomalies. Other details are given in the appropriate footnotes to Table 23.

526. *Summary of risk estimates obtained using the doubling dose method.* At present, there are no reasons to alter either the doubling dose estimate of 1 Gy (for chronic low-LET irradiation conditions) or the estimates of spontaneous prevalence of autosomal dominant, X-linked, autosomal recessive and chromosomal disorders. Consequently, the estimates of risk for these disorders are the same as those made in 1982 and these are reproduced in Table 24. However, the situation is different with respect to disorders of complex aetiology (congenital anomalies and other multifactorial disorders). In particular, new data on the latter (these disorders are predominantly of late onset) suggest that their spontaneous prevalence is much higher than was estimated in 1982 (1982: 4.7%; now estimated at about 60%). This difference is due to the fact that disorders that become manifest up to age 70 have now been included (in contrast with the inclusion of only those that become manifest up to age 21 in the 1982 report). Considerable uncertainty still remains on the following questions: (a) whether the doubling dose estimate of 1 Gy (based on clear-cut genetic end-points in the mouse, such as specific locus mutations, dominant visibles and reciprocal translocations) is applicable to disorders of complex aetiology; and (b) whether the estimate of 5% mutation component used in the 1977 and 1982 reports is a realistic figure for these disorders. In the absence of further information, and particularly on the mechanisms of maintenance of these disorders in the population and the effect of radiation on their prevalence, the Committee is not in a position to provide risk estimates for these disorders.

IX. ESTIMATES OF DETRIMENT FOR SPONTANEOUSLY ARISING MENDELIAN, CHROMOSOMAL AND OTHER DISORDERS

527. The 1982 UNSCEAR report reviewed the information available then on the approaches to the estimation of detriment associated with spontaneously arising Mendelian, chromosomal and other disorders and provided some tentative estimates using years of life lost and impaired as indicators. The results of studies that have since been carried out are summarized below.

A. THE EFFECTS OF MENDELIAN DISORDERS ON HUMAN HEALTH

528. Costa et al. [C74] and Hayes et al. [H61] conducted a literature survey to estimate the impact of Mendelian disorders on human health and their response to medical treatment. The asterisked entries (i.e., those with a confirmed mode of inheritance) in McKusick's 1978 catalogue [M79] were used as a basis for disorder selection (every third asterisked entry). From these (after exclusion of conditions due to neutral polymorphisms and of those for which insufficient information was available), the authors selected a total of 351 conditions (147 autosomal dominants, 170 autosomal recessives and 34 X-linked ones) for further analysis. Published information on each of these was collected and examined to determine age at onset, impact on longevity, reproduction and social handicap. However, no prevalence estimates are given for any of these conditions.

529. About 75% of these conditions were found to be disadaptive, impairing one or more of the following: life span, reproduction, development and/or social adjustment. Of these, 25% manifest themselves at birth, 70% by age three years and over, 90% by the end of puberty. With regard to age at onset, autosomal recessives and X-linked disorders show a unimodal distribution and almost all are expressed by reproductive age. Autosomal dominants, on the other hand, showed a trimodal age distribution with modes occurring during morphogenesis, infancy and early adult life.

530. About 58% of the conditions affect more than one bodily system and these are most often recessives and autosomal dominants and are, in general, associated with a single system involvement. Of the 351 conditions, 42.5% are compatible with a normal life span, as reported in the source literature and the remainder lead to premature death, most often in the pre- and intra-reproductive age groups. Autosomal recessives and X-linked ones have a more severe effect on longevity than autosomal dominants. Prognosis also differs with the system involved: among the conditions selected by the authors, those affecting the immune system carry the most severe prognosis, none being compatible with a normal life span and 64% causing death before 20 years of age. Involvement of the respiratory system, blood and blood-forming tissues, the nervous system and intermediary metabolism follow the immune system (in descending order) for their degree of impact on longevity.

531. Of all the conditions examined, 69% are associated with decreased reproductive capacity, the major contributors being autosomal recessives and X-linked conditions. The largest impact on reproductive capacity is seen in those phenotypes that affect the immune system, followed by the endocrine, the genitourinary and the nervous systems. About 75% of the conditions compatible with life beyond infancy affect schooling and/or ability to work. A severe handicap is most often associated with phenotypes involving (in descending order of severity) the nervous system, metabolic function, the musculoskeletal system, ears and eyes.

532. With respect to amenability to medical treatment, Hayes et al. [H61] estimate that the response is slight in the whole sample of 351 conditions: life span could be prolonged in 15% of the conditions, reproductive capacity in 11% and social adaptation in 6%. Among the 65 inborn errors of metabolism, treatment gives relief in 12%, partial response in 40% and none in the remaining 48%. The authors suggest that these findings have implications for prognosis, genetic counselling and medical care of patients with Mendelian disease.

B. DETRIMENT ASSOCIATED WITH CHROMOSOMAL ANOMALIES ASSESSED IN TERMS OF PSYCHOLOGICAL DISTURBANCES, LEARNING PROBLEMS, GROWTH AND DEVELOPMENT

533. Bancroft et al. [B21], Ratcliffe [R8], Ratcliffe and Field [R9] and Ratcliffe et al. [R10, R11] presented their results on the assessment of psychological disturbances and educational problems in children with sex-chromosomal anomalies. Eighteen XYY, 23 XXY and 16 XXX children aged between 2 and 13.5 were examined as part of a long-term follow-up study of these children. All three conditions were found to have a significant degree of language delay, the XXY and XXX conditions being more affected. Likewise, the children exhibited significant deficits in cognitive ability with the XXX being more severely affected in this respect. Furthermore, all three condi-

tions showed disturbances and delay in the development of social behaviour: the XXX girls and XXY boys had difficulty in forming relationships, the XXY and XYY boys had excess negative moods and XYY boys had a greater incidence of maladjustment than the other two groups or controls. Nonetheless, no individual in this series had any serious mental retardation or abnormality. Although the sample sizes are small, it is worth stressing that the group studied represents an unbiased sample (the children were those included in the Edinburgh new-born cytogenetic survey) and the conclusions, therefore, are of greater general relevance than those derived from selected groups (e.g., cytogenetic surveys of mentally retarded individuals and inmates of penitentiaries).

534. In another paper, Tierney et al. [T14] reported the results of a longitudinal study of growth and development on 30 (of the 36) children who were identified as having structural chromosome rearrangements in the Edinburgh new-born survey. In addition, 4 siblings who had structural chromosomal anomalies were included. The breakdown is: 7 de novo and 7 familial reciprocal translocations, 3 de novo and 9 familial Robertsonian translocations, 3 Y-autosome translocations and 5 inversions of chromosomes other than chromosome 9 (children with inversion of chromosome 9 were considered to have a normal variant). Two hundred and twenty children with normal karyotype (220) from the same new-born population were used as controls.

535. The principal findings were the following: (a) the IQ scores of the 10 children with de novo Robertsonian or reciprocal translocations were significantly lower than those of 20 children with familial translocations, but not lower than those of normal controls; however, there were 3 children in the de novo group of above-average intelligence; (b) 7 children with familial reciprocal translocations had significantly higher IQ scores than those with familial Robertsonian translocations (n = 9) and control groups; (c) with the exception of one child with a de novo reciprocal translocation who died (and who was characterized as mentally retarded), all other children attended normal schools. These limited data are consistent with the view that balanced structural rearrangements are probably not as harmful (based on cytogenetic studies in primarily mentally retarded populations; reviewed in the 1982 UNSCEAR report; see also chapter I) as previous reports have implied.

C. DETRIMENT ASSOCIATED WITH SPONTANEOUSLY ARISING CONGENITAL ANOMALIES IN MAN ESTIMATED USING YEARS OF LIFE LOST OR IMPAIRED AS INDICATORS

536. In chapter I, the results of Hungarian studies [C13] on birth prevalences of isolated and multiple congenital anomalies in man were presented and compared with those for the United States and Canada. It was pointed out that the Hungarian prevalence of 597.4 per 10^4 live births (of which about 43% is due to congenital dislocation of the hip) may

be an underestimate of the true prevalence rate and that the underestimation relates primarily to the less serious major congenital anomalies. However, the fact that in Hungary systematic records of the mortality of individuals with congenital anomalies are kept and organized according to ICD codes, provided the possibility for their use, in conjunction with prevalence data, to construct mortality profiles for each of the different congenital anomalies and to make reliable estimates of detriment.

537. Some of the essential aspects of the analysis carried out by Czeizel and Sankaranarayanan [C13] are the following:

(a) The birth prevalences for congenital anomalies in conjunction with the total number of births (1,975,524) for the study period 1970-1981 permitted estimates of the total numbers of individuals with given congenital anomalies;

(b) The Central Statistical Office, Budapest, provided data on the mortality of individuals with congenital anomalies who died at specific ages/age-intervals (a total of 23 age-groups/age-intervals); these data were used to construct a mortality profile and to estimate mean ages at death. For the sake of brevity and convenience in presentation, the mortality data were grouped into three age groups: infant death (from day 0 to 365th day), early death (ages 1-19), late death (ages 20-69);

(c) In calculations on the mean number of years of lost life for any given congenital anomaly, the average life expectancy for the general population was assumed to be 70 years (in fact, for the study period, the mean life expectancy for the general population was 66.8 years for males and 73.1 years for females in Hungary);

(d) Since, in the case of congenital anomalies, one is dealing with birth defects, individuals with congenital anomalies were considered to have potentially impaired life for the duration of their life span;

(e) Since the degree of impairment depends on the nature of the handicap and the efficacy of medical procedures, actual life impairment was considered to exist if the proportion of handicapped individuals (even after appropriate medical help) with a given congenital anomaly was equal to or more than 15%; this was an arbitrary cut-off point, based on consultations with a number of specialists in Hungary;

(f) The total number of years of lost life was computed by multiplying live birth prevalence by the average number of years of life lost; similarly, the total number of potentially impaired years of life for each kind of congenital anomaly was calculated by multiplying the live birth prevalence by the mean life expectancy of individuals;

(g) The total number of actually impaired years of life was calculated by multiplying the estimate for potentially impaired life years (entry (f) above) by the percentage of individuals with the persistent handicap.

538. Table 25 presents an overall summary of the results (see [C13] for details). It can be seen that, with a total prevalence of about 600 per 10^4 live births (i.e., 600 individuals affected with one or another kind of isolated or multiple congenital anomaly per 10^4 live births) used in the calculations, about 4800 years of life are lost, 37,000 years of life are potentially impaired (of which about one-half is due to congenital dislocation of the hip) and 4500 years of life are actually impaired per 10^4 live births. In terms of the average number of years of lost life (an index of detriment at the individual level), the CNS anomalies cause the greatest amount of detriment, followed by anomalies of the respiratory and cardiovascular systems, chromosomal anomalies, and others. Anomalies of the ear, face and neck, of genital organs and of the musculoskeletal system and cleft lip, with or without cleft palate, have a small or negligible effect in this regard. When the ranking is done according to the total number of years of life lost (an index of detriment at the population level), however, anomalies of the cardiovascular system are associated with the highest amount of detriment, followed by those of the central nervous system and others.

539. The total number of potentially impaired years of life—a measure of the upper limit of impairment that would be expected when suitable medical facilities are unavailable and a reflection of the contribution of some of the less serious anomalies—is highest for musculoskeletal anomalies; this is due to the fact that in Hungary congenital dislocation of the hip has a very high birth frequency (257.7 per 10^4 as compared to about 10 per 10^4 for many other European and European-derived populations; see Carter [C25]).[aa] If the latter figure is used, the number of potentially

[aa]Czeizel and Tusnády [C32] have extensively discussed the possible reasons for the high prevalence of congenital dislocation of the hip in Hungary. Among these, the following four deserve mention: (a) a genuinely high rate of incidence in the Hungarian population; (b) owing to the low birth rate in Hungary, the proportion of first-born is high (in Budapest, 64.3% of live births in 1962-1967 were first-born) and this condition is more common among first-born; (c) relaxation of selection: in earlier generations, a severe congenital dislocation of the hip was a serious obstacle for marriage, pregnancy and childbirth and thus interfered with the transmission of genetic liability. However, this condition can now be successfully treated with no adverse effects on fitness; this means that the genes involved are being transmitted without hindrance and therefore the liability for this condition may increase in the future; and (d) the high prevalence is most probably a reflection of widespread adoption of neo-natal and infantile orthopaedic screening and the consequent high rate of detection. Because of this early and extensive screening, a large number of cases of diagnosed dysplasia of the hip joint of lesser severity are subjected to treatment together with true congenital dislocation of the hip. While undoubtedly a considerable proportion of congenital dislocation of hip cases of lesser severity heal spontaneously, there is evidence [F19] that, in a certain percentage of these cases, osteo-arthrosis of the hip develops in adult life. Thus, the large number of cases of congenital dislocation of the hip that undergo treatment may lead to a reduction in the prevalence of osteo-arthrosis in adults. However, it is likely that some infants with merely an unstable hip or with adduction contracture are unnecessarily subjected to treatment. It is worse, of course, not to recognize and treat congenital dislocation of the hip than to place a presumably normal child in the Pavlik stirrup. Sometimes, it is impossible to draw a sharp line between conditions requiring treatment and those likely to recover spontaneously among the dysplasias observed in infants 3-4 months old. Furthermore, unjustified delay may mean that one misses the most adequate time for treatment and by treating a less severe dysplasia one may prevent osteo-arthrosis in adult life.

impaired life years for musculoskeletal conditions will be reduced from about 18,000 to 3100 years. (The total birth prevalence of all congenital anomalies will also be reduced from 597.4 per 10^4 to 349.7 per 10^4).

540. An index of detriment based on years of actually impaired life provides a good perspective of the situation under modern medical conditions. As will be clear from Table 25, with this criterion anomalies of the cardiovascular system are associated with the highest amount of detriment, followed by those involving the genital organs, chromosomal anomalies and others.

541. There are at least two reasons why the estimates of detriment presented in Table 25 may be underestimates. Firstly, it is clear that these figures are heavily dependent on the Hungarian birth prevalences, which, as mentioned earlier, may be underestimates. Secondly, the frequencies of chromosomal disorders are certainly underestimated in Hungary, at least by a factor of 3. This is clear not only from the results of chromosome surveys of new-born children (summarized in [U1]) but also from the fact that partial deletions and duplications involving every chromosome of the human complement are now known (but we do not yet have estimates of prevalences), and from the ongoing studies on the relationship between mental retardation and the fragile site on the X-chromosome (see chapter I).

D. COMPARISON OF THE ESTIMATES OF DETRIMENT FOR MENDELIAN, CHROMOSOMAL AND OTHER DISORDERS

542. Table 26 compares the estimates of detriment for Mendelian and chromosomal disorders made by Carter [C26] (see also [U1]) with those made by Czeizel and Sankaranarayanan [C13] for congenital anomalies. It is clear that monogenic disorders with a total birth prevalence of 125 per 10^4 live births account for about 1900 years of lost life, 3000 years of potentially impaired life and 1500 years of actually impaired life, per 10^4 live births. Congenital anomalies, on the other hand, account for over 4500 years of lost life, 37,000 years of potentially impaired life (about half of which is due to congenital dislocation of the hip) and 4000 years of actually impaired life per 10^4 live births. The estimates of Carter for chromosomal disorders per 10^4 live births (prevalence, 40; lost life-years, 900; potentially impaired life-years, 1800; and actually impaired life-years, 900) are probably more reliable, for reasons mentioned earlier, although, here too, partial deletions and duplications of chromosomes and X-linked mental retardation due to fragile-X have not been included.

E. FREQUENCY AND ECONOMIC BURDEN OF GENETIC DISEASE IN A PAEDIATRIC HOSPITAL

543. Carnevale et al. [C75] surveyed a total of 2945 admissions to the National Institute of Paediatrics in Mexico City to assess the frequency of admission and the economic burden due to disorders with a genetic basis. The patients were classified into five categories: (a) single-gene disorders; (b) chromosomal disorders; (c) complex genetic aetiology; (d) unknown aetiology; and (e) non-genetic disorders. Of all the admissions studied, 126 or 4.3% fell into the first two categories (61 autosomal dominants, 20 autosomal recessives, 20 X-linked recessives and 25 chromosomal), 998 (33.5%) into the complex aetiology group, 406 (13.8%) into the group with unknown causes and 1425 (48.4%) into the group of non-genetic disorders. In terms of economic burden, patients of categories (a)-(c) came more frequently from outside the city and had more admissions for longer durations with a higher number of surgeries. On the basis of all the data, the authors suggest that Mendelian and chromosomal disorders and those of complex aetiology, although less frequent than environmentally caused diseases, impose a considerable financial burden on the hospital and affected families.

F. SUMMARY AND CONCLUSIONS

544. A literature survey has been conducted to estimate the impact of Mendelian disorders on human health and their response to medical treatment. About 75% of the 351 conditions (autosomal dominant, autosomal recessive and X-linked) included in the analysis were found to be harmful, impairing one or more of the following: life span, reproduction, development and/or social adjustment. About 42% are compatible with a normal life span and the remainder lead to premature death, most often in the pre- and intra-reproductive age groups. Autosomal recessives and X-linked disorders have a more severe effect on longevity than autosomal dominants. Medical treatment can help to prolong life span in 15% of the conditions, reproductive capacity in 11% and social adaptation in 6%.

545. In a long-term follow-up of children with numerical sex-chromosomal anomalies and autosomal structural anomalies (ascertained in the Edinburgh new-born survey), the detriment associated with these anomalies was assessed using psychological development, learning and cognitive abilities, social behaviour and growth and development as end-points. While children with sex-chromosomal anomalies (XXY, XXX, XYY) had some problems (language delays, deficits in cognitive ability, higher incidence of maladjustment, etc.), none of them had any serious mental retardation or other handicap that could be characterized as really adverse. Likewise, there were no really adverse effects associated with balanced autosomal translocations. Children with familial translocations had significantly higher IQ scores than those with de novo ones and all children attended normal schools. The sample sizes involved in these studies, however, are small.

546. The detriment associated with spontaneously arising isolated and multiple congenital anomalies has been assessed on the basis of data available from Hungary. In these calculations, the average life expectancy for the general population was assumed to be 70 years. It has been found that, with a total estimated

prevalence of about 600 per 10^4 live births, these congenital anomalies may cause, per 10^4 live births, about 4800 years of life loss, about 37,000 years of potentially impaired life and about 4500 years of actually impaired life. However, one-half of the total potentially impaired years of life is due to congenital dislocation of the hip, which is known to have a high birth prevalence in Hungary.

547. Estimates of detriment for congenital anomalies made in the present report are much higher than those for Mendelian and chromosomal disorders (in terms of years of lost life or impaired life) made in the 1982 UNSCEAR report. Mendelian and chromosomal disorders as well as those of complex aetiology impose a considerable burden on medical care facilities and on affected families.

Table 1

Cytogenetic abnormalities and embryonic and fetal death
by gestational age
(from Hook [H1])

	Gestational age in completed weeks					
	5-7	8-11	12-15	16-19	20-27	All known (pooled)
Proportion abnormal among those karyotyped a/	24/137	488/965	625/1330	156/475	49-456	1342/3363
Per cent abnormal a/	17.5	50.6	47.0	32.8	10.7	39.9
95% confidence interval b/	12.4-23.8	47.7-53.5	44.6-49.4	29.2-36.7	8.4-13.4	
Range (in %) among studies	14.0-25.8	40.4-64.4	39.1-56.2	18.5-69.6	6.6-27.0 c/	

a/ Calculated from data from 5 specific studies (in Honolulu, Geneva, Hiroshima, London, New York) presented by Warburton et al. [W1].
b/ Assuming homogeneity among populations studied. In fact the ranges suggest that at least for the 16-19 week group this is unlikely.
c/ Excluding extremes of 0 and 40% in two studies in which only small numbers of fetuses were studied.

T a b l e   2

Proportion of recognized conceptuses
with cytogenetic abnormalities by interval
(from Hook [H1])

Gestational interval (weeks)	Per cent cytogenetically abnormal in those lost in intervals a/	x	Proportion of recognized conceptuses lost in interval (%)	=	Proportion of embryos or fetuses that have cytogenetic abnormality detected during interval (%)
5-7	17.5	x	6.3	=	1.1
8-11	50.6	x	3.3	=	1.7
12-15	47.0	x	2.5	=	1.2
16-10	32.8	x	1.0	=	0.3
20-27	10.7	x	1.4	=	0.14
>28 (stillbirths)	5.7	x	1.0	=	0.06
Total			15.5		4.5

Total of all recognized pregnancies that
  (a) result in fetal or embryonic death
  (b) have cytogenetic abnormality   =   4.5%

Live births with recognized chromosome abnormality
(0.6%) x proportion of eventual live births among
recognized conceptions (84.5%)   =   0.5%

Total = estimated proportion of recognizable
conceptions with chromosome abnormality   =   5.0%

a/ Calculated using data from Harlap et al. [H62] on fetal and embryonic
    death rates from 5 to 27 weeks, and assuming a 1% fetal death rate
    (still birth rate) thereafter, and using data from Warburton et al. [W2]
    on abnormalities in those from 5 to 28 weeks; from Sutherland et al. [S1]
    on still birth; and from Hook and Hamerton [H2] on live births.
    Note that ages are in completed weeks, so interval 20-27, for example,
    is from day 140 to day 195 inclusive.

T a b l e   3

A comparison of the frequencies of chromosomal anomalies in new-borns
(anomalies detected using chromosome banding methods)
in surveys carried out in Norway [H13] and Denmark [N1]
with those in other surveys (summarized in [U1])
in which banding techniques were not used

Aberration type	Norway (1830 children; banded preparations of chromosomes)		Denmark (3658 children; banded preparations of chromosomes)		(11,148 children; no banding of chromosomes)		Pooled studies a/ (59,465 children; no banding of chromosomes)	
	No.	Frequency (%)	No.	Frequency (%)	No.	Frequency (%)	No.	Frequency (%)
Sex-chromosomal anomalies	5 b/	0.27	15 g/	0.41	29	0.26	134	0.23
Autosomal trisomies	5 c/	0.27	7 h/	0.19	18	0.16	88	0.15
Robertsonian translocations	4 d/	0.22	3 i/	0.08	17	0.15	57	0.10
Reciprocal translocations	5	0.27	7	0.19	15	0.13	61	0 10
Autosomal inversions excluding those of chromosome 9	1	0.05	2	0.05	1	0.01	9	0.02
Others	4 e/	0.22	5 f/	0.13	13 j/	0.12	23	0.04
Subtotal	24	1.30	39	1.05	93	0.83	372	0.64
Inversions, chromosome 9	12	0.66	35	0.96	-	-	-	-
Total	36	1.96	74	2.01	93	0.83	372	0.64

a/   Results of 7 surveys; see [U1] for details.
b/   One case of 47,XYY, one case of 47,XXY and 3 inversions of Y.
c/   One case of +18, 3 cases of +21 and one case of +21 mosaic.
d/   2 cases of t(13q;14q) and 1 case of t(14q;21q).
e/   2 cases of small supernumerary chromosomes and 2 cases of small
     supernumerary/mosaics.
f/   1 case of +mar, 2 cases of +ring and 2 cases of duplications.
g/   3 cases of 47,XXY, 2 cases of 47,XYY, 3 cases of 47,XXX, 4 cases of
     45,X and 2 cases of inversion Y.
h/   One case of +18, 5 cases of +21 and 1 case of +8.
i/   2 cases of t(13;14) and 1 case of t(14;21).
j/   6 cases of +mar, 1 deletion and 6 cases of unbalanced Y-autosome
     translocations.

Table 4

Comparison of the results of surveys of mentally retarded patients
(From Rasmussen et al. [R1])

Total examinations	Down's syndrome (%)	Autosomal other than Down's (%)	Sex-chromosomal anomalies (%)	Total (%)	Ref.
6163	9.7	1.3	0.9	11.8	[J1]
512	8.2	1.9	1.0	11.1	[A1]
756	12.0	0.8	0.8	13.6	[F1]
449	7.3	0.6	0.2	8.2	[K2]
7880	9.7	1.2	0.8	11.7	
1905 a/	14.7	2.4	1.8	18.8	[R1]

a/ In banded chromosome preparations.

Table 5

Major chromosome aberrations in patients with
multiple congenital anomalies (MCA) / mental retardation (MR) syndromes
(from Coco and Penchaszadeh [C1])

	Sex chromosome aberrations		Autosomal aneuploidy (excl.21)		Deletions and rings		Extra markers or rings		Structural rearrangement a/		Other		Total		Ref.
	No.	%	No.	%	No.	%	No.	%	No.	%	No.	%	No.	%	
50			1	2.0	1	2.0	1	2.0			1	2.0	4	8.0	[S3]
50	1	2.0			2	4.0			2	4.0			5	10.0	[D1]
170	1	0.6	2	1.2	1	0.6	3	1.8	4	2.4	2	1.2	13	7.6	[A2,A3]
50					1	2.0					2	4.0	3	6.0	[W3]
121	1	0.8	9	7.2	5	4.1			4	3.3			19	15.7	[C2]
15b/									2	13.3	1	6.7	3	20.0	[L1]
50					1	2.0			2	4.0			3	6.0	[T2]
50					2	4.0	1	2.0	3	6.0			6	12.0	[M2]
90	1	1.1			2	2.2			1	1.1	1	1.1	5	5.5	[D2]
51	1	2.0	1	2.0	2	3.9	1	2.0					5	9.8	[E2]
199c/	4	2.0	9	4.5	14	7.0	1	0.5	12	6.0			40	20.1	[O1]
200							1	0.5	4	2.0			5	2.5	[T1]
200	5	2.5	11	5.5	10	5.0	3	1.5	13	6.5			42	21.0	[C1]
Total: 1296	14	0.8	33	1.7	41	2.8	11	0.8	47	3.7	7	1.2	153	11.0	

a/ Includes unbalanced rearrangements (duplications and/or deficiencies) and apparently balanced interchanges.
b/ MR and MCA individuals from a total of 54 patients with mental retardation studied.
c/ After sorting out individuals with Down syndrome and other known conditions among 384 patients with MCA/MR syndromes and not taking into account two individuals with minor familial chromosome variants.

113

T a b l e   6

Chromosomal anomalies in 958 infertile males
[D24]

Autosome anomalies		Sex chromosome anomalies	
Type	Number	Type	Number
45, XY, t(DqDq)	1	47, XXY	21
45, XY, t(13q14q)	4	46, XX	3
45, XY, t(14q21q)	1	47, XXY/46, XX	1
45, XY, t(14q22q)	1	47, XYY	1
46, XY, t(11;22)(q23;q11)	3	46, X, inv(Y)	5
46, XY, t(3;11)(q24;q24)	1	46, X, ter rea(Y)	1
46, XY, t(6;11)(q26;q22)	1	46, X, del(Yq)	2
46, XY, t(6;20)(q16;p13)	1	46, Y, t(X;1)(q27;q31)	1
46, XY, t(5;8)(p14;q11)	1	46, X, t(Y;5)(q11;p15)	1
46, XY, t(10;14)(q25;q13)	1		
46, XY, inv(1)(p22;q32)	1		
46, XY, inv(7)(p22;q21)	1		
46, XY, inv(10)(p11;q21)	1		
47, XY, +mar	1		
48, XY, +mar, +mar	2		
46, XY, 11qfra	1		
Total	22	Total	36

a/   del = deletion; ter rea = end to end translocation; inv = inversion; t = translocation; p = short arm of chromosome; q = long arm of chromosome; fra = fragile site; +mar = additional small marker chromosome. Except for 3 cases of inv(Y), all sex-chromosome anomalies were found among azoospermics. Among autosome anomalies, only two cases of t(13q14q), the t(3;11) and the inv(1) were found in azoospermics.

T a b l e   7

A comparison of the prevalence of chromosomal anomalies in subfertile men as a whole and in azoospermics alone with those in surveys of new-borns
[D24]

Anomaly	Prevalence per 10^3 males in		
	Newborns	All subfertiles a/	Azoospermics a/
XXY	1.24 b/	34 (x30)	129 (x100)
XX (males)	0.05	1 (x20)	8 (x160)
XYY	0.92	1	3 (x3)
In(Y)	0.24	1.4 (x 5)	4 (x16)
Robertsonian translocations c/	0.92	7.2 (x 8)	2.7 (x3)
Reciprocal translocations c/	1.05 d/	8.3 (x 8) e/	3.6 (x3) e/
Autosomal inversions	0.62	3.5 (x 6) d/	2.4 (x4) d/
Supernumeraries	0.32	1.9 (x 6)	2.7 (x9)

a/   Prevalence estimates based on all studies summarized by Dutrillaux et al., unless otherwise stated. The factor by which these are higher in the first two groups relative to the new-borns is given in parenthesis.

b/   Includes mosaics with an XXY cell line.

c/   Note that the situation is different from that of sex-chromosomal anomalies in which the magnitude of increase (relative to new-borns) is higher among azoospermics than among subfertiles as a whole.

d/   Includes only studies done with chromosome banding.

e/   Includes only the data of Dutrillaux et al. since this study is the largest one carried out using chromosome banding.

T a b l e   8

Chromosomal anomalies in 820 infertile males

Type	Patients No.	Patients %	Sperm count/ml
Sex chromosomal abnormalities (3.4%)			
47,XXY	21	2.5	Azoospermia
47,XYY	1	0.1	Azoospermia
46,XY/47,XXY	4	0.5	Azoospermia
47,XXY/48,XXXY	1	0.1	Azoospermia
46,XX	1	0.1	Azoospermia
Autosomal translocations (1.0%)			
13/14	4	0.5	$(0.8-12)\ 10^6$
14/21	2	0.2	$(1.0-3)\ 10^6$
1/3 (p34/q21)	1	0.1	Azoospermia
3/5 (q24/q13)	1	0.1	$1,0\ 10^6$
6/10 (q14/q22)	1	0.1	Azoospermia
Inversion 9 (p11q12)	22	2.7	9 azoospermia 13 oligozoospermia
Inversion 9 (p23/q33)	1	0.1	$6\ 10^6$
Chromosomal variants (9.3%)			
Yq+	27	3.3	18 azoospermia 9 oligozoospermia
Yq-	17	2.1	7 azoospermia 10 oligozoospermia
21h+	12	1.5	7 azoospermia 5 oligozoospermia
22h+	6	0.7	6 oligozoospermia
1h+	2	0.2	2 oligozoospermia
13h+	3	0.4	3 oligozoospermia
14h+	2	0.2	1/1 azoo/oligozoospermia
15h+	6	0.7	1/5 azoo/oligozoospermia
16h+	2	0.2	1/1 azoo/oligozoospermia

The prevalence of fra(X) in different groups of individuals studied

Authors' group designation	Males			Females			Refs.
	Number	fra(X)	%	Number	fra(X)	%	
Neonates (Australia)	1810	0	–	1648	0	–	[S5, S86]
Institutionalized retarded (Australia)	444	7	1.6	80	0	–	[S5]
Males with mental retardation of unknown origin in an institution (Finland)	150	6	4.0	–	–	–	[K10]
Institutionalized retarded (moderate to severe) (Belgium)	354	57	16.1	30	1	3.3	[F29]a/
Severely retarded boys (IQ< 50) from various registers (Sweden)	96	7	7.3	–	–	–	[B2, B25]
Less severely retarded children from various registers (Sweden)	110	5	4.5	61	0	–	[B25]
Sheltered workshops for mentally handicapped (Australia)	84	0	–	44	0	–	[S86]
Special schools for mentally handicapped (Australia)	328	11	3.4	174	2	1.1	[S86]
	–	–	–	128	5	3.9	[T31]
Retarded individuals in community placement (Hawaii, United States)	274	5	1.8	278	1	0.4	[J12, M54]
Referral patients (Australia)	2283	13	5.3	1890	3	1.6	[S86]

a/ The 58 fra(X) positive individuals were found to belong to 37 different families.

T a b l e   10

Break-points in constitutional chromosome rearrangements: a summary
[H28, H29]

Origin of rearrangement	Break-points in rearrangements a/			
	In bands with fragile site			
	Number	Observed	Expected	Ratio of observed to expected
Maternal	269	56	29.6	1.9
Paternal	202	40	22.2	1.8
Unknown b/	701	128	77.1	1.7
Total	1172	224	128.9	1.8

a/ Includes data from amniocentesis studies [H28] and those
    from spontaneous abortions, still births and new-borns.

b/ Includes de novo rearrangements.

117

Specific chromosomal changes associated with particular types of cancers
involving bands where fragile sites have been assigned
or located near such bands
(General references [B43, L11, Y4, Y11])

Chromosome and fragile site	Chromosomal abnormality and break-points	Cancer	References
2q13	t(2;8)	Burkitt's lymphoma	[L11, Y4]
3p14	t(3;18)(p21;q12)	Mixed salivary gland tumour	[M55]
	t(3;11)(p13-14;p15)	Renal cell carcinoma	[P31]
	t(3;9)(p21;q24)	Renal cell carcinoma	[C60]
	del(3)(p14;p23)	Small cell lung carcinoma	[W38]
	del(3)(p14)	Breast carcinoma	[A16]
6p23	t(6;9)(p23;q34)	Acute non-lymphocytic leukaemia	[S88]
7p11	del(7q)	Acute non-lymphocytic leukaemia	[L11, Y4]
8q22	t(8;21)(q22;q22)	Acute myeloblastic leukaemia-M2	[R49, S89]
9p21	t(9;11)(p21;q23)	Acute monoblastic leukaemia	[H44]
	del(9)(p21)	Acute lymphocytic leukaemia	[K36]
11q13	t(11;14)(q13;q32)	Non-Hodgkin lymphoma	[F30]
	t(11q); del(11q)	Acute myeloid and lymphoid leukaemias and lymphomas	[L11, Y4]
11q23	t(11;12)(q23 or q24; q12)	Ewing's sarcoma	[L11, Y4]
	t(9;11)(p21;q23)	Acute myeloblastic leukaemia-M5	[H44]
	t(4;11)(q21;q23)	Acute lymphocytic leukaemia	[V12]
12q13	+12	Chronic lymphocytic leukaemia	[L11, Y4]
	t(9;12)(p12;q13)	Mixed salivary gland tumour	[M56]
16q22	inv(16)(p13;q22)	Acute myeloblastic leukaemia-M4	[L11]
	del(16)(q22)	Acute non-lymphocytic leukaemia	[A17]
17p12	t(15;17); inv(17q)	Acute promyelocytic leukaemia; chronic myelogenous leukaemia (blast crisis)	[L11, Y4]
20p11	del(20q)	Myeloproliferative disorder	[L11, Y4]

Note: some fragile sites (2q13, 7p11, 12q13, 17p12 and 20p11) may or may not
coincide with the break-points of the chromosomal changes involved in the
different cancers shown in the Table.

**A comparison of birth prevalences of congenital anomalies
in the United States [M12], Hungary [C13] and British Columbia [T9]
(based on ref. [C13])**

ICD code	Congenital anomaly	Prevalence[a]/ per 10^4			
		United States	Hungary		British Columbia
		Total births	Total births	Live births	Live births
740–741	Anencephaly and spina bifida	17.4 (42) [b]/	16.6	10.3	9.2
742	Other anomalies of the nervous system	35.2 (85)	14.6	11.4	7.9
743	Anomalies of the eye	23.6 (57)	3.2	3.2	7.8
744	Anomalies of the ear, face and neck	14.9 (36)	4.7	4.6	6.0
745–747	Cardiovascular anomalies	86.5 (209)	80.8	79.2	42.6
748	Anomalies of the respiratory system	14.1 (34)	2.8	2.8	1.5
749	Cleft palate and cleft lip	27.3 (66)	14.8	14.5	17.5
750–751	Anomalies of the digestive system	61.7 (149)	27.8	27.8	17.6
752–753	Anomalies of the genital organs and urinary system	115.5 (279)	93.7	90.9	27.5
754–756	Musculoskeletal and skeletal anomalies excluding congenital dislocation of the hip	364.7 (881)	56.5	55.0	52.0
757	Anomalies of the integument	101.4 (245)	7.6	7.4	2.4
758	Chromosomal anomalies	16.1 (39)	12.6	12.6	14.1
759	Other and unspecified anomalies	12.8 (31)	21.5	20.0	1.9
	Subtotal CAs	891.2 (2153)	–	–	–
	Subtotal, affected births	632.1–775.0 [c]/	357.2	339.7	208.0 [d]/

ICD code	Congenital anomaly	Prevalence[a]/ per 10^4			
		United States	Hungary		British Columbia
		Total births	Total births	Live births	Live births
754.1	Congenital dislocation of the hip	73.3 (177)	257.7	257.7	14.2
	Total CAs (ICD 740-759)	964.5(2330)	-	-	-
	Total, affected births (ICD 740-759)	704.0-846.1 e/	614.9	597.4	222.0 f/ 374.0 g/ 428.0 h/
550	Inguinal hernia	127.9 (309)	110.4	110.4	1.4
553	Umbilical hernia	10.8 (26)	9.4	8.8	3.2
227-228	Congenital tumours	6.2 (15) (350)	1.2	1.2	9.6
	Grand total, CAs	1109.6(2680)	-	-	-
	Grand total, affected births	849.2(2051) i/	735.9	717.8	236.4

a/ Unless otherwise stated, the United States prevalence figures refer to the number of congenital anomalies (and not to the number of affected births); in the other two studies, the figures are based on the numbers of affected individuals.

b/ The figures given in parentheses (column 4) refer to the number of congenital anomalies on which the prevalence estimates given in column 3 are based.

c/ The estimate of 632.1 is arrived at by assuming that the number of births with congenital dislocation of the hip, hernias and tumours is the same as the number of these CAs (= 527) and that a total of 2051-527 = 1524 births have 2153 CAs or roughly 1.41 CAs per affected births. Therefore, 891.2/1.41 = 632.1 births are affected by CAs. The estimate of 775.0 is arrived at by a similar procedure, assuming that the affected births = 2051-177 = 1874. These had 2153 CAs or roughly 1.15 CAs per affected birth; 891.2/1.15 = 775.0.

d_/ The figure of $208.0/10^4$ is for the period 1952-1972 (excluding congenital dislocation of the hip).

e/ The estimate of 704.0 is arrived at by assuming that the number of cases affected with hernias and congenital tumours is the same as the number of these CAs (= 350) and that a total of 2051-350 = 1701 cases had 2330 CAs or 1.37 CAs per affected case. Therefore, 946.5/1.37 = 704.0. The value of 846.1 is arrived at by assuming that 2051 affected births had 2330 CAs or roughly 1.14 per affected birth. Thus the number of affected births is 964.5/1.14 = 846.1.

f/ The figure of 222.0 is applicable to the total period of 1962-1972, including the congenital dislocation of the hip.

g/ The minimal estimate of Trimble and Doughty [T9] for the total prevalence of CAs (ICD entries 740-759).

h/ The corrected or adjusted estimate of Trimble and Doughty [T9] for the total prevalence of CAs (ICD entries 740-759).

q/ The number of malformed births in a total of 24,153 [M12].

Some epidemiological features of selected multifactorial disorders in man a/

ICD	Disorder	Population prevalence per 10^4		Sex-ratio M : F	Onset (yrs)		Herita-bility	References	
		Hungary	Other countries		Mean	Range		Hungarian studies	Others
242	Thyrotoxicosis with or without goitre (Grave's disease)	65	100 b/ (25–500) c/	1:4	42	13–62	0.47	[S116]	[B70, O19]
250.0	Diabetes mellitus (adult onset; non-insulin dependent, type II)	407	480 (190–1600)	1:2	60	20–	0.65	[B71]	[K50, W49, N34, R63, K51]
250.1	Diabetes mellitus (juvenile onset; insulin-dependent, type I)	20	20 (8–56)	1:1	11	1–19	0.30		
274	Gout	18	30 (13–37)	15:1	25	18–55	0.50	[M74]	[C70]
295	Schizophrenic psychoses	85	100 (70–200)	1:1	25	15–45	0.80	[P46,U8 a/]	[G56, K52, P47, S117]
296	Affective psychoses (uni- and bi-polar depression)	110	131 (40–500)	1:2	40	20–60	0.80	[R64]	[A22, E27, G57, S117, W50]
340	Multiple sclerosis	4	5 (1–13)	1:2	33	10–50	0.58	[P48]	[B72, S118, S119, S120]
345	Epilepsy	60	170 (33–429)	1:1	4	0–70	0.50	[R65]	[A23, D63, G58, N35]
365	Glaucoma	160	160 (80–220)	1:1	55	20–	0.32	[L51]	[F39, H55]
401	Essential hypertension	850	500 (200–1000)	1:1	60	10–	0.75	[U9]	[N36, N37]
410–441	Acute and sub-acute myocardial infarction	359	500 (300–2000)	3:1	50	30–	0.65	[C71,G59]	[M75, S121]
454	Varicose veins of lower extremities	1250	500 (200–3560)	1:3	30	20–	0.70	[L52]	[H56]
477	Allergic rhinitis	360	400 (300–500)	1:1	25	5–50	0.48		
493	Asthma	249	500 (50–900)	1:1	35	1–70	0.70	[S122]	[R66]
531–533	Gastric ulcer, duodenal ulcer, peptic ulcer, site unspecified	460	500 (150–900)	2:1	45	30–60	0.65	[N38]	[D64, R63]
556	Idiopathic proctocolitis (colitis ulcerosa)	3	5 (4–10)	1:1	35	20–60	0.60	[P49]	[B73]
574	Cholelithiasis	94	100 (40–120)	1:3	35	25–	0.63	[H57, R67]	[V18, W51]
579.0	Coeliac disease	13	12 (3–25)	1:1	1	1–10	0.80		[D65]
592	Calculus of kidney and ureter	90	60 (10–150)	2:1	45	30–60	0.70	[B74]	
691	Atopic dermatitis and related conditions, mainly eczema	60	70 (50–80)	1:1	18	10–25	0.50	[M76]	[M77]
696	Psoriasis and related disorders	39	130 (10–400)	1:1	20	10–60	0.75	[B75]	[R68]
710.0	Systemic lupus erythematosus	4	4 (2– 7)	1:9	34	13–45	0.90	[N39,S123]	[H58, K53, L53]
714.0	Rheumatoid arthritis	131	179 (50–500)	1:2	40	35–64	0.83	[S124]	[L54, L55, L56, O20, P50]
720.0	Ankylosing spondylitis	19	18 (5–23)	5:1	23	18–35	0.79	[G60]	[E28]
732.0	Juvenile osteochondrosis of spine	1100	900 (400–1500)	1:2	12	8–18	0.56	[B76]	[H59, F40]
737.3	Adolescent idiopathic scoliosis	41	33 (13–64)	1:2	13	10–18	0.88	[B77, C72]	[S125]
	Total	6051	5607						

a/ Preliminary data (Czeizel et al.).
b/ Best estimate.
c/ Range of prevalences reported in different studies.

Table 14

<u>Some restriction endonucleases and their recognition and cleavage sites (*)</u>
(from [E18]; a more exhaustive list is given in [R19])

Enzyme	Organism	Cleavage site (*) 5' .... 3'
TETRANUCLEOTIDES (4)		
AluI	Arthrobacter luteus	A G * C T
HaeIII	Haemophilus aegyptius	G G * C C
HpaII	Haemophilus parainfluenzae	C * C G G
MboI	Moraxella bovis	* G A T C
TaqI	Thermus aquaticus	T * C G A
MspI	Moraxella species	C * C G G
PENTANUCLEOTIDES (5)		
AvaII	Anabaena variabilis	G * G (A/T) C C
DdeI	Desulfovibrio desulfuricans	C * T N A G
EcoRII	Escherichia coli R.245	* C C (A/T) G G
HinfI	Haemophilus influenzae Rf	G * A N T C
HEXANUCLEOTIDES (6)		
AvaI	Anabaena variabilis	C * Py C G Pu G
BalI	Brevibacterium albidum	T G G * C C A
BamHI	Bacillus amyloliquefaciens H	G * G A T C C
BglII	Bacillus globigii	A * G A T C T
EcoRI	Escherichia coli RY13	G * A A T T C
HaeII	Haemophilus aegyptius	Pu G C G C * Py
HincII	Haemophilus influenzae Rc	G T Py * Pu A C
HindIII	Haemophilus influenzae Rd	A * A G C T T
HpaI	Haemophilus parainfluenzae	G T T * A A C
HsuI	Haemophilus suis	A * A G C T T
PstI	Providencia stuartii	C T G C A * G
SacI	Streptomyces achromogenes	G A G C T * C
SalI	Streptomyces albus	G * T C G A C
SmaI	Serratia marcescens	C C C * G G G
XmaI	Xanthomonas malvacearum	C * C C G G G
SphI	Streptomyces phaeochromogenes	G C A T G * C
HEPTANUCLEOTIDES (7)		
MstII	Microcoleus species	C C * T N A G G

Note: some enzymes (isoschizomers) recognize the same sequence
(e.g., HindIII and HsuI; HpaII and MspI).
Py = pyrimidine, Pu = purine, N = any base.

Table   15

Analysis of human genetic disease by means of recombinant DNA technology
(based on [C35] with some additions)

Disease	Gene probe	Ref.
A. DIRECT ANALYSIS OF GENETIC DISEASE USING GENE PROBES TO DETECT INTRAGENIC DEFECTS		
Antithrombin III deficiency	Antithrombin III	[P17]
α-Antitrypsin deficiency	Synthetic oligonucleotide	[K19]
Atherosclerosis	Apolipoprotein A-1	[K20]
Diabetes	Insulin	[H31]
Ehlers-Danlos syndrome	α(1) Collagen	[P18]
Growth hormone deficiency	Growth hormone	[P19]
Haemophilia B	Factor IX	[G26]
Hereditary persistance of fetal haemoglobin	β-Globin	[F20,T22]
Hypoxanthine-guanine phosphoribosyl-transferase (HPRT) deficiency	HPRT	[W20]
Lesch-Nyhan syndrome	HPRT	[Y7, N16]
Osteogenesis imperfecta	Pro α1(1) collagen	[C36, P18]
Retinoblastoma	Chromosome 13 DNA segments	[C37]
Sickle cell anaemia	β-Globin	[G19]
	Synthetic oligonucleotide	[C38]
Thalassaemia	α- and β-globin	[O11, L12]
	Synthetic oligonucleotide	[O10]
B. INDIRECT ANALYSIS OF GENETIC DISEASE USING GENE PROBES TO DETECT LINKED POLYMORPHISMS		
Atherosclerosis	Apolipoprotein A-1	[K21]
Diabetes (type II)	Insulin	[R22,R23]
Growth hormone deficiency type I	Growth hormone	[P20]
Hypertriglyceridaemia	Apolipoprotein A-1	[R24]
Sickle cell anaemia	β-Globin	[K13, P21, B27]
Lesch-Nyhan syndrome	HPRT	[N16, Y7]
Osteogenesis imperfecta	pro α2(1) Collagen	[T23]
Phenylketonuria	Phenylalanine hydroxylase	[W21]
Thalassaemia	β-Globin	[B27]

Disease	Probe	Distance between probe and disease locus (cM)	Ref.
C. INDIRECT ANALYSIS OF GENETIC DISEASE USING CLONED DNA SEGMENTS TO DETECT LINKED DNA POLYMORPHISMS			
Fragile-X mental retardation syndrome	Factor IX	<12	[C29]
Huntington's chorea	G8	<10	[G27]
Menkes kinky hair	LI.28	16	[W22]
Muscular dystrophy			
Becker	LI.28	16	[K12]
	LI.28	19	
	RC8	20	[K22]
	pDP34	38	
Duchenne	λRC8	17	[D18]
	LI.28	17	[D18]
Myotonic dystrophy [D16]	Complement C3 gene	7	
Retinoschisis	λRC8	15	[W24]
Steroid-sulphatase-X-linked ichthyosis	λRC8	25	[W23]
Retinitis pigmentosa	LI.28	3	[B28]

123

Table 16

Identified oncogenes and their viral prototypes
(from references [B13, C3, D11])

Gene a/	Prototype virus	Isolation source	Protein products		Cancer in animals			Transformation in cell culture	
			Biochemical function	Subcellular location	Sarcoma	Carcinoma	Acute leukaemia	Fibroblasts	Blood cells
v-src	Rous sarcoma virus	Chicken	PK(tyr)b/	Plasma membrane	+	-	-	+	?
v-fps c/	Fujinami sarcoma virus	Chicken	PK(tyr)	Plasma membrane	+	-	-	+	-
v-fes c/	Snyder-Theilin feline sarcoma virus	Cat	PK(tyr)	Plasma membrane	+	+	-	+	-
v-yes	Y-73 Yamaguchi sarcoma virus	Chicken	PK(tyr)	?	+	-	-	+	-
v-ros	Rochester-2 sarcoma virus	Chicken	PK(tyr)	?	+	-	-	+	-
v-myc	Myelocytomatosis virus strain MC29	Chicken	DNA binding	Nucleus	+	+	+	+	+
v-erb-A v-erb-b	Avian erythroblastosis virus	Chicken	?	Cytoplasm/ membranes	+	+	+	+	+
v-myb	Avian myeloblastosis virus	Chicken	?	Nucleus	-	-	+	-	+
v-rel	Avian reticuloendotheliosis virus strain T	Turkey	?	?	-	-	+	-	+
v-mos	Moloney murine sarcoma virus	Mouse	?	Cytoplasm	+	-	-	+	-
v-abl	Abelson leukaemia virus	Mouse,cat	PK(tyr)	Plasma membrane	-	-	+	+	+
v-fos	FBJ murine osteosarcoma virus	Mouse	?	?	+d/	-	-	+	?
v-Ha-ras v-bas e/	Harvey rat sarcoma virus	Rat/mouse	Binds GTP; PK(thr)f/	Plasma membrane	+	+	-	+	?
v-Ki-ras	Kirsten rat sarcoma virus	Rat		Plasma	+	+	-	+	?
v-fms	SM feline sarcoma virus	Cat	?	Membranes	+	-	-	+	-
v-sis	Simian sarcoma virus	Woolly monkey/cat	?	?	+	-	-	+	-

a/ The names of viral genes are treated here as generic terms, although, in most instances, several separate viral isolates are known and the proteins encoded by the homologous oncogenes in the different isolates may differ in size.

b/ PK denotes protein kinase; the aminoacid subject to phosphorylation is given in parentheses.

c/ The genes fps and fes are homologous genes of viruses from different species.

d/ Osteosarcoma.

e/ Names assigned before adoption of a standard nomenclature; homologous genes transduced from different species are now given the same name. Examples include abl from mice and cats and sis from woolly monkeys and cats.

f/ Binds guanine nucleotides and carries out autophosphorylation on threonine.

124

Table 17

Candidate oncogenes detected as transforming genes in the NIH/3T3 cells
[V13 a/]

Genes	Examples of cell types in which transforming activity is found b/
c-Ha-ras1	Bladder carcinoma cell line (human) Urinary tract tumours (human) Lung carcinoma cell line (human) DMBA and MNU-induced mammary carcinomas (rat) DMBA/TPA-induced skin papillomas, benign and malignant (mice) Melanoma cell line (human) Mammary carcinosarcoma line (human) MC, BP, DEN and MNNG-transformed primary cells (guinea pig) Myeloid tumour cell line (mouse)
c-Ki-ras2	Lung carcinomas and cell lines (human) Colon carcinomas and cell lines (human) Pancreatic carcinoma cell line (human) Gall bladder carcinoma cell line (human) Rhabdomyosarcoma cell line (human) Ovarian carcinoma, primary (human) Acute lymphocytic leukemia line (human) MC-induced fibrosarcomas and MC-transformed fibroblasts (mouse) γ-irradiation induced thymoma (mouse) MC-induced thymic lymphoma and macrophage tumour lines (mouse) BP-induced fibrosarcoma (mouse)
N-ras	Neuroblastoma cell line (human) Burkitt lymphoma line (human) Fibrosarcoma and rhabdomyosarcoma cell lines (human) Promyelocytic leukaemia line (human) T cell leukaemia line (human) Melanoma cell lines (human) Teratocarcinoma line (human, late passage) Lung carcinoma line (human) Acute and chronic myeloblastic leukaemia (human) Lung carcinoma cell line (mouse) Carcinogen-induced thymoma (mouse)
c-mos	Plasmocytoma cell lines (mouse)
c-erbB-related	ENU-related neuroblastoma cell lines (rat)
Blym	ALV-induced bursal lymphomas (chickens) Burkitt lymphoma lines (human)
Tlym	Intermediate T cell lymphoma lines (human) MLV-induced T cell lymphomas (mouse)
tx-1	Mammary carcinoma cell line (human) MMTV and DMBA-induced mammary carcinomas (mouse)
tx-2	Pre B tumour cell lines (human) AbMLV-induced pre B tumour cell lines (mouse)
tx-3	Myeloma and plasmocytoma cell lines (human, mouse)
tx-4	Mature T cell lymphoma lines (human, mouse)
Unnamed Unnamed	Pre B cell leukaemia cell line (human) MNNG-treated osteosarcoma cell line

a/ To be consulted for detailed references.
b/ Abbreviations: MC, methylcholanthrene; DMBA, dimethylbenzanthracene;
   TPA, tetradecanoyl-13-phorbol acetate; MNU, methylnitrosourea;
   MNNG, N-methyl-N-nitro-nitroguanidine; BP, benz(a)pyrene;
   DEN, diethylnitrosamine; ENU, ethylnitrosourea.

T a b l e   18

Mutations in transforming ras genes
[V13]

Source of allele	ras allele	Codons 12	Codons 59	Codons 61	References
Normal	Human c-Ha-ras1	GGC gly	GCC ala	CAG gln	[C16]
Normal	Rat c-Ha-ras1	GGA gly	?	?	[S94]
Ha-MSV	v-Ha-ras	AGA arg	ACA thr	CAA gln	[D47]
RaSV	v-Ra-ras a/	AGA arg	GCA ala	CAA gln	[R54]
Bladder Ca lines	Human EJ/T24-Ha-ras1	GTC val	GCC ala	CAG gln	[T5, S65, R2, C16, T11]
Lung Ca line	Human HS242-Ha-ras1	GGC gly	GCC ala	CTG leu	[Y5]
Mammary Ca	Rat NMU-Ha-ras1	GAA glu	?	?	[S94]
Normal	Human c-Ki-ras2	GGT gly	GCA ala	CAA gln	[M13]
Ki-MSV	v-Ki-ras	AGT ser	ACA thr	CAA gln	[T36]
Lung Ca line	Human Calu-Ki-ras2	TGT cys	GCA ala	CAA gln	[S63, C17]
Colon Ca line	Human SW480-Ki-ras2	GTT val	GCA ala	CAA gln	[C17]
Lung Ca	Human LL-10-Ki-ras2	CGT arg	?	?	[S95]
Lung Ca line	Human A2182-Ki-ras2	CGT arg	?	?	[S95]
Bladder Ca line	Human A1698-Ki-ras2	CGT arg	?	?	[S95]
Lung Ca line	Human PR371-Ki-ras2	TGT lys	?	?	[N21]
Lung Ca line	Human PR310-Ki-ras2	GGT gly	GCA ala	CAT his	b/
Normal	Human N-ras	GGT gly	GCT ala	CAA gln	[T24]
Neuroblastoma line	Human SK-N-ras	GGT gly	GCT ala	AAA lys	[T24]
Teratocarcinoma line, late passage	Human PA1-N-ras	GAT asp	?	?	[T37]
Fibrosarcoma line	Human HT1080-N-ras	?	?	AAA lys	b/
Malignant melanoma line	Human Mel N-ras	GGT gly	GCT ala	AAA lys	b/
Lung Ca line	Human SW1271 N-ras	GGT gly	GCT ala	CGA arg	[Y10]

a/ Amino acid positions aligned with those of other ras proteins.
b/ Personal communications to [V13].

Table 19

Localization of cellular oncogenes to human chromosomes
(Based on [B13, G29, R12, Y4])

Cellular oncogene	Chromosomal location	Ref.
N-ras	1p11→p13	[H15, M14, R14, R26]
c-src	1p34→p36	[L14]
c-fos	2	[B13]
c-myb	6q22→24	[D14, H16]
	6q21→qter	[Z2]
c-Ki-ras1	6	[O5]
c-mos	8q22	[N12, P12]
c-myc	8q24	[D14, N12, T12]
c-abl	9q34.1	[D5, H5, J16]
c-Ha-ras1	11p11→15	[M15, O5, F22]
	11p14.1	[J17]
c-ets a/	11q23→24	[D31]
c-Ha-ras2	X	[O5]
c-Ki-ras2	12	[O5, S36]
c-fes	15q26.1	[H5, H16, D14, J16]
c-erb-A	17	[G29 W25]
c-src	20q12→13	[L14]
c-sis	22q13.1	[J16]

a/ Cellular counterpart located 3' to v-myb in the acute E26 acute leukaemia avian virus.

Table 20

Induction by x rays of heritable reciprocal translocations in mouse spermatogonia
[G16]

Exposure (R)	Number of male progeny tested	Number of translocation heterozygotes a/	Frequency (%)	Expected frequency (%) b/
0	5433	1	0.018	
150	3078	19	0.62	0.63
300	3342	46	1.38	2.04
600	1075	20	1.86	4.18
1200	1038	6	0.58	0.94
500x4 c/	1135	84	7.40	10.42
600x2 d/	1198	64	5.34	7.23

a/ The frequencies for the irradiated groups are based on all partially sterile males plus the steriles that have been cytologically confirmed; in the controls, the frequency is based on partially steriles only.
b/ The expected frequencies were estimated from cytogenetic data using the assumptions employed by Ford et al [F7].
c/ Fractionated exposures. Interval between doses, 4 weeks.
d/ Fractionated exposures. Interval between doses, 8 weeks.

Table 21

Induction of reciprocal translocations in primate species,
studied cytogenetically through spermatocyte analysis of irradiated males

Species	Number of animals	Radiation	Dose (Gy)	Dose rate (Gy/min)	Number of cells	Translocation yield (%) Definite plus possible	Definite	Ref.
Macaca mulatta	1	x	1.00	0.63	1815	1.4	0.8	[L40]
(Rhesus monkey)	2	x	2.00	0.63	1130	1.5	1.2	[L40]
	2	x	3.00	0.63	478	1.0	1.0	[L40]
Macaca mulatta	22	none	–	–	3600	–	0.08	[V14]
(Rhesus monkey)	6	x	0.25	0.30	5940	–	0.19	and
	6	x	0.50	0.30	2750	–	0.36	[V15]
	7	x	1.00	0.30	4650	–	0.86	
				(Rate of induction up to 1 Gy: 0.86 10^{-2}/Gy)				
	7	x	2.00	0.30	3350	–	0.99	
	4	x	3.00	0.30	1475	–	0.68	
	4	x	1.00	0.002	3870	–	0.34	
	6	γ	1.00	0.0002	15900	–	0.43	
	3	γ	1.00	0.14	7700	–	0.43	
	3	x	4.00	0.30	1450		0	
	3	x		0.30	560	–	0.71	
			2.00+2.00 Gy (24 h interval)					
Saguinus	2	none	–	–	600	–	0	[B61]
fusicollis	2	x	0.25	a/	600	–	2.80	
(marmoset)	2	x	0.50	a/	600	–	3.30	
	2	x	1.00	a/	600	–	7.80	
	1	x	2.00	a/	200	–	7.50	
	2	x	3.00	a/	600	–	7.00	
			(Rate of induction up to 1 Gy: 7.44 10^{-2}/Gy)					
Callithrix	4	none	–	–	230	–	0	[V5]
jacchus	2	x	0.50	0.35	260		0.80	and
(marmoset)	4	x	1.00	0.35	420		1.20	[V11]
	4	x	2.00	0.35	880		0.80	
Macaca	6	none	–	–	4700		0.09	[M27]
fascicularis	3	γ	0.25	0.25	4500	0.56	0.53	and
(Crab-eating	3	γ	0.50	0.25	4500	1.16	1.07	[M69]
monkey)	4	γ	1.00	0.25	3500	1.91	1.86	
	3	γ	2.00	0.25	3000	2.67	2.47	
	3	γ	3.00	0.25	3000	1.50	1.33	
			(Rate of induction up to 1 Gy: 1.79 10^{-2}/Gy)					
	2	γ	1.00	0.18 10^{-4}	4000	–	0.28	[T45]
	2	γ	1.50	0.18 10^{-4}	4000	–	0.33	
			(Rate of induction up to 1.5 Gy: 0.16 10^{-2}/Gy)					
Human	2	none	–	–	200	–	0	[B61]
	2	x	0.78	a/	371		4.00	
	2	x	2.00	a/	300	–	7.00	
	2	x	6.00	a/	180	–	6.10	
			(Rate of induction up to 2 Gy: 3.41 10^{-2}/Gy) (Rate of induction up to 1 Gy and including Saguinus fusicollis data: 7.7 10^{-2}/Gy)					

a/ Not given.

Mutagen-induced survival and mutagenesis (experiments using a viral probe)
[H53]

Virus (DNA)	Host	Host treatment	Maximal reactivation treatment	Induced mutagenesis	Ref.
λ	E.coli	UV	26	8-10 (clear plaques)	[D53]
λ	E.coli	UV	20	8-10 (clear plaques)	[B65]
λ(r)	E.coli	UV	4	4 (clear plaques)	[B65]
HSV	Monkey kidney (CV-1)	UV	2	-	[B66]
HSV	Monkey kidney (CV-1)	γ ray	10(0 d), 4(3 d)	-	[B67]
HSV	Monkey kidney (CV-1)	HU	3	-	[L43]
HSV	Monkey kidney (CV-1)	Aflatoxin B₁3(0 h)-10(40 h) AAAF		-	[L44]
HSV	Monkey kidney (Vero)	UV	2(16 h)	2.7 (tk→tk-)(16 h)[1]	[D54]
HSV	Human kidney (NBK)	UV	2(36 h)	-	[G51]
HSV	Normal human fibroblasts(KD)	UV	2(4 d)	-	[L45]
HSV	Xeroderma pigmentosum	UV	2-3(4 d)	-	[L45]
SV40	Monkey kidney (CV-1)	UV	2.4(0 d, 4 d)	-	[B67]
SV40	Monkey kidney (CV-1P)	UV	7(1 d)[10⁻²]	-	[S108]
SV40	Monkey kidney (CV-1P)	UV	10(1 d)	10-100 (ts→wt)(1 d)[10⁻⁴]	[S109]
SV40	Monkey kidney (CV-1)	γ ray	6-8(0 d, 4 d)	-	[B67]
SV40	Monkey kidney (CV-1P)	AAAF	6(1 d)	20-25(ts→wt)(1 d)[1 10⁻³]	[S110]
SV40	Monkey kidney (CV-1P)	AAAF		27[5 10⁻⁴]	[D55]
SV40	Monkey kidney (CV-1P)	Aflatoxin B1 AAAF MMF EMS	4-20(1 d-3 d)[10⁻²]	-	[S108]
SV40	Monkey kidney (CV-1P)	Mitomycin C	100(1 d)	8-16(ts→wt)(1 d)[6 10⁻⁴]	[S110]
SV40	Monkey kidney (BSC-1)	UV	3(3 d)	1(ts→wt)(3 d)[10⁻³] a/	[C65]
SV40-DNA	Monkey kidney (CV-1P)	UV	4.9(1 d)	1(ts→wt)(1 d) a/	[G52]
SV40-DNA	Monkey kidney (CV-1P)	Mitomycin C	3(1 d)	1(ts→wt)(1 d) a/	[G52]
SV40-DNA	Monkey kidney (BSC-1)	UV	5(3 d)	-	[C65]
Simian adenovirus 7	Monkey kidney (CV-1)	UV	2(0 d)-15(4 d)	-	[B67]
Simian adenovirus 7	Monkey kidney (CV-1)	γ ray	1.3(0 d)-10(5 d)	-	[B67]
Adeno 5	Normal human fibroblasts	UV	-	1(ts→wt)20 h [1] a/	[D56]
Adeno 2	Normal human fibroblasts	γ ray	3- 5 b/	-	[J25]
Adeno 2 (γ) c/	Normal human fibroblasts	γ ray	5-15 b/	-	[J26]
Minute-virus of mice d/	Mouse A9	UV	4(30 h)[0.5-30]	-	[R60]
Parvovirus LuIII	Human kidney (NBK)	UV	2(0 d, 2 d)	-	[G51]
Kilham rat virus	Rat cells	UV	2(0 d, 2 d)	-	[G51]
Vaccinia	Monkey kidney (CV-1)	UV	1(0 d, 4 d)	-	[B67]
Polio	Monkey kidney (CV-1)	UV	1(0 d, 4 d)	-	[B67]

Reactivation factor: $\dfrac{\text{Survival of irradiated virus on treated host}}{\text{Survival of irradiated virus on non-treated host}}$

Induced mutagenesis: $\dfrac{\text{Mutation frequency of the irradiated virus in treated host}}{\text{Mutation frequency of the irradiated virus in non-treated host}}$

The virus is UV-irradiated, except when stated otherwise. In some experiments, the time elapsed between host cell treatment and infection is indicated in parentheses, the multiplicity of infection is given in square brackets. The type of mutation screened for is also indicated. The list is incomplete, particularly for the bacterial systems described.
HU, hydroxyurea: AAAF, acetoxyacetylaminofluorene; MMS, methylmethanesulfonate; EMS, ethylmethanesulfonate

a/ Irradiated viral DNA could itself fully induce a mutation mechanism in the host cell.
b/ Here survival is calculated from V antigen positive cells.
c/ Extremely high γ dose of 3 Mrad.
d/ Single-strand DNA virus.

Table 23

Risk of induction of genetic damage in man per 0.01 Gy
at low dose rates of low-LET irradiation, according to the direct method
(see Table 24 for risk estimates using the doubling dose method)

Genetic damage	Expected frequency (per 10^6 live birth) of genetically abnormal children in the first generation after irradiation	
	Males	Females
Mutations having dominant effects a/ b/	~ 10 to ~ 20 c/	0 to ~ 9 d/
Recessive mutations e/	0	0
Unbalanced products of reciprocal translocations	~ 1 to ~ 15 f/	0 to ~ 5 g/

a/ Includes risk from the induction of dominant mutations, deletions and balanced reciprocal translocations with dominant effects and from that of the most detrimental effects of recessives.

b/ Does not include the risk of induction of genetic changes with dominant sub-lethal effects which may kill between birth and early life (between 5 and 10 cases per 10^6 live births per 0.01 Gy of paternal irradiation; estimated on the basis of data on litter size reduction in mice; see VII.A.3 for details). For maternal irradiation, a comparable estimate is not available.

c/ The lower limit of ~ 10 is derived from the data on dominant cataract mutations and the upper limit of ~ 20 from those on dominant skeletal mutations (both in mice). The latter is the same as that arrived at in the 1977 report [U2]. A multiplication factor of 2 has been used in the estimate based on skeletal data, but not in the one based on cataract data. This factor is an attempt to allow for the likelihood that many dominant mutations (especially those affecting bodily systems other than the skeleton) remain to be detected. A correction factor of 0.5, which allows for skeletal mutations that are not clinically significant, is not required for the estimate based on cataract data. See the 1982 report [U1] for details.

d/ The lower limit of zero is based on the assumption that the mutational sensitivity of human immature oocytes is similar to that of mouse immature oocytes; the upper limit of ~ 9 is based on the assumption that the sensitivity of the human oocytes is similar to that of the mature and maturing mouse oocytes and that the latter is 0.44 times that of spermatogonia. See the 1982 report [U1] for details.

e/ Although the risk of recessive disease from the induction of recessive mutations is zero in the first generation, about 1 extra case per million live births would be expected in the following ten generations from partnership effects and, on certain assumptions, about 10 extra cases per million would be expected by the tenth generation from effects due to identity by descent. See [S126] for further details.

f/ The lower limit of ~ 1 per million is based on combined cytogenetic data from chronic low-LET irradiation experiments involving the rhesus monkey and the crab-eating monkey (see paragraphs 522-523) and the upper limit of ~ 15 per million is based on the combined human and marmoset Saguinus fuscicollis cytogenetic data [U2]. It has been assumed that 9% of unbalanced products of reciprocal translocations will result in the birth of congenitally malformed children (paragraph 502), while the remaining 91% lead to intra-uterine death, often at a very early embryonic stage.

g/ The lower limit of zero is based on the assumption that the sensitivity of the human immature oocytes to the induction of heritable reciprocal translocations will be similar to that of the mouse immature oocytes with respect to the induction of chromosome aberration phenomena. The upper limit of ~ 5 per million is based on the assumptions: (a) that the sensitivity of the human immature oocytes to the induction of reciprocal translocations will be one-half of that of human and marmoset spermatogonia (based on results with mice on heritable translocations); (b) that the frequency of unbalanced products will be six times that of recoverable balanced translocations; and (c) that about 9% of unbalanced products will result in congenitally malformed children (paragraph 502). See the 1982 report [U1] for details.

Estimated effect of 0.01 Gy per generation of low dose
or low dose rate low-LET irradiation
on a population of one million live-born, according to the doubling dose method
[The doubling dose assumed in these calculations is 1 Gy
(see Table 23 for risk estimates using the direct method)]

Disease classification	Current incidence	Effect of 0.01 Gy per generation	
		First generation	Equilibrium
a/	b/	c/	
Autosomal dominant and X-linked diseases d/	10000	15	100
Autosomal recessive diseases	2500 e/	Slight	Slow increase
Chromosomal diseaes due to:			
Structural anomalies	400 f/	2.4	4
Numerical anomalies	3400 g/	Probably very small	Probably very small

a/ Follows that given in the BEIR Report [B79], except that chromosomal diseases are divided into those with structural and those with numerical anomalies.

b/ Based on the results of the British Columbia survey and other studies; for details see the 1977 Report [U2]; note that the new data on congenital anomalies and other multifactorial disorders are not used (see paragraphs 73-93 and 526).

c/ The first generation increment is assumed to be 15% of the equilibrium value for autosomal dominant and X-linked diseases and about 3/5 of the equilibrium value for structural anomalies. See the 1977 and 1982 reports [U2, U1] for details.

d/ Includes diseases with both early and late onset, but excludes the fragile-X syndrome.

e/ Also includes diseases maintained by heterozygous advantage.

f/ Unbalanced structural rearrangements.

g/ Excludes mosaics.

T a b l e   25

Summary of birth prevalences and detriment estimates for congenital anomalies
(from [C13])

ICD code	Congenital anomaly	Prevalence per 10^4 live births	Average years of lost life	Total years lost per 10^4 live births	Total years per 10^4 live births	
					Potentially impaired	Actually impaired
740-742	CNS anomalies	21.7	55.1	1191.8	327.2	287
743	Eye anomalies	3.2	13.4	43.4	180.6	100
744	Anomalies of ear, face and neck	4.6	0	0	322.0	97
745-747	Cardiovascular system anomalies	79.2	23.5	1838.5	3722.2	981
748	Anomalies of respiratory system	2.8	24.5	65.9	130.1	72
749	Cleft palate, cleft lip ± cleft palate	14.5	2.1	33.3	981.7	224
750-751	Anomalies of the alimentary system	27.8	16.1	433.1	1512.1	69
752	Anomalies of genital organs	75.2	0	0	5264.0	720
753	Anomalies of the urinary organs	15.7	13.2	207.1	891.9	399
754	Anomalies of the muscoloskeletal system (excluding congenital dislocation of the hip)	34.3	0	0	2399.9	101
754.3	Congenital dislocation of the hip	257.7	0	0	18039.0	180
755-756.5	Anomalies of skeletal system	20.7	13.0	268.1	1180.9	268
758	Chromosomal anomalies	12.6	24.8	312.7	569.3	560
756.6-757.9 and 759	Miscellaneous (including multiple) congenital anomalies	27.4	15.9	434.4	1483.6	432
		597.4	8.1	4828.3	37004.5	4490

T a b l e   26

Summary of detriment estimates for spontaneously-arising Mendelian, chromosomal and other disorders

All estimates are per 10^4 individuals and an assumed life expectancy
at birth of 70 years for the general population.
(The estimates for monogenic and chromosomal disorders are those
of Carter discussed in the 1982 Report [U1]
and those for congenital anomalies, of Czeizel and Sankaranarayanan, [C13])

Category	Prevalence	Total years of lost life	Total years of potentially impaired life	Total years of actually impaired life
Monogenic	125	1900	3000	1500
Chromosomal a/	40	890	1800	900
Congenital anomalies b/	585	4515	37000 c/	3930

a/ Does not include the fragile site on the X-chromosome which is associated with mental retardation.
b/ Excluding chromosomal anomalies.
c/ One-half of this is due to congenital dislocation of the hip.

REFERENCES

A1   Ally, F.E. and H.J. Grace. Chromosome abnormalities in South African mental retardates. S. Afr. Med. J. 55: 710-712 (1979).

A2   Atnip, R.L., J.D. Williams and R.L. Summitt. A controlled cytogenetic study of mentally defective children with other anomalies. Excerpta Medica Int. Cong. Ser. 233: 18-19 (1971).

A3   Atnip, R.L. 1977; cited in A.T. Tharapel and R.L. Summitt, Ref. T1.

A4   Ananiev, E.V., V.A. Gvozadev, Yu.V. Ilyin et al. Reiterated genes with varying location in intercalary heterochromatin of Drosophila melanogaster polytene chromosomes. Chromosoma 70: 1-17 (1978).

A5   Aurias, A., M. Prieur, B. Dutrillaux et al. Systematic analysis of 95 reciprocal translocations of autosomes. Hum. Genet. 45: 259-282 (1982).

A6   Albertini, R.J. Drug-resistant lymphocytes in man as indicators of somatic cell mutation. Teratog., Carcinog., Mutag. 1: 25-48 (1980).

A7   Alwine, J.C., D.J. Kemp and G.R. Stark. Method for detection of specific RNAs in agarose gels by transfer to diazogenzyloxymethyl paper and hybridization with DNA probes. Proc. Natl. Acad. Sci. U.S.A. 74: 5350-5354 (1977).

A8   Antonarakis, S.E., C.D. Boehm, P.J.V. Giardina et al. Non-random association of polymorphic restriction sites in the beta-globin gene cluster. Proc. Natl. Acad. Sci. U.S.A. 79: 137-141 (1982).

A9   Angell, R.R., R.J. Aitken, P.F.A. van Look et al. Chromosome abnormalities in human embryos after in vitro fertilization. Nature 303: 336-338 (1983).

A10 Altukhov, Yu. P. Monitoring of human populations for genetic load: theoretical and experimental considerations. Paper presented at the Joint Expert Consultation Meeting (UNEP/WHO) on Genetic Monitoring. 1978, Moscow.

A11 Alitalo, K., M. Schwab, C.C. Lin et al. Homogeneously-staining chromosomal regions contain amplified copies of an abundantly expressed cellular oncogene (c-onc) in malignant neuroendocrine cells from a human colon carcinoma. Proc. Natl. Acad. Sci. U.S.A. 80: 1707-1711 (1983).

A12 Antoniades, H.N., C.D. Scher and C.D. Stiles. Purification of human platelet-derived growth factor. Proc. Natl. Acad. Sci. U.S.A. 76: 1809-1813 (1979).

A13 Alstein, A.D. Oncogenes of tumour viruses. Zh. Vsesojuzn Chim. Ob-Va-Im Mendeleeva 18: 630-635 (1973) (in Russian).

A14 Albertini, R.J., K.L. Castle and W.R. Borchording. T-cell cloning to detect mutant 6-thioguianine resistant lymphocytes present in human peripheral blood. Proc. Natl. Acad. Sci. U.S.A. 79: 6617-6621 (1982).

A15 Aymes, S and A. Lippman-Hand. Maternal age effect in aneuploidy: does altered embryonic selection play a role? Am. J. Hum. Genet. 34: 558-565 (1982).

A16 Ayraud, N., J.C. Lambert, K. Hufferman-Tribollet et al. Etude de cytogenetique comparative de sept carcinomes d'origine mammaire. Ann. Genet. 20: 171-177 (1977).

A17 Arthur, D.C. and C.D. Bloomfield. Partial deletion of the long arm of chromosome 16 and bone marrow eosinophilia in acute non-lymphocytic leukaemia. A new association. Blood 61: 994-998 (1983).

A18 Antonarakis, S.E., H.H. Kazazian and S.H. Orkin. DNA polymorphism and molecular pathology of the human globin clusters. Hum. Genet. 69: 1-14 (1985).

A19 Antonarakis, S.E., S.D. Kittur, C. Metaxotou et al. Analysis of DNA haplotypes suggests a genetic predisposition to trisomy 21 associated with DNA sequences on chromosome 21. Proc. Natl. Acad. Sci. U.S.A. 82: 3360-3364 (1985).

A20 Albertini, R.J. Somatic gene mutations in vivo as indicated by the 6-thioguanine resistant T-lymphocytes in human blood. Mutat. Res. 150: 411-422 (1985).

A21 Albertini, R.J., J.P. O'Neill, J.N. Nicklas et al. Alteration of the hprt gene in human in vivo derived 6-thioguanine resistant T lymphocytes. Nature 316: 369-371 (1985).

A22 Angst, J., R. Frey, B. Lohmeyer et al. Bipolar manic depressive psychosis. Results of a genetic investigation. Hum. Genet. 55: 237-254 (1980).

A23 Anderman, E. Multifactorial inheritance of generalized and focal epilepsy. p. 355-374 in: Genetic Basis of Epilepsy (N.E. Anderson et al., eds.). Raven Press, New York, 1982.

A24 Abrahamson, S. Risk estimates for genetic effects. p. 223-250 in: Assessment of Risk from Low Level Exposure to Radiation and Chemicals: A Critical Overview (A.D. Woodhead et al., eds.) Plenum Press, New York, 1985.

B1   Bishop, M.J. Oncogenes. Sci. Am. 246: 68-78 (1982).

B2   Blomquist, H.K., K.H. Gustavson, G. Holmgren et al. Fragile site X chromosomes and X-linked mental retardation in severely retarded boys in a northern Swedish study. Clin. Genet. 21: 209-214 (1982).

B3   Bishop, M.J. Enemies within: the genesis of retrovirus oncogenes. Cell 23: 5-6 (1981).

B4   Bukhari, A.I., J.A. Shapiro and S.L. Adhya (eds.). Insertion elements, plasmids and episomes. Cold Spring Harbor Laboratory, New York, 1977.

B5   Bregliano, J.C., G. Picard et al. Hybrid dysgenesis in Drosophila melanogaster. Science 207: 606-611 (1980).

B6   Berg, R.L. A simultaneous mutability rise at the singed locus in two out of three Drosophila melanogaster populations studied in 1973. Dros. Inf. Serv. 51: 100-102 (1974).

B7   Brewen, J.G. The induction of chromatid lesions by cystosine arabinoside in post-DNA synthetic human lymphocytes. Cytogenetics 4: 28-36 (1965).

B8   Brewen, J.G. and N.T. Christie. Studies on the induction of chromosomal aberrations in human leucocytes by cytosine arabinoside. Ext. Cell Res. 46: 276-291 (1977).

B9   Bender, M.A. and R.J. Preston. Role of DNA base damage in aberration formation: interaction of aphidicolin and x-rays. p. 37-46 in: Progress in Mutation Research, Vol. 4, 1982.

B10   Benjamin, R.C. and D.M. Hill. Poly(ADP-ribose) synthesis in vitro programmed by damaged DNA. A comparison of DNA molecules containing different types of strand breaks. J. Biol. Chem. 255: 10502-10508 (1980).

B12   Berenblum, I. and N. Trainin. Possible two-stage mechanism in experimental leukemogenesis. Science 132: 40-41 (1960).

B13   Bishop, M.J. Cellular oncogenes and retroviruses. Ann. Rev. Biochem. 52: 301-354 (1983).

B14   Balmain, A. and I.B. Pragnell. Mouse skin carcinomas induced in vivo by chemical carcinogens have a transforming Harvey-rat oncogene. Nature 303: 72-74 (1983).

B15   Battey, J., C. Moulding, R. Taub et al. The human c-myc oncogene: structural consequences of translocation into the IgH locus in Burkitt lymphoma. Cell 34: 779-787 (1983).

B16   Brown, D.D. Gene expression in eukaryotes. Science 211: 667-674 (1981).

B17   Botstein, D., R.L. White, M. Skolnick et al. Construction of a genetic map in man using restriction fragment length polymorphisms. Am. J. Hum. Genet. 32: 314-331 (1980).

B18   Banbury Report 14. Recombinant DNA Applications to Human Disease (C.T. Caskey and R.L. White, eds.). Cold Spring Harbor Laboratory, New York, 1983.

B19   Bishop, D.T. and M.K. Skolnick. Genetic markers and linkage analysis. p. 251-259 in: Banbury Report 14. Recombinant DNA Applications to Human Disease (C.T. Caskey and R.L. White, eds.). Cold Spring Harbor Laboratory, New York, 1983.

B20   Beaudet, A.L., T.S. Su, H.G.O. Bock et al. The human arginosuccinate synthetase locus: overview and analysis of citrullinemia fibroblasts. p. 97-103 in: Banbury Report 14. Recombinant DNA Applications to Human Disease (C.T. Caskey and R.L. White, eds.). Cold Spring Harbor Laboratory, New York, 1983.

B21   Bancroft, J., D. Axworthy and S. Ratcliffe. The personality and psychosexual development of boys with 47,XXY chromosome constitution. J. Child Pyschol. Psychiat. 23: 169-180 (1982).

B22   Brandriff, B., L. Gordon, L. Ashworth et al. Chromosomes of human spermatozoa: variability among individuals. Hum. Genet. 70: 18-24 (1985).

B23   Brookwell, R. and G. Turner. High resolution banding and the locus of the Xq fragile site. Hum. Genet. 63: 77 (1983).

B24   Brondom-Nielsen, K., N. Tommerup, H. Poulsen et al. Carrier detection and x-inactivation studies in the fragile-X syndrome. Cytogenetic studies in 63 obligate and potential carriers of the fragile-X. Hum. Genet. 64: 240-245 (1983).

B25   Blomquist, K.K., K.H. Gustavson, G. Holmgren et al. Fragile-X syndrome in mildly mentally retarded children in a Northern Swedish county. A prevalence study. Clinical Genet. 24: 393-398 (1983).

B26   Brookwell, R., A. Daniel, G. Turner and J. Fishburn. The fragile-X (q27) form of mental retardation. FudR as an inducing agent for Fra(X)(q27) expression in lymphocytes, fibroblasts and amniocytes. Am. J. Hum. Genet. 13: 139-148 (1982).

B27   Boehm, C.D., S.E. Antonarakis, J.A. Phillips et al. Prenatal diagnosis using DNA polymorphisms. Report on 95 pregnancies at risk for sickle-cell disease or beta-thalassemia. New Engl. J. Med. 308: 1054-1058 (1983).

B28   Bhattacharya, S.S., A.E. Wright, J.F. Clayton et al. Close linkage between X-linked retinitis pigmentosa and a restriction fragment length polymorphism identified by recombinant DNA probe L1.28. Nature 309: 253-255 (1984).

B29   Brennand, J., A.C. Chinnault, D.S. Konecki et al. Cloned cDNA sequences of HPRT gene from a mouse neuroblastoma cell line found to have amplified genomic sequences. Proc. Natl. Acad. Sci. U.S.A. 79: 1950-1954 (1982).

B30   Blair, D.G., M. Oskarsson, T.G. Wood et al. Activation of transforming potential of a normal cell sequence. A molecular model for oncogenesis. Science 212: 941-943 (1981).

B31   Benedict, W.F., A.L. Murphee, A. Banerjee et al. Patients with chromosome 13 deletion: evidence that the retinoblastoma gene is a recessive cancer gene. Science 219: 973-975 (1983).

B32   Bryant, P.E. Enzymatic restriction of in situ mammalian cell DNA using PuvII and BamHI. Evidence for the double strand break origin of chromosomal aberrations. Int. J. Radiat. Biol. 46: 57-65 (1984).

B33   Brooks, J.D., R.G. Gosden and A.C. Chandley. Maternal ageing and aneuploid embryos. Evidence from the mouse that biological and not chronological age is the important influence. Hum. Genet. 66: 41-45 (1984).

B34   Brewen, J.G. and R.J. Preston. Chromosomal interchanges induced by radiation in spermatogonial cells and leukocytes of mouse and Chinese hamster. Nature 244: 111-113 (1973).

B35   Brewen, J.G., R.J. Preston, K.P. Jones et al. Genetic hazards of ionizing radiation: cytogenetic extrapolation from mouse to man. Mutat. Res. 17: 245-254 (1983).

B36   Balanov, M.I. and O.V. Kudritskaya. Mutagenic action of tritium upon the germ cells of male mice. I. Induction of dominant lethal mutations by tritium oxide and estimation of RBE. Genetika 20: 224-232 (1984) (in Russian).

B38   Brandriff, B., L. Gordon, L. Ashworth et al. Chromosomal abnormalities in human sperm: comparisons among four healthy men. Hum. Genet. 66: 193-201 (1984).

B39   Blomquist, H.K., M. Bohman, S.O. Edvinsson et al. Frequency of the fragile-X syndrome in infantile autism. Clin. Genet. 27: 113-117 (1985).

B40   Brown, W.T., E. Friedman, E.C. Jenkins et al. Association of fragile-X syndrome with autism. Lancet i: 100 (1982).

B41   Brown, W.T., E.C. Jenkins, E. Friedman et al. Autism is associated with the fragile-X syndrome. J. Autism Dev. Dis. 12: 303-308 (1982)

B42   Braekeleer, M De., Fragile sites and chromosome breakpoints in constitutional rearrangements. Clin. Genet. 27: 523-524 (1985).

B43   Braekeleer, M De., B. Smith and C.C. Lin. Fragile sites and structural rearrangements in cancer. Hum. Genet. 69: 112-116 (1985).

B44 Bénézech, M. and B. Nöel. Fra(X) syndrome and autism. Clin. Genet. 28: 93 (1985).

B45 Beaudet, A.L. Bibliography of cloned human and other selected DNAs. Am. J. Hum. Genet. 37: 386-406 (1985).

B46 Bunn, H.F., B. Forget and H.M. Ramney. Human Haemoglobins. Saunders, Philadelphia, 1977.

B47 Bernards, R., P.F.R. Little, G. Annison et al. Structure of the human $^{G\gamma-A\gamma}\delta-\beta$-globin gene locus. Proc. Natl. Acad. Sci. 76: 4827-4832 (1979).

B48 Bell, G.I., R.L. Picket, W.J. Rutter et al. Sequence of the human insulin gene. Nature 284: 26-32 (1980).

B49 Bell, G.I. and J.H. Karan. The polymorphic locus flanking the human insulin gene. Is there an association with diabetes mellitus? p. 317-324 in: Recombinant DNA: Applications to Human Disease (C.T. Caskey and R.L. White, eds.). Banbury Report 14, Cold Spring Harbor Laboratory, 1983.

B50 Bell, G.I., S. Horita and J.H. Karan. A polymorphic locus flanking the human insulin gene is associated with insulin-dependent diabetes mellitus. Diabetes 33: 176-183 (1984).

B51 Bishop, C.E., G. Guellaën, D. Geldwerth et al. Single copy DNA sequences specific for the human Y chromosome. Nature 303: 831-832 (1983).

B52 Bishop, J.M., J.D. Rowley and M. Greaves (Eds.) Genes and Cancer. UCLA Symposium on Molecular and Cellular Biology. New Series. Vol. 17. Alan R. Liss Inc., New York, 1984.

B53 Bos, J.L., D. Toksoz, C.J. Marshall et al. Aminoacid substitutions at codon 13 of the N-ras oncogene in human acute myeloid leukaemia. Nature 315: 726-730 (1985).

B54 Brodeur, G., C. Seeger, M. Schwab et al. Amplification of N-myc in untreated neuroblastoma correlates with advanced disease stage. Science 224: 1121-1124 (1984).

B55 Bingham, P.M., M.G. Kidwell and G.M. Rubin. The molecular basis of P-M hybrid dysgenesis: the role of the P element, a P strain-specific transposon family. Cell 29: 995-1004 (1982).

B56 Bregliano, J.C. and M.G. Kidwell. Hybrid dysgenesis determinants. p. 363-410 in: Mobile Genetic Elements (J.A. Shapiro, ed.). Academic Press, New York, 1983.

B57 Bingham, P.M., R. Levis and G.M. Rubin. The cloning of DNA sequences from the white locus of D. melanogaster using a novel and general method. Cell 25: 693-704 (1981).

B58 Boeke, J.D., D.J. Garfinkel, C.A. Styles et al. Ty elements transpose through an RNA intermediate. Cell 40: 491-500 (1985).

B59 Baltimore, D. Retroviruses and retrotransposons. The role of reverse transcription in shaping the eukaryotic genome. Cell 40: 481-482 (1985).

B60 Britten, R. and D.E. Kohne. Repeated sequence in DNA. Science 161: 529-540 (1968).

B61 Brewen, J.G., R.J. Preston and N. Gengozian. Analysis of x-ray-induced chromosomal translocations in human and marmoset spermatogonial cells. Nature 253: 468-470 (1975).

B62 Brewen, J.G. and R.J. Preston. Cytogenetic effects of environmental mutagens in mammalian cells and the extrapolation to man. Mutat. Res. 26: 297-305 (1974).

B63 Balonov, M.I., M.D. Pomerantseva and L.K. Ramaiya. The mutagenic effects of tritium on germ cells of male mice. Consequences of ^{3}H-glucose incorporation. Radiobiology 24: 753-757 (1984). (in Russian)

B64 Baker, T.G. and A. McLaren. The effect of tritiated thymidine on the developing oocytes of mice. J. Reprod. Fertil. 34: 121-130 (1973).

B65 Bresler, S.E., V.L. Kalinin and V.N. Shelegedin. W-reactivation and W-mutagenesis of gamma-irradiated phage lambda. Mutat. Res. 49: 341-355 (1978).

B66 Bockstahler, L.E. and D. Lytle. UV-light enhanced reactivation of a mammalian virus. Biochem. Biophys. Res. Commun. 41: 184-189 (1970).

B67 Bockstahler, L.E. and D. Lytle. Radiation-enhanced reactivation of nuclear replicating mammalian virus. Photochem. Photobiol. 25: 477-482 (1977).

B68 Bockstahler, L.E. Induction and enhanced reactivation of mammalian viruses by light. Prog. Nucleic Acids Res. Mol. Biol. 26: 303-308 (1981).

B69 Brown, C.S., P.L. Pearson et al. Linkage analysis of a DNA polymorphism proximal to the Duchenne and Becker muscular dystrophy loci on the short arm of the X-chromosome. J. Med. Genet. 22: 179-181 (1985).

B70 Barker, D.J.P. and D.I.W. Phillips. Current incidence of thyrotoxicosis and past prevalence of goitre in 12 British towns. Lancet 2: 567-570 (1984).

B71 Bodnár, O. Screening of diabetes mellitus in district X of Budapest in 1976. Népegészségügy 60: 1-3 (1979). (in Hungarian)

B72 Baum, H.M. and B.B. Rothschild. The incidence and prevalences of reported multiple sclerosis. Ann. Neurol. 10: 420-428 (1981).

B73 Binder, V., E. Weeks, I.H. Olson et al. Genetic study of ulcerosa colitis. Scand. J. Gastroenterol. 1: 49-56 (1966).

B74 Berényi M. Urolithiasis. Medicina Kiadó. Budapest, 1981.

B75 Berecz, M., A. Czeizel and I. Varga. Epidemiological and family study of psoriasis. Orrosi Hetilap 115: 1039-1044 (1974).

B76 Bellyei, A. A study on Scheuermann's disease. (in press)

B77 Bellyei, A., A. Czeizel, O. Barta et al. Prevalence of adolescent idiopathic scoliosis in Hungary. Acta Orthop. Scand. 48: 177-180 (1977).

B78 Boué, A., A. Gropp and J. Boué. Cytogenetics of pregnancy wastage. p. 1-57 in: Advances in Human Genetics (H. Harris and K. Hirschhorn, eds.). Vol. 14. Academic Press, New York, 1985.

B79 BEIR Report. The effects on populations of exposure to low levels of ionizing radiation. National Academy of Sciences, National Research Council, Washington, 1972.

B80 BEIR Report. The effects on populations of exposure to low levels of ionizing radiation. National Academy of Sciences, National Research Council, Washington, 1980.

B81 Batchelor, A.L., R.J.S. Philipps and A.G. Searle. A comparison of the mutagenic effectiveness of chronic neutron and gamma irradiation of mouse spermatogonia. Mutat. Res. 3: 218-229 (1966).

C1 Coco, R. and V.B. Penchaszadeh. Cytogenetic findings in 200 children with mental retardation and multiple congenital anomalies of unknown cause. J. Med. Genet. 12: 155-173 (1982).

C2 Carrel, R.E., R.S. Sparkes and S.W. Wright. Chromosome survey of moderately to profoundly retarded patients. Am. J. Ment. Defic. 77: 616-622 (1973).

C3 Cooper, G.M. Cellular transforming genes. Science 218: 801-806 (1982).

C4 Cold Spring Harbor Symposia on Quantitative Biology. Volume 44. Viral Oncogenes, Parts 1 and 2. Cold Spring Harbor, New York, 1980.

C5 Cooper, G.M., S. Okenquist and L. Silverman. Transforming activity of DNA of chemically transformed and normal cells. Nature 284: 418-421 (1980).

C6 Cold Spring Harbor Symposia on Quantitative Biology. Volume 45. Movable Genetic Elements. Parts 1 and 2. Cold Spring Harbor Laboratory, New York, 1981.

C7 Cohen, S.S., J.G. Flaks, H.D. Barner et al. The mode of action of 5-fluorouracil and its derivatives. Proc. Natl. Acad. Sci. U.S.A. 44: 1004-1012 (1958).

C8 Creissen, D. and S. Shall. Regulation of DNA ligase activity by poly (ADP-ribose). Nature 296: 271-272 (1982).

C9 Cleaver, J.E., W.I. Bodell, C. Borek et al. Poly(ADP-ribose): spectator or protagonist in excision repair of various kinds of DNA damage. p.195-207 in: ADP-ribosylation, DNA Repair and Cancer, (M. Miwra et al., eds.) Japan Scientific Societies Press, Tokyo, 1983.

C10 Croci, C. BrdU-sensitive fragile site on long arm of chromosome 16. Am. J. Hum. Genet. 35: 530-533 (1983).

C11 Czeizel, A. The base-line data of the Hungarian congenital malformation Registry. 1970-1976. Acta Paediatr. Acad. Sci. Hungaricae 19: 149-156 (1978).

C12 Czeizel, A. The Hungarian congenital monitoring system. Acta Paediatr. Acad. Sci. Hungaricae 19: 225-238 (1978).

C13 Czeizel, A. and K. Sankaranarayanan. The load of genetic and partially genetic disorders in man. I. Congenital anomalies. Estimates of detriment in terms of years of life lost and years of impaired life. Mutat. Res. 128: 73-103 (1984).

C14 Chen, I.S.Y., K.C. Wilhelmsen and H.M. Temin. Structure and expression of c-rel, the cellular homologue to the oncogene of reticuloendotheliosis virus strain T. J. Virol. 45: 104-113 (1983).

C15 Colby, W.W., E.Y. Chen, D.H. Smith et al. Identification and nucleotide sequence of a human locus homologous to the v-myc oncogene of avian myelocytomatosis virus MC29. Nature 301: 722-725 (1983).

C16 Capon, D.J., E.Y. Chen, A.D. Levinson et al. Complete nucleotide sequences of the T24 human bladder carcinoma oncogene and its normal homologue. Nature 302: 33-37 (1983).

C17 Capon, D.J., P.H. Seeburg, J.P. McGrath et al. Activation of Ki-ras,2 gene in human colon and lung carcinomas by two different point mutations. Nature 304: 507-513 (1983).

C18 Canani, E., K.C. Robbins and S.A. Aaronson. The transforming gene of Moloney murine sarcoma virus. Nature 282: 378-383 (1979).

C19 Cox, D.W., V.D. Markovic and I.E. Teshima. Genes for immunoglobulin heavy chains and for alpha-antitrypsin are localized to specific regions of chromosome 14q. Nature 297: 428-430 (1982).

C20 Calame, K., S. Kim, P. Lalley et al. Molecular cloning of translocations involving chromosome 15 and immunoglobulin alpha chain from chromosome 12 in two murine plasmocytomas. Proc. Natl. Acad. Sci. U.S.A. 79: 6994-6998 (1982).

C21 Chang, J.C. and Y.W. Kan. A sensitive new test for sickle cell anaemia. New Engl. J. Med. 307: 30-32 (1982).

C22 Chan, H.W., T. Bryan, J.L. Moore et al. Identification of ecotropic proviral sequences in inbred mouse strains with a cloned subgenomic DNA fragment. Proc. Natl. Acad. Sci. U.S.A. 77: 5779-5783 (1980).

C23 Chattopadhyay, S.K., M.R. Lander, E. Rands et al. Structure of endogenous murine leukaemia virus DNA in mouse genomes. Proc. Natl. Acad. Sci. U.S.A. 77: 5774-5778 (1980).

C24 Calabretta, B., D.L. Robberson, H.A. Barrera-Saldana et al. Genomic instability in a region enriched in Alu repeat sequences. Nature 296: 219-225 (1982).

C25 Carter, C.O. Genetics of common single malformations. Brit. Med. Bull. 32: 21-26 (1976).

C26 Carter, C.O. The relative contribution of mutant genes and chromosomal abnormalities to genetic ill-health in man. p. 1-8 in: Chemical Mutagenesis, Human Population Monitoring and Genetic Risk Assessment (K.C. Bora et al., eds.). Prog. Mut. Res., Vol. 3. Elsevier Biomedical Press, Amsterdam, 1982.

C27 Crompton, N.E.A., J. Kiefer, E. Schneider et al. Mutations in continuous cultures of Chinese hamster cells induced by low dose-rate gamma irradiation. Proc. VII Int. Cong. Rad. Res. Abstract B4-10 (Book B). (J.J. Broerse et al., eds.). Martinus Nijhoff, The Hague, 1983.

C28 Crandall, B.F., T.B. Lebherz, L. Rubinstein et al. Chromosome findings in 2500 second trimester amniocentesis. Am. J. Med. Genet. 5: 345-356 (1980).

C29 Camerino, G., M.G. Mattei, J.F. Mattei et al. Close linkage of fragile-X mental retardation syndrome to haemophilia B and transmission through a normal male. Nature 306: 701-704 (1983).

C30 Côte, G.B., S. Papadakou-Lagayanni and S. Pantelakis. A cascade of chromosome aberrations in three generations. A fragile 16q, an extra fragment and a rearranged 20. Ann. Genet. 21: 209-214 (1978).

C31 Chudley, A.E., J. Knoll, J.W. Gerrard et al. Fragile X-linked mental retardation. I. Relationship between age and intelligence on the frequency of expression of fragile (X)(q28). Am. J. Med. Genet. 14: 699-712 (1983).

C32 Czeizel, A. and G. Tusnády. Aetiological Studies of Isolated Common Congenital Abnormalities in Hungary. Akadémiai Kiadó, Budapest, 1984.

C33 Clevell, D.B. Nature of ColE plasmid replication in Escherichia coli in the presence of chloramphenicol. J. Bacteriol. 110: 667 (1972).

C34 Collins, J. and B. Hohn. Cosmids: a type of plasmid gene cloning vector that is packageable in vitro in bacteriophage lambda heads. Proc. Natl. Acad. Sci. U.S.A. 75: 4242-4246 (1978).

C35 Cooper, D.N. and J. Schmidtke. DNA restriction fragment length polymorphisms and heterozygosity in the human genome. Hum. Genet. 66: 1-16 (1984).

C36 Chu, M.L., C.J. Williams, G. Pepe et al. Internal deletion in a collagen gene in a perinatal lethal form of osteogenesis imperfecta. Nature 304: 78-80 (1983).

C37 Cavenee, W.K., T.P. Dryja, R.A. Phillips et al. Expression of recessive alleles by chromosomal mutation in retinoblastoma. Nature 305: 779-784 (1983).

C38 Conner, B.J., A.A. Reyes, C. Morin et al. Detection of sickle cell beta-s-globin allele by hybridization with synthetic oligonucleotides. Proc. Natl. Acad. Sci. U.S.A. 80: 278-282 (1983).

C39 Cleary, M.L., J. Chao, R. Warner et al. Immuno-globulin gene rearrangements as a diagnostic criterion of B-cell lymphoma. Proc. Natl. Acad. Sci. U.S.A. 81: 593-597 (1984).

C40 Copper, G.M. Activation of transforming genes in neoplasms. Br. J. Cancer 50: 137-142 (1984).

C41 Chang, E.H., M.E. Furth, E.M. Skolnick et al. Tumorogenic transformation of mammalian cells induced by a normal human gene homologous to the oncogene of Harvey murine sarcoma virus. Nature 297: 479-483 (1982).

C42 Collins, S. and M. Groudine. Amplification of endogenous myc-related DNA sequences in a human myeloid leukaemia cell line. Nature 298: 679-681 (1982).

C43 Cooper, C.S., M. Park, D.G. Blair et al. Molecular cloning of a new transforming gene from a chemically transformed human cell line. Nature 311: 29-33 (1984).

C45 Cairns, J. and J. Logan. Step by step into carcino-genesis. Nature 304: 582-583 (1983).

C46 Carpenter, G. and S. Cohen. Epidermal growth factor. Ann. Rev. Biochem. 48: 193-216 (1979).

C47 Cooper, J.A., D.F. Bowen-Pope, E. Raines et all. Similar effects of platelet-derived growth factor and epidermal growth factor on the phosphorylation of tyrosine in cellular proteins. Cell 31: 263-273 (1983).

C48 Campisi, J., H.E. Gray, A.B. Pardec et al. Cell-cycle control of c-myc but not c-ras expression is lost following chemical transformation. Cell 36: 241-247 (1984).

C49 Campbell, A., D. Berg, D. Botstein et al. Nomenclature of transposable elements in procaryotes. p. 15-22 in: DNA Insertion Elements, Plasmids and Episomes (A.I. Bukhari et al., eds.). Cold Spring Harbor Laboratory, New York, 1977.

C50 Campbell, A., D. Berg, D. Botstein et al. Nomenclature of transposable elements in procaryotes. Plasmids 2: 466-473 (1979).

C51 Cameron, J.R., E.Y. Loh and R.W. Davis. Evidence for transposition of repetitive DNA families in yeast. Cell 24: 625-627 (1979).

C52 Collins, A., C.S. Downes and R.T. Johnson (eds). DNA Repair and its Inhibition. p. 371 in: Nucleic Acids Symposium Series No. 13, IRL Press, Oxford, 1984.

C53 Cattanach, B.M., D. Papworth and M. Kirk. Genetic tests for autosomal non-disjunction and chromosome loss in mice. Mutat. Res. 126: 189-204 (1984).

C54 Cattanach, B.M. and A.J.M. Crocker. Modified genetic response to x-irradiation of mouse spermatogonial cells surviving treatment with TEM. Mutat. Res. 70: 211-220 (1980).

C55 Cawood, A.H. and G. Breckon. Synaptonemal complexes as indicators for structural change in chromosomes after irradiation of spermatogonia. Mutat. Res. 122: 149-154 (1983).

C56 Cox, R., W.K. Masson, P.G. Debenham et al. The use of recombinant DNA plasmids for the determination of DNA-repair and recombination in cultured mammalian cells. Br. J. Cancer 49 (Suppl. VI): 67-72 (1984).

C57 Choo, K.H., K.G. Gould, D.J.G. Rees et al. Molecular cloning of the gene for human anti-haemophilic factor IX. Nature 299: 178-180 (1982).

C58 Camerino, G., K.H. Grzeschik, M. Jaye et al. Regional localization on the human X chromosome and polymorphism of the coagulation (haemophilia B locus). Proc. Natl. Acad. Sci. 81: 498-502 (1984).

C59 Choo, K.H., D. George, G. Fillby et al. Linkage analysis of X-linked mental retardation with and without fragile-X using factor IX gene probe. Lancet i: 349 (1984).

C60 Cohen, A.J., F.P. Li, S. Berg et al. Hereditary renal cell carcinoma associated with a chromosome translocation. New Eng. J. Med. 301: 592-595 (1979).

C61 Croce, C.M. and G. Klein. Chromosome translocation and human cancer. Sci. Am. 252: 44-50 (1985).

C62 Calos, M.P. and J.H. Miller. Transposable elements. Cell 20: 579-595 (1980).

C63 Cacheiro, N.L.A., L.B. Russell and M.S. Swartout. Translocations, the predominant cause of total sterility in sons of mice treated with mutagens. Genetics 76: 73-91 (1974).

C64 Crocker, M. Metaphase I delay as a factor influencing translocation yield from spermatogonial irradiation in mice carrying Robertsonian translocations. Mutat. Res. 103: 339-343 (1982).

C65 Cornelis, J.J., J.H. Lupker and A.J. van der Eb. UV-reactivation, virus production and mutagenesis of SV40 in UV-irradiated monkey kidney cells. Mutat. Res. 71: 139-146 (1980).

C66 Cornelis, J.J., B. Klein, J.H. Lupker et al. The use of viruses to study DNA repair and induced mutagenesis in mammalian cells. p. 337-350 in: Prog. Mut. Res. (A.T. Natarajan et al., eds.). Vol.4. Elsevier, Amsterdam, 1982.

C67 Cleaver, J.E. Absence of interaction between x-rays and uv light in inducing ouabain- and thioguanine-resistant mutants in Chinese hamster cells. Mutat. Res. 52: 247-253 (1978).

C68 Cairns, J. Efficiency of the adaptive response of E. coli to alkylating agents. Nature 286: 176-179 (1980).

C69 Cox, R. and W.K. Masson. The isolation and preliminary characterization of 6-thioguanine resistant mutants of human diploid fibroblasts. Mutat. Res. 36: 93-104 (1976).

C70 Carter, C.O. and T.J. Fairbank. The Genetics of Locomotor Disorders. p. 59-61. Oxford University Press, London, 1974.

C71 Czeizel, A. and T. Kadar. Family study of patients affected by acute myocardial infarctus. Orvosi Hetilap 119: 1841-1844 (1978).

C72 Czeizel, A., A. Bellyei, O. Barta et al. Genetics of adolescent idiopathic scoliosis. J. Med. Genet. 15: 424-427 (1978).

C73 Carr, D.H. Chromosomes and abortion. p. 201-257 in: Advances in Human Genetics (H. Harris and K. Hirschhorn, eds.). Vol. 2. Plenum Press, New York, 1971.

C74 Costa, T., C.R. Scriver and B. Childs. The effect of Mendelian disease on human health: a measurement. Am. J. Med. Genet. 21: 231-242 (1985).

C75 Carnevale, A., M. Hernández, R. Reyes et al. The frequency and economic burden of genetic disease in a pediatric hospital in Mexico City. Am. J. Med. Genet. 20: 665-675 (1985).

C76 Copeland, N.G., K.W. Hutchison and N.A. Jenkins. Escision of the DBA ecotropic provirus in dilute coat colour revertants of mice occurs by homologous recombination involving viral LTRs. Cell 33: 379-387 (1983).

C77 Cattanach, B. and M. Kirk. Differential activity of maternally and paternally-derived chromosome regions in mice. Nature 315: 496-498 (1985).

D1 Daly, R.F. Chromosome aberrations in 50 patients with idiopathic mental retardation and in 50 control subjects. J. Pediatr. 77: 444-453 (1970).

D2 Doyle, C.T. The cytogenetics of 90 patients with idiopathic mental retardation/malformation syndromes and in 90 normal subjects. Hum. Genet. 33: 131-146 (1976).

D3 Dykes, J. Ten thousand severely handicapped children in New South Wales and the Australian Capital Territory. Australian Government Publishing Service, Canberra, 1978.

D4 Der, C.J., T.G. Krontiris and G.M. Cooper. Transforming genes of human bladder and lung carcinoma cell lines are homologous to the ras genes of Harvey and Kirsten sarcoma virus. Proc. Natl. Acad. Sci. U.S.A. 79: 3637-3640 (1982).

D5 De Klein, A., A.G. van Kessel, G. Grosveld et al. A cellular oncogene is translocated to the Philadelphia chromosome in chronic myelocytic leukaemia. Nature 300: 765-767 (1982).

D6 Dhar, R., W.L. McClements et al. Nucleotide sequences of integrated Moloney sarcoma provirus long terminal and their host and viral junctions. Proc. Natl. Acad. Sci. U.S.A. 77: 3937-3941 (1980).

D7 Downes, C.S., A.R.S. Collins and R.T. Johnson. International workshop on inhibitors of DNA repair. Mutat. Res. 112: 75-83 (1983).

D8 Durkacz, B.W., O. Omidiji, D. Gray et al. (ADP-ribose)$_n$ participates in DNA excision repair. Nature 283: 593-596 (1980).

D9 Dutrillaux, B., E. Viegas-Pequignot, A. Aurias et al. Tentative estimate of the risk of chromosomal disease due to radiation-induced translocations in man. Mutat. Res. 82: 191-200 (1981).

D10 Dutrillaux, B., E. Viegas-Pequignot, M. Mouthuy et al. Risk of chromosomal disease due to radiation: tentative estimate from the study of radiation-induced translocations in human fibroblasts. Mutat. Res. 119: 343-350 (1983).

D11 Duesberg, P.H. Retroviral transforming genes in normal cells? Nature 304: 219-226 (1983).

D12 Duesberg, P.H. and P.K. Vogt. Differences between the ribonucleic acids of transforming and non-transforming avian tumour viruses. Proc. Natl. Acad. Sci. U.S.A. 67: 1673-1680 (1970).

D13 Diamond, A., G.M. Cooper, J. Ritz et al. Identification and molecular cloning of the human Blym transforming gene activated in Burkitt lymphomas. Nature 305: 112-115 (1983).

D14 Dalla-Favera, R., G. Franchini, S. Martinotti et al. Chromosomal assignment of the human homologues of feline sarcoma virus and avian myeloblastosis virus oncogenes. Proc. Natl. Acad. Sci. U.S.A. 79: 4714-4717 (1982).

D15 Davies, K.E. The application of DNA recombinant technology to the analysis of the human genome and genetic disease. Hum. Genet. 58: 351-357 (1981).

D16 Davies, K.E., J. Jackson, R. Williamson et al. Linkage analysis of myotonic dystrophy and sequences on chromosome 19 using a cloned complement 3 gene probe. J. Med. Genet. 20: 259-263 (1983).

D17 Davies, K.E., D.A. Hartley, J.M. Murray et al. The characterization of sequences from a human X-chromosome library for the study of X-linked diseases. p. 279-290 in: Banbury Report. 14. Recombinant DNA Applications to Human Diseases (C.T. Caskey and R.L. White, eds.). Cold Spring Harbor Laboratory, New York, 1983.

D18 Davies, K.E., P.L. Pearson, P.S. Harper et al. Linkage analysis of two cloned DNA sequences flanking the Duchenne muscular dystrophy locus on the short arm of the human X-chromosome. Nucleic Acids Res. 11: 2303-2312 (1983).

D19 Davies, K.E. A comprehensive list of cloned eukaryotic genes. p. 143-173 in: Genetic Engineering Vol. 3. (R. Williamson, ed.). Academic Press, New York, 1982.

D20 Dausset, J. The major histocompatibility complex in man. Past, present and future. Science 213: 1469-1473 (1981).

D21 Das, H.K., B. Duceman, A.K. Sood et al. Molecular studies of the genes of the human major histocompatibility. p. 41-51 in: Banbury Report 14 (C.T. Caskey and R.L. White, eds.). Cold Spring Harbor Laboratory, New York, 1983.

D22 Driscoll, M.C., M. Baird., A. Bank et al. A new polymorphism in the human beta-globin gene useful in antenatal diagnosis. J. Clin. Invest. 68: 915-918 (1981).

D23 Dubinin, N.P. and Yu. P. Altukhov. Gene mutations (de novo) found in electrophoretic studies of blood proteins of infants with anomalous development. Proc. Natl. Acad. Sci. U.S.A. 76: 5226-5229 (1979).

D24 Dutrillaux, B., J. Rotman and J. Gueguen. Chromosomal factors in the infertile male. p. 89-102 in: Int. Perspectives in Urology, Vol. 4 (J.A. Liberto, Series ed.), Aspects of Male Infertility (R. de Vere White, ed.) Williams & Wilkins, Baltimore & London, 1982.

D25 Donti, E., G. Venti, V. Bucchini et al. The constitutional fragility of chromosome 12 in a case of 46, XX var(12)qh, RHG, GAG, CBG. Hum. Genet. 48: 53-59 (1979).

D26 Dunn, H.G., H. Rennpenning, J.W. Gerrard et al. Mental retardation as a sex-linked defect. Am. J. Men. Def. 67: 827-848 (1963)

D27 Daniel, A., L. Ekblom and S. Phillips. Constitutional fragile sites 1p31, 3p14, 6q26 and 16q23 and their use as controls for false negative results with the fragile (X). Am. J. Med. Genet. 18: 483-491 (1983).

D28 Denhardt, D.J., D. Dressler and D.S. Ray (eds.) The single-stranded DNA phages. Cold Spring Harbor Laboratory, New York, 1978.

D29 Davies, K.E., K. Harper, D. Bonthron et al. Use of a chromosome 21 cloned DNA probe for the analysis of non-disjunction in Down syndrome. Hum. Genet. 66: 54-56 (1984).

D30 Dalla-Favera, R.D., F. Wong-Staal and R.G. Gallo. One gene amplification in promyelocytic leukaemia cell lines HL-60 and primary leukaemia cells of the same patient. Nature 299: 61-63 (1982).

D31 de Taisne, C., A. Gegonne, D. Stehlin et al. Chromosomal localization of the human proto-oncogene c-ets. Nature 310: 581-583 (1984).

D32 Dryja, T.P., W. Cavenee, R. White et al. Homozygosity of chromosome 13 in retinoblastoma. New Engl. J. Med. 310: 550-553 (1984).

D33 Doolittle, R.F., M.F. Hunkapiller, L.E. Hood et al. Simian sarcoma virus onc gene v-sis is derived from the gene (or genes) encoding a platelet-derived growth factor. Science 221: 275-277 (1983).

D34 Downward, J., Y. Yarden, E. Mayes et al. Close similarity of epidermal growth factor and v-erb-B oncogene protein sequences. Nature 307: 521-527 (1984).

D35 Deuel, T.F., J.S. Huang, R.T. Proffitt et al. Human platelet-derived growth factors. Purification and resolution into two active protein fractions. J. Biol. Chem. 256: 8896-8899 (1981).

D36 de Boer, P. and A.D. Tates. Radiation-induced nondisjunction. p.299-325 in: Radiation-induced Chromosome Damage in Man (T. Ishihara and M.S. Sasaki, eds.), Alan R. Liss Inc., New York, 1983.

D37 Dobson, R.L., and J.S. Felton. Female germ cell loss from radiation and chemical exposures. Am. J. Industrial Med. 4: 175-190 (1983).

D39 Dobson, R.L., T.C. Kwan and T. Straume. p. 1-8 in: Tritium effects on germ cells and fertility. UCRL-88376 (1982).

D40 Dobson, R.L. The toxicity of tritium. p. 203-211 in: Biological Implications of Radionuclides Released from Nuclear Industries, Vol. I. IAEA, Vienna, 1979.

D41 Dawson, R.L. and T. Straume. Mutagenesis in primordial mouse oocytes could be masked by cell-killing: Monte-Carlo analysis. Abstract, 15th Ann. Meeting of Environmental Mutagen Society, Montreal, Canada (1984).

D42 Debenham, P.G., M.B.T. Wegg, W.K. Masson et al. DNA-mediated gene transfer into human diploid fibroblasts derived from normal and ataxia telangiectasia donors: parameters for DNA transfer and properties of DNA transformants. Int. J. Radiat. Biol. 45: 525-536 (1984).

D43 Davies, K.E., M.G. Mattei, J.F. Mattei et al. Linkage studies of X-linked mental retardation: high frequency of recombination in the telomeric region of the human C-chromosome. Hum. Genet. 70: 240-255 (1985).

D44 De Martinville, B., L.M. Kunkel, G. Bruns et al. Localization of DNA sequences in region Xp21 of the human X-chromosome. Search for molecular markers close to the Duchenne muscular dystrophy locus. Am. J. Hum. Genet. 37: 235-249 (1985).

D45 Duesberg, P.H. Activated proto-onc genes: sufficient or necessary for cancer? Science 228: 669-677 (1985).

D46 DeFeo-Jones, D., E.H. Scolnick, R. Koller et al. Ras-related gene sequences identified and isolated from Saccharomyces cerevisiae. Nature 306: 707-709 (1983).

D47 Dhar, R. R. Ellis, T.Y. Shih et al. Nucleotide sequence of the p21 transforming protein of Harvey murine sarcoma virus. Science 217: 934-937 (1982).

D48 Dawid, I.B., E.O. Long, P.P. Di Nocora et al. Ribosomal insertion-like elements in Drosophila melanogaster are interspersed with mobile sequences. Cell 25: 399-408 (1981).

D49 Dobson, R.L., T.C. Kwan and T. Straume. Tritium effects in germ cells and fertility. In: Radiation Protection: European Seminar on the Risks of Tritium Exposure (G. Gerber and C. Myttenaere, eds.). CEC, Brussels, 1984.

D50 Dobson, R.L. Delayed reproductive consequences of low level irradiation early in life. American Nuclear Safety Meeting, 1985. UCRL-92866 (1985).

D51 Dobson, R.L. and M.F. Cooper. Tritium toxicity: effect of low level ^3HOH exposure on developing female germ cells in the mouse. Radiat. Res. 58: 91-100 (1974).

D52 Dobson, R.L. and T.C. Kwan. The tritium RBE at low level exposure: variation with dose, dose-rate and exposure duration. Curr. Top. Radiat. Res. 12: 44-62 (1977).

D53 DeFais, M.J., P. Fauquet et al. Ultraviolet reactivation and ultraviolet mutagenesis of lambda in different genetic systems. Virology 43: 495-503 (1971).

D54 DasGupta, U.B. and W.C. Summers. Ultraviolet reactivation of herpes simplex virus is mutagenic and inducible in mammalian cells. Proc. Natl. Acad. Sci. 75: 2378-2381 (1978).

D55 DeFais, M.J., P.C. Hanwalt and A.R. Sarasin. Viral probes for DNA repair. Adv. Radiat. Biol. 10: 1-37 (1982).

D56 Day, R.S. and C.H.J. Ziolkowski. UV-induced reversion of adenovirus 5ts2 infecting human cells. Photochem. Photobiol. 34: 403-406 (1981).

D57 D'Ambrosio, S.M. and R.B. Setlow. Enhancement of post-replication repair in Chinese hamster cells. Proc. Natl. Acad. Sci. 73: 2396-2400 (1976).

D58 Demple, B.P., P. Karran and T. Lindahl. Isolation of O^6-methylguanine DNA methyl transferase from E. coli. p. 41-52 in: DNA Repair: A Laboratory Manual of Research Procedures (E.C. Friedberg and P.C. Hanawalt, eds.). Decker, New York, 1983.

D59 Dutrillaux, B. Chromosomal evolution in primates: tentative phylogeny from Microcebus murinus (prosimian) to man. Hum. Genet. 48: 251-314 (1979).

D60 Dutrillaux, B., M. Muleris and M. Paravatou-Petosota. Diagrammatic representation for chromsomal mutagenesis studies. I. Karyotypes most similar to that of man. Mutat. Res. 126: 81-92 (1984).

D61 Decat, G., A. Léonard and W. de Meurichy. Anomalies chromosomiques induites par les rayons x dans les lymphocytes du Gorille. C. R. Soc. Biol. 174: 851-855 (1980).

D62 De Ruijter, Y.C.E.M. and J.W.I.M. Simons. Determination of expression time and the dose-response relationship for mutation at the HG-PRT locus induced by x-irradiation of human diploid fibroblasts. Mutat. Res. 69: 325-332 (1980).

D63 Doose, H., H. Gerken, R. Leonhardt et al. Centrocephalic myoclonic astatic petit mal: clinical and genetic investigations. Neuropaediatrie 2: 59-78 (1970).

D64 Damon, A. and A.P. Polednak. Constitution, genetics and body form in peptic ulcer. A review. J. Chronic Dis. 20: 787-802 (1967).

D65 David, T.J. and A.B. Ajudukiewicz. A family study of coeliac disease. J. Med. Genet. 12: 79-82 (1975).

D66 Duckett, D.P. and S.H. Roberts. Adjacent-2 meiotic disjunction. Report of a case resulting from familial 13qf15q balanced reciprocal translocation and review of the literature. Hum. Genet. 58: 377-386 (1981).

D67 Davis, J.R., B.B. Rogers, R.M. Hagman et al. Balanced reciprocal translocations: risk factors for aneuploid segregant viability. Clin. Genet. 27: 1-19 (1985).

E2 Erdtman, B., F.M. Salzano and M.S. Mattevi. Chromosome studies in patients with congenital malformation and mental retardation. Hum. Genet. 26: 297-306 (1975).

E3 Eeken, J.C.J. The stability of mutator (MR)-induced-X-chromosome recessive visible mutations in Drosophila melanogaster. Mutat. Res. 96: 213-224 (1982).

E4 Eeken, J.C.J. and F.H. Sobels. The effect of biochemical mutagens ENU and MMS on MR-mediated reversion of an unstable insertion-sequence mutations in Drosophila melanogaster. Mutat. Res. 110: 297-310 (1983).

E5 Eeken, J.C.J. and F.H. Sobels. Modification of MR mutator activity in repair-deficient strains of Drosophila melanogaster. Mutat. Res. 83: 191-200 (1981).

E6 Eeken, J.C.J. and F.H. Sobels. The influence of deficiencies in DNA repair on MR-mediated reversion of unstable mutations in Drosophila melanogaster. Mutat. Res. 110: 287-295 (1983).

E7 Evans, H.J. and A. Adams. X-ray-induced chromosome aberrations in human lymphocytes irradiated in vitro: the influence of exposure conditions, genotype and age on aberrations yields. p. 335-348 in: Advances in Radiation Research, Vol. I (J.F. Duplan et al., eds.). Gordon and Breach, London, 1970.

E11 Emery, A.E.H. Recombinant DNA technology. Lancet ii: 1406-1409 (1981).

E12 Erlich, H., D. Stetler and C. Grumet. Restriction length polymorphism analysis of HLA-typed families using cloned HLA probes. p. 327-334 in: Banbury Report 14. Recombinant DNA Applications to Human Disease (C.T. Caskey and R.L. White, eds.). Cold Spring Harbor Laboratory, New York, 1983.

E13 Eva, A. and S.A. Aaronson. Frequency activation of c-kis as a transforming gene in fibrosarcomas induced by methylcholoranthrene. Science 220: 955-956 (1983).

E14 Eva, A., S.R. Tronick, R.A. Gol et al. Transforming genes of human haematopoietic tumours: frequent detection of ras-related onc genes whose activation appears to be independent of tumour phenotype. Proc. Natl. Acad. Sci. U.S.A. 80: 4926-4930 (1983).

E15 Ek, B., B. Westermark, A. Wasteson et al. Stimulation of tyrosine-specific phosphorylation by platelet-derived growth factor. Nature 295: 419-420 (1982).

E16 Errede, B., T.S. Cardillo, F. Sherman et al. Mating signal control expression of mutations resulting from insertion of transposable repetitive element adjacent to diverse yeast genes. Cell 25: 427-436 (1980)

E17 Evans, E.P. Cytological method for the study of meiotic properties in mice. Genetics 92: s97-s103 (1979).

E18 Emery, A.E.H. An Introduction to Recombinant DNA. John Wiley & Sons, Chichester, 1984.

E19 Embury, S.H., R. Lebo, V. Dezy et al. Organization of alpha-globin genes in the Chinese alpha-thalassemia syndromes. J. Clin. Invest. 63: 1307-1310 (1979).

E20 Efstradiatis, A., J.W. Posakony, T. Maniatis et al. The structure and evolution of the human beta globin gene family. Cell 21: 653-668 (1980).

E21 Eiberg, H., J. Mohr, L.S. Nielsen et al. Genetics and linkage relationships of the C3 polymorphism: discovery of C3-Se-linkage and assignment of LE5-C3-DM-Se-PEPO-Lu synteny to chromosome 19. Clin. Genet. 24: 159-170 (1983).

E22 Eighth International Human Gene Mapping Workshop. Book of Abstracts. Helsinki, 1985.

E23 Eva, A. and S.A. Aaronson. Isolation of a new human oncogene from a diffuse B-cell lymphoma. Nature 316: 273-275 (1975).

E24 Engels, W.R. Hybrid dysgenesis in Drosophila melanogaster. Rules of inheritance of female sterility. Genet. Res. 33: 219-223 (1979).

E25 Engels, W.R. The P family of transposable elements in Drosophila. Ann. Rev. Genet. 17: 315-344 (1983).

E26 Eeken, J.C.J., F.H. Sobels, V. Hyland et al. Distribution of MR-induced sex-linked recessive lethal mutations in Drosophila melanogaster. Mutat. Res. 150: 261-275 (1985).

E27 Essen-Möller, E. and O. Hagrell. The frequency and risk of depression within a rural population group in Scania. Acta Physiol. Scand. 162 (Suppl): 28-35 (1961).

E28 Emery, A.E.H. and I.S. Lawrence. Genetics of ankylosing spondylitis. J. Med. Genet. 4: 239-245 (1967).

E29 Ehling, U.H. Induction and manifestation of hereditary cataracts. p. 354-367 in: Assessment of Risk from Low Level Exposure (A.D. Woodhead et al. eds.). Plenum Press, New York, 1985.

E30 Ehling, U.H. Schätzung des strahlengenetischen Risikos. p. 70-72 in: Strahlung und Radionuklide in der Umwelt, Tagung der Arbeitsgemeinschaft der Großforschungseinrichtungen (AGF). Bonn-Bad Godesberg, 1984.

E31 Eeken, J.C.J., R.J. Romeyn and A.W.M. de Jong. An analysis of X-linked recessive lethals induced by MR and x-rays in Drosophila melanogaster carrying P-elements. Mutat. Res. (1986) (in press).

E32 Evans, J.S., D.W. Moeller and D.W. Cooper. Health Effects Model for Nuclear Power Plant Accident Consequence Analysis. p. II-139 to II-180 in: Chapter III: Genetic Effects. Prepared for the U.S. Nuclear Regulatory Commission. U.S. Government Printing Office, Washington, D.C., 1985.

E33 Ehling, U.H. and A. Neuhäuser-Klaus. Dose-effect relationships of germ-cell mutations in mice. p. 15-25 in: Problems of Threshold in Chemical Mutagenesis (Y. Tazima et al., eds.). The Environmental Mutagen Society of Japan, Tokyo, 1984.

F1 Faed, M.J.W., J. Robertson et al. A chromosome survey of a hospital for the mentally subnormal. Clin. Genet. 16: 191-204 (1979).

F2 Forman, D. and J. Rowley. Chromosome and cancer. Nature 300: 403-404 (1982).

F3 Fiandt, M., W. Szybalski and M.H. Malamy. Polar mutations in lac, gal and phage lambda consist of a few DNA sequences inserted in either orientation. Mol. Gen. Genet. 199: 223-231 (1972).

F4 Finnegan, D.J., G.M. Rubin, M.W. Young et al. Repeated gene families in Drosophila melanogaster. Cold Spring Harbor Symp. Quant. Biol. 42: 1053-1063 (1978).

F5 Farabaugh, P.J. and G.R. Fink. Insertion of the eukaryotic transposable element Ty1 creates a 5-base pair duplication. Nature 286: 352-354 (1980).

F6 Farzaneh, F., R. Zalin, D. Brill et al. DNA strand-breaks and ADP-ribosyl transferase activation during cell differentiation. Nature 300: 362-366 (1982).

F7 Ford, C.A., A.G. Searle, E.P. Evans et al. Differential transmission of translocations induced in spermatogonia of mice by x-irradiation. Cytogenetics 8: 4470-4479 (1969).

F8 Frankel, A. and P.J. Fischinger. Nucleotide sequences in mouse DNA and RNA specific for Moloney sarcoma virus. Proc. Natl. Acad. Sci. U.S.A. 73: 3705-3709 (1976).

F9 Frankel, A., H.J. Gilbert, K.J. Porzig et al. Nature and distribution of feline sarcoma virus nucleotide sequences. J. Virol. 30: 821-827 (1979).

F10 Fuchs, R. and R. Blakesley. Guide to the use of type II restriction endonucleases. p. 3-38 in: Methods in Enzymology, Vol.. 100, Recombinant DNA, Part B (R. Wu et al., eds.). Academic Press, New York, 1983.

F11 Flavell, R.A. The use of genomic libraries for the isolation and study of eukaryotic genes. p. 49-127 in: Genetic Engineering (R. Williamson, ed.). Vol. 2, Academic Press, New York, 1981.

F12 Forget, B.G., E.J. Benz and S.M. Weissman. Normal human globin and mutations causing the beta-thalassemia. p. 3-17 in: Banbury Report 14. Recombinant DNA Applications to Human Disease (C.T. Caskey and R.L. White, eds.). Cold Spring Harbor Laboratory, New York, 1983.

F13 Friedmann, T., A. Esty, D. Filpula et al. Characterization of an expressible human hypoxanthin phosphoribosyl transferase cDNA. p. 91-96 in: Banbury Report 14. Recombinant DNA Applications to Human Disease (C.T. Caskey and R.L. White, eds.). Cold Spring Harbor Laboratory, New York, 1983.

F14 Francke, U., B. de Martiniville. Mapping of DNA sequences to chromosomal regions in somatic cell hybrids. p. 175-187 in: Banbury Report 14. Recombinant DNA Applications to Human Disease (C.T. Caskey and R.L. White, eds.). Cold Spring Harbor Laboratory, New York, 1983.

F15 Filippi, G., A. Rinaldi, N. Archidiacono et al. Brief Report: linkage between G6-PD and fragile-X syndrome. Am J. Med. Genet. 15: 113-119 (1983).

F16 Fishburn, J., G. Turner, A. Daniel et al. The diagnosis and frequency of X-linked conditions in a cohort of moderately retarded males with affected carriers. Am. J. Med. Genet. 14: 713-724 (1983).

F17 Fryns, J.P. and H. van der Berghe. Transmission of fragile (X)(q27) from normal male(s). Hum. Genet. 61: 262-263 (1982).

F18 Fonatsch, C. A simple method to demonstrate the fragile X chromosome in fibroblasts. Hum. Genet. 59: 186 (1981).

F19 Francillon, M.R. Prevention of hip arthrosis deformans: diagnosis and therapy of epiphysiolysis capitis femoris. Schweiz. Med. Wochenschr. 86: 167-177 (1984).

F20 Farquar, M., R. Gelinas, B. Tatsis et al. Restriction endonuclease mapping of gamma, delta-beta globin region in Ggamma(beta)+HPEF and a Chinese Agamma HPFG variant. Am. J. Hum. Genet. 35: 611-620 (1983).

F21 Fung, Y.K.T., W.G. Lewis, L.B. Crittenden et al. Activation of cellular oncogene c-erb-B by LTR insertion: molecular basis for induction of erythroblastosis by avian leukosis virus. Cell 33: 357-368 (1983).

F22 Fearson, E.R., S.E. Antonarakis, D.A. Meyers et al. c-Ha-ras1 oncogene lies between beta-globin and insulin loci on human chromosome 11p. Am. J. Hum. Genet. 36: 329-337 (1984).

F23 Fisher, J.H., Y.E. Miller, R.S. Sparkes et al. Wilms' tumour-aniridia association: segregation of affected chromosome in somatic cell hybrids, identification of cell surface antigen associated with deleted area and regional mapping of c-Ha-ras1 oncogene, insulin gene and beta-globin gene. Somatic Cell Mol. Genet. 10: 455-464 (1984).

F24 Fearson, E.R., B. Vogelstein and A.P. Feinberg. Somatic deletion and duplication of genes on chromosome 11 in Wilms' tumour. Nature 309: 176-178 (1984).

F25 Fran, R.J. and D.W. Kufe. The effect of inhibitors of DNA synthesis on DNA repair. p. 95-107 in: DNA Repair and its Inhibition (A. Collins et al., eds.) IRL Press, Oxford, 1983.

F26 Fabrikant, J.D. and E.L. Schneider. Studies on the genetic and immunological components of the maternal age effect. Devel. Biol. 66: 337-343 (1978).

F27 Fuscoe, J.C., R.G. Fenwick, D.H. Ledbetter et al. Deletion and amplification of the HG-PRT locus in Chinese hamster cells. Mol. Cell. Biol. 3: 1086-1096 (1983).

F28 Fenwick, R.G., J.C. Fuscoe and C.T. Caskey. Amplification versus mutation as a mechanism for reversion of an HG-PRT mutation. Somatic Cell Mol. Genet. 10: 71-84 (1984).

F29 Fryns, J.P. The fragile-X chromosome. A study of 83 families. Clin. Genet. 26: 497-528 (1984).

F30 Fleischmann, E.W. and E.L. Prigogina. Karyotype peculiarities of malignant lymphomas. Hum. Genet. 35: 269-279 (1977).

F31 Flavell, R.A., J.M. Koeter, E. De Boer et al. Analysis of the human beta-delta globin gene loci in normal and Hb Lepore DNA. Direct determination of gene linkage and intergenic distance. Cell 15: 25-41 (1978).

F32 Fritsch, E.F., R.M. Lawn and T. Maniatis. Characterization of deletions which affect the expression of fetal globin genes in man. Nature 279: 598-603 (1979).

F33 Fritsch, E.F., R.M. Lawn and T. Maniatis. Molecular cloning and characterization of the human beta-like globin gene cluster. Cell 19: 959-972 (1980).

F34 Francke, U., H.D. Ochs, B. De Martinville et al. Minor Xp21 chromosome deletion with expression of Duchenne muscular dystrophy, chronic granulomatosis disease, retinitis pigmentosa and McLeod syndrome. Am. J. Hum. Genet. 37: 250-267 (1985).

F35 Fasano, O., T. Aldrich, F. Tamanoi et al. Analysis of transforming potential of the human H-ras gene by random mutagenesis. Proc. Natl. Acad. Sci. 81: 4008-4012 (1984).

F36 Foster, T.J., M.A. Davis, D.E. Roberts et al. Genetic organization of transposon Tn10. Cell 23: 201-213 (1981).

F37 Friedberg, E.C. DNA damage tolerance in eukaryotic cells. Chapter 8 in: DNA Repair. W.H. Freeman & Co., New York, 1985.

F38 Frosina, G. and A. Abbondandolo. The current evidence for an adaptive response to alkylating agents in mammalian cells with special reference to experiments with in vitro cell cultures. Mutat. Res. 154: 85-100 (1985).

F39 Francois, J. Genetic predisposition to glaucoma. Dev. Ophthal. 3: 1-45 (1981).

F40 Fisk, J.W., M.L. Baigent, P.D. Gill et al. Incidence of Scheuerman disease. Am. J. Phys. Med. 61: 32-35 (1982).

G1 Glover, T.W. FUdR induction of the X chromosome fragile site. Evidence for the mechanism of folic acid and thymidine inhibition. Am. J. Hum. Genet. 33: 234-242 (1981).

G2 Graham, F.L. and J. van der Eb. A new technique for the assay of infectivity of human adenovirus DNA. Virology 52: 456-467 (1973).

G3 Green, M.M. Transposable elements in Drosophila and other diptera. Ann. Rev. Genet. 14: 109-120 (1980).

G4 Green, M.M. The case for DNA insertion mutations in Drosophila. p. 437-445 in: Insertion elements, plasmids and episomes (A.I. Bukhari et al., eds.). Cold Spring Harbor Laboratory, 1977.

G5 Golubovsky, M.D., Yu.N. Ivanov and M.M. Green. Genetic instability in Drosophila melanogaster. Putative multiple insertions mutants at the singed bristle locus. Proc. Natl. Acad. Sci. U.S.A. 74: 2973-2975 (1977).

G6 Green, M.M. Genetic instability in Drosophila melanogaster. De novo induction of putative insertions mutants. Proc. Natl. Acad. Sci. U.S.A. 74: 3490-3493 (1977).

G7 Green, M.M. The genetic control of mutation in Drosophila. Stadler Symp. 10: 95-104 (1978).

G8 Green, M.M. The genetics of a mutable gene at the white locus of Drosophila melanogaster. Genetics 61: 423-428 (1969).

G9 Green, M.M. Mapping a Drosophila melanogaster "controlling element" by interallelic crossing over. Genetics 61: 423-482 (1967).

G10 Green, M.M. Controlling element mediated transpositions of the white gene in Drosophila melanogaster. Genetics 61: 429-441 (1969).

G11 Gehring, W.J. and R. Paro. Isolation of a hybrid plasmid with homologous sequences to a transposing element of Drosophila melanogaster. Cell 79: 897-904 (1980).

G12 Gafner, J. and P. Philippsen. The yeast transposon Ty1 generates duplications of target DNA on insertion. Nature 286: 414-418 (1980).

G15 Generoso, W.M., K.T. Cain and S.W. Huff. Dose-effects of acute x-rays on induction of heritable reciprocal translocations in mouse spermatogonia. p. 138-139 in: ORNL-4993 (1974).

G16 Generoso, W.M., K.T. Cain, N.L.A. Cacheiro et al. Response of mouse spermatogonial stem cell to x-ray induction of heritable translocations. Mutat. Res. 126: 177-187 (1984).

G17 Goldfarb, M., K. Shimizu, M. Perucho et al. Isolation and preliminary characterization of a human transforming gene from T24 bladder carcinoma cells. Nature 296: 404-409 (1982).

G18 Goubrin G., D. Goldman, J. Nice et al. Molecular cloning and nucleotide sequence of a transforming gene detected by transfection of chicken B-cell lymphoma DNA. Nature 302: 114-119 (1983).

G19 Geever, R.F., L.B. Wilson, F.S. Nallaseth et al. Direct identification of sickle cell anemia by blot hybridization. Proc. Natl. Acad. Sci. U.S.A. 78: 5081-5085 (1981).

G20 Ginter, E.K., A.K. Revazov, K.D. Krasnopolskaya et al. Medico-genetic studies of the population of Turkmenia. I. Hereditary pathology of 5 regions of the Askhabad province. Genetika 8: 1487-1494 (1980) (in Russian).

G21 Ginter, E.K., A.K. Revazov, K.D. Krasnopolskaya et al. Medio-genetic studies of the population of Turkmenia. II. Hereditary pathology of 5 regions of the Tashauz province. Genetika 6: 1018-1023 (1982) (in Russian).

G22 Ginter, E.K., Sh. M. Turaeva, A.A. Revasov et al. Medico-genetic studies of the Turkmenia population. III. Hereditary disorders among the Turkmen-Nochurli. Genetika 8: 1344-1352 (1983).

G23 Golbus, M.S., W.D. Loughman, C.J. Epstein et al. Prenatal genetic diagnosis in 3000 amniocentesis. New Engl. J. Med. 300: 157-163 (1979).

G24 Giraud, F., S. Ayme and M.G. Mattei. Constitutional chromosome breakage. Hum. Genet. 34: 125-136 (1976).

G25 Glover, T.W., C. Berger, J. Coyle et al. DNA polymerase alpha-inhibition by aphidicolin induces gaps and breaks at common fragile sites in human chromosomes. Hum. Genet. 67: 136-142 (1984).

G26 Gianelli, F., K.H. Choo, D.J.G. Rees et al. Gene deletions in patients with haemophilia B and anti-factor IX antibodies. Nature 303: 181-182 (1983).

G27 Gusella, J.F., W.S. Wexler, P.M. Conneally et al. A polymorphic DNA marker genetically linked to Huntington disease. Nature 306: 234-238 (1983).

G28 Gianelli, F., D.S. Anson, K.H. Choo et al. Characterization and use of an intragenic polymorphic marker for detection of carriers of haemophilia B (factor IX deficiency). Lancet 1: 239-241 (1984).

G29 Gilbert, F. Chromosomal aberrations and oncogenes. Nature 303: 475 (1983).

G30 Gerhard, D.S., K.K. Kidd, D. Housman et al. Abstract. Los Angeles 7th Int. Workshop on Human Gene Mapping. Cited in [R28].

G31 Greenberg, M.E. and E.B. Ziff. Stimulation of 3T3 cells induce transcription of the c-fos proto-oncogene. Nature 311: 433-437 (1984).

G32 Georgiev, G.P. On mechanisms of oncogenesis: the promotor hypothesis. Mol. Bilogia 15: 261-273 (1981) (in Russian).

G33 Grimaldi, G. and M.F. Singer. A monkey Alu sequence is flanked by 13-basepair direct repeats of an interrupted alpha-satellite DNA sequence. Proc. Natl. Acad. Sci. U.S.A. 79: 1497-1500 (1982).

G34 Gosden, R.G. Chromosome anomalies of preimplantation mouse embryos in relation to maternal age. J. Repro. Fert. 35: 351-354 (1973).

G35 Goncalves, O., E. Drobetsky and M. Meuth. Structure of the aprt locus induced by deoxyribonucleoside triphosphate pool imbalances in Chinese hamster ovary cells. Mol. Cell. Biol. 4: 1792-1799 (1984).

G36 Graf, L.H. and L.A. Chasin. Direct demostration of genetic alterations at the dihydrofolate reductase locus after gamma irradiation. Mol. Cell Biol. 2: 93-96 (1982).

G37 Gillberg, C. Identical triplets with infantile autism and the fragile X-chromosome. Br. J. Psychiatry 143: 256-260 (1983).

G38 Gillberg, C. and J. Wahlström. Chromosome abnormalities in infantile autism and other childhood psychoses. A population study of 66 cases. Dev. Med. Child. Neurol. (Cited in ref. [B39]).

G39 Guichaoua, M., M. G. Mattei, J.F. Mattei et al. Aspécts génétiques des sites fragiles autosomiques. A propos de 40 cas. J. Génét. Hum. 30: 180-197 (1982).

G40 Gosden, J.R., C.M. Gosden, S. Christie et al. Rapid fetal sex determination in first trimester prenatal diagnosis by dot hybridization of DNA probes. Lancet i: 540-541 (1984).

G41 Goeddel, D.V., D.G. Kleid, F. Bolivar et al. Expression in E. coli of chemically synthesized genes for human insulin. Proc. Natl. Acad. Sci. 76: 106-110 (1979).

G42 Goeddel, D.V., H.L. Heyneker, T. Hozumi et al. Direct expression in E. coli of a DNA sequence coding for human growth hormone. Nature 281: 544-548 (1979).

G43 Goeddel, D.V., E. Yelverton, A. Ullrich et al. Human leukocyte interferon produced by E. coli is biologically active. Nature 287: 411-416 (1980).

G44 Gallwitz, D., C. Donath and C. Sander. A yeast gene encoding a protein homologous to the human c-has/bas protooncogene product. Nature 306: 704-707 (1983).

G45 Guerrero, I., O. Calzada, A. Mayer et al. A molecular approach to leukaemogenesis: mouse lymphomas contain an activated c-ras oncogene. Proc. Natl. Acad. Sci. 81: 202-205 (1984).

G46 Groffen, J., J.R. Stephenson, N. Heisterkamp et al. Philadelphia chromosomal breakpoints are clustered within a limited region, ber, on chromosome 22. Cell. 36: 93-99 (1984).

G47 Gill, G., F. Heffron, G. Dougan et al. Analysis of sequences transposed by complementation of transposition deficient mutants of Tn3. J. Bacteriol. 136: 742-756 (1978).

G48 Green, M.M. Genetic instability in Drosophila melanogaster. On the identity of the MR and P-M mutator systems. Biol. Zentralbl. 103: 1-8 (1984).

G49 Georgiev, G.P. Mobile genetic elements in animal cells and their biological significance. Eur. J. Biochem. 145: 203-220 (1984).

G50 Goldberg, M.L., R. Paro and W.J. Gehring. Molecular cloning of the gene of the white locus region of Drosophila melanogaster using a large transposable element. EMBO J. 1: 93-98 (1982).

G51 Gunther, M., R. Wicker et al. Enhanced survival of uv-damaged parvovirus Lu III and herpes virus in carcinogen-pretreated transformed human cells. p. 605-609 in: Chromosome Damage Repair (E. Seeberg and K. Kleppe, eds.). Plenum Press, New York, 1980.

G52 Gentil, A., A. Margot and A. Sarasin. Enhanced reactivation and mutagenesis after transfection of carcinogen-treated monkey cells with UV-irradiated Simian virus-40 DNA. Biochimie 64: 693-696 (1982).

G53 Gerchman, L., D.B. Ludlum. The properties of O^6-methylguanine in templates for DNA polymerase. Biochim. Biophys. Acta. 308: 310-316 (1973).

G54 Goth, R. and M.F. Rajewsky. Persistence of O^6-ethylguanine in rat brain DNA. Correlation with nervous system specific carcinogens by ENU. Proc. Natl. Acad. Sci. 71: 639-643 (1974).

G55 Generoso, W.M., K.T. Cain et al. ^{239}Pu-induced heritable translocation in male mice. Mutat. Res. 152: 49-52 (1985).

G56 Garfield, E. What do we know about the group of disorders called schizophrenia? I and II. Current Contents 25: 5-13 (1983), Current Contents 27: 5-16 (1983).

G57 Garfield, E. What do we know about depression? Part I. Etiology. Current Contents 19: 5-12 (1981).

G58 Goodridge, D.M.G. and S.D. Shorvon. Epileptic seizures in a population of 6000. Br. Med. J. 287: 641-644 (1983).

G59 Gyárfás, I. and A. Czukás-ne. Epidemiologic study of acute myocardial infarction with the population of South Pest. Népegészégügy 56: 149-159 (1975).

G60 Gömör, B., M. Andor and L. Bakos. Screening of rheumatoid arthritis and ankylosing spondylitis in a district of Budapest. Orvosi Hetilap 115: 1463-1466 (1974).

G61 Ginter, E.K., A.A. Revasov, M.I. Talanov et al. Medical genetic studies of the Kostroma district population. I. The load of hereditary disorders in population. Genetika 21: 153-160 (1985) (in Russian).

G62 Ginter, E.K., A.A. Revasov, M.I. Talanov et al. Medical genetic studies of the Kostroma district population. II. The diversity of hereditary pathology in five regions. Genetika 21: 1372-1379 (1985). (in Russian)

G63 Ginter, E.K., K.A. Budagove, A.A. Revasov et al. Medical genetic studies of the population of Uzbekistan. VII. The diversity of hereditary pathology in four regions of Khorezm province. Genetika 22: 312-320 (1986). (in Russian)

H1 Hook, E.B. Contribution of chromosome abnormalities to human morbidity and some comments upon surveillance of chromosome mutation rates. p. 9-38 in: Progress in Mutation Research (K.C. Bora et al., eds.), Elsevier Biomedical Press, Amsterdam, 1982.

H2 Hook, E.B. and J.L. Hamerton. The frequency of chromosome abnormalities detected in consecutive newborn studies—differences between studies—results by sex and by severity of phenotypic involvement. p. 63-79 in: Population Cytogenetics, Studies in Humans (E.B. Hook and I.H. Porter, eds.), Academic Press, New York, 1977.

H3 Hecht, F., P.B. Jacky and G.R. Sutherland. The fragile X-chromosome: current methods. Am. J. Med. Genet. 11: 489-495 (1982).

H4 Herbst, D.S., H.G. Dunn, F.J. Dill et al. Further delineation of X-linked mental retardation. Hum. Genet. 58: 366-372 (1981).

H5 Heisterkamp, N., Groffen, J.R. Stephenson et al. Chromosomal localization of human cellular homologues of two viral oncogenes. Nature 299: 747-749 (1982).

H6 Hiraizumi, Y. Spontaneous recombination in Drosophila melanogaster males. Proc. Natl. Acad. Sci. U.S.A. 68: 268-270 (1971).

H7 Hartman, K.U. and C. Heidelberger. Studies on fluorinated pyrimidines. XIII. Inhibition of thymidylate synthetase. J. Biol. Chem. 236: 3006-3013 (1961).

H8 Hansson, K. and B. Hartley-Asp. Potentiation by hydroxyurea in G_2 prophase of thitepa and bleomycin induced chromosome aberrations in Chinese hamster cells. Hereditas 94: 21-27 (1981).

H9 Hansson, K., F. Palitti, B.A. Hihman et al. Potentiation of x-ray and streptonigrin induced chromosome aberrations in human lymphocytes by post-treatments with hydroxyurea and caffeine. Hereditas 97: 51-58 (1982).

H10 Hubermann, J.A. New views on the biochemistry of eukaryotic DNA replication revealed by aphidicolin an unusual inhibitor of the DNA polymerase alpha. Cell 23: 647-648 (1980).

H11 Hayaishi, O. and K. Ueda. Poly(ADP-ribose) and ADP-ribosylation of proteins. Ann. Rev. Biochem. 46: 95-116 (1977).

H12 Hori, T. High incidence of sister chromatid exchanges and chromatid interchanges in the conditions of lowered activity of poly(ADP-ribose) polymerase. Biochem. Biophys. Res. Commun. 102: 38-45 (1981).

H13 Hansteen, I.L., K. Varslot, J.S. Johnsen et al. Cytogenetic screening of a newborn population. Clin. Genet. 21: 309-314 (1982).

H14 Herbst, D.S. and J.R. Miller. Non-specific X-linked mental retardation. II. The frequency in British Columbia. Am. J. Med. Genet. 7: 461-470 (1980).

H15 Hall, Ac., C.J. Marshall, N.K. Spurr et al. Identification of transforming genes in two human sarcoma lines as a new member of the ras gene family. Nature 303: 396-400 (1983).

H16 Harper, M.E., G. Franchini, J. Love et al. Chromosomal sublocalization of human c-myb and c-fes cellular onc genes. Nature 305: 638-641 (1983).

H17 Huerre, C., S. Despoisse, S. Gilgenkrantz et al. c-Ha-ras1 is not deleted in aniridia-Wilms' tumour association. Nature 305: 638-641 (1983).

H18 Hill, M.E.E., K.E. Davies, P.S. Harper et al. The Mendelian inheritance of a human X-chromosome-specific DNA sequence polymorphism and its use in linkage studies of genetic disease. Hum. Gen. 60: 222-226 (1982).

H19 Harper, P.S., T. O'Brien, J.M. Murray et al. The use of linked DNA polymorphisms for genotypic prediction in families with Duchenne muscular dystrophy. J. Med. Genet. 20: 252-254 (1983).

H20 Harper, M.E. Chromosome mapping of single-copy sequences in in situ hybridization. p. 159-165 in: Banbury Report 14. Recombinant DNA Applications to Human Disease (C.T. Caskey and R.L. White, eds.). Cold Spring Harbor Laboratory, New York, 1983.

H21 Hori, T.A., T. Shiomi and K. Sato. Human chromosome 13 compensates a DNA repair defect in UV-sensitive mouse cells by mouse-human cell hybridization. Proc. Natl. Acad. Sci. U.S.A. 80: 5655-5659 (1983).

H22 Hunt, A. and R.H. Lindenbaum. Tuberous sclerosis; a new estimate of prevalence within the Oxford region. J. Med. Genet. 21: 272-277 (1984).

H23 Hassold, T., D. Chiu and J.A. Yamane. Parental origin of autosomal trisomies. Ann. Hum. Genet. 48: 129-144 (1984).

H24 Hook, E.B. Rates of chromosome abnormalities at different maternal ages. Obstet. Gynecol. 58: 282-285 (1981).

H25 Hook, E.B., D.M. Schreinemachers, A.M. Willey et al. Rates of mutant structural chromosome rearrangements in human fetuses: data from prenatal cytogenetic studies and associations with maternal age and parental mutagen exposure. Am. J. Hum. Genet. 35: 96-109 (1983).

H26 Howard-Peebles, P.N. and A.J. Carroll. Letter to the Editor: recombination between the fragile-X and G6-PD. Am. J. Med. Genet. 17: 275-276 (1984).

H27 Holden, J.A., H. Wang and B. White. The fragile-X syndrome. IX. Progress towards the identification of linked restriction fragment length variants. Am. J. Med. Genet. 17: 259-273 (1984).

H28 Hecht, F. and B.K. Hecht. Fragile sites and chromosome breakpoints in constitutional rearrangements. I. Amniocentesis. Clin. Genet. 26: 169-173 (1984).

H29 Hecht, F. and B.K. Hecht. Fragile sites and chromosome breakpoints in constitutional rearrangements. II. Spontaneous abortions, stillbirths and new borns. Clin. Genet. 26: 174-177 (1984).

H30 Howard-Peebles, P.N. and G.R. Stoddard. Familial X-linked mental retardation with a marker X-chromosome and its relationship to macroorchidism. Clin. Genet. 17: 125-128 (1980).

H31 Haneda, M., S.J. Chan, S.C.M. Kwok et al. Studies on mutant human insulin gene. Identification and sequence analysis of a gene encoding (ser^{B24})insulin. Proc. Natl. Acad. Sci. U.S.A. 80: 6366-6370 (1983).

H32 Heldin, C.H. and B. Westermark. Growth factors: mechanism of action and relation to oncogenes. Cell 37: 9-20 (1984).

H33 Hayward, W.S., B.S. Neel and S.M. Astrin. Activation of a cellular oncogene by promotor insertion in ALV-induced lymphoid leukosis. Nature 290: 475-480 (1981).

H34 Hunter, T. and J.A. Cooper. Epidermal growth factor induces rapid tyrosine phosphorylation of proteins in A431 tumour cells. Cell 24: 741-752 (1981).

H35 Heldin, C.H., B. Westermark and A. Wasteson. Platelet-derived growth factors: purification and partial characterization. Proc. Natl. Acad. Sci. U.S.A. 76: 3722-3726 (1979).

H36 Heffron, F. Tn3 and its relatives. p. 223-260 in: Mobile Genetic Elements (J.A. Shapiro, ed.) Academic Press, New York, 1983.

H37 Haynes, R., T.P. Toomey, L. Leinward et al. The Chinese hamster Alu-equivalent sequence: a conserved highly repetitious, interspersed DNA sequence in mammals has a structure suggestive of a transposable element. Mol. Cell Biol. 1: 573-583 (1981).

H38 Hittelman, W.N. and P.N. Rao. Premature chromosome condensation. I. Visualization of x ray induced chromsome damage in interphase cells. Mutat. Res. 23: 251-258 (1974).

H39 Hittelman, W.N. and P.N. Rao. Bleomycin-induced damage in prematurely condensed chromosomes and its relationship to cell cycle progression in CHO cells. Cancer Res. 34: 3433-3439 (1974).

H40 Hittelman, W.N. and P.N. Rao. The nature of adriamycin-induced cytotoxicity in Chinese hamster cells as revealed by premature chromosome condensation. Cancer Res. 35: 3027-3035 (1975).

H41 Hittelman, W.N. Prematurely condensed chromosomes: a model system for visualizing effects of DNA damage, repair and inhibition at the level of chromosome structure. p. 341-371 in: DNA Repair and its Inhibition (A. Collins et al., eds.). IRL Press, Oxford, 1983.

H42 Henderson, S.A. and R.G. Edwards. Chiasma frequency and maternal age in mammals. Nature 218: 22-28 (1968).

H43 Hassold, T. and D. Chiu. Maternal age-specific rates of numerical chromosome abnormalities with specific reference to trisomy. Hum. Genet. 70: 11-17 (1985).

H44 Hagemeijer, A., K. Hahlen, W. Sizoo et al. Translocation (9;11) (p21;q23) in three cases of acute monoblastic leukaemia. Cancer Genet. Cytogenet. 5: 95-105 (1982).

H45 Harper, P.S. Myotonic Dystrophy. W.B. Saunders, Philadelphia, 1979.

H46 Hofker, M.H., M.C. Wapenaar, W.C. Goor et al. Isolation of probes detecting restriction fragment length polymorphisms from X-chromosome-specific libraries: potential use for diagnosis of Duchenne muscular dystrophy. Hum. Genet. 70: 148-156 (1985).

H47 Hagemeijer, A. and E.M.E. Smit. Partial trisomy 21. Further evidence that trisomy of band 21q22 is essential for Down's phenotype. Hum. Genet. 38: 15-23 (1977).

H48 Hunter, T. The proteins of oncogenes. Sci. Am. 251: 60-69 (1984).

H49 Heisterkamp, N., J.R. Stephenson, J. Groffen et al. Localization of the c-abl oncogene adjacent to a translocation breakpoint in chronic myelocytic leukaemia. Nature 306: 239-242 (1983).

H50 Heisterkamp, N., J.R. Stephenson, G. Grosveld et al. The involvement of human c-abl and bcr in the Philadelphia translocation. p. 547-567 in: Genes and Cancer (J.M. Bishop et al. eds.). UCLA Symposium on Molecular and Cellular Biology. New Series. Vol. 17. Alan R. Liss Inc., New York, 1984.

H51 Heartlein, M.W. and R.J. Preston. An explanation of interspecific differences in sensitivity to x-ray-induced chromosomal aberrations and a consideration of dose-response curves. Mutat. Res. 150: 299-305 (1985).

H52 Holmberg, M. and E. Gumauskas. The role of short-lived DNA lesions in the production of chromosome-exchange aberrations. Mutat. Res. 160: 221-229 (1986).

H53 Herrlich, P., U. Mallick et al. Genetic changes in mammalian cells reminiscent of an SOS response. Hum. Genet. 67: 360-368 (1984).

H55 Hollow, F.C. and P.A. Graham. Intraocular pressure glaucoma and glaucoma suspects in a defined population. Br. J. Ophthalmol. 50: 570-586 (1966).

H56 Hauge, M. and J. Gundersen. Genetics of varicose veins of the lower extremities. Hum. Hered. 19: 579-580 (1969).

H57 Hüttl, F. and G. Ecsedy. Is there an increasing trend in prevalence of cholelithiasis or gall bladder disorders? Magyar Sebészet 33: 159-162 (1980).

H58 Hughes, G.R.V. and J.R. Batchelor. Genetics of systemic lupus erythematosus. Br. Med. J. 286: 416-417 (1983).

H59 Holal, F., R. Gledhill and F.C. Fraser. Dominant inheritance of Scheuermann juvenile kyphosis. Am. J. Dis. Child. 132: 1105-1107 (1978).

H60 Hassold, T. and P. Jacobs. Trisomy in man. Ann. Rev. Genet. 18: 69-97 (1984).

H61 Hayes, A., T. Costa et al. The effect of Mendelian disease on human health. II. Response to treatment. Am. J. Med. Genet. 21: 243-255 (1985).

H62 Harlap, S., P.H. Shiono and S. Ramcharan. A life table of spontaneous abortions and the effects of age, parity and other variables. p. 145-158 in: Human Embryonic and Foetal Death (I.H. Porter and E.B. Hook, eds.), Academic Press, New York, 1980.

H63 Harrison, C.J., E.M. Jack, T.D. Allen et al. The fragile X: a scanning electron microscope study. J. Med. Genet. 20: 280-283 (1983).

H64 Hutchison, K.W., N.G. Copeland and N.A. Jenkins. Dilute coat colour locus of mice. Nucleotide sequence analysis of the d^{+25} and d^{+Ha} revertant alleles. Mol. Cell. Biol. 4: 2899-2904 (1984).

I1 Ising, G. and C. Ramel. The behaviour of a transposing element in Drosophila melanogaster. p. 947-954 in: The Genetics and Biology of Drosophila (M. Ashburner and E. Novitski, eds.). Vol. 1b. Academic Press, New York, 1976.

I2 Ising, G. and K. Block. Derivation-dependent distribution sites for a Drosophila transposon. Cold Spring Harbor Symp. Quant. Biol. 45: 527-544 (1981).

I3 Ilyin, Yu.V., N.A. Tchurikov, E.V. Ananiev et al. Studies on the DNA fragments of mammals and Drosophila containing structural genes and adjacent sequences. Cold Spring Harbor Symp. Quant. Biol. 42: 959-969 (1978).

I4 Ikegami, S., T. Taguchi, M. Ohashi et al. Aphidicolin prevents mitotic cell division by interfering with the activity of DNA polymerase alpha. Nature 275: 458-460 (1978).

I5 International Classification of Diseases. Manual of the International Classification of Diseases, Injuries and Causes of Death. Volumes 1 and 2. 1975 Revision. World Health Organization, Geneva, 1977.

I6 ISCN. An International System for Human Cytogenetic Nomenclature: high resolution banding. Cytogenetics and Cell Genetics 31: 1-23 (1981).

I7 Ikkala, E. Haemophilia: a study of its laboratory, clinical, genetic and social aspects based on known haemophiliacs in Finland. Scand. J. Clin. Lab. Invest. 12 (Suppl. 76): 1-144 (1960).

I8 Iida, S., J. Meyer and W. Arber. Prokaryotic IS elements. p.159-221 in: Mobile Genetic Elements (J.A. Shapiro, ed.) Academic Press, New York 1983.

I9 Ishihara, T. and M.S. Sasaki (eds). Radiation-induced Chromosome Damage in Man. Prog. and Topics in Cytogenetics Vol. 4 (A.A. Sandberg, ed.) Alan R. Liss Inc., New York, 1983.

I10 Ingle, C., R. Williamson, A. de La Chapelle et al. Mapping of DNA sequences in a human X-chromosome deletion which extends across the region of the Duchenne muscular dystrophy mutation. Am. J. Hum. Genet. 37: 451-462 (1985).

I11 Itakura, K., T. Hirose, R. Crea et al. Expression in Escherichia coli of a chemically synthesized gene for the hormone somatostatin. Science 198: 1056-1063 (1977).

I12 Ismailov, Z.F., S.P. Smirnov and V.A. Tarasov. The isolation of mutants with a high frequency of translocation of Tn1 transposon in E. coli cells. Genetika 18: 1938-1944 (1982). (in Russian)

I13 Iliakis, G. and P.E. Bryant. Effects of nucleoside analogs—araA, araB and araC—on cell growth and repair of potentially lethal damage and DNA double-strand breaks in mammalian cell cultures. Anticancer Res. 3: 143-150 (1983).

I14 Iselius, L., J. Lindsten, A. Aurias et al. The 11q;22q translocation. A collaborative study of 20 new cases and analysis of 110 families. Hum. Genet 64: 343-355 (1983).

J1 Jacobs, P.A., J.S. Matsuura, M. Mayer et al. A cytogenetic survey of an institution for the mentally retarded. Clin. Genet. 13: 37-60 (1978).

J2 Jordan, E., H. Saedler and P. Starlinger. O^c and strong polar mutations in the gal operon are insertions. Mol. Gen. Genet. 102: 353-363 (1968).

J3 Jordan, E., H. Saedler and P. Starlinger. Strong polar mutations in the transferase gene of the galactose operon in E. coli. Mol. Gen. Genet. 100: 296-306 (1967).

J4 Jaskunas, S.R., L. Lindahl and M. Nomura. Isolation of polar insertion mutants and the direction of transcription of ribosomal protein genes in E. coli. Nature 256: 183-187 (1975).

J5 Johnstones, A.P. and G.T. Williams. Role of DNA breaks and ADP-ribosyl transferase activity in eukaryotic differentiation demonstrated in human lymphocytes. Nature 300: 368-370 (1982).

J6 Jeffreys, J.A. DNA sequence variants in the G$_r$, Arδ and beta-globin genes of man. Cell 18: 1-10 (1979).

J7 Jenkins, N.A., N.G. Copeland, B.A. Taylor et al. Dilute (d) coat colour mutation of DBA/2J mice is associated with the site of integration of an ecotropic MuLV genome. Nature 293: 370-374 (1981).

J8   Jaenisch, R., K. Harbers, A. Schnieke et al. Germline integration of Moloney leukaemia virus at the Mov 13 locus leads to recessive lethal mutation and early embryonic death. Cell 32: 209-216 (1983).

J9   Jelnick, W.R. and C.W. Schmid. Repetitive sequences in eukaryotic DNA and their expression. Ann. Rev. Biochem. 51: 813-844 (1982).

J10   Jacobs, P.A. Mutation rates of structural chromosome rearrangements in man. Am. J. Hum. Genet. 33: 44-54 (1981).

J11   Jacobs, P.A., T.W. Glover, M. Mayer et al. X-linked mental retardation: a study of 7 families. Am. J. Med. Genet. 7: 471-489 (1980).

J12   Jacobs, P.A., M. Mayer, J. Matsuura et al. A cytogenetic study of a population of mentally retarded males with special reference to the marker (X) syndrome. Hum. Genet. 63: 139-148 (1983).

J13   Jacobs, P.A., M. Mayer, E. Rudak et al. Note on marker-X chromosomes, mental retardation and macroorchidism. New Engl. J. Med. 300: 737-738 (1979).

J14   Jeanpierre, M. and C. Junien. DNA analysis as clinical investigation. When and how? Ann. Genet. 27: 134-147 (1984).

J15   Jolly, P.D., A.C. Esty, H.U. Bernard et al. Isolation of a genomic clone partially encoding human HPRT. Proc. Natl. Acad. Sci. U.S.A. 79: 5038-5041 (1982).

J16   Jhanwar, S.C., B.G. Neel, W.S. Hayward et al. Localization of the cellular oncogenes ABL, SIS and FES on human germ-line chromosomes. Cytogenetics and Cell Genetics 38: 73-75 (1984).

J17   Jhanwar, S.C., B.G. Neel, W.S. Hayward et al. Localization of c-ras oncogene family on human germ-line chromosomes. Proc. Natl. Acad. Sci. U.S.A. 80: 4794-4797 (1983).

J18   Johnson, R.T. and P.N. Rao. Mammalian cell fusion: induction of premature chromosome condensation in interphase nuclei. Nature 226: 717-722 (1970).

J19   Jagadeeswaran, P., D.E. Lavelle, R. Kaul et al. Isolation and characterization of human factor IX cDNA: identification of TaqI polymorphism and regional assignment. Somatic Cell Mol. Genet. 10: 465-473 (1984).

J20   Jaye, M., De La Salle, F. Schamaker et al. Isolation of human anti-haemophilic factor IX cDNA clone using a unique 52 base synthetic oligonucleotide probe deduced from the aminoacid sequence of bovine factor IX. Nucleic Acids Res. 11: 2325-2335 (1983).

J21   Jagadeeswaran, P., J. Pan, B.G. Forget et al. Sequences of human repetitive DNA, non-alpha globin genes in man. Cold Spring Harbor Symposium. Quant. Biol. 47: 1079-1086 (1982).

J22   Jeffreys, A.J. and R.A. Flavell. The rabbit beta globin gene contains a large insert in the coding sequence. Cell 12: 1097-1108 (1977).

J23   Jorgensen, R.A. and S.N. Reznikoff. Organization of structural and regulatory genes that mediate tetracycline resistance of transposon Tn10. J. Bacteriol. 138: 705-714 (1979).

J24   Jagadeeswaran, P., B.G. Forget and S.M. Weissman. Short interspersed repetitive DNA elements in eukaryotes. Transposable DNA elements generated by reverse transcription of RNA pol III transcripts. Cell 26: 141-143 (1981).

J25   Jeeves, W.P. and A.J. Rainbow. Gamma-ray-enhanced reactivation of uv-irradiated adenovirus in normal human fibroblasts. Mutat. Res. 60: 33-41 (1979).

J26   Jeeves, W.P. and A.J. Rainbow. Gamma-ray-enhanced reactivation of gamma-ray irradiated adenovirus in human cells. Biochem. Biophys. Res. Commun. 90: 567-574 (1979).

J27   Jeggo, P., M. Defais, L. Samson et al. An adaptive response of E. coli to low levels of alkylating agent. Comparison with previously characterized DNA repair pathways. Mol. Gen. Genet. 157: 1-9 (1977).

K1   Kuleshov, N.P., N.I. Alekhin et al. Frequency of chromosome abnormalities among infants dying during the perinatal period. Genetika 11: 107-110 (1975).

K2   Kondo, I., H. Hamaguchi et al. A cytogenetic survey of 449 patients in a Japanese institution for the mentally retarded. I. Chromosome abnormalities. Clin. Genet. 17: 177-182 (1980).

K3   Klein, G. The role of gene dosage and genetic transposition in carcinogenesis. Nature 294: 313-318 (1981).

K4   Kleckner, N. Translocatable elements in prokaryotes. Cell 11: 11-23 (1977).

K5   Kidwell, M.G., J.F. Kidwell and J.A. Sved. Hybrid dysgenesis in Drosophila melanogaster. A syndrome of aberrant traits including mutations, sterility and male recombination. Genetics 86: 813-833 (1977).

K6   Kihlman, B.A., K. Hansson, F. Palitti et al. Potentiation of chromosome alterations by inhibitors of DNA repair. p. 319-339 in: DNA repair and its inhibition (A. Collins et al., eds.). IRL Press, Oxford, 1983.

K7   Kihlman, B.A., K. Hansson, F. Palitti et al. Potentiation of induced chromatid-type aberrations by hydroxyurea and caffeine in G_2. p. 11-24 in: Progress in Mutation Research (A.T. Natarajan et al., eds.). Vol. 4, Elsevier Biomedical Press, Amsterdam, 1982.

K8   Kihlman, B.A., W.W. Nichols and A. Levan. The effect of deoxyadenosine and cytosine arabinoside on the chromosome of human leucocytes in vitro. Hereditas 50: 139-144 (1963).

K10   Kähkönen, M., J. Leisti, M. Wilska et al. Marker-X-associated mental retardation. A study of 150 retarded males. Clin. Gent. 23: 397-404 (1983).

K11   Kirsch, I.R., C.C. Morton, K. Nakahara et al. Human immunoglobulin heavy chain genes map to a region of translocations in malignant B lymphocytes. Science 216: 301-303 (1982).

K12   Kingston, H.M., N.S.T. Thomas, P.L. Pearson et al. Genetic linkage between Becker muscular dystrophy and a polymorphic DNA sequence on the short arm of the X-chromosome. J. Med. Genet. 20: 255-258 (1983).

K13   Kan, Y.W. and A.M. Dozy. Polymorphism of DNA sequence adjacent to the human beta-globin structural gene. Relationship to sickle cell mutation. Proc. Natl. Acad. Sci. U.S.A. 75: 5631-5635 (1978).

K14   Kazazian, H.H., S.Y. Antonarakis, T. Cheng et al. DNA polymorphism in the beta-globin gene cluster: use in discovery of mutations and prenatal diagnosis. p. 29-39 in: Banbury Report 14. Recombinant DNA Applications to Human Disease (C.T. Caskey and R.L. White, eds.). Cold Spring Harbor Laboratory, New York, 1983.

K15   Kurachi, K., T. Chandra, S.J.F. Degen et al. Cloning and sequence of cDNA coding for alpha-l-antitrypsin. Proc. Natl. Acad. Sci. U.S.A. 78: 6826-6830 (1981).

K16 Kirk, M. and F. Lyon. Induction of congenital anomalies in offspring of female mice exposed to varying doses of X-rays. Mutat. Res. 106: 73-83 (1982).

K17 Kirk, M. and M.F. Lyon. Induction of congenital malformations in the offspring of male mice treated with X-rays at pre-meiotic and post-meiotic stages. Mutat. Res. 125: 75-85 (1984).

K19 Kidd, V.J., R.B. Wallace, K. Itakura et al. Alpha-antitrypsin deficiency detection by direct analysis of the mutation in the gene. Nature 304: 230-234 (1983).

K20 Karathanasis, S.K., V.I. Zannis and J.L. Breslow. A DNA insertion in the apolipoprotein A-I gene of patients with premature atherosclerosis. Nature 305: 823-825 (1983).

K21 Karathanasis, S.K., R.A. Norum, V.I. Zannis et al. An inherited polymorphism in the human apolipoprotein A-I gene locus related to the development of atherosclerosis. Nature 301: 718-720 (1983).

K22 Kingston, H.M., N. Safarazi, N.S.T. Thomas et al. Localization of the Becker muscular dystrophy gene on the short arm of the X chromosome by linkage to cloned DNA sequences. Hum. Genet. 67: 6-17 (1984).

K23 Krontiris, T. The emerging genetics of human cancer. New Engl. J. Med. 309: 404-409 (1983).

K24 Khoury, G. and P. Gruss. Enhancer elements. Cell 33: 313-314 (1983).

K25 Koufos, A., M.F. Hansen, B.C. Lampkin et al. Loss of alleles at loci on human chromosome 11 during genesis of Wilms' tumour. Nature 309: 170-172 (1984).

K26 Kasuga, M., Y. Zick, D.L. Blithe et al. Insulin stimulates tyrosine phosphorylation of the insulin receptor in the cell-free system. Nature 298: 667-669 (1982).

K27 Kelly, K., B.H. Cochran, C.D. Stiles et al. Cell specific regulation of the c-myc gene by lymphocyte mitogens and platelet-derived growth factor. Cell 35: 603-610 (1983).

K28 Kleckner, N. Transposon Tn10, p. 261-298 in: Mobile Genetic Elements (J.A. Shapiro, ed.) Academic Press, New York, 1983.

K29 Kleckner, N. Transposable elements in prokaryotes. Ann. Rev. Genet. 15: 341-404 (1981).

K30 Kuff, E.L., A. Feenstra, K. Lucdors et al. Intracisternal A-particle genes as movable elements in the mouse genome. Proc. Natl. Acad. Sci. U.S.A. 80: 1992-1996 (1983).

K31 Kamiguchi, Y., K. Funaki and K. Mikamo. Chromosomal anomalies caused by preovulatory overripeness of the primary oocyte. Proc. Jap. Acad. 55 (Series B): 398-402 (1979).

K32 Kamuguchi, Y., K. Funaki and K. Mikamo. A new technique for chromosome study of murine oocytes. Proc. Jap. Acad. 52: 316-319 (1976).

K33 Kamiguchi, Y. and K. Mikamo. Dose-response relationship for induction of structural chromosome aberrations in Chinese hamster oocytes after x-irradiation. Mutat. Res. 103: 33-37 (1982).

K34 Krawczun, M.S., E.C. Jenkins and W.T. Brown. Analysis of the fragile-X chromosome: localization and detection of the fragile site in high resolution preparations. Hum. Genet. 69: 209-211 (1985).

K35 Kurachi, K. and E.W. Davie. Isolation and characterization of a cDNA coding for human factor IX. Proc. Natl. Acad. Sci. U.S.A. 79: 6461-6464 (1982).

K36 Kowalczyk, J. and A.A. Sandberg. A possible subgroup of ALL with 9p-. Cancer Genet. Cytogenet. 9: 383-385 (1983).

K37 Kessler, C., P.S. Neumaier and W. Wolff. Recognition sequences of endonucleases and methylases. A review. Gene 33: 1-101 (1985).

K38 Kelly, T.J., and H.O. Smith. A restriction enzyme from Haemophilus influenzae II. Base sequence of the recognition site. J. Mol. Biol. 51: 393-409 (1970).

K39 Karathanasis, S.K., V.I. Zannis and J.L. Breslow. Isolation and characterization of human apolipoprotein A-I gene. Proc. Natl. Acad. Sci. U.S.A. 80: 6147-6151 (1983).

K40 Klein, G. and E. Klein. Evolution of tumours and the impact of molecular oncology. Nature 315: 190-195 (1985).

K41 Kahn, S.A. and R.P. Novick. Terminal nucleotide sequence of Tn551, a transposon specifying erythromycin resistance in Staphylococcus aureus. Homology with Tn3. Plasmids 4: 148-154 (1980).

K42 Kubaneishwili, M.G., S.P. Smirnov and V.A, Tarasov. Induction of transposon Tn1 translocation under the action of different mutagens. Genetika 19: 903-911 (1983) (in Russian).

K43 Kleckner, N., R.K. Chan, B.K. Tye et al. Mutagenesis by insertion of a drug-resistance element carrying an inserted repetition. J. Mol. Biol. 97: 561-575 (1975).

K44 Kidwell, M.G. and J.F. Kidwell. Selection for male recombination in Drosophila melanogaster. Genetics 84: 333-351 (1976).

K45 Karess, R. and G.M. Rubin. A small tandem duplication is responsible for the unstable white-ivory mutation in Drosophila. Cell 30: 63-69 (1982).

K46 Krayev, A.S., D.A. Kramerov, K.G. Skryabin et al. The nucleotide sequence of the ubiquitous repetitive DNA sequence B1 complementary to the most abundant class of mouse foldback DNA. Nucleic Acids Res. 8: 1201-1215 (1980).

K47 Krayev, A.S., T.V. Markusheva, D.A. Kramerov et al. Ubiquitous transposon-like repeats B1 and B2 of the mouse genome. B2 sequencing. Nucleic Acids Res. 10: 7461-7476 (1982).

K48 Kenyon, C.J. The bacterial response to DNA damage. TIBS 8: 84-87 (1983).

K49 Kaplan, J.C., G.B. Zamansky and P.H. Black. Parallel induction of sister chromatid exchanges and infectious virus from SV40-transformed cells by alkylating agents. Nature 271: 662-663 (1978).

K50 Köbberling, J. and H. Tillil. Empirical risk figures for first degree relatives of non-insulin-dependent diabetes. p. 201-209 in: The Genetics of Diabetes Mellitus (J. Köbberling and T. Tattersall, eds.). Academic Press, London, 1982.

K51 Keen, H. and J.M. Ekoe. The geography of diabetes mellitus. Brit. Med. Bull. 40: 359-365 (1984).

K52 Karlsson, J.L. The Biological Basis of Schizophrenia. C.C. Thomas, Springfield, Illinois. 1966.

K53 Koffler, D. Systemic lupus erythematosus. Sci. Am. 243: 40-49 (1980).

K54 Korobko, V.G., V.N. Dobrynin, E.F. Boldyreva et al. Synthesis of oligo- and polynucleotides. XXVIII. The chemical and enzymatic synthesis and closing of an artificial structural gene for bradykinin. Bioorg. Khim. 5: 1802-1814 (1979).

K55 Kalikinskaya, E.I., O.L. Kolomiets, V.A. Shevchenko et al. Chromosome aberrations in F_l from irradiated male mice studied by their synaptenemal complexes. Mutat. Res. 174: 59-65 (1986).

L1 Lubs, H.A. and M.L. Lubs. New cytogenetic techniques applied to a series of children with mental retardation. p. 241-250 in: Chromosome Identification. Nobel Symp. 23 (T. Caspersson and L. Zech, eds.). Academic Press, New York, 1973.

L2 Logan, J. and J. Cairns. The secrets of cancer. Nature 300: 104-105 (1982).

L3 Loeb, L.A., S.S. Agarwal et al. Inhibitors of mammalian DNA polymerase: possible chemotherapeutic approaches. p. 27-45 in: Inhibitors of DNA and RNA Polymerases (P.S. Sarin and R.C. Gallo, eds.). Pergamon Press, Oxford, 1980.

L6 Lee, W.H., C.P. Lin and P.J. Duesberg. DNA clone of avian Fujinami sarcoma virus with temperature-sensitive transforming function in mammalian cells. J. Virol. 44: 401-412 (1982).

L7 Land, H., L.F. Parada and R.A. Weinberg. Tumorigenic conversion of primary embryo fibroblasts requires at least two co-operating genes. Nature 304: 596-602 (1983).

L8 Lange, K. and M. Boehnke. How many polymorphic genes will it take to span the human genome? Am. J. Hum. Genet. 34: 842-845 (1982).

L9 Lin, P.F. and F.H. Ruddle. Murine DNA repair gene. Located on chromosome 4. Nature 289: 191-194 (1981).

L10 Lalley, P.A., J.A. Diaz, A.A. Francis et al. DNA repair: genetic dissection and chromosomal location of the genes required for ultraviolet radiation-induced DNA damage in man using human x mouse somatic cell hybrids. in: Proc. VII Int. Cong. Rad. Res. Abstract B2-22. Book B (J.J. Broerse et al., eds.). Martinus Nijhoff, The Hague, 1983.

L11 LeBeau, M.M. and J.D. Rowley. Heritable fragile sites in cancer. Nature 308: 607-608 (1984).

L12 Little, P.F.R., G. Annison, S. Darling et al. Model for antenatal diagnosis of beta-thalassemia and other monogenic disorders by molecular analysis of linked DNA polymporphisms. Nature 285: 144-147 (1980).

L13 Lin, P., M. Yamaizumi, P.D. Murphy et al. Partial purification and characterization of the mRNA for human TK and HPRT. Proc. Natl. Acad. Sci. U.S.A. 79: 4290-4294 (1982).

L14 LeBeau, M.M., C.A. Westbrook, M.O. Diaz et al. Evidence for two distinct c-src loci on human chromosome 1 and 20. Nature 312: 70-71 (1984).

L15 Land, H., L.F. Parada and R.A. Weinberg. Cellular oncogenes and multistep carcinogenesis. Science 222: 771-778 (1983).

L16 Lyon, M.F. The use of Robertsonian translocations for studies on non-disjunction. p.327-346 in: Radiation Induced Chromosome Damage in Man (T. Ishihara and M.S. Sasaki, eds.) Alan R. Liss Inc., New York, 1983.

L17 Lehman, A.R. Minireview: use of recombinant DNA techniques in cloning DNA repair genes and in the study of mutagenesis in mammalian cells. Mutat. Res. 150: 61-67 (1985).

L18 Lowy, I., A. Pellicer, J.F. Jackson et al. Isolation of transforming DNA: cloning the hamster aprt gene. Cell 22: 817-823 (1980).

L19 Leck, I. Descriptive epidemiology of common malformations. Brit. Med. Bull. 32: 45-52 (1976).

L20 Leck, I. The geographical distribution of neural tube defects and oral clefts. Brit. Med. Bull. 40: 390-395 (1984).

L21 Lejeune, J. Is the fragile X syndrome amenable to treatment? Lancet i: 273-274 (1982).

L22 Levitas, A., R.J. Hagerman, M. Braden et al. Autism and the fragile X syndrome. J. Dev. Behavioral Pediatr. 3: 151-158 (1983).

L23 Leck, I. Congenital malformations and childhood neoplasms. J. Med. Genet. 14: 321-326 (1977).

L25 Leary, J.J., D.J. Brigati and D.C. Ward. Rapid and sensitive calorimetric method for visualizing biotin-labeled DNA probes hybridized to DNA or RNA immobilized on nitrocellulose: bioplots. Proc. Natl. Acad. Sci. 80: 4045-4049 (1983).

L26 Lauer, J., C.K.J. Shen and T. Maniatis. The chromosomal arrangement of human alpha-like globin genes. Sequence homology and alpha globin gene deletions. Cell 20: 119-130 (1980).

L27 Lawn, R.M., E.F. Fritsch, R.C. Parker et al. The isolation and characterization of linked delta and beta globin genes from a cloned library of human DNA. Cell 15: 1157-1174 (1978).

L28 Little, P.F.R., R. Williamson, G. Annison et al. Polymorphisms of human gamma globin genes in Mediterranean populations. Nature 282: 316-318 (1979).

L29 Lebo, R.V., A. Chakravarti, K.H. Beutow et al. Recombination within and between the human insulin and beta globin gene loci. Proc. Natl. Acad. Sci. U.S.A. 80: 4804-4812 (1983).

L30 Levanon, D., J.L. Lieman-Hurwitz, N. Dafni et al. Architecture and anatomy of the chromosome locus in human chromosome 21 encoding the Cu/Zn superoxide dismutase. EMBO J. 4: 77-84 (1985).

L31 Lieman-Hurwitz, J., N. Dafni, V. Lavie et al. Human cytoplasmic superoxide dismutase cDNA clone: a probe for studying the molecular biology of Down syndrome. Proc. Natl. Acad. Sci. U.S.A. 79: 2808-2811 (1982).

L32 Lewis, S., A. Gifford and D. Baltimore. DNA elements are asymmetrically joined during the site-specific recombination of kappa immunoglobin genes. Science 228: 677-685 (1984).

L33 Leder, P. The genetics of antibody diversity. Sci. Am. 246: 72-83 (1982).

L34 Little, C.D., M.M. Nau, D. Carney et al. Amplification and expression of the c-myc oncogene in human lung cancer cell lines. Nature 306: 194-196 (1983).

L35 Livak, K.J., R. Freund, M. Schweber et al. Sequence organization and transcription of two heat shock loci in Drosophila. Proc. Natl. Acad. Sci. U.S.A. 75: 5613-5617 (1978).

L36 Levis, R., P.M. Bingham and G.M. Rubin. Physical map of the white locus of Drosophila melanogaster. Proc. Natl. Acad. Sci. U.S.A. 79: 564-568 (1982).

L37 Levis, R. M. Collins and G.M. Rubin. FB elements are the common basis for the instability of the w^{DZL} and w^c Drosophila mutations. Cell 30: 551-565 (1982).

L38 Lyon, M.F., C.H. Ward and G.M. Simpson. A genetic method for measuring non-disjunction in mice with Robertsonian translocations. Genet. Res. 26: 283-295 (1976).

L39 Lyaginskaya, A.M., S.N. Sinitsina and P.G. Nisimov. Late effects in the offspring of rats exposed to Plutonium-238 nitrate. p. 69-70 in: Urgent Problems of Health Physics. Abstracts of Report at the All Union Conference. Moscow, 1983.

L40 Lyon, M.F., B.D. Cox and J.H. Marston. Dose-response data for x-ray-induced translocations in spermatogonia of rhesus monkey. Mutat. Res. 35: 429-436 (1976).

L41 Lyon, M.F., B.D. Cox. The induction by x-rays of chromosomal aberrations in male guinea pigs, rabbits and golden hamsters. III. Dose response relationship after single doses of x-rays to spermatogonia. Mutat. Res. 29: 407-422 (1975).

L42 Little, J.W. and D.W. Mount. The SOS regulatory system of E. coli. Cell 29: 11-22 (1982).

L43 Lytle, C.D. and J.D. Goddard. UV-enhanced virus reactivation in mammalian cells. Effects of metabolic inhibitors. Photochem. Photobiol. 29: 959-962 (1979).

L44 Lytle, C.D., J. Coppey and W.D. Taylor. Enhanced survival of uv-irradiated herpes simplex virus in carcinogen-pretreated cells. Nature 272: 60-62 (1978).

L45 Lytle, C.D., R.S. Day et al. Infection of uv-irradiated xeroderma pigmetosum fibroblasts by herpes simplex virus: study of capacity and Weigle reactivation. Mutat. Res. 36: 257-264 (1976).

L46 Lytle, C.D. Radiation-enhanced virus reactivation in mammalian cells. Natl. Cancer Inst. Monograph. 50: 145-149 (1978).

L47 Loveless, A. Possible relevance of 0^6-alkylation of de-oxyguanosine to the mutagenicity and carcinogenicity of nitrosamines and nitrosamides. Nature 223: 206-207 (1969).

L48 Lindahl, T., B. Rydberg, T. Hjelmgren et al. Cellular defense mechanisms against alkylation of DNA. p. 89-99 in: Molecular and Cellular Mechanisms of Mutagenesis (J.F. Lemont and W.M. Generoso, eds.). Plenum Press, New York, 1981.

L49 Léonard, A., G. Decat and L. Fabry. The lympho-cytes of small mammals. A model for research in cytogenetics? Mutat. Res. 95: 31-44 (1982).

L50 Lüning, K.G. and A.G. Searle. Estimates of genetic risks from ionizing radiation. Mutat. Res. 12: 291-304 (1971).

L51 Lakatos, I. and I. Pandi. Screening of glaucoma. Szemészet 117: 121-128 (1980).

L52 Lakos, T. Morbidity study of varicosity, deep venous thrombosis and post thrombosis syndrome among grown-up population of Hajdu-Bihar county. Népegészségügy 57: 277-278 (1976).

L53 Lowenstein, M.B. and N.F. Rothfield. Family study of systemic lupus erythematosus. Arthritis Rheum. 20: 1293-1303 (1977).

L54 Lawrence, J.S. and I. Ball. Genetic studies on rheumatoid arthritis. Ann. Rheum. Dis. 17: 160-169 (1958).

L55 Lawrence, J.S. Prevalence of rheumatoid arthritis. Ann. Rheum. Dis. 20: 11-17 (1961).

L56 Lawrence, J.S. Epidemiology of rheumatoid arthritis. Ann. Rheum. 6: 166-172 (1963).

L57 Lyon, M.F. and T. Morris. Gene and chromosome mutation after large fractionated or unfractionated radiation doses to mouse spermatogonia. Mutat. Res. 8: 191-198 (1969).

L58 Lefevre, G. The distribution of randomly-recovered x-ray-induced sex-linked genetic effects in Drosophila melanogaster. Genetics 99: 461-480 (1981).

L59 Lüning, K.G. Studies of irradiated mouse populations. IV. Effects on productivity in the 7th to 18th generations. Mutat. Res. 14: 331-344 (1972).

M1 Méhes, K. and K. Bajnoczky. Incidence of major chromosomal abnormalities. Clin. Genet. 9: 75-76 (1981).

M2 Magnelli, N.C. Cytogenetics of 50 patients with mental retardation and multiple congenital anomalies and 50 normal subjects. Clin. Genet. 9: 169-182 (1976).

M3 McClintock, B. Mutable loci in maize. Carnegie Inst. Wash. Year Book 47: 155-163 (1948).

M4 McClintock, B. The origin and behaviour of mutable loci in maize. Proc. Natl. Acad. Sci. U.S.A. 36: 344-355 (1950).

M5 McClintock, B. Chromosome organization and genic expression. Cold Spring Harbor Symp. Quant. Biol. 16: 13-47 (1952).

M6 McClintock, B. Controlled mutations in maize. Car-negie Inst. Wash. Year Book 54: 245-258 (1955).

M7 McClintock, B. Intranuclear systems controlling gene action and mutation. Brookhaven Symp. Biol. 8: 58-72 (1956).

M8 Matthews, K.A., B.E. Slatko et al. A consideration of the negative correlation between transmission ration and recombination frequency in a male recombination system of Drosophila melanogaster. Jap. J. Genet. 53: 13-25 (1978).

M9 McClements, W.L., R. Dhar et al. The long terminal repeat of Moloney sarcoma provirus. Cold Spring Harbor Symp. Quant. Biol. 45: 699-705 (1981).

M10 Mouthuy, M. and B. Dutrillaux. Cytogenetic study of skin fibroblasts in a case of accidental acute irradia-tion. Mutat. Res. 95: 19-30 (1982).

M11 Martin, R.H., C.C. Lin et al. The chromosome constitution of 1000 spermatozoa. Hum. Genet. 63: 305-309 (1983).

M12 Myrianthopoulos, N.C. and C.S. Chung. Congenital Malformations in Singletons: Epidemiological Survey. Birth Defects Original Article Series, Vol. 10. National Foundation for the March of Dimes, 1974.

M13 McCoy, M.S., J.J. Toole, J.M. Cunningham et al. Characterization of a human colon/lung carcinoma oncogene. Nature 302: 79-81 (1983).

M14 Murray, M.J., J.M. Cunningham, L.F. Parada et al. The HL-60 transforming sequence: a ras oncogene coexisting with altered myc genes in haematopoietic tumours. Cell 33: 749-757 (1983).

M15 McBride, O.W., D.C. Swan, E. Santos et al. Localiza-tion of the normal allele of T24 human bladder carcinoma oncogene to chromosome 11. Nature 300: 773-774 (1982).

M16 Martinville, B., J. Giacalone, C. Shih et al. Oncogene from human EJ bladder carcinoma is located on the short arm of chromosome 11. Science 219: 498-501 (1983).

M17 Mittelman, F. and G. Levan. Clustering of aberrations to specific chromosomes in human neoplasms. Here-ditas 95: 79-139 (1981).

M18 Marcu, K., L.J. Harris, L.W. Stanton et al. Trans-criptionally active c-myc oncogene contained with NIARD, a DNA sequence associated with chromo-some translocation in B-cell neoplasia. Proc. Natl. Acad. Sci. U.S.A. 80: 518-523 (1983).

M19 Malcolm, S., P. Barton, C. Murphy et al. Localization of human immunoglobulin K-light chain variable region genes to the short arm of chromosome 2 by in situ hybridization. Proc. Natl. Acad. Sci. U.S.A. 79: 4957-4961 (1982).

M20 Martinville, B. de and U. Francke. The c-Ha-rasl, insulin and beta-globin loci map outside the deletion associated with aniridia-Wilms' tumour association. Nature 305: 641-643 (1983).

M21 McKusick, V.A. Mendelian Inheritance in Man. Catalogs of Autosomal Dominant, Autosomal Recessive and X-linked Phenotypes. Sixth Edition. Johns Hopkins University Press, Baltimore, 1983.

M22 Maniatis, T., R.C. Hardison, E. Lacy et al. The isolation of structural genes from libraries of eukaryotic DNA. Cell 15: 687-701 (1978).

M23 Murray, J.M., K.E. Davies, P.S. Harper et al. Linkage relationships of a cloned DNA sequence on the short arm of the X-chromosome to Duchenne muscular dystrophy. Nature 300: 69-71 (1982).

M24 McKusick, V.A. The human genome through the eyes of a clinical geneticist. Cytogenet. Cell Genet. 32: 7-23 (1982).

M25 Marotta, C.A., J.T. Wilson, B.G. Forget et al. Human beta-globin messenger RNA. III. Nucleotide sequence derived from complementary DNA. J. Biol. Chem. 252: 5040-5053 (1977).

M27 Matsuda, Y., I. Tobari, T. Utsugi et al. Gamma-ray induced reciprocal translocation in stem-cell spermatogonia of the crab-eating monkey (Macaca fascicularis). Mutat. Res. 129: 373-380 (1984).

M28 Moric-Petrovic, S. and Z. Laca. Fragile site at 12q13 associated with phenotypic abnormalities. Am. J. Med. Genet. 21: 216-217 (1984).

M29 Martin, J.P. and J. Bell. A pedigree of mental defect showing sex-linkage. J. Neurol. Psychiat. 6: 154-157 (1943).

M30 Morton, N.E. and C.S. Chung. Formal genetics of muscular dystrophy. Am. J. Hum. Genet. 11: 360-379 (1959).

M31 Morton, N.E. Effect of inbreeding on IQ and mental retardation. Proc. Natl. Acad. Sci. U.S.A. 75: 3906-3908 (1978).

M32 Maniatis, T., E.F. Fritsch and J. Sambrook. Molecular cloning. A Laboratory Manual. Cold Spring Harbor Laboratory, New York, 1982.

M33 Murray, N.E. and K. Murray. Manipulation of restriction targets in phage lambda to form receptor chromosomes for DNA fragments. Nature 251: 476-481 (1974).

M34 Maniatis, T., A. Jeffrey and D.G. Kleid. Nucleotide sequence of the rightward operator of phage lambda. Proc. Natl. Acad. Sci. U.S.A. 72: 1184-1188 (1975).

M35 Maxam, A.M. and W. Gilbert. A new method for sequencing DNA. Proc. Natl. Acad. Sci. U.S.A. 74: 560-564 (1977).

M36 Maxam, A.M. and W. Gilbert. Sequencing end-labeled DNA with base-specific chemical cleavages. Methods Enzymol. 65: 499 (1980).

M37 Melton, D.W., D.S. Konecki, J. Brennand et al. Structure, expression and mutation of the hypoxanthine phosphoribosyl transferase gene. Proc. Natl. Acad. Sci. U.S.A. 81: 2147-2151 (1984).

M38 Miwa, M., O. Hayaishi, S. Shall et al. (eds.). ADP-ribosylation, DNA repair and Cancer. Proc. 13th Int. Symp. Princess Takamatsu Cancer Res. Fund, Tokyo, 1982. Japan Scientific Societies Press, Tokyo, 1983.

M39 Mikamo, K. and H. Hamaguchi. Chromosomal disorders caused by preovulatory overripeness of oocytes. p. 72-97 in: Ageing Gametes (R.J. Blandau, ed.). S. Karger, Basel, 1975.

M40 Mikamo, K. Overripeness of the egg of Xenopus laevis. D.Sc. Thesis, Hokkaido Univ., Japan, 1961.

M41 Mikamo, K. and Y. Kamiguchi. A new assessment system for chromosomal mutagenicity using oocytes and early zygotes for the Chinese hamster, p. 411-432 in: Radiation-induced Chromosome Damage in Man (T. Ishihara and M.S. Sasaki, eds.). Alan R. Liss, Inc., New York 1983.

M42 Mikamo, K. and Y. Kamiguchi. Primary incidence of spontaneous chromosomal anomalies and their origins and causal mechanisms in the Chinese hamster. Mutat. Res. 108: 265-278 (1983).

M43 Mikamo, K. Y., Kamiguchi, K. Funaki et al. Stage-dependent changes in chromosomal radiosensitivity in primary oocytes of the Chinese hamster. Cytogenetics and Cell Genetics 30: 174-178 (1981).

M44 Mikamo, K. Meiotic chromosomal radiosensitivity in primary oocytes of the Chinese hamster. Cytogenet. Cell Genet. 33: 88-94 (1982).

M45 Mandl, A.M. A quantitative study of the sensitivity of oocytes to x-irradiation. Proc. R. Soc. (London), Ser. B. 150: 53-69 (1959).

M46 Morley, A.A., K.J. Trainor and R. Seshadri. Cloning of human lymphocytes using limited dilution. Exp. Hem. 11: 418-424 (1983).

M47 Moretta, A., G. Pantaleo, L. Moretta et al. Direct demonstration of the clonogenic potential of evey peripheral blood T cell. Clonal analysis of HLA-DR expression and cytological activity. J. Exp. Biol. 157: 743-754 (1983).

M48 Morley, A.A., K.J. Trainor, R. Seshadri et al. Measurements of in vivo mutations in human lymphocytes. Nature 302: 155-156 (1983).

M49 MacInnes, M.A., J.M. Bingham, L.H. Thompson et al. DNA-mediated co-transfer of excision repair capacity and drug resistance into Chinese hamster ovary mutants cell line UV-135. Mol. Cell Biol. 4: 1152-1158 (1984).

M50 Meuth, M. and J.E. Arrand. Alterations of gene structure in EMS-induced mutants of mammalian cells. Mol. Cell Biol. 2: 1459-1462 (1982).

M51 Micic, M., S. Micic and V. Diklic. Chromosomal constitution of infertile men. Clin. Genet. 25: 33-36 (1984).

M52 Moreau, N. and M. Teyssier. Variant D and G chromosomes in male related infertility. Arch. Androl. 9: 307-310 (1982).

M53 Martin, R.H., A. Rademaker, M. Barnes et al. Analysis of human sperm complements after radiation treatment. European Society of Human Genetics. Book of Abstracts. Budapest, 1985.

M54 Mayer, M. M.A. Abruzzo, P.A. Jacobs et al. A cytogenetic study of a population of retarded females with special reference to the fragile-X syndrome. Hum. Genet. 69: 206-208 (1985).

M55 Mark, J. R. Dahlenfors, C. Ekedahl et al. Chromosomal pattern in a benign neoplasm, the mixed salivary gland tumour. Hereditas 96: 141-148 (1982).

M56 Mark, J., R. Dahlenfors and C. Ekedahl. Chromosomal deviations and their specificity in human mixed salivary gland tumours. Anticancer Res. 1: 49-57 (1981).

M57 McKusick, V.A. The human gene map, 1 December 1984. Clin. Genet. 27: 207-239 (1985).

M58 Mekler, Ph., J.T. Delehanty, P.H.M. Lohman et al. The use of recombinant DNA technology to study gene alteration. Mutation Res. 153: 13-15 (1985).

M59 Malcolm, A.D.B. The use of restriction enzymes in genetic engineering. p. 129-173 in: Genetic Engineering (R. Williamson, ed.). Vol. 2. Academic Press, New York, 1981.

M60 Mulligan, L.M., M.A. Phillips et al. Genetic mapping of DNA segments relative to the locus for the fragile-X syndrome at Xq27.3. Am. J. Hum. Genet. 37: 463-472 (1985).

M61 Maniatis, T., E.F. Fritsch, J. Lauer et al. The molecular genetics of human haemoglobins. Ann. Rev. Genet. 14: 45-78 (1980).

M62 Mears, J.G., F. Ramires et al. Organization of human delta and beta globin in cellular DNA and the presence of intragenic inserts. Cell 15: 15-23 (1978).

M63 Myklebost, R., A. Williamson, F. Markham et al. The isolation and characterization of cDNA clones for human apolipoprotein CII. J. Biol. Chem. 259: 4401-4404 (1984).

M64 Moser, H. Duchenne muscular dystrophy: pathogenetic aspects and genetic prevention. Hum. Genet. 66: 17-40 (1983).

M65 Michalopoulos, E.E., P.J. Bevilacqua et al. Molecular analysis of gene deletion in aniridia-Wilms' tumour association. Hum. Genet. 70: 157-162 (1985).

M66 Meselson, M., P. Dunsmuir, M. Schweber et al. Unstable DNA elements in the chromosomes of Drosophila. p. 88-92 in: Genes, Cells and Behaviour: A View of Biology 50 Years Later (H. Horowitz and E. Hutchings, eds.). Caltech., Pasadena, 1983.

M67 Mikamo, K. Intrafollicular over-ripeness and teratologic development. Cytogenetics 7: 212-233 (1968).

M68 Masui, Y. and R.A. Pedersen. Ultraviolet-induced unscheduled DNA synthesis in mouse oocytes during meiotic maturation. Nature 257: 705-706 (1975).

M69 Matsuda, Y., I. Tobari, Y. Yamagiwa et al. Dose-response relationship of gamma-ray induced reciprocal translocations at low doses in spermatogonia of crab-eating monkey (Macaca fascicularis). Mutat. Res. 151: 121-127 (1985).

M70 Miller, J.H. Mutational specificity in bacteria. Ann. Rev. Genet 17: 215-238 (1983).

M71 Moustacchi, E., U.K. Ehmann and E.C. Friedberg. Defective recovery of semiconservative DNA synthesis in XP cells following split-dose uv-irradiation. Mutat. Res. 62: 159-171 (1979).

M72 Muleris, M., M. Paravatou-Petsota and B. Dutrillaux. Diagrammatic representation for chromosomal mutagenesis studies. II. Radiation-induced rearrangements in Macaca fascicularis. Mutat. Res. 126: 93-103 (1984).

M73 Messing, K. and W.E.C. Bradley. In vivo mutant frequency rises among breast cancer patients after exposure to high doses of gamma-irradiation. Mutat. Res. 152: 107-112 (1985).

M74 Mituszova, M., B. Banyai and M. Nagy. Serum urea studies with a healthy population. III. Rheumatológia, Balneológia Allergológia 18: 66-71 (1977).

M75 Moriyama, I.M., D.E. Krueger and I. Stamler. Cardiovascular disease in the United States. Harvard University Press, Cambridge, 1971.

M76 Mezei, G., Cserháti and I. Kelemen. Bedeutung des Ekzems der Bronchialasthmas im Kindesalter. Gyermekgyógyászer 32: 255-260 (1981).

M77 Marsch, D.G., D.A. Meyers and W.B. Bias. The epidemiology and genetics of atopic allergy. New Engl. J. Med. 305: 1551-1559 (1981).

M78 Miller, J.F., E. Williamson, J. Glue et al. Fetal loss after implantation. Lancet ii: 554-556 (1980)

M79 McKusick, V.A. Mendelian Inheritance in Man: Catologs of Autosomal Dominant, Autosomal Recessive and X-linked Phenotypes (5th edition). Johns Hopkins University Press, Baltimore, 1978.

M80 Morris, T. and S.E. O'Grady. Dose-response curve for x-ray induced translocations in mouse spermatogonia. II. Fractionated doses. Mutat. Res. 9: 411-415 (1970).

M81 Martin, M.H. Chromosomal abnormalities in human sperm. p. 91-102 in: Aneuploidy, Etiology and Mechanisms (V.L. Dellarco et al., eds.). Plenum Press, New York, 1985.

N1 Nielsen, J., M. Wohlert et al. Incidence of chromosome abnormalities in newborn children. Comparison between incidences in 1969-1974 and 1980-1982 in the same area. Human Genet. 61: 98-101 (1982).

N2 Natarajan, A.T., A.A. van Zeeland and T.S.B. Zwanenburg. Influence of inhibitors of poly(ADP-ribose) polymerase on DNA repair, chromosomal alterations and mutations. p. 227-242 in: ADP-ribosylation, DNA Repair and Cancer (M. Miwa et al., eds.). Japan Scientific Societies Press, Tokyo, 1983.

N3 Natarajan, A.T., G. Obe et al. Molecular mechanisms involved in the production of chromosomal aberrations. II. Utilization of neurospora endonuclease for the study of aberration production by x-rays in G_1 and G_2 stages of the cell cycle. Mutat. Res. 69: 293-305 (1980).

N4 Natarajan, A.T. and T.S.B. Zwanenburg. Mechanisms for chromosomal aberrations in mammalian cells. Mutat. Res. 95: 1-6 (1982).

N5 Natarajan, A.T., I. Csukas, F. Degrasse et al. Influence of inhibition of repair enzymes on the induction of chromosomal aberrations by physical and chemical agents. p. 47-59 in: Progress in Mutation Research (A.T. Natarajan et al., eds.). Vol. 4. Elsevier Biomedical Press, Amsterdam, 1982.

N6 Natarajan, A.T., I. Csukas and A.A. van Zeeland. Contribution of incorporated 5-bromodeoxyuridine in DNA to the frequencies of SCEs induced by inhibition of poly(ADP-ribose) polymerase. Mutat. Res. 84: 125-132 (1981).

N7 Nomura, T. Parental exposure to x-rays and chemicals induces heritable tumours and anomalies in mice. Nature 296: 575-577 (1982).

N8 Nomura, T. X-ray-induced germ-line mutation leading to tumours: its manifestation by post-natally given urethane in mice. Mutat. Res. 121: 59-65 (1983).

N9 Nomura, T. Changed urethane and radiation response of the mouse germ cells to tumour induction. p. 873-891 in: Tumours of Early Life in Man and Animals. (L. Severi, ed.), Perugia Univ. Press, Perugia, 1978.

N10 Nashed, N. The peritoneal cells carcinogenecity test: a new short-term test system in rats. Mutat. Res. 85: 207-214 (1981).

N11 Nielsen, J. and I. Sillesen. Incidence of chromosome aberrations among 11148 newborn children. Humangenetik 30: 1-12 (1975).

N12 Neel, B.G., S.C. Jhanwar, R.S.K. Chaganti et al. Two human c-oncogenes are located on the long arm of chromosome 8. Proc. Natl. Acad. Sci. U.S.A. 79: 7842-7846 (1982).

N13 Newbold, R.F. and R.W. Overell. Fibroblast immortality is a prerequisite for transformation by EJ c-Ha-ras oncogene. Nature 304: 648-651 (1983).

N14 Newbold, R.F., R.W. Overell and J.R. Connell. Induction of immortality is an early event in malignant transformation of mammalian cells by carcinogens. Nature 200: 633-635 (1982).

N15 Nussbaum, R.L., J. Brennand, C. Chinault et al. Molecular analysis of the hypoxanthine phosphoribosyl-transferase locus. p. 81-89 in: Banbury Report 14. Recombinant DNA Applications to Human Disease. (C.T. Caskey and R.L. White, eds.). Cold Spring Harbor Laboratory, New York, 1983.

N16 Nussbaum, R.L., W.E. Crowder, W.L. Nyhan et al. A three-allele restriction-fragment length polymorphism at the hypoxanthine phosphoribosyl-transferase locus in man. Proc. Natl. Acad. Sci. U.S.A. 80: 4035-4039 (1983).

N17 Neel, J.V., H.M. Mohrenweiser and M.H. Meisler. Rate of spontaneous mutation at human loci encoding protein structure. Proc. Natl. Acad. Sci. U.S.A. 77: 6037-6041 (1980).

N18 Nielsen, K.B., N. Tommerup, H. Poulsen et al. X-linked mental retardation with fragile-X. A pedigree showing transmission by apparently unaffected males and partial expression in female carriers. Hum. Genet. 59: 23-25 (1981).

N19 Novick, R.P., R.C. Clowes, S.N. Cohen et al. Uniform nomenclature for bacterial plasmids: a proposal. Bacterial. Rev. 40: 168-189 (1976)

N20 Neri, G. Some questions on the significance of chromosome alterations in leukaemias and lymphomas: a review. Am. J. Med. Genet. 18: 471-481 (1984).

N21 Nakano, H., F. Yamamato, C. Neville et al. Isolation and characterization of transforming sequences of two human lung carcinomas: structural and functional analysis of the activated c-K-ras oncogenes. Proc. Natl. Acad. Sci. U.S.A. 81: 71-75 (1984)

N22 Nishimura, J., J.S. Huang and T.F. Deuel. Platelet-derived growth factor stimulated tyrosine-specific protein kinase activity in Swiss mouse 3T3 cell membranes. Proc. Natl. Acad. Sci. U.S.A. 79: 4303-4307 (1982).

N23 Natarajan, A.T. and G. Obe. Molecular mechanisms involved in the production of chromosomal aberrations. I. Utilization of neurospora endonuclease for the study of aberration production in G_2 stage of the cell cycle. Mutat. Res. 52: 137-149 (1978).

N24 Natarajan, A.T. and G. Obe. Molecular mechanisms involved in the production of chromosomal aberrations. III. Restriction endonucleases. Chromosoma 90: 120-127 (1984).

N25 Natarajan, A.T. Mutagenesis and chromosome changes: Review. p. 239-247 in: Radiation Research, Proc. 7th Int. Cong. Rad. Res. (J.J. Broerse et al., eds.). Martinus Nijhoff, The Hague, 1983.

N26 Nalbantogly, J., P. Goncalves and M. Meuth. Structure of mutant alleles at the aprt locus of Chinese hamster ovary cells. J. Mol. Biol. 167: 575-594 (1983).

N27 Niebuhr, E. Down's syndrome: the possibility of a pathogenetic segment on chromosome No. 21. Hum. Genet. 21: 99-101 (1974).

N28 Nagata, S., H. Taira, A. Hall et al. Synthesis in E. coli of a polypeptide with human leukocyte interferon activity. Nature 284: 316-320 (1984).

N29 Natarajan, A.T., F. Darroudi, L.H.F. Mullenders et al. The nature and repair of DNA lesions that lead to chromosomal aberrations induced by ionizing radiation. Mutat. Res. 160: 231-236 (1986).

N30 Nomura, T. Further studies on x-ray and chemically-induced germ-line alterations causing tumours and malformations in mice. in: Proc. IV. Intl. Conf. Env. Mutagens. Stockholm. 1985.

N31 Novikova, V. Effects of radioactive material on the reproductive function and the offspring. In: Meditsinskaya Literatura (D.I. Zakutinsky, ed.). Moscow, 1963. (in Russian)

N32 Nifhoff, J.H. and P. de Boer. A first exploration of a Robertsonian translocation heterozygote in the mouse for its usefulness in cytological evaluation of radiation-induced meiotic autosomal non-disjunction. Mutat. Res. 61: 77-86 (1979).

N34 Notkins, A.L. The causes of diabetes. Sci. Am. 241: 62-73 (1979).

N35 Newmark, M.E. and J.K. Penry. Genetics of Epilepsy. A Review. Raven Press, New York, 1980.

N36 National Center for Health Statistics, II, No. 4, 1964.

N37 National Health Survey. Blood pressure of adults by age and sex. United States, 1960-1962.

N38 Nyekita, S., L. Zsiga, K. Tobias et al. Clinical epidemiological study on young adult population. Honvédorvos 31: 225-231 (1979).

N39 Németh, C.S., T. Joó-Sabados and J. Kovacs. The role of genetic and age- and sex-connected immunological factors in the morbidity of systemic lupus erythematosus. Ann. Immun. Hung. 18: 57-85 (1974).

N40 Neel, J.V. and H.M. Mohrenweiser. Failure to demonstrate mutations affecting protein structure or function in children with congenital defects or born prematurely. Proc. Natl. Acad. Sci. U.S.A. 81: 5499-5503 (1984).

N41 Nomura, T. Quantitative studies in mutagenesis, teratogenesis and carcinogenesis in mice. p. 27-33 in: Problems of Threshold in Chemical Mutagenesis (Y. Tazima et al., eds.). The Environmental Mutagen Society of Japan, Tokyo, 1984.

O1 Opitz, J.M. Diagnostic genetic studies in severe mental retardation. p. 417-445 in: Genetic Counselling (H.A. Lubs and F. de la Cruz, eds.). Raven Press, New York, 1977.

O2 Obe, G., A.T. Natarajan and F. Palitti. Role of DNA double-strand breaks in the formation of radiation-induced chromosomal aberrations. p. 1-9 in: Progress in Mutation Research, Vol. 4 (A.T. Natarajan et al., eds.). Elsevier Biomedical Press, 1982.

O3 Oikawa, A., H. Thoda, M. Kanai et al. Inhibitors of poly(ADP-ribose) polymerase induced sister chromatid exchanges. Biochem. Niophy. Res. Commun. 97: 1311-1316 (1980).

O4 Oskrasson, M., W.L. McClements, D.G. Blair et al. Properties of a normal mouse cell sequence (src) homologous to the src sequence of Moloney sarcoma virus. Science 207: 1222-1224 (1980).

O5 O'Brien, S.J., W.G. Nash, J.L. Goodwin et al. Dispersion of the ras family of transforming genes to four different chromosomes in man. Nature 302: 839-842 (1983).

O6 O'Brien, T., P.S. Harper, K.E. Davies et al. Absence of genetic heterogeneity in Duchenne muscular dystrophy shown by a linkage study using two cloned DNA sequences. J. Med. Genet. 20: 249-251 (1983).

O7   Orkin, S.H. A review of beta-thalassemias: the spectrum of gene mutations. p. 19-28 in: Banbury Report 14. Recombinant DNA Applications to Human Disease (C.T. Caskey and R.L. White, eds.). Cold Spring Harbor Laboratory, New York, 1983.

O8   Orkin, S.H., H.H. Kazazian, S.E. Antonarakis et al. Linkage of beta-thalassemia mutations and beta-globin gene polymorphisms with DNA polymorphisms in the human beta-globin gene cluster. Nature 296: 627-631 (1982).

O9   Opitz, J.M. and G.R. Sutherland. Conference report. International Workshop on the Fragile-X and X-linked Mental Retardation. Am. J. Med. Genet. 17: 5-94 (1984).

O10   Orkin, S.H., A.F. Markham and H.H. Kazazian. Direct detection of the common mediterranean beta thalassemia gene with synthetic probes: an alternative approach for prenatal diagnosis. J. Clin. Invest. 71: 775-779 (1983).

O11   Orkin, S.H., B.P. Alter, C. Altay et al. Application of endonuclease mapping to the analysis and prenatal diagnosis of thalassemias caused by globin gene deletion. New Engl. J. Med. 299: 166-172 (1978).

O12   Orkin, S.H., D.S. Goldman and S.E. Sallan. Development of homozygosity for chromosome 11p markers in Wilms' tumour. Nature 309: 172-174 (1984).

O13   Oakberg, E.F. Gamma ray sensitivity of oocytes in immature mice. Proc. Soc. Exp. Biol. Med. 109: 763-767 (1962).

O14   Orkin, S.H. and H.H. Kazazian. The mutation and polymorphism of the human beta globin gene and its surrounding DNA. Ann. Rev. Genet. 18: 131-171 (1984).

O15   Orkin, S.H. The duplicated human alpha globin genes lie close together in cellular DNA. Proc. Natl. Acad. Sci. U.S.A. 75: 5950-5954 (1978).

O16   O'Brien, T., S. Ball, M. Safarazi et al. Genetic linkage between the loci for myotonic dystrophy and peptidase. D. Am. J. Hum. Genet. 47: 117-121 (1983).

O17   O'Hare, K. and G.M. Rubin. Structures of P transposable elements of D. melanogaster and their sites of insertion and excision. Cell 34: 25-35 (1983).

O18   Olivieri, G., J. Bodycote and S. Wolff. Adaptive response of human lymphocytes to low concentrations of radioactive thymidine. Science 223: 594-597 (1984).

O19   Obezdisse, K. and E. Klein. Krankheiten der Schilddrüse. Thieme Verlag, Stuttgart, 1967.

O20   O'Brien, W.M. The genetics of rheumatoid arthritis. Clin. Exp. Immunol. 2 (Suppl): 785-802 (1967).

O21   Obe, G., F. Palitti, C. Tanzarella et al. Chromosomal aberrations induced by restriction endonucleases. Mutat. Res. 150: 359-368 (1985).

O22   Oftedal, P. and A.G. Searle. An overall genetic risk assessment for radiological protection purposes. J. Med. Genet. 17: 15-20 (1980).

P1   Parada, L.F., C.J. Tabin, C. Shih et al. Human bladder carcinoma oncogene is homologue of Harvey sarcoma virus ras gene. Nature 297: 474-478 (1982).

P2   Pulciani, S., E. Santos, A.V. Lauver et al. Oncogenes in solid tumours. Nature 300: 539-542 (1982).

P3   Peto, R. and M. Schneiderman (eds.). Quantification of occupational cancer. p. 269-284 in: Banbury Report 9. Cold Spring Harbor Laboratory, New York.

P4   Picard, G. Non-mendelian female sterility in Drosophila melanogaster: Hereditary transmission of I factor. Genetics 83: 107-123 (1976).

P5   Picard, G., J.C. Bregliano et al. Non-mendelian female sterility and hybrid dysgenesis in Drosophila melanogaster. Genet. Res. 32: 275-287 (1978).

P6   Preston, R.J. The use of inhibitors of DNA repair in the study of the mechanisms of induction of chromosome aberrations. Cytogenet. Cell Genet. 33: 20-26 (1982).

P7   Preston, R.J. The effects of cytosine arabinoside on the frequency of x-ray-induced chromosome aberrations in normal leucocytes. Mutat. Res. 69: 71-79 (1980).

P8   Preston, R.J. and P.C. Gooch. The induction of chromosome-type aberrations in G_1 by menthyl methanesulphonate and 4-nitroquinoline-N-oxide and the non-requirement of an S phase for their production. Mutat. Res. 83: 393-402 (1981).

P11   Pulciani, S., E. Santos, A. Lauver et al. Oncogenes in human tumour cell lines. Molecular cloning of a transforming gene from human bladder carcinoma cells. Proc. Natl. Acad. Sci. U.S.A. 79: 2845-2849 (1982).

P12   Prakash, K., O.W. McBride, D.C. Swan et al. Molecular cloning and chromosomal mapping of a human locus related to the transforming gene of Moloney murine sarcoma virus. Proc. Natl. Acad. Sci. U.S.A. 79: 5210-5214 (1982).

P13   Phillips III, J.A. The growth hormone (hgH) gene and human disease. p. 305-315 in: Banbury Report 14. Recombinant DNA Applications to Human Disease. (C.T. Caskey and R.L. White, eds.). Cold Spring Harbor Laboratory, New York, 1983.

P14   Pious, D., H. Erlich, P. Gladstone et al. Analysis of the HLA regions using somatic cell mutants. p. 61-68 in: Banbury Report 14. Recombinant DNA Applications to Human Disease. (C.T. Caskey and R.L. White, eds.). Cold Spring Harbor Laboratory, New York, 1983.

P15   Pöting, A., C. Lücke-Hule, M. Pech et al. Transfection of human genomic wild-type DNA into xeroderma pigmentosum group A. in: Proc. VII Int. Cong. Rad. Res. Abstract B4-29 (Book B) (J.J. Broerse et al., eds.). Martinus-Nijhoff, The Hague, 1983.

P16   Pohl-Rüling, J., P. Fisher, O. Haas et al. Effects of low-dose acute x-irradiation on the frequencies of chromosomal aberrations in human peripheral lymphocytes in vitro. Mutat. Res. 110: 71-82 (1983).

P17   Prochwnick, E.V., S. Antonarakis, K.A. Bauer et al. Molecular heterogeneity of inherited antithrombin III deficiency. New Engl. J. Med. 308: 1549-1552 (1983).

P18   Pope, F.M., A.C. Nicholls and F.G. Grosveld. Similar alpha1(1)-like gene deletions cause some type of Ehlers Danlos syndrome type II and lethal osteogenesis imperfecta. Clin. Genet. 24: 303 (1983).

P19   Phillips, J.A., B.L. Hjelle, P.H. Seeberg et al. Molecular basis for familial isolated growth hormone deficiency. Proc. Natl. Acad. Sci. U.S.A. 78: 6372-6375 (1981).

P20   Phillips, J.A., J.S. Parks, B.L. Hjelle et al. Genetic analysis of familial isolated growth hormone deficiency type I. J. Clin. Invest. 70: 489-495 (1982).

P21   Phillips, J.A., S.R. Panny, H.H. Kazazian et al. Prenatal diagnosis of sickle cell anaemia by restriction endonuclease analysis. HindIII polymorphisms in gamma globin genes extend test applicability. Proc. Natl. Acad. Sci. U.S.A. 77: 2853-2856 (1980).

P22 Patel, P.I., R.L. Nussbaum, P.E. Framson et al. Organization of the HPRT gene and related sequences in the human genome. Som. Cell Mol. Genet. 10: 483-493 (1984).

P23 Peake, I.R., B.L. Furlong and A.L. Bloom. Carrier detection by direct gene analysis in a family with haemophilia B (factor IX deficiency). Lancet i: 242-243 (1984).

P24 Petruzzelli, L.M., S. Ganguli, C.J. Smith et al. Insulin activates a tyrosine-specific protein kinase in extracts of 3T3-L1 adipocytes and human placenta. Proc. Natl. Acad. Sci. U.S.A. 79: 6792-6796 (1982).

P25 Pledger, W.J., C.D. Stiles, H.N. Antoniades et al. Induction of DNA synthesis in BALB/c3T3 cells by serum component: reevaluation of the commitment process. Proc. Natl. Acad. Sci. U.S.A. 74: 4481-4485 (1977).

P26 Preston, R.J. DNA repair and chromosome aberration: interactive effects of radiation and chemicals. p. 25-35 in: DNA Repair, Chromosome Alterations and Chromatin Structure (A.T. Natarajan et al., eds.). Elsevier Biomedical Press, Amsterdam, 1982.

P27 Patterson, M.C. and R.B. Setlow. Endonucleolytic activity from Micrococcus luteus that acts on gamma-ray induced damage in plasmid DNA of Escherichia coli mini cells. Proc. Natl. Acad. Sci. U.S.A. 69: 2927-2931 (1972).

P28 Polani, P.E., J.H. Briggs, C.E. Ford et al. A mongol girl with 46 chromosomes. Lancet i: 721-724 (1960).

P29 Pomerantseva, M.D., L.K. Ramaiya, G.A. Vilkina et al. Genetic effects of radiocarbon in reproductive cells of male mice. Mutat. Res. 122: 341-346 (1983).

P31 Pathak, S., L.C. Strong, R.E. Ferrel et al. Familial renal cell carcinoma with a 3;11 chromosomal translocation limited to tumour cells. Science 217: 939-941 (1982).

P32 Paterson, B.M., B.E. Roberts and E.L. Kuff. Structural gene identification and mapping by DNA-mRNA hybrid arrested cell-free translation. Proc. Natl. Acad. Sci. 74: 4370-4374 (1977).

P33 Proudfoot, W.J. and F.E. Baralle. Molecular cloning of human ε-globin gene. Proc. Natl. Acad. Sci. U.S.A. 76: 5435-5439 (1979).

P34 Proudfoot, W.J., A. Gil and T. Maniatis. The structure of the human zeta gene and a closely-linked nearly identical pseudogene. Cell 31: 553-563 (1982).

P35 Phillip, T., J. Fraisse, P.M. Sinet et al. Confirmation of the assignment of the human SODs gene to chromosome 21q22. Cytogenet. Cell. Genet. 22: 521-523 (1978).

P36 Parada, L.F. and R.A. Weinberg. Presence of a Kirsten murine sarcoma virus ras oncogene in cells transformed by 3-methyl chloranthrene. Mol. Cell Biol. 3: 2298-2301 (1983).

P37 Pelicci, P.G., L. Lanfrancone, M.D. Brathwaite et al. Amplification of the c-myb oncogene in a case of human acute myelogenous leukaemia. Science 224: 1117-1121 (1984).

P38 Potter, S.S., W.J. Brorein, P. Dunsmuir et al. Transposition of elements of the 412, copia and 297 dispersed repeated gene families in Drosophila. Cell 17: 415-427 (1979).

P39 Pierce, D.A. and J.C. Lucchesi. Analysis of a dispersed repetitive DNA sequence in isogenic lines of Drosophila. Chromosoma 82: 471-492 (1981).

P40 Potter, S.S., M. Truett, M. Philips et al. Eukaryotic transposable elements with inverted terminal repeats. Cell 20: 639-647 (1980).

P41 Pantelias, G. and S. Wolff. Cytosine arabinoside is a potent clastogen and does not affect the repair of x-ray-induced chromosome fragments in unstimulated human lymphocytes. Mutat. Res. 151: 65-72 (1985).

P42 Pomerantseva, M.D., P.V. Goloshchapov et al. Genetic effects of chronic exposure of male mice to gamma rays. Mutat. Res. 141: 195-200 (1984).

P43 Pomerantseva, M.D., M.I. Balonov et al. Mutagenic effects of tritium in the germ cells of male mice. II. Genetic damages in stem spermatogonia induced by tritiated water and gamma irradiation. Genetika 20: 782-787 (1984). (in Russian)

P44 Pomerantseva, M.D. and L.K. Ramaiya. Relative genetic efficiency of some radionuclides in mammals. Mutat. Res. 147: 314-315 (1985).

P45 Paravatou-Petsota, M., M. Muleris et al. Diagrammatic representation of chromosomal mutagenesis studies. III. Radiation-induced rearrangements in Pan troglodytes (Chimpanzee). Mutat. Res. 149: 57-66 (1985).

P46 Pethö, B. and A. Czeizel. Heredity of schizophrenia, particularly hebephrenic and cycloid types. Orvosi Hetilap 114: 2949-2954 (1973).

P47 Propping, P. Genetic disorders presenting as schizophrenia: Karl Bonhoffer's early views of the psychoses in the light of medical genetics. Hum. Genet. 65: 1-10 (1983).

P48 Pálfy, G., E. Gyódi, M. Benczur et al. Erstmalige klinische und immunogenetische Untersuchung gesicherter multipler Sklerose bei einem Zigeuner. Ideggrógyaszati Szemle 34: 194-199 (1981).

P49 Pronay, G., L. Ujszászy and G. Nagy. Prevalence of colitis ulcerosa in Borsod county. Orvosi Hetilap 116: 1929-1931 (1975).

P50 Panayi, G.S., P. Wooley and J.R. Batchelor. Genetic basis of rheumatoid disease. HLA antigens, disease manifestation and toxic reaction to drugs. Brit. Med. J. ii: 1326-1328 (1978).

P51 Piratsu, M., Y.W. Kan, A. Cao et al. Prenatal diagnosis of beta thalassemia: detection of a single mutation in DNA. New Engl. J. Med. 309: 284-287 (1983).

P52 Parker, D.R. and J.H. Williamson. Aberration induction and segregation in oocytes. p.1251-1268 in: Genetics and Biology of Drosophila (M. Ashburner and E. Novitski, eds.). Vol. 1C, Chapter 27, Academic Press, New York, 1976.

Q1 Quack, B., Y. Nantois, J. Mottet et al. Lacune stéréotypée constitutionelle des chromosomes humains. J. Génét. Hum. 26: 56-67 (1978).

R1 Rasmussen, K., J. Nielsen and G. Dahl. The prevalence of chromosome abnormalities among mentally retarded persons in a geographically delimited area of Denmark. Clin. Genet. 22: 244-255 (1982).

R2 Reddy, E.P., R.K. Reynolds, E. Santos et al. A point mutation is responsible for the acquisition of transforming properties by T24 human bladder carcinoma oncogene. Nature 300: 149-152 (1982).

R3 Rasmuson, R., I. Montell et al. Genetic instability in Drosophila melanogaster. Evidence for regulation, excision and transposition at the white locus. Mol. Gen. Genet. 177: 567-570 (1980).

R4 Rasmuson, B., B.M. Westerberg et al. Transpositions, mutable genes and the dispersed gene family Dm 225 in Drosophila melanogaster. Cold Spring Harbor Symp. Quant. Biol. 45: 545-551 (1981).

R5 Rubin, G.M., D.J. Finnegan and D.S. Hogness. The chromosomal arrangement of coding sequences in a family of repeated genes. Prog. Nucl. Acid Res. Mol. Biol. 19: 221-226 (1976).

R6 Rubin, G.M., W.J. Brorein, A.J. Flavell et al. Copia-like transposable elements in the Drosophils genome. Cold Spring Harbor Symp. Quant. Biol. 45: 619-628 (1981).

R7 Rudak, E., P.A. Jacobs and R. Yamagimachi. Direct analysis of the chromosome constitution of human spermatozoa. Nature 274: 911-913 (1978).

R8 Ratcliffe, S.G. Speech and learning disorders in children with sex-chromosome abnormalities. Developmental Medicine and Child Neurology 24: 80-84 (1982).

R9 Ratcliffe, S.G. and M.A.S. Field. Emotional disorders in XYY children: four cases reports. J. Child Psycho. Psychiatr. 23: 401-406 (1982).

R10 Ratcliffe, S.G., I. Tierney, L. Smith et al. Psychological and educational progress in children with sex-chromosome abnormalities in the Edinburgh longitudinal survey. p. 31-34 in: Human Behaviour and Genetics (W. Schmid and J. Nielsen, eds.). Elsevier-North Holland Biomedical Press, Amsterdam, 1981.

R11 Ratcliffe, S.G., I. Tierney, J. Nshaho et al. The Edinburgh study of growth and development of children with sex-chromosome abnormalities. Birth Defects, Original Article Series 18: 41-60 (1982).

R12 Rowley, J.D. Human oncogene locations and chromosome aberrations. Nature 301: 290-291 (1983).

R13 Rechavi, G., D. Givol and E. Cananni. Activation of a cellular oncogene by DNA rearrangement: possible involvement of an IS-like element. Nature 300: 607-611 (1982).

R14 Ryan, J., P.E. Barker, K. Shimizu et al. Chromosomal assignment of a family of human oncogenes. Proc. Natl. Acad. Sci. U.S.A. 80: 4460-4463 (1983).

R15 Ruley, H.E. Adenovirus early region 1A enables viral and cellular transforming genes to transform primary cells in culture. Nature 304: 602-606 (1983).

R16 Ruddle, F.H. A new era in mammalian gene mapping: somatic cell genetics and recombinant DNA methodologies. Nature 294: 115-120 (1981).

R17 Roberts, R.J. Restriction and modification enzymes and their recognition sequences. Nucleic Acids Res. 10: r117-r144 (1982).

R18 Ryder, L.P., A. Svejgaard and J. Dauset. Genetics of HLA disease association. Ann. Rev. Genet. 15: 169-187 (1981).

R19 Roberts, R.J. Directory of restriction endonucleases. p. 27-41 in: Methods in Enzymology. Vol. 68, Recombinant DNA (R. Wu, ed.). Academic Press, New York, 1979.

R20 Rhoads, F.A., A.C. Oglesby, M. Mayer et al. Marker X syndrome in an oriental family with probable transmission by a normal male. Am. J. Med. Genet. 12: 205-217 (1982).

R21 Rambach, A. and P. Tiollais. Bacteriophage lambda having EcoRI endonuclease site only in the non-essential region of the genome. Proc. Natl. Acad. Sci. U.S.A. 71: 3927-3930 (1974).

R22 Rotwein, P., R. Chyn, J. Chirgwin et al. Polymorphism in the 5'-flanking region of the human insulin gene and its possible relationship to type 2 diabetes. Science 213: 1117-1120 (1981).

R23 Rotwein, P.S., J. Chirgwin, M. Province et al. Polymorphism in the 5'-flanking region of the human insulin gene. A genetic marker for non-insulin dependent diabetes. New Engl. J. Med. 308: 65-71 (1983).

R24 Rees, A., C.C. Shoulders, J. Stocks et al. DNA polymorphism adjacent to human apolipoprotein A-1 gene: relation to hypertriglyceridemia. Lancet i: 444 (1983).

R25 Radman, M., P. Jeggo and R. Wagner. Chromosomal rearrangement and carcinogenesis. Mutat. Res. 98: 249-264 (1982).

R26 Rabin, M., M. Watson, P.E. Barker et al. N-ras transforming gene maps to region p11-p13 on chromosome 1 by in situ hybridization. Cytogenetics and Cell Genetics 38: 70-72 (1984).

R27 Rabbits, T.H., A. Forster, P. Hamlyn et al. Effect of somatic mutation within translocated c-myc genes in Burkitt's lymphoma. Nature 309: 592-597 (1984).

R28 Reeve, A.E., P.J. Housiaux, R.J.M. Gardner et al. Loss of a Harvey ras allele in sporadic Wilms' tumour. Nature 309: 174-176 (1984).

R29 Robinson, M.K., P.M. Bennett and M.H. Richmond. Inhibition of TnA translocation by TnA. J. Bacteriol. 29: 407-414 (1977).

R30 Roeder, G.S. and G.R. Fink. Transposable elements in yeast. p. 299-328 in: Mobile Genetic Elements (J.A. Shapiro, ed.) Academic Press, New York, 1983.

R31 Roeder, G.S. and G.R. Fink. DNA rearrangements associated with a transposable element in yeast. Cell 21: 239-249 (1980).

R32 Roeder, G.S., P.J. Farabaugh, D.T. Chaleff et al. The origins of gene instability in yeast. Science 209: 1375-1380 (1980).

R33 Rubin, G.R. Dispersed repetitive DNAs in Drosophila. p. 329-361 in: Mobile Genetic Elements (J.A. Shapiro, ed.) Academic Press, New York, 1983.

R34 Russell, L.B. Personal communication.

R35 Russell, L.B. Numerical sex-chromosome anomalies in mammals: their spontaneous occurrence and use in mutagenesis studies. p. 55-91 in: Chemical Mutagens: Principles and Methods for Their Detection, Vol. 4 (A. Hollaender, ed.). Plenum Press, New York, 1976.

R36 Russell, L.B. Meiotic non-disjunction in the mouse. Methodology for genetic testing and comparison with other methods. Env. Health Persp. 31: 113-118 (1979).

R37 Reichert, W., W. Buselmaier and F. Vogel. Elimination of x-ray-induced chromosomal aberrations in the progeny of female mice. Mutat. Res. 139: 87-94 (1984).

R38 Reichert, W., I. Hansmann and G. Röhrborn. Chromosome anomalies in mouse oocytes after irradiation. Humangenetik 28: 25-38 (1979).

R39 Russell, L.B. Quantitative analysis of mouse specific locus mutations: information on genetic organization, gene expression and the chromosomal nature of induced lesions. p. 241-258 in: Utilization of Mammalian Specific Locus Studies in Hazard Evaluation and Estimation of Genetic Risk (F. J. de Serres, ed.). Plenum Press, New York, 1983.

R40 Russell, L.B. Genetic and functional mosaicism in the mouse. p. 153-181 in: The Role of Chromosome in Development (M. Locke, ed.). Academic Press, New York, 1964.

R41 Russell, L.B. Analysis of the albino locus region of the mouse. II. Fractional mutants. Genetics 91: 141-147 (1979).

R42 Russell, L.B. and W.L. Russell. Genetic analysis of induced deletions and of spontaneous non-disjunction involving chromosome 2 of the mouse. J. Cell Comp. Physiol. 56: (Suppl.1), 169-188 (1960).

R43 Russell, L.B. Definition of functional units in a small chromosomal segment of the mouse and its use in interpreting the nature of spontaneous mutations. Mutat. Res. 11: 107-123 (1971).

R47 Rubin, J.S., A.L. Joyner, A. Bernstein et al. Molecular identification of a human DNA repair gene following DNA-mediated gene transfer. Nature 306: 206-208 (1983).

R48 Raoul (1970); cited in Quack et al. [Q1].

R49 Rowley, J.D. Identification of a translocation with quinacrine flourescence in a patient with acute leukaemia. Ann. Genet. 16: 109-112 (1973).

R50 Rodríguez, R.L. and R.C. Tait. Recombinant DNA Techniques. An Introduction. Addison-Wesley, Massachusetts, 1983.

R51 Ramires, F., A.L. Burns, J.G. Mears et al. Isolation and characterization of human foetal globin genes. Nucleic Acids Res. 7: 1147-1162 (1979).

R52 Roncuzzi, L., S. Fadda, M. Mochi et al. Mapping of X-linked muscular dystrophy through crossovers identified by DNA polymorphisms and by haplotype characterization in somatic cell hybrids. Am. J. Hum. Genet. 37: 407-417 (1985).

R53 Robertson, M. Gene rearrangement and the generation of diversity. Nature 297: 184-186 (1982).

R54 Rasheed, S., G.L. Norman and G. Heidecker. Nucleotide sequence of the Rasheed rat sarcoma virus oncogene: new mutations. Science 221: 155-157 (1983).

R55 Rowley, J.D. Implications of consistent chromosome rearrangements. p. 503-524 in: Genes and Cancer (J.M. Bishop et al., eds.). UCLA Symposium on Molecular and Cellular Biology. New Series. Vol. 17. Alan R. Liss Inc., New York, 1984.

R56 Rubin, G.M., M.G. Kidwell and P.M. Bingham. The molecular basis of P-M hybrid dysgenesis. The nature of induced mutation. Cell 29: 987-994 (1982).

R57 Rogers, J. Retroposons defined. Nature 301: 460 (1983).

R58 Russell, W.L. Positive genetic hazard predictions for short term tests have proved false positive results in mammalian spermatogonia with all environmental chemicals. In: Proc. Int. Conf. Env. Mutagens. Stockholm, 1985.

R59 Radman, M. Phenomenology of an inducible mutagenic DNA repair pathway in E. coli. SOS repair hypothesis. In: Molecular and Environmental Aspects of Mutagenesis (L. Prakash et al. eds.). Thomas, Springfield, 1974.

R60 Romnelaere, J., J.M. Vos et al. UV-enhanced reactivation of minute-virus of mice. Stimulation of a late step in the viral life cycle. Photochem. Photobiol. 33: 845-854 (1981).

R61 Robins, P.E. and J. Cairns. Quantitation of the adaptive response to alkylating agents. Nature 280: 74-76 (1979).

R62 Rees, D.J., C.R. Rizza and G.G. Brownlee. Haemophilia B caused by a point mutation in a donor splice junction of the human factor IX gene. Nature 316: 643-645 (1985).

R63 Rimoin, D.L. and J.I. Potter. Genetic heterogeneity in common disease. p. 97-109 in: Human Genetics, Part B, Medical Aspects (B. Bonné-Tamir et al., eds.). Alan R. Liss Inc., New York, 1982.

R64 Rihmer, Z. Nosology of endogenous depression. Orvosi Hetilap 122: 2519-2525 (1981).

R65 Rajna, P. and P. Halász. General problem of treatment and care of epilepsy. Orvosi Hetilap 120: 133-139 (1979).

R66 Rees, I. ABC of asthma. Brit. Med. J. 288: 1370-1372 and 1441-1442 (1984).

R67 Rosdy, E. An epidemiological study on nephrolithiasis. Ann. Report of Municipal Bajcsi-Zsilinsky Hospital, 347-354 (1982).

R68 Romanus, T. Psoriasis from a Prognostic and Hereditary Points of View. Thesis, Uppsala, 1945.

R69 Russell, W.L. An error in the calculation of the percentage of conceptions with an unbalanced chromosome rearrangement that survive birth. Mutat. Res. 142: 217 (1985).

R69a Russell, W.L. and E.M. Kelly. Specific locus mutation frequencies in mouse stem cell spermatogonia at very low radiation dose rates. Proc. Natl. Acad. Sci. U.S.A. 79: 539-541 (1982).

R70 Russell, W.L. and E.M. Kelly. Mutation frequencies in male mice and the estimation of genetic hazards of radiation in man. Proc. Natl. Acad. Sci. U.S.A. 79: 542-544 (1982).

R71 Rinchik, E.M., L.B. Russell, N.G. Copeland et al. Molecular genetic analysis of the dilute-short-ear (d-se) region of the mouse. Genetics 112: 321-342 (1986).

R72 Russell, W.L. Effects of the interval between irradiation and conception on mutation frequency in female mice. Proc. Natl. Acad. Sci. U.S.A. 54: 1552-1557 (1965).

R73 Russell, W.L. The genetic effects of radiation. p. 487-500 in: Peaceful Uses of Atomic Energy. United Nations, New York, 1972.

S1 Sutherland, G.R., R.F. Carter, R. Bauld et al. Chromosome studies at the pediatric necropsy. Ann. Hum. Genet. 42: 173-181 (1978).

S2 Sutherland, G.R., P.B. Jackey, E. Baker et al. Heritable fragile sites on human chromosomes. X. New folate-sensitive fragile sites: 6p23, 9p21, 9q32 and 11q23. Am. J. Hum. Genet. 35: 432-437 (1983).

S3 Summit, R.L. Cytogenetics in mentally defective children with anomalies. A controlled study. J. Pediatr. 74: 58-66 (1969).

S4 Sutherland, G.R. Heritable fragile sites on human chromosomes. III. Detection of fra(X)(q27) in males with X-linked mental retardation and their female relatives. Hum. Genet. 53: 23-27 (1979).

S5 Sutherland, G.R. Heritable fragile sites on human chromosomes. VIII. Preliminary population cytogenetic data on the folic acid sensitive fragile sites. Am. J. Hum. Genet. 34: 452-458 (1982).

156

S6   Sutherland, G.R. Heritable fragile sites on human chromosomes. IX. Population cytogenetics and segregation analysis of the BrdU-requiring fragile site at 10q25. Am. J. Hum. Genet. 34: 753-756 (1982).

S7   Santos, E., S.R. Tronick, S.A. Aaronson et al. T24 human bladder carcinoma oncogene is an activated form of the normal human homologue of BALB- and Harvey-MSV transforming genes. Nature 298: 343-347 (1982).

S8   Starlinger, P. and H. Saedler. Insertion mutations in microorganisms. Biochemie 54: 177-185 (1972).

S9   Starlinger, P. and H. Saedler. IS-elements in microorganisms. Curr. Topics in Microbiol. Immunol. 75: 111-152 (1976).

S10   Starlinger, P. DNA rearrangements in prokaryotes. Ann. Rev. Genetc. 11: 103-126 (1977).

S11   Sved, J.A. The hybrid dysgenesis syndrome in Drosophila melanogaster. Bioscience 29: 659-664 (1979).

S12   Slatko, B.E. Evidence for newly-induced genetic activity responsible for male recombination induction in Drosophila melangaster. Genetics 90: 105-124 (1978).

S13   Slatko, B.E. and Y. Hiraizumi. Elements causing male crossing over in Drosophila melanogaster. Genetics 81: 313-324 (1975).

S14   Slatko, B.E. and M.M. Green. Genetic instability in Drosophila melanogaster. Mapping the mutator activity of an MR strain. Biol. Zentralblat 99: 149-155 (1980).

S15   Sobels, F.H. and J.C.J. Eeken. Influence of MR(mutator) factor on x-ray-induced genetic damage. Mutat. Res. 83: 201-206 (1981).

S16   Strobel, E., P. Dunsmuir and G.M. Rubin. Polymorphism in the chromosomal location of elements of the 412, copia and 297 dispersed repeated gene families in Drosophila. Cell 17: 429-439 (1979).

S17   Shimotohno, K., S. Mizutani and H.M. Temin. Sequence of retrovirus provirus resembles that of bacterial transposable elements. Nature 285: 550-554 (1980).

S21   Shall, S. ADP-ribosylation, DNA repair, cell differentiation and cancer. p. 3-25 in: ADP-ribosylation, DNA Repair and Cancer (M. Miwra et al., eds.). Japan Scientific Societies Press, Tokyo, 1983.

S23   Strauss, G.H. and R.J. Albertini. Enumeration of 6-thioguanine resistant peripheral blood lymphocytes in man as a potential test for somatic cell mutations arising in vivo. Mutat. Res. 61: 353-359 (1979).

S24   Shabtai, F., D. Klar and I. Halbrecht. A new familial fragile site on chromosome 16 (q23-24). Cytogenetic and clinical considerations. Human Genet. 64: 273-276 (1983).

S25   Schmid, M., C. Klett and A. Niederhofer. Demonstration of a heritable fragile site in human chromosome 16 with distamycin. Cytogenet. Cell Genet. 28: 87-94 (1980).

S26   Sutherland, G.R. Heritable fragile sites on human chromosomes. VII. Children homozygous for the BrdU-requiring fra(10) (q25) are phenotypically normal. Am. J. Hum. Genet. 33: 946-949 (1981).

S27   Sutherland, G.R. Heritable fragile site on human chromosomes. I. Factors affecting expression in lymphocyte cultures. Am. J. Hum. Genet. 31: 125-135 (1979).

S28   Sutherland, G.R. The population cytogenetics of fragile sites (abstract). Sixth Int. Cong. Hum. Genet. Jerusalem, Israel (1981).

S29   Solnick, E.M., E. Rands, D. Williams et al. Studies on the nucleic acid sequence of Kirsten sarcoma virus: a model for studies of a mammalian RNA-containing sarcoma virus. J. Virol. 12: 458-463 (1973).

S30   Solnick, E.M. and W.P.J. Parks. Harvey sarcoma virus. A second murine type C sarcoma virus with rat genetic information. J. Virol. 13: 1211-1219 (1974).

S31   Stehlin, D., H.E. Varmus, J.M. Bishop et al. DNA related to the transforming gene(s) of avian sarcoma viruses is present in normal avian DNA. Nature 260: 170-173 (1976).

S32   Spector, D.H., K. Smith, T. Padgett et al. Uninfected avian cells contain RNA related to the transforming genes of avian sarcoma virus. Cell 13: 371-379 (1978).

S33   Shilo, B.Z. and R.A. Weinberg. DNA sequences homologous to vertebrate oncogenes are conserved in Drosophila melanogaster. Proc. Natl. Acad. Sci. U.S.A. 78: 6789-6792 (1981).

S34   Shih, K. and R.A. Weinberg. Isolation of a transforming sequence from a human bladder carcinoma cell line. Cell 29: 161-169 (1982).

S35   Shimizu, K., M. Goldfarb, Y. Suard et al. Three human transforming genes are related to the viral ras oncogenes. Proc. Natl. Acad. Sci. U.S.A. 80: 2112-2116 (1983).

S36   Sakaguchi, A.Y., S.L. Naylor, T.B. Shows et al. Human c-Ki-ras 2 proto-oncogene on chromosome 12. Science 219: 1081-1083 (1983).

S37   Shen-Ong, G.L.C., E.J. Keath, S.P. Piccoli et al. Novel myc oncogene RNA from abortive immunoglobulin gene recombination in mouse plasmocytomas. Cell 31: 443-452 (1982).

S38   Sheer, D. et al. in: Chromosomes and Cancer. Bristol Meyer Cancer Symposium. Series 5 (in press).

S39   Sinsheimer, R.L. Recombinant DNA. Ann. Rev. Biochem. 46: 415-438 (1977).

S40   Shows, T.B., A.Y. Sakaguchi and S.L. Naylor. Mapping the human genome, cloned genes, DNA polymorphisms and inherited disease. Adv. Hum. Genet. 12: 341-452 (1982).

S41   Skolnick, M.H. and R.L. White. Strategies for detecting and characterising restriction fragment length polymorphisms (RFLPs). Cytogenet. Cell Genet. 32: 58-67 (1982).

S42   Southern, E.M. Detection of specific sequences among DNA fragments separated by gel electrophoresis. J. Mol. Biol. 98: 503-517 (1975).

S43   Shows, T.B. The human molecular map of cloned genes and DNA polymorphisms. p. 347-356 in: Banbury Report 14. Recombinant DNA Applications to Human Disease (C.T. Caskey and R.L. White, eds.). Cold Spring Harbor Laboratory, New York, 1983.

S44   Schmidtke, J. and D.N. Cooper. A list of cloned human DNA sequences. Hum. Genet. 65: 19-26 (1983).

S45   Spritz, R.A. and B.G. Forget. The thalasemias: molecular mechanisms of human genetic disease. Am. J. Hum. Genet. 35: 333-361 (1983).

S46   Southern, E.M. Application of DNA analysis to mapping the human genome. Cytogenet. Cell Genet. 32: 52-57 (1982).

S47 Schlager, G. and M.M. Dickie. Spontaneous mutation rates in mice. Annual Report (1968-1969). The Jackson Laboratory, Bar Harbor, Maine, 1969.

S48 Shiraishi, Y., T. Yosida and A.A. Sandberg. Analysis of single and twin sister chromatid exchanges in endoreduplicated normal and Bloom syndrome B-lymphoid cells. Chromosoma 87: 1-8 (1982).

S49 Shiraishi, Y., T. Yosida and A.A. Sandberg. Analyses of bromodeoxyuridine-associated sister chromatid exchanges (SCEs) in Bloom syndrome based on cell fusion: single and twin SCEs in endoreduplication. Proc. Natl. Acad. Sci. U.S.A. 80: 4369-4373 (1983).

S50 Schreinemachers, D.M., P.K. Cross and E.B. Hook. Rates of trisomies 21, 18, 13 and other chromosomal abnormalities in about 20 000 prenatal studies compared with estimated rates in livebirths. Hum. Genet. 61: 318-324 (1983).

S51 Sutherland, G.R. and L. Hinton. Heritable fragile sites on human chromosomes. Hum. Genet. 57: 217-219 (1981).

S52 Soresnson, K., J. Nielsen, V. Holm et al. Fragile site on long arm of chromosome 16. Hum. Genet. 48: 131-134 (1979).

S53 Sutherland, G.R. and F. Hecht. Fragile Sites on Human Chromosomes. Oxford University Press, 1984.

S54 Sherman, S.L., N.E. Morton, P.A. Jacobs et al. The marker (X) syndrome: a cytogenetic and genetic analysis. Ann. Hum. Genet. 48: 21-37 (1984).

S55 Sutherland, G.R. The fragile X chromosome. Int. Rev. Cytol. 81: 107-143 (1983).

S56 Sutherland, G.R., P.B. Jacky and E.G. Baker. Heritable fragile sites on human chromosomes. XI. Factors affecting expression of fragile sites at 10q25, 16q22 and 17p12. Am. J. Hum. Genet. 36: 110-122 (1984).

S57 Sutherland, G.R., M.I. Parslow and E. Baker. New classes of common fragile sites induced by 5-azacytidine and BrdU. Hum. Genet. 69: 233-237 (1985).

S58 Shabtai, F., D. Klar and I. Halbrecht. Chromosome 17 has a real fragile site at p12. Hum. Genet. 61: 177-179 (1982).

S59 Sutherland, G.R., P.B. Jacky and E.G. Baker. Heritable fragile sites on human chromosomes. XI. Factors affecting expression of fragile sites at 10q25, 16q22 and 17p12. Am. J. Hum. Genet. 36: 110-122 (1984).

S60 Scheres, J.M.J.C. and T.W.J. Hustinx. Heritable fragile sites and lymphocyte culture medium containing BrdU. Am. J. Hum. Genet. 32: 628-629 (1980).

S61 Sutherland, G.R., E. Baker and R.S. Seshadri. Heritable fragile sites on human chromosomes. V. A new class of fragile site requiring BrdU for expression. Am. J. Hum. Genet. 32: 542-548 (1980).

S62 Sasaki, M.S. Role of chromosomal mutation in the development of cancer. Cytogenetics and Cell Genetics 33: 160-168 (1982).

S63 Shimizu, K., D. Birnbaum, M.A. Ruley et al. Structure of the ki-ras gene of the human lung carcinoma cell line Calu-1. Nature 304: 497-500 (1983).

S64 Shimizu, K., M. Goldfarb, M. Perucho et al. Isolation and preliminary characterization of the transforming gene of a neuroblastoma cell line. Proc. Natl. Acad. Sci. U.S.A. 80: 383-387 (1983).

S65 Santos, E., E.P. Reddy, S. Pulciani et al. Spontaneous activation of a tumour proto-oncogene. Proc. Natl. Acad. Sci. U.S.A. 80: 4679-4683 (1983).

S66 Schwab, M., K. Alitalo, H.E. Varmus et al. A cellular oncogene (c-ki-ras) is amplified, overexpressed and located within karyotype abnormalities in mouse adrenocortical tumour cells. Nature 303: 497-501 (1983).

S67 Stiles, C.D. The molecular biology of platelet-derived growth factor. Cell 33: 653-655 (1983).

S68 Stiles, C.D., G.T. Capone, C.D. Scher et al. Dual control of cell growth by somatomedins and platelet-derived growth factor. Proc. Natl. Acad. Sci. U.S.A. 76: 1279-1283 (1979).

S69 Scher, C.D., S.L. Hendrickson, A.P. Whipple et al. Cold Spring Harbor Conf. Cell Proliferation 9: 289-303 (1982).

S70 Singh, J.P., M.A. Chaikin, W.J. Pledger et al. Persistence of the mitogenic response to platelet-derived growth factor (competence) does not reflect a long term interaction between the growth factor and the target cell. J. Cell Biol. 96: 1497-1502 (1983).

S71 Sandberg, A.A. A chromosomal hypothesis of onco-genesis. Cancer Genet. Cytogenet. 8: 277-285 (1983).

S72 **Shapiro, J.A. (ed.) Mobile Genetic Elements. p. 688. Academic Press, New York, 1983.**

S73 Schmid, C.W. and W.R. Jelinek. The Alu family of dispersed repetitive sequences. Science 216: 1065-1074 (1982).

S74 Schmookler-Reis, R.J., C.K. Lumpkin, J.R. McGill et al. Extrachromosomal circular copies of an "inter-Alu" unstable sequence in human DNA are amplified during in vitro and in vivo ageing. Nature 301: 394-398 (1983).

S75 Sharp, P.A. Conversion of RNA to DNA in mammals. Alu-like elements and pseudogenes. Nature 301: 471-472 (1983).

S76 **Shall, S. Inhibition of DNA repair by inhibitors of nuclear ADP-ribosyl transferase. p. 143-191 in: DNA Repair and Its Inhibition (A. Collins et al., eds.). IRL Press, Oxford.**

S77 Speed, R.M. and A.C. Chandley. Meiosis in the foetal mouse ovary. II. Oocyte development and age-related aneuploidy. Does a production line exist? Chromosoma 88: 184-189 (1983).

S78 Speed, R.M. Meiosis in the foetal mouse ovary. I. Analysis at the light microscope level using surface spreading. Chromosoma 85: 427-437 (1982).

S79 Sugawara, S. and K. Mikamo. Absence of correlation between univalent formation and meiotic non-disjunction in aged female Chinese hamsters. Cytogenetics and Cell Genetics 35: 34-40 (1983).

S80 Sugawara, S and K. Mikamo. An experimental approach to the analysis of mechanisms of meiotic non-disjunction and anaphase lagging in primary oocytes. Cytogenetics and Cell Genetics 28: 251-264 (1980).

S81 Searle, A.G. Cytogenetic effects of incorporated radionuclides on mammalian germ cells. p. 347-367 in: Radiation-induced Chromosome Damage in Man (T. Ishihara and M.S. Sasaki, eds.). Alan R. Liss Inc., New York, 1983.

S82 Straume, T. Biological Effectiveness of Neutron Irradiation on Animals and Man. Ph. D. Thesis, Univ. California, Davis, 1982.

S83 Sanderson, B.J.S., J.L. Dempsey and A.A. Morley. Mutations in human lymphocytes: effects of x and uv irradiation. Mutat. Res. 140: 223-227 (1984).

S84 Stevenson, A.C., H.A. Johnston, M.I.P. Steward et al. Congenital malformations: a report of a study of series of consecutive births in 24 centres. WHO, Geneva, 1966.

S85 Sherman, S.L., P.A. Jacobs, N.E. Morton et al. Further segregation analysis of the fragile-X syndrome with special reference to transmitting males. Hum. Genet. 69: 289-299 (1985).

S86 Sutherland, G.R. Heritable fragile sites on human chromosomes. XII. Population cytogenetics. Ann. Hum. Genet. 49: 153-161 (1985).

S87 Sanfilipo, S., G. Neri, N. Tedeschi et al. Chromosomal fragile sites: preliminary data of a population survey. Clin. Genet. 24: 295 (1983).

S88 Sandberg, A.A., R. Morgan, J.A. MacCallister et al. Acute myeloblastic leukaemia (AML) with t(6;9) (p23;q34): a specific subgroup of AML? Cancer Genet. Cytogenet. 10: 139-142 (1983).

S89 Second International Workshop on Chromosomes in Leukaemia. Cancer Res. 40: 4826-4827 (1980).

S91 Smith, H.O. and K.W. Wilcox. A restriction enzyme from Haemophilus influenzae. I. Purification and general properties. J. Mol. Biol. 51: 379-391 (1970).

S92 Shaw, D.J., A.L.Meredith, M. Sarfarazi et al. The apolipoprotein CII gene. Sub-chromosomal localization and linkage to the myotonic dystrophic locus. Hum. Genet. 70: 271-273 (1985).

S93 Sinet, P.M., J. Counturier, B. Dutrillaux et al. Trisomie 21 et superoxyde dismutase-I (IPO-A). Tentative de localisation sur la sous bande 21q22.1. Exp. Cell. Res. 97: 47-55 (1976).

S94 Sukumar, S., V. Notario, D. Martin-Zanca et al. Induction of mammary carcinomas in rats by nitrosomethylurea involves malignant activation of H-ras-1 locus by single point mutations. Nature 306: 658-661 (1983).

S95 Santos, E., D. Martin-Zanca, E. Reddy et al. Malignant activation of a K-ras oncogene in lung carcinoma but not in normal tissue of the same patient. Science 223: 661-664 (1984).

S96 Schwab, M., H.E. Varmus and J.M. Bishop. Human N-myc gene contributes to neoplastic transformation of mammalian cells in culture. Nature 316: 160-163 (1985).

S97 Shtivelman, E., B. Lifshitz, R. Gale et al. Fused transcripts of abl and bcr genes in chronic myelogenous leukaemia. Nature 315: 550-554 (1985).

S98 Smirnov, S.P. and V.A. Tarasov. Induction of transposon Tn1 translocation in uv-irradiated E. coli cells. Genetika 18: 420-423 (1981). (in Russian)

S99 Syvanen, M. The evolutionary implications of mobile genetic elements. Ann. Rev. Hum. Genet. 18: 271-293 (1984).

S100 Sved, J. Hybrid dysgenesis in D. melanogaster. A possible explanation in terms of spatial organization of chromosomes. Aust. J. Biol. Sci. 29: 375-388 (1976).

S101 Simmons, M.J. and J.K. Lim. Site specificity of mutation arising in dysgenic hybrids of D. melanogaster. Proc. Natl. Acad. Sci. U.S.A. 77: 6042-6046 (1980).

S102 Spralding, A.C. and G.M. Rubin. Drosophila genome organization: conserved and dynamic aspects. Ann. Rev. Genet. 15: 219-264 (1981).

S103 Strobel, E., P. Dunsmuir and G.M. Rubin. Polymorphism in the chromosomal locations of elements of the 412, copia and 297 dispersed repeated gene families in Drosophila. Cell 17: 429-439 (1979).

S104 Saigo, K., W. Kugimiya, Y. Matsuo et al. Identification of the coding sequence for a reverse transcriptase-like enzyme in a transposable genetic element in Drosophila melanogaster. Nature 312: 659-661 (1984).

S105 Searle, A.G. and C.V. Beechey. The use of Robertsonian translocations in the mouse for studies on non-disjunction. Cytogenet. Cell Genet. 33: 81-87 (1982).

S106 Strel'tsova, V.N., Yu. N. Pavlenko-Mikhailov and A.B. Oshepkov. A study of mammary gland tumours in rats born of parents exposed to pre-conception irradiation. Questions in Oncology 28: 45-48 (1982). (in Russian)

S107 Searle, A.G., C.V. Beechey and E.P. Evans. Meiotic effects in chromosomally derived male sterility of mice. Ann. Biol. Anim. Biochim. Biophys. 18 (2B): 391-398 (1978).

S108 Sarasin, A. and P.C. Hanawalt. Carcinogens enhance survival of uv-irradiated simian virus 40 in treated monkey kidney cells. Induction of a recovery pathway? Proc. Natl. Acad. Sci. U.S.A. 75: 346-350 (1980).

S109 Sarasin, A. and A. Benoit. Induction of an error-prone mode of DNA repair in uv-irradiated monkey kidney cells. Mutat. Res. 70: 71-81 (1980).

S110 Sarasin, A., F. Bourre and A. Benoit. Error-prone replication of uv-induced SV-40 in carcinogen-treated monkey kidney cells. Biochimie 64: 815-821 (1982).

S111 Sarasin, A., F. Bourre and A. Benoit. Molecular analysis of mutagenesis in mammalian cells. Int. J. Rad. Biol. 47: 479-488 (1985).

S112 Samson, L. and J. Cairns. A new pathway for DNA repair in E. coli. Nature 267: 281-283 (1977).

S113 Samson, L. and L. Schwartz. The induction of resistance to alkylation damage in mammalian cells. p. 291-309 in: Induced Mutagenesis. Molecular Mechanisms and Their Implications for Environmental Protection (C.W. Lawrence, ed.). Plenum Press, New York, 1983.

S114 Schendel, P.F. and P.E. Robins. Repair of O^6-methylguanine in adapted E. coli. Proc. Natl. Acad. Sci. U.S.A. 75: 6017-6020 (1978).

S115 Schendel, P.F., M. DeFais, P. Jeggo et al. Pathway of mutagenesis and repair in E. coli exposed to low levels of simple alkylating agents. J. Bacteriol. 135: 466-477 (1978).

S116 Stenszky, V., C. Balázs, L. Kozma et al. Identification of subjects of patients with Graves' disease by cluster analysis. Clin. Endocrinl. 18: 335-345 (1983).

S117 Shields, J. The major psychoses. J. Med. Genet. 14: 327-329 (1977).

S118 Sadovnick, A.D. and P.A. Baird. Reproductive counselling for MS patients. Am. J. Med. Genet. 20: 349-354 (1985).

S119 Spielman, R.S. and N. Nathanson. The genetics of susceptibility to multiple sclerosis. Epidemiol. Rev. 4: 45-65 (1982).

S120 Sweeney, V.P., A.D. Sadovnick and V. Brandejs. The multiple sclerosis program for British Columbia: preliminary report on prevalence (abstract). Can. J. Neurol. Sci. 10: 151-152 (1983).

S121 Stallones, R.A. The rise and fall of ischaemic heart disease. Sci. Am. 243: 43-49 (1980).

S122 Schweiger, O. and E. Stolmar. Epidemiologic data of patients with bronchial asthma recorded in TB dispensaries. Orvosi Hetilap 124: 2861-2863 (1983).

S123 Stenszky, V., L. Kozma, I. Sonkely et al. HLA and systemic lupus erythematosus. Tissue Antigen 16: 20 (1980).

S124 Siró, B., G. Csoban, I. Gyarmati et al. Mode of heredity in the rheumatoid arthritis in adulthood. Orvasi Hetilap 124: 1555-1558 (1983).

S125 Shands, A.R. and H.B. Eisberg. The incidence of scoliosis in the state of Delaware. A study of 50,000 minifilms of the chest made during a survey of tuberculosis. J. Bone Joint Surg. 37A: 1243-1249 (1955).

S126 Searle, A.G. and J.H. Edwards. The estimation of risks from the induction of recessive mutations after exposure to ionizing radiation. J. Med. Genet. (1985).

S127 Selby, P.B. and W.L. Russell. First generation litter-size reduction following irradiation of spermatogonial stem cells in mice and its use in risk estimation. Environ. Mutagen. 7: 451-469 (1985).

S128 Schull, W.J., M. Otake and J.V. Neel. Genetic effects of the atomic bombs: a re-appraisal. Science 213: 1220-1227 (1980).

S129 Searle, A.G. Some growing points in mammalian radiation genetics. p. 367-372 in: Radiation Research: Proc. VII Intl. Cong. Rad. Res. (J.J. Broerse et al., eds.). Reviews and Summaries. Martinus Nijhoff, The Hague, 1983.

S130 Shapiro, J.A. Mutations caused by the insertion of genetic material into the galactose operon of E.coli. J. Mol. Biol. 40: 93-105 (1969).

S131 Schull, W.J., M. Otake and J.V. Neel. Hiroshima and Nagasaki: a re-assessment of the mutagenic effects of exposure to ionizing radiation. p. 277-303 in: Population and Biological Aspects of Human Mutation (E.B. Hook and I.J. Porter, eds.). Academic Press, New York, 1981.

S132 Sankaranarayanan, K. Transposable genetic elements, spontaneous mutations and the doubling dose method of radiation genetic risk evaluation in man. Mutat. Res. 160: 73-86 (1986).

S133 Schnieke, A., K. Harbers and R. Jaenisch. Embryonic lethal mutation in mice induced by retrovirus insertion into the alpha 1(I) collagen gene. Nature 304: 315-319 (1983).

S134 Searle, A.G. and C.V. Beechey. Non-complementation phenomena and their bearing on non-disjunctional effects. p. 363-376 in: Aneuploidy, Etiology and Mechanisms (V.L. Dellarco et al., eds.). Plenum Press, New York, 1985.

S135 Searle, A.G. and C.V. Beechey. The influence of mating status and age on the induction of chromosome aberrations and dominant lethals in irradiated female mice. Mutat. Res. 147: 357-362 (1985).

S136 Searle, A.G. Mutation induction in mice. Advances in Rad. Biol. 4: 131-207 (1974).

S137 Searle, A.G. and D.G. Papworth. Analysis of pre- and post-natal mortality after spermatogonial irradiation of mice. Personal communication (1986).

S138 Shevchenko, V.A. and M.D. Pomerantseva. Genetic Effects of Ionizing Radiations. Nauka, Moskow, 1985. (in Russian)

T1 Tharapel, A.T. and R.L. Summitt. Acytogenetic survey of 200 unclassifiable mentally retarded children with congenital anomalies and 200 normal controls. Hum. Genet. 37: 329-338 (1977).

T2 Tipton, R.E. and R.L. Summitt. Cytogenetic studies in mentally retarded subjects using banding techniques. Clin. Genet. 23: 64A (1975).

T3 Tariverdian, G. and B. Weck. Non-specific X-linked mental retardation—a review. Hum. Genet. 62: 95-109 (1982).

T4 Tommerup, N., K.B. Nielsen and M. Mikkelsen. Marker X chromosome induction in fibroblasts by FUdR. Am. J. Med. Genet. 9: 263-264 (1981).

T5 Tabin, C.F., S.M. Bradley et al. Mechanism of activation of a human oncogene. Nature 300: 143-149 (1982).

T6 Thompson, J.N. and R.C. Woodruff. Mutator genes—pacemakers of evolution. Nature 274: 317-321 (1978).

T8 Turner, G. and B. Turner. X-linked mental retardation. J. Med. Genet. 11: 109-113 (1974).

T9 Trimble, B.K. and J.H. Doughty. The amount of hereditary disease in human populations. Ann. Hum. Genet. (Lond.) 38: 199-229 (1974).

T10 Tsuchida, N., R.V. Gilden and M. Hatenada. Sarcoma-virus-related RNA sequences in normal rat cells. Proc. Natl. Acad. Sci. U.S.A. 71: 4503-4507 (1974).

T11 Taporowsky, E., Y. Suard, O. Fasano et al. Activation of the T24 bladder carcinoma transforming gene is linked to a single amino acid change. Nature 300: 762-765 (1982).

T12 Taub, R., I. Kirsch, C. Morton et al. Translocation of the c-myc gene into the immunoglobulin heavy chain locus in human Burkitt lymphoma and murine plasmacytoma cells. Proc. Natl. Acad. Sci. U.S.A. 79: 7837-7841 (1982).

T13 Tuan, D., P.A. Biro, J.K. de Riel et al. Restriction endonuclease mapping of the human beta globin gene loci. Nucleic Acids Res. 6: 2519-2525 (1979).

T14 Tierney, I., Axworthy, L. Smith et al. Balanced rearrangements of the autosomes. Results of longitudinal study of a newborn survey population. J. Med. Genet. 21: 45-51 (1984).

T15 Thacker, J., P. Debenham, A. Stretch et al. Use of a cloned gene to study mutation in mammalian cells. in: Proc. VII. Int. Cong. Rad. Res. Abstract B4-39 (J.J. Broerse et al., eds.). Martinus Nijhoff, The Hague, 1983.

T17 Tease, C. Similar dose-related chromosome non-disjunction in young and old female mice after x-irradiation. Mutat. Res. 95: 287-296 (1982).

T18 Tease, C. Radiation-induced chromosome non-disjunction in oocytes stimulated by different doses of superovulating hormones. Mutat. Res. 105: 95-100 (1983).

T19 Turner, G. and P.A. Jacobs. Marker (X)-linked mental retardation. Chapter 2. Advances in Human Genetics, 13: 83-112 (1984).

T20 Turner, G., A. Daniel and M. Frost. X-linked mental retardation, macroorchidism and the Xq27 fragile site. J. Pediat. 96: 837-841 (1980).

T21 Thomas, M., J.R. Cameron and R.W. Davis. Viable molecular hybrids of bacteriophage lambda and eukaryote DNA. Proc. Natl. Acad. Sci. U.S.A. 71: 4579-4583 (1974).

T22 Tuan, D., P.A. Biro, J.K. de Riel et al. Restriction endonuclease mapping of gamma globin gene loci. Nucleic Acids Res. 6: 2519-2544 (1979).

T23 Tsipouros, P., J. Myers, D. Prockop et al. Genetic analysis of the mild autosomal dominant osteogenesis imperfecta with RFLP associated with the pro-alpha 2(1) collagen gene. p. 182A in: Abstracts, 34th Meeting, Am. Soc. of Hum. Genet., 1983.

T24 Taporowsky, E., K. Shimizu, M. Goldfarb et al. Structure and activation of the human N-ras gene. Cell 34: 581-586 (1980).

T25 Tateno, H. and K. Mikamo. Neonatal oocyte development and selective oocyte killing by x-rays in the Chinese hamster Cricetulus griseus. Int. J. Rad. Biol. 45: 139-149 (1984).

T26 Trainor, K.J., D. Wigmore, A. Chrysostomou et al. Mutation frequency in human lymphocytes increases with age. Cited in ref. S83.

T27 Tindall, K.R., L.F. Stannkowski, R. Machanoff and A.W. Hsie. Analysis of mutations in DNA transformed Chinese hamster ovary cells. Abstract. Env. Mutagenesis 5: 415 (1983).

T28 Thacker, J. The molecular nature of mutations in cultured mammalian cells: a review. Mutat. Res. 150: 431-442 (1985).

T29 Thompson, L.H., K. Busch, C.L. Brookman et al. Genetic diversity of ultraviolet sensitive DNA repair mutants of Chinese hamster ovary cells. Proc. Natl. Acad. Sci. U.S.A. 78: 3734-3737 (1981).

T30 Tommerup, N., J. Nielsen and M. Mikkelsen. A folate-sensitive heritable fragile site at 19p13. Clin. Genet. 27: 510-514 (1985).

T31 Turner, G., R. Brookwell, A. Daniel et al. Heterozygous expression of X-linked mental retardation and X-chromosome marker fra(X)(q27). New Engl. J. Med. 303: 662-664 (1980).

T32 Tuan, D., P.A. Biro, J.K. de Riel et al. Restriction endonuclease mapping of human gamma globin loci. Nucleic Acids Res. 6: 2519-2544 (1979).

T33 Tilghman, S.M., D.C. Tiemeier, B. Seidman et al. Intervening sequence of DNA identified in the structural portion of a mouse beta globin gene. Proc. Natl. Acad. Sci. U.S.A. 75: 725-729 (1978).

T34 Taniguchi, T., L. Guarente, T.M. Roberts et al. Expression of the human fibroblast interferon gene in E. coli. Proc. Natl. Acad. Sci. U.S.A. 77: 5230-5233 (1980).

T35 Tonegawa, S. Somatic generation of antibody diversity. Nature 302: 575-581 (1983).

T36 Tsuchida, N., T. Ryder and E. Ohtsubo. Nucleotide sequence of the oncogene encoding the p21 transforming protein of Kirsten murine sarcoma virus. Science 217: 937-938 (1982).

T37 Tainsky, M.A., C.S. Cooper, B.C. Giovanella et al. An activated ras[N] gene is detected in late but not in early passage human PAI teratocarcinoma of the human N-ras gene. Cited by Varmus [V13]. Nature.

T38 Tease, C. Dose-related chromosome non-disjunction in female mice after x-irradiation of dictyate oocytes. Mutat. Res. 151: 109-119 (1985).

T39 Thompson, L.H., C.L. Mooney and K.W. Brokman. Genetic complementation between uv-sensitive CHO mutant and xeroderma pigmentosum fibroblasts. Mutat. Res. 150: 423-429 (1985).

T40 Thacker, J. The nature of mutants induced by ionizing radiation in cultured hamster cells. III. Molecular characterization of HPRT-deficient mutants induced by gamma rays or alpha particles showing that the majority have deletions of all or part of the HPRT gene. Mutat. Res. 160: 267-275 (1985).

T41 Turner, D.R., A.A. Morley, M. Haliandros et al. In vivo somatic mutations in human lymphocytes frequently result from major alterations. Nature 315: 343-345 (1985).

T42 Tease, C. and G. Fisher. X-ray-induced chromosomal aberrations in immediately pre-ovulatory oocytes. Mutat. Res. 173: 211-215 (1986).

T43 Tease, C. and G. Fisher. Oocytes from young and old female mice respond directly to colchicine. Mutat. Res. 173: 31-34 (1986).

T44 Tease, C. X-ray-induced chromosome aberrations in dictyate oocytes of young and old mice. Mutat. Res. 119: 191-194 (1983).

T45 Tobari, I., Y. Matsuda, T. Utsugi et al. Personal communication (1986).

U1 United Nations. Ionizing Radiation: Sources and Biological Effects. United Nations Scientific Committee on the Effects of Atomic Radiation, 1982 Report to the General Assembly, with annexes. United Nations Sales Publication, No. E.82.IX.8. New York, 1982.

U2 United Nations. Sources and Effects of Ionizing Radiation. United Nations Scientific Committee on the Effects of Atomic Radiation, 1977. Report to the General Assembly, with annexes. United Nations Sales Publication, No. E.77.IX.I. New York, 1977.

U3 United Nations. Ionizing Radiation. Levels and Effects. A report of the United Nations Scientific Committee on the Effects of Atomic Radiation to the General Assembly, with annexes. United Nations Sales Publication, No. E.72.IX.17 and 18. New York, 1972.

U5 Uchida, I.A. and E.M. Joyce. Activity of the fragile-X in heterozygous carriers. Am. J. Hum. Genet. 34: 286-293 (1982).

U6 Uchida, I.A., V.C.P. Freeman, H. Jamro et al. Additional evidence for fragile X activity in heterozygous carriers. Am. J. Hum. Genet. 35: 861-868 (1983).

U7 Ushiro, H. and S. Cohen. Identification of phosphotyrosine as a product of epidermal growth-factor-activated protein kinase in A-431 cell membranes. J. Biol. Chem. 255: 8363-8365 (1980).

U8 Ungvari, G. Clinical genetic studies on schizophrenic psychoses. I and II. Ideggyógyászati Szemle 35: 481-489 (1982) and 36: 105-113 (1983).

U9 Unoka, I., G. Hollósi, I. Marticsek. Prevalence and causes of hypertension. Orvosi Hetilap 115: 616-623 (1974).

V1 Van Dyke, D.L., L. Weiss, J.R. Robertson et al. The frequency and mutation rate of balanced autosomal rearrangements in man estimated from prenatal genetic studies for advanced maternal age. Am. J. Hum. Genet. 35: 301-308 (1983).

V2 Vijayalaxmi, H.J. Evans, J.H. Ray et al. Bloom's syndrome: evidence for an increased mutation frequency in vivo. Science 221: 851-853 (1983).

V3 Venter, P.A. and J. Op't Hof. Cytogenetic abnormalities including the marker X-chromosome in patients with severe mental retardation. S.A. Med. J. 62: 947-950 (1982).

V4 Vijayalaxmi and H.J. Evans. Measurement of spontaneous and x-ray-induced 6-thioguanine resistant human blood lymphocytes using a T-cell cloning technique. Mutat. Res. 125: 87-94 (1984).

V5 Van Buul, P.P.W. p. 950-952 in: EURATOM Progress Report 1982. EUR-8486 (1983).

V7 Vogel, A., E. Raines, B. Kariya et al. Coordinate control of 3T3 cell proliferation by platelet-derived growth factor and plasma components. Proc. Natl. Acad. Sci. U.S.A. 75: 2810-2814 (1978).

V8 Van Buul, P.P.W. and A. Léonard. Evidence of a threshold x-ray dose for sensitizing stem cell spermatogonia of the mouse to the induction of chromosomal translocations by a second larger dose. Mutat. Res. 70: 95-101 (1980).

V9 Van Buul, P.P.W. and A. Léonard. Effects of unequally fractionated x-ray exposures on the induction of chromosomal rearrangements in mouse spermatogonia. Mutat. Res. 127: 65-72 (1984).

V10 Van Buul, P.P.W. Induction of chromosome aberrations by ionizing radiation in stem cell spermatogonia of mammals. p. 369-400 in: Radiation-induced Chromosome Damage in Man (T. Ishihara and M.S. Sasaki, eds.). Alan R. Liss Inc., New York, 1983.

V11 Van Buul, P.P.W. X-ray-induced translocations in marmoset (Callithrix jacchus) stem cell spermatogonia. Mutat. Res. 129: 234-239 (1984).

V12 Van den Berghe, H., G. David, A. Broekaert-van Orshoven et al. A new chromosome anomaly in acute lymphoblastic leukaemia (ALL). Hum. Genet. 46: 173-180 (1979).

V13 Varmus, H.E. The molecular genetics of cellular oncogenes. Ann. Rev. Genet. 18: 553-612 (1984).

V14 Van Buul, P.P.W. X-ray-induced reciprocal translocations in stem cell spermatogonia of the rhesus monkey: dose and fractionation responses. Mutat. Res. 107: 337-345 (1983).

V15 Van Buul, P.P.W., J.F. Richardson and J.H. Goudzwaard. The induction of reciprocal translocations in rhesus monkey stem-cell spermatogonia: effects of low doses and low dose rates. Radiat. Res. 105: 1-7 (1986).

V16 Vijayalaxmi, E. Wunder and T.M. Schroeder. Spontaneous 6-thioguanine resistant lymphocytes in Fanconi anaemia patients and their heterozygous parents. Hum. Genet. 70: 264-270 (1985).

V17 Vrieling, H., J.W. Simons, F. Arwert et al. Mutations induced by x-rays at the HPRT locus in cultured Chinese hamster cells are mostly large deletions. Mutat. Res. 144: 281-286 (1985).

V18 Van der Linden, W. and N. Simonson. Familial occurrence of gallstone disease. Hum. Hered. 23: 123-127 (1973).

V19 Vauhkonen, A.E., E.M. Sankila, K.O.J. Simola et al. Segregation and fertility analysis in an autosomal reciprocal translocation t(1;8)(q41;q23.1). Am. J. Hum. Genet. 37: 533-542 (1985).

W1 Warburton, D., Z. Stein, J. Kline et al. Chromosome abnormalities in spontaneous abortions: data from New York City study. p. 261-287 in: Human Embryonic and Foetal Death (I.H. Porter and E.B. Hook, eds.). Academic Press, New York, 1980.

W2 Warburton, D.Z., Z. Stein, J. Kline et al. Environmental influences on rates of chromosome anomalies in spontaneous abortions. Am. J. Hum. Genet. 32: 27A (1980).

W3 Williams, J.D. Cytogenetic studies in subjects with mental retardation and congenital anomalies. M.S. Thesis, University of Tennessee. Cited in A.T. Tharapel and R.L. Summitt, 1977, ref. T1.

W4 Weiss, R.A., N.M. Teich, H. Varmus et al. The molecular biology of tumour viruses. Cold Spring Harbor Laboratory, New York, 1973.

W5 Westin, W.H., R.C. Gallo, S.K. Arya et al. Differential expression of the amv gene in human haematopoietic cells. Proc. Natl. Acad. Sci. U.S.A. 79: 2194-2198 (1982).

W6 Weinberg, R.A. Fewer and fewer oncogenes. Cell 30: 3-4 (1982).

W7 Weinberg, R.A. A molecular basis of cancer. Sci. Am. 249: 102-116 (1983).

W8 Wu, R. (ed). Methods of Enzymology. Vol. 68. Recombinant DNA. Academic Press, New York, 1979.

W9 Wu, R., L. Grossman and K. Moldave (eds.). Methods in Enzymology, Vol. 100. Recombinant DNA, Part B. Academic Press, New York, 1983.

W10 Wu, R., L. Grossman and K. Moldave (eds.). Methods of Enzymology, Vol. 101. Recombinant DNA, Part C. Academic Press, New York, 1983.

W11 Williams, J.G. The preparation and screening of cDNA clone bank. in: Genetic Engineering I (R. Williamson, ed.). Academic Press, New York, 1981.

W12 White, R.L., D. Barker, T. Holm et al. Approaches to linkage analysis in the human. p. 235-250 in: Banbury Report 14. Recombinant DNA Applications to Human Disease (C.T. Caskey and R.L. White, eds.). Cold Spring Harbor Laboratory, New York, 1983.

W13 Waldemann, T.A., S.J. Korsmeyer, P.A. Heiter et al. Immunoglobin gene rearrangements in human lymphatic leukemia. p. 53-60 in: Banbury Report 14. Recombinant DNA Applications to Human Disease (C.T. Caskey and R.L. White, eds.). Cold Spring Harbor Laboratory, New York, 1983.

W14 Woo, S.L.C., V.J. Kidd, Z.K. Pam et al. Alpha-1-antitrypsin deficiency and pulmonary emphysema: identification of recessive homozygotes by direct analysis of the mutation site in the chromosomal gene. p. 105-112 in: Banbury Report 14. Recombinant DNA Applications to Human Disease (C.T. Caskey and R.L. White, eds.). Cold Spring Harbor Laboratory, New York 1983.

W15 Wilson, J.T., P.F. Milner, M.E. Summer et al. Use of restriction endonucleases for mapping the allele for beta-globin. Proc. Natl. Acad. Sci. U.S.A. 79: 3628-3631 (1982).

W17 Weatherall, D. New Genetics and Clinical Practice. Nuffield Provincial Hospitals Trust. 1982.

W18 Williams, B.G. and F.R. Blattner. Bacteriophage lambda vectors for DNA cloning. p. 201 in: Genetic Engineering, Vol.2 (J.K. Setlow and A. Hollaender, eds.). Plenum Press, New York, 1980.

W20 Wilson, J.M., A.B. Young and W.N. Kelley. Hypoxanthine guanine-phosphoribosyltransferase deficiency: the molecular basis of clinical syndromes. New Engl. J. Med. 309: 900-910 (1983).

W21 Woo, S.L.C., A.S. Lidsky, F. Güttler et al. Cloned human phenylalanine hydroxylase gene allows prenatal diagnosis and carrier detection of classical phenylketonuria. Nature 306: 151-155 (1983).

W22 Wieacker, P., N. Horn, P. Pearson et al. Menkes Kinky hair disease. A search for closely linked RFLP. Hum. Genet. 64: 139-142 (1983).

W23 Wieacker, P., K.E. Davies, B. Mevorah et al. Linkage studies in a family with X-linked recessive icthyosis employing a cloned DNA sequence from the distal short arm of the X-chromosome. Hum. Genet. 63: 113-116 (1983).

W24 Wieacker, P., T.E. Wienker, B. Dallapiccola et al. Linkage relationships between retinoschisis, Xg and a cloned sequence from the distal short arm of the X chromosome. Hum. Genet. 64: 143-145 (1983).

W25 Willecke, K. and R. Schäffer. Human oncogenes. Hum. Genet. 66: 132-142 (1984).

W26 Watson, R., M. Oskarsson and V.D. Woude. Human DNA sequence homologous to the transforming gene (mos) of Moloney murine sarcoma virus. Proc. Natl. Acad. Sci. U.S.A. 79: 4078-4082 (1982).

W27 Westermark, B., C.H. Heldin, E.B. Johnsson et al. Biochemistry and biology of the platelet-derived growth factor. p. 73-115 in: Growth and Maturation Factors I (G. Guroff, ed.). John Wiley, New York, 1983.

W28 Waterfield, M.D., T. Scrarce, N. Whittie et al. Platelet-derived growth factor is structurally related to the putative transforming protein p28^{sis} of simian sarcoma virus. Nature 304: 35-39 (1983).

W29 Weiss, R.A. Transmission of cellular genetic elements by RNA tumour viruses. p. 130-141 in: Possible Episomes in Eukaryotes (L. Silvestri, ed.). North-Holland, Amsterdam, 1973.

W30 Weiss, R.A. and C.J. Marshall. Oncogenes. Lancet ii: 1138-1142 (1984).

W31 Williamson, V.M., E.T. Young and M. Ciriacy. Transposable elements associated with constitutive expression of yeast alcohol dehydrogenase-II. Cell 23: 605-614 (1981).

W32 Whish, W.J.D., M.I. Davies and S. Shall. Stimulation of poly(ADP-ribose) polymerase activity by anti-tumour antibiotics streptozotocin. Biochem. Biophy. Res. Comm. 65: 722-730 (1975).

W33 Waldren, C.A. and R.T. Johnson. Analysis of inter-phase chromosome damage by means of premature chromosome condensation after x- and ultraviolet-irradiation. Proc. Natl. Acad. Sci. U.S.A. 71: 1137-1141 (1974).

W34 Westerveld, A., J.H.J. Hoeijmakers, M. van Duin et al. Molecular cloning of a human repair gene. Nature 310: 425-429 (1984).

W35 World Health Organization. Genetic factors in con-genital malformations. WHO Tech.R/438. WHO, Geneva, 1970.

W36 Warburton, D., Z. Stein and J. Kline. In utero selection against fetuses with trisomy. Am. J. Hum. Genet. 35: 1059-1064 (1983).

W37 Warren, S.T., T.W. Glover, R.L. Davidson et al. Linkage and recombination between fragile-X linked mental retardation and the factor IX gene. Hum. Genet. 69: 44-46 (1985).

W38 Whang-Peng J., P.A. Bunn, C.S. Kao-Shan et al. A non-random chromosomal abnormality, del 3p(14-23) in human small cell lung cancer (CTCL). Cancer Genet. Cytogenet. 6: 119-134 (1982).

W40 Walker, J.M. and W. Gaestra (eds.). Techniques in Molecular Biology. Croom Helm/Macmillan, 1983.

W42 Weatherall, D.J. and J.B. Clegg. Recent developments in the molecular genetics of human haemoglobin. Cell 16: 467-479 (1979).

W43 Westerveld, A. and S. Naylor. Report of the Com-mittee on the genetic constitution of chromosomes 18, 19, 20, 21 and 22. Cytogenet. Cell Genet. 37: 155-175 (1984).

W44 White, R., M. Leppert, T. Bishop et al. Construction of linkage maps with DNA markers for human chromosomes. Nature 313: 101-105 (1985).

W45 Williams, J.D., R.L. Summit, P.R. Martens et al. Familial Down syndrome due to t(10;21) transloca-tion: evidence that the Down phenotype is related to trisomy of a specific segment of chromosome 21. Am. J. Hum. Genet. 27: 478-485 (1975).

W46 West, J.D., M. Kirk, Y. Goyder et al. Discrimination between the effects of x-irradiation of the mouse oocytes and uterus on the induction of dominant lethals and congenital anomalies. I. Embryo transfer experiments. Mutat. Res. 149: 221-230 (1985).

W47 West, J.D., M. Kirk, Y. Goyder et al. Discrimination of the effects of x-irradiation of the mouse oocytes and uterus on the induction of dominant lethals and congenital anomalies. II. Localized irradiation experi-ments. Mutat. Res. 149: 231-238 (1985).

W48 Witkin, E.M. Ultraviolet mutagenesis and inducible DNA repair in E. coli. Bacteriol. Rev. 40: 869-907 (1976).

W49 World Health Organization. Expert Committee on Diabetes mellitus. Second report. WHO Tech. R/646. WHO, Geneva, 1980.

W50 World Health Organization. Report of the Collabora-tive Study on Standardized Assessment of Depressive Disorders. p. 1-150 (1983).

W51 Weiss, K., R.E. Ferrell, C.L. Hanis et al. Genetics and epidemiology of gall bladder disease. Am. J. Hum. Genet. 36: 1259-1278 (1984).

W52 World Health Organization. Effects of Nuclear War on Health and Health Services. Report of the Inter-national Committee of Experts in Medical Sciences and Public Health to Implement Resolution WHO 34.38. WHO, Geneva, 1984.

W53 Winegar, R.A. and R.J. Preston. Environmental Mutagenesis 8 (Suppl. 6), 246 (1986).

Y1 Yannopoulos, G. Ability of male recombinant factor 31.1 MRF to be transposed to another chromosome in Drosophila melanogaster. Mol. Gen. Genet. 176: 247-253 (1979).

Y2 Young, M.W. Middle repetitive DNA. A fluid com-ponent of the Drosophila genome. Proc. Natl. Acad. Sci. U.S.A. 76: 6274-6278 (1979).

Y3 Young, M.W. and H.E. Schwartz. Nomadic gene families in Drosophila. Cold Spring Harbor Symp. Quant. Biol. 45: 629-640 (1981).

Y4 Yunis, J.J. The chromosomal basis of human neo-plasia. Science 221: 227-236 (1983).

Y5 Yuasa, Y., S.K. Shrivatsava, C.Y. Dunn et al. Acquisition of transforming properties by alternative point mutations within c-bas/has proto-oncogene. Nature 303: 775-779 (1983).

Y6 Yasuda, N. Geographical variations in inborn errors of metabolism. Hum. Hered. 34: 1-8 (1984).

Y7 Yang, T.P., P.I. Patel, J. Brennand et al. Molecular analysis of the human HPRT locus. Abstracts of the 34th Ann. Meeting, Am. Soc. Hum. Genet. 185A (1983).

Y8   Yokayoma, S. Polymorphism in the 5'-flanking region of the human insulin gene and the incidence of diabetes. Am. J. Hum. Genet. 35: 193-200 (1983).

Y9   Yang, T.P., P.I. Patel, A.C. Chinault et al. Molecular evidence for new mutation at the HPRT locus in Lesch-Nyhan patients. Nature 310: 412-414 (1984).

Y10   Yuasa, Y., R.A. Gol, A. Chang et al. Mechanism of activation of an N-ras oncogene of SW-1271 human lung carcinoma cells. Proc. Natl. Acad. Sci. U.S.A. 81: 3670-3674 (1984).

Y11   Yunis, J.J. and A.L. Soreng. Constitutive fragile sites and cancer. Science 226: 1199-1204 (1984).

Y12   Yankner, B.A. and E.M. Shooter. The biology and mechanism of action of nerve growth factor. Ann. Rev. Biochem. 51: 845-868 (1982).

Z1   Zeeland, A.A.V., C.J.M. Bussman, F. Degrassi et al. Effects of aphidicolin on repair replication and induced chromosomal aberration in mammalian cells. Mutat. Res. 92: 379-392 (1982).

Z2   Zabel, B.U., S.L. Naylor, K.H. Grzeschik et al. Regional assignment of human proto-oncogene c-myb to 6q21-qter. Somatic Cell Mol. Genet. 10: 105-108 (1984).

Z3   Zapt, J., E.R. Froesch and R.E. Humbel. The insulin-like growth factors (IGF) of human serum: chemical and biological characterization and aspects of their possible physiological role. Curr. Topics Cell Reg. 19: 257-309 (1981).

Z4   Zaborovsky, E.R., I.M. Chumakov and L.L. Kissler. Tight linkage of retroviral-like sequences to a variant human c-mos gene in the human genome. Cell 23: 379-384 (1983).

Z5   Zaleski, M.B., S. Dubiski, E.G. Niles et al. Immunogenetics. Pitman, Boston, 1983.

Z6   Zarbl, H., S. Sukumar, A.V. Arthur et al. Direct mutagenesis of Ha-ras-1 oncogenes by N-nitroso-N-methylurea during initiation of mammary carcinogenesis in rats. Nature 315: 382-385 (1985).

Z7   Zamansky, G.B., L.F. Kleinman et al. Reactivation of herpes simplex virus in a cell line inducible for simian virus 40. Mutat. Res. 70: 1-9 (1980).

ANNEX B

Dose-response relationships for radiation-induced cancer

CONTENTS

Introduction

1. It has long been recognized by UNSCEAR that radiation-induced malignant diseases are the most important late somatic effect in human populations exposed at high doses for which direct observations are available [U6, U7, U9-U12, U24]. For evaluation of radiological risk or detriment [I2] this importance derives from the fact that these diseases are often lethal and they are the only statistically verifiable cause of radiation-induced life shortening at intermediate and low doses [B17, B18, J1, K39, K40, U24]. Radiation-induced cancer belongs to those radiobiological effects whose frequency of occurrence (but not severity) is believed—as a rule—to correlate with dose.[a] The postulated probabilistic nature of the relationship between dose and frequency of malignancy[b] has led to the acceptance of the term "stochastic" for effects of such type.

2. Assessment of risk, from environmental and occupational radiation sources in the dose region from fractions of mGy to a few tens of mGy, would be greatly facilitated by knowledge of the shapes of the dose-response relationships for radiation-induced cancers in humans. This knowledge is not available at present and is not likely to be obtained by direct observation. Two features of the dose-response relations are most important for evaluation of the risk at low doses: the possible presence of a threshold dose below which the effects would not occur, and the shape of the dose-response curve.

3. Lack of threshold for a given effect is usually assumed if the response for this effect, plotted against the independent variable (causal factor, or, specifically, dose), permits extrapolation by eye to the origin of the coordinate system, or when the calculated regres-

sion line intercepts the abscissa at values that are not significantly different from zero. Conversely, a threshold is usually assumed when the fitted regression function crosses the abscissa at a value significantly greater than zero. However, proving or disproving a threshold below the levels of direct observation may be impossible, due to statistical fluctuations of the spontaneous level and of the presumably induced response. Therefore, assumptions regarding a threshold are based essentially on theoretical considerations of the mechanisms of radiation interaction with the biological targets for initiation of neoplasia, supplemented by empirical observations to support the hypothesis. Although absence of the threshold is often assumed, this has not been proved for any form of radiation-induced malignancy [U6] and must be regarded as a working hypothesis.

4. In annex I of the 1977 UNSCEAR report [U6], the available data concerning experimental radiation carcinogenesis in numerous animal species were reviewed. The large variation of susceptibility to cancer induction in different tissues was emphasized. Physical and biological factors modifying the frequency of induction were discussed in great detail and interactions of other agents (e.g., viruses) with radiation were also reviewed. The extreme complication and unsatisfactory understanding of the pathogenesis of all forms of cancer, including those induced by radiation, were particularly stressed.

5. Various physical factors, such as dose, dose rate, and quality of radiation, were also considered, and general patterns could be recognized in cases where such factors were systematically studied in a given strain of animals, and for specific tumour types. Among the patterns identified, were a sparing effect of dose fractionation and protraction of low-LET radiation (x or gamma rays) upon the frequency of induced cancer and the absence, or even reversal, of such an effect for high-LET radiation (neutrons, alpha particles).

6. Current theories of cancer induction by radiation and some other agents (viruses, chemicals) were also briefly reviewed in the 1977 UNSCEAR report [U6]. None of these was able to accommodate all the known facts and to allow development of a theory or of

---

[a]For brevity, the term "dose" is used here instead of the more correct "absorbed dose".

[b]In this annex, the term "carcinogenesis" is used to include carcinoma, leukaemia or any other form of malignancy (sarcoma, lymphoma, etc.). The word "malignancy" is used when the reference is to all such malignant conditions, while "cancer" or "malignant tumour" refer only to solid or focal malignancies. The term "tumour" is used without qualification when it is either clear from the context, or unimportant, whether a malignant or a benign tumour is intended.

comprehensive models of cancer induction by ionizing radiation. It was recognized, however, that known carcinogens have a common target within the susceptible cells, which is most likely the nuclear DNA or genome.

7. Since the 1977 report [U6], new information has been published on experimental induction of cancer by radiation. Some of it refers to observations at intermediate and low doses. Of particular importance is the information dealing with high-LET particles (mostly neutrons). This is reviewed here when it appears relevant to models of radiation-induced malignancies.

8. In annex I of the 1977 report [U6], the response relationships as a function of single acute doses for various forms of experimental radiation-induced cancer—both after whole-body and localized irradiation—were reviewed thoroughly. Tumours could be broadly subdivided into three categories:

(a) Those showing an increasing incidence with increasing dose up to a maximum, with a decline following that maximum (most forms);

(b) Those displaying a negative correlation between incidence and dose, as observed in tumours with an unusually high spontaneous frequency;

(c) Those showing no clear rise with increasing dose up to several Gy.

For occupational and environmental exposure of man, type (a) is the most relevant. Schematic examples of dose-response curves are shown in Figure I.

9. UNSCEAR [U6] also identified a large variability of the net incidence of various tumour types at intermediate to high doses between different species and, within species, between inbred strains. It was also found that in many cases a particular tumour could be induced by radiation in only one or two strains of a given species, an observation that must raise questions

as to whether such tumours may represent adequate models of corresponding human diseases. Similar doubts would also apply to some observed forms of dose-response relationships. In some cases, dose-response relationships differ from species to species, although in many cases consistent patterns have been found. For these reasons, the increased incidence per unit dose of a given form of cancer cannot—as a rule—be extrapolated between species.

10. For dose-response relationships of category (a) some regularities were pointed out that appeared to conform to other radiobiological phenomena occurring in single cells (e.g., cell killing, induction of mutations and chromosome aberrations). These common features were as follows:

(a) The RBE values for densely-ionizing radiation relative to x and gamma rays are higher than 1 and decrease as doses increase;

(b) With acute doses of high-LET radiation the dose-response relationship is closer to linearity than for sparsely-ionizing radiation, for which upward concave curvilinearity is usually observed;

(c) The tumour yield often shows little dependence on dose protraction and fractionation for high-LET radiation, while for x and gamma rays the yield usually declines.

11. Since publication of the 1977 report [U6], additional information has appeared on tumour induction and life shortening in the low and intermediate dose region. It shows that after acute (high dose rate) high-LET exposure, in some cases at intermediate and in most cases at high doses, the incidence of tumours per unit dose decreases with increasing dose. For low-LET acute exposures, such a decline is usually observed only at high doses (above several Gy). These and other observations, together with some notable exceptions, will be discussed in detail in chapter IV.

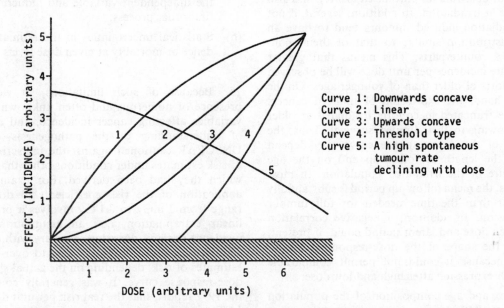

Curve 1: Downwards concave
Curve 2: Linear
Curve 3: Upwards concave
Curve 4: Threshold type
Curve 5: A high spontaneous tumour rate declining with dose

Figure I. Typical dose-response curves for radiation-induced tumours. Curve 1: Downwards concave; Curve 2: Linear; Curve 3: Upwards concave; Curve 4: Threshold type; Curve 5: A high spontaneous tumour rate declining with dose. The shaded area represents the spontaneous (control) incidence.

12. In annex G of the 1977 report [U6], UNSCEAR presented a comprehensive review of epidemiological data on radiation-induced cancer in man. Absolute risk estimates of mortality per unit dose were examined in detail for malignant diseases of various organs, and confidence limits were attached to these estimates, derived in most cases from irradiation with doses at or above 1 Gy. Also, an approximate life-time risk of mortality from cancer at all sites per unit dose was estimated from the ratio of incidence of all non-leukaemic malignancies to the incidence of leukaemias in several groups (atomic bomb survivors, American radiologists, and patients treated for ankylosing spondylitis and metropathia haemorrhagica). However, the previously available dosimetry at Hiroshima and Nagasaki has been questioned, and the new dosimetric system (DS86) is expected to yield improved risk coefficients for atomic bomb survivors, who are one of the most important sources of information.

13. The merit of such risk estimates lies in the fact that they are derived directly from human data and thus avoid interspecies extrapolations of doubtful validity. The precision of the 1977 risk estimates was the best possible under the conditions of exposure and follow-up then available, but many limitations of the estimates were discussed extensively.

14. Uncertainties regarding the shape of the dose-response relationships for radiation-induced malignancies, and the related risk estimates in man, derive mostly from the following conditions:

(a) The short duration of follow-up of irradiated populations compared to the length of latent period of most tumours. Whereas 20 to 30 years may be sufficient for manifestation of leukaemias and bone sarcomas after short-term irradiation, it is not so for other cancers. At present, the time distribution of their latent periods is not known in detail, and for some cancers it depends upon dose (or dose rate for chronic exposure), and also on age at irradiation. In addition, several, if not all, radiation-induced tumours tend to have an age distribution similar to that of their spontaneous counterparts. This means that greater absolute incidence per unit dose will be observed in cohorts of older than of younger ages. On the other hand, the expression of induced cancers will be truncated in cohorts irradiated at older ages, owing to their limited survival. Thus, the shape of the dose-response curve may depend upon the length of follow-up and on the age structure of the irradiated population. In most studies, the mean follow-up period is substantially shorter than the time needed for full tumour expression. In addition, a negative correlation between dose and latent period could, if present, affect the shape of the dose-response relationship, because it could not permit comparable tumour expression after high and low dose;

(b) The sex and age composition of the population under study. Since for certain tumours the age at irradiation and sex have a pronounced effect upon the risk of later development of the malignancy, a given dose-response relationship

may not be representative of populations of different composition;

(c) There is a pronounced geographical, socio-economic and ethnic variation of the spontaneous incidence of cancers in most organs. (For a review of this point see [D17, W9].) This suggests that epidemiological observations on radiation-induced cancer cannot be applied indiscriminately to populations of different ethnic, socio-economic or geographic characteristics. On the other hand, such differences are not necessarily reflected in the value of the absolute risk or the shape of the dose-response relationship. For instance, in spite of large differences in the age-specific incidence, the age-corrected excess risk of breast cancer and dose-response curves in Japanese atomic bomb survivors are very similar to those in women irradiated in the United States for medical reasons;

(d) Deficiencies of tumour ascertainment in retrospective studies from available records of incidence or specific mortality;

(e) Difficulties in the selection of suitable comparison groups for the calculation of the expected (control) incidence or mortality due to a given tumour;

(f) Presence of confounding variables and modifying factors (promoters, inhibitors) that, if correlated with dose, or per se, could modify the shape of the dose-response relation;

(g) Questionable accuracy of dosimetric estimates, particularly when these involve retrospective reconstructions of complex situations. Numerous examples of such uncertainties are given in chapter V. In this category belongs also the very narrow range of doses to which a population may have been exposed, as well as the non-uniformity of dose distribution in the target organs. The latter condition may distort the relationship when the mean organ dose is used as the independent variable and induction is not a first-order process;

(h) Statistical uncertainties in the estimates of incidence or mortality at given dose levels.

15. Because of such limitations, in view of the presence of numerous and often unknown biological variables affecting cancer incidence, and of the lack of understanding of the pathogenesis of cancer, UNSCEAR cautioned against the indiscriminate use of risk estimates under conditions other than those for which they had been derived. For example, direct application of the risk coefficients to doses in the range from 1 mGy to 0.1 Gy involves a procedure of linear extrapolation, i.e., an assumption that the incidence per unit dose does not vary with dose. Such a procedure could, however, lead to over- or under-estimates of risk, depending on the actual shape of the dose-response curve. It was generally concluded, in the 1977 report, that the real risk per unit dose of low-LET radiation at low doses and/or dose rates would be unlikely to be higher, but could be substantially lower, than the values derived for the range of a few tens of mGy. The derivation was based essentially on

observations made above 1 Gy, but some reduction of the effect at low doses was already assumed (e.g., for leukaemia by a factor of about 2).

16. The wide confidence limits on the data from man allow various mathematical functions to be fitted to the same epidemiological series [B17, B20, B24, C29, M31, R21, S50]. Consequently, the probability of being able to discriminate between the statistical goodness of fit of various alternatives, or to reject some of them, is too low. In addition, the extrapolation of a relationship beyond the region of direct observation is always questionable when the underlying mechanism is not well understood.

17. In view of all these difficulties UNSCEAR has followed another approach in preparing the present annex. It has reviewed evidence at the subcellular and cellular level, from which inferences could be made as to the possible nature of the dose-response for cancer initiation by radiation. It has also examined how initiation of cancerous clones, and their progression to clinical tumours, may affect the shape of the dose-response relationship. Finally, it has reviewed published models of cancer induction and tested them for compatibility with epidemiological and experimental findings. It is hoped that this complex exercise may help to establish, with some confidence, the shape of dose-response relationships, and thereby limit the uncertainty in the extrapolation of the risk to low doses.

18. Thus, the objectives of this annex may be summarized as follows:

(a) To review the critical assumptions involved in the formulation of models linking radiation-induced cancer to dose;

(b) To review and discuss dose-response relationships for effects at the cellular level that could conceptually be linked with malignant transformation;

(c) To discuss models of cancer induction by radiation from the standpoint of resulting dose-response relationships for tumours of some organs and tissues;

(d) To review the effects of the mode of dose delivery (dose rate, fractionation) and quality of radiation upon the dose-response relationships;

(e) To identify possible general trends, and interspecies similarities, brought about by changes in the above variables upon the dose-response relationships for various types of cancer.

UNSCEAR wishes to stress that in pursuing this exercise it does not intend to give more weight or credit to one or another model of tumour induction, nor to depart from previously established policies in risk estimation adopted within the Committee. This review is meant to be a purely scientific analysis of data aiming at an assessment of systematic errors in the risk estimates derived from existing epidemiological evidence when one or another model is assumed in interpreting such evidence.

I. DOSE-RESPONSE RELATIONSHIPS FOR RADIATION-INDUCED CANCER

19. Radiation-induced cancer, as a stochastic phenomenon, can be analysed in terms of probabilistic concepts such as the distribution function of the time from irradiation to the occurrence of cancer. Depending on the data, the event may be assumed to occur at the time of diagnosis for readily apparent tumours, or at the time of death for rapidly lethal ones. The definitions and procedures of estimation are similar, but the two cases should not be confused because this could lead to serious errors, particularly with cancers for which effective therapy is available.

20. In experimental work, the populations under study consist generally of inbred animals standardized for species, strain, sex and age. They are irradiated under controlled conditions and followed for a specified time or up to death. Appropriately matched control groups are followed concurrently under similar conditions. The time of death and, at least in some experiments, the cause of death, can be ascertained for each animal. Such data may undergo sophisticated statistical treatments.

21. Easily diagnosed or rapidly lethal tumours are readily discovered. For such "manifest" neoplasms, established mathematical procedures can be applied to correct for competing risks, e.g., intercurrent mortality not related to the tumour incidence. Under these conditions, the time to the expression of the tumour is known only for some of the individuals in the collective, while others die or disappear from observation due to unrelated causes before a tumour is observed. For these latter individuals one knows only that the hypothetical time to the tumour would have been longer than the observation time, i.e., it would lie to the right on the time scale. Hence one speaks of "right censored" data.

22. If tumours are "occult", in the sense that they are discovered only incidentally in animals killed or dying for other reasons, one speaks of "double censored" data. In this case, one knows either that the time to the expression of the tumour is shorter than the observed time of death or that the hypothetical time would be longer than the time of death, according to whether the dead animals carry a tumour, or not. Under these conditions the expression "double censored data" is used (meaning that the data are both "left and right censored") and the methods for a competing-risk-corrected analysis are more complex (see paragraph 31). There are special difficulties for partly lethal tumours, but a four-point grading of the tumours is usually practicable and sufficient for the analysis; it ranges from "definitively incidental" to "definitively manifest (e.g., lethal)" [P18, P19].

23. In epidemiological work on human populations, the situation is quite different. The series are, in most cases, retrospective; the final data on morbidity and mortality are frequently incomplete; and the composition of the group is often heterogeneous with respect

to sex, age, socio-economic status, health conditions and exposure to carcinogenic or promoting agents other than radiation. Also, the control population is seldom fully adequate; follow-up to extinction is rarely achieved owing to the long life span of man; and dosimetry is frequently uncertain. The statistical treatment of such data must obviously follow methods different from those applying to prospective experiments.

A. THE INDEPENDENT VARIABLE

24. Dose-response curves are functional relationships between an independent variable, the radiation dose in a given organ or tissue, and a dependent variable represented by a suitable measure of the response. The specific energy, z, absorbed in a cell or in its critical structures, is a random variable. The mean value of z, i.e., the absorbed dose, D, is commonly used as the quantity of reference, but at equal values of absorbed dose the distribution of the values of specific energy can vary greatly, depending on the tissue volume for which the specific energy is determined and the value of the absorbed dose, as well as the radiation quality (see III.B.2). Furthermore, the same dose may be delivered at different dose rates. In the present context, the following terminology will be adopted for sparsely-ionizing radiation: low doses, < 0.2 Gy; intermediate doses, 0.2-2.0 Gy; and high doses, > 2.0 Gy. For densely-ionizing radiation (e.g., fast neutrons) doses < 0.05 and > 0.5 Gy will be referred to as low or high, respectively, with intermediate doses falling between the figures quoted. Low dose rates for all radiations are < 0.05 mGy min^{-1}; high dose rates are > 0.05 Gy min^{-1}; and intermediate dose rates fall between these limits. Other quantities will at times be used as the independent variable, such as the injected activity of a specified radionuclide, or the time-integrated concentration of alpha-energy of short-lived radon daughters ultimately to be released in air. With some oscillations, such quantities are proportional to dose.

B. THE DEPENDENT VARIABLES IN EXPERIMENTAL WORK

25. In experimental work on radiation carcinogenesis, various expressions of the response may be adopted (see annex I in [U6]). The simplest, and most commonly used, is the fraction of animals incurring a tumour after irradiation with a given dose (crude incidence). It has been stressed repeatedly [F1, G17-G19, H15, M32, R9, S37, U2-U5, U20-U22] that such way of expressing the response leads to erroneous results. The reason is the interference of competing risks and of the different duration of life between animals receiving different doses. Actually, animals receiving the highest doses tend to die earlier and thus have less chance of expressing the tumours that may be induced.

26. Corrections for differences in the distribution of survival times between control and irradiated animals may be made by approximate methods, as, for example, in studies by Ullrich and Storer [U2-U5, U20, U21, U23-U26]. In this approach, the data are truncated at the time when the group is extinguished through natural death and the observed incidence in the treated group is corrected by a factor equal to the ratio of the mean lifetime for the control and the irradiated groups. This approach can provide approximate age corrections, but it may be misleading when the frequency of tumour appearance varies considerably with time after exposure.

27. Rigorous corrections for age and intercurrent mortality may be made by following the response of irradiated and control individuals throughout their life after irradiation or during a pre-selected post-irradiation period, with appropriate methods of investigation, including careful post-mortem pathology. The relevant parameter is then the age- or time-dependent rate of tumour appearance [C18, C19, H15, K8, S37] or a related cumulative quantity that can be more readily determined in the experiment. The basic quantities in this approach and their competing-risk-corrected estimates for manifest tumours are:

(a) The tumour rate, r(t), as a function of age or time (t) after irradiation. It is the probability at time t per individual to develop a tumour per unit time. This quantity, r(t), is to be interpreted as a mean value for the population under study. Since, for tumours diagnosed during the lifetime, the actual time of origin of the tumour is unknown, the time of its first observation is generally used; the time of death is used for rapidly developing, lethal tumours. In experimental work one derives r(t) as an average value in a group of animals at time t. If N animals are observed (i.e., are at risk) over the interval $t - \Delta t/2$ to $t + \Delta t/2$, and n tumours appear within the interval, the estimate of the tumour rate is $\hat{r}(t) = \Delta n/N\Delta t$. For incidentally observed tumours a direct estimate of the tumour rate is impossible; the tumour prevalence can, however, be estimated (see paragraph 31);

(b) The cumulative tumour rate, R(t). Estimates of this quantity are less affected by statistical fluctuations and are therefore more readily derived. The quantity is defined as the integral of the tumour rate from the time of exposure (t = 0) up to time t:

$$R(t) = \int_0^t r(t) \, dt \qquad (1.1)$$

R(t) is the number of tumours per animal up to time t under the hypothetical condition that one could keep the number of animals at risk constant in spite of intercurrent mortality and the occurrence of tumours. R(t) exceeds, therefore, not only the crude incidence, but also the incidence I(t), corrected for competing risks (see paragraphs 29 and 30). A competing-risk-corrected estimate of the integral tumour rate is [A1, N3, S37]:

$$\hat{R}(t) = \sum_i (n_i/N_i\Delta t) \, \Delta t = \sum_i n_i/N_i \qquad (1.2)$$

for all i with $i\Delta t < t$, where n_i is the number of tumours appearing within the time interval $(i - 1)\Delta t$ to $i\Delta t$, and N_i is the actual number of individuals still at risk at this time, i.e., individuals still without a tumour. The standard error for equation (1.2) can be obtained by the relationship [S37]

$$\sigma_{R(t)} = \sqrt{(\sum_i n_i/N_i^2)} \qquad (1.3)$$

28. If multiple non-lethal tumours occur, estimates of the tumour rate or the integral tumour rate can be based also on all observed tumours [S37]. In this case all animals still at risk are included in N_i (equation 1.2), regardless of whether these animals had developed a tumour or not. With this modification, similar estimates are obtained, provided that the animals without previous tumour had experienced the same tumour rate as the animals that had already incurred a tumour. This is so because both the numerator and the denominator in equation (1.2) are increased. If, on the other hand, there are inherent variations of the tumour rate within a population, or if the occurrence of a tumour increases the probability of subsequent tumours, the tumour rate estimated from all tumours will be larger than the rate estimated from first tumours only. It is mandatory, therefore, to specify whether the estimates of the integral tumour rate are based on the first or on all observed tumours. For partly lethal or rapidly developing lethal tumours the estimate can be based only on first tumours.

29. A frequently used quantity, related to the cumulative tumour rate, is the actuarial incidence, or incidence corrected for competing risks, $I(t)$. It is the probability of an animal at risk up to time t to have incurred a tumour. In the absence of competing risks, the actuarial incidence equals the crude incidence (see paragraph 25). In the presence of competing risks, and for manifest tumours, a quantity can be obtained in terms of the product limit estimate [K1]:

$$\hat{I}(t) = 1 - \prod_{i=1} [1 - n_i/N_i] \qquad t_1 \le t \qquad (1.4)$$

where the product extends over a number of time intervals (i) up to time t; n_i is the number of animals with tumours appearing within the time interval $t_{i+1} - t_i$; and N_i is the number of animals without tumours still at risk at time t_i. The standard error of the product limit estimate is expressed by the so-called Greenwood formula:

$$\hat{\sigma}_{I(t)} = [1 - \hat{I}(t)] \sqrt{\sum_i n_i/N_i^2} \qquad t_i \le 1 \qquad (1.5)$$

When N is very small the log-rank test is preferable (see paragraph 33).

30. If few individuals incur the tumour, the actuarial incidence and the integral tumour rate, based on first tumours only, are nearly equal. At high frequencies, the actuarial incidence can approach 1, and the integral tumour rate may exceed 1. The sum limit estimate (equation 1.2) is largely equivalent to the product limit estimate (equation 1.4), i.e., the integral tumour rate can also be obtained from the product limit estimate by the relationship:

$$R(t) = -\ln[1 - I(t)] \qquad (1.6)$$

Similarly, the actuarial incidence can be obtained from the sum limit estimate by the relationship:

$$I(t) = 1 - \exp[-R(t)] \qquad (1.7)$$

31. For occult tumours (see paragraph 22), which frequently occur in short-lived animals, the actuarial incidence (which is then usually called prevalence) or the integral tumour rate are more difficult to estimate. Theoretical analyses have shown that a combination of serial killing and survival data is required for such estimates in the case of tumours with unknown degree of lethality or life shortening [C36, M22, N4, R8]. If occult tumours are definitely non-lethal, estimates can be obtained by serial sacrifices at specified times after irradiation. However, this approach requires large numbers of animals. As Hoel and Walburg have pointed out [H29], the method of isotonic regression (see also [B84, K38]) may be used to estimate the competing-risk-corrected incidence from survival experiments. This provides a maximum likelihood solution with the constraint of monotonicity of the incidence. The algorithm for isotonic regression is straightforward and has been utilized for the analysis of radiation carcinogenesis [C36]. At present, however, there are no methods to derive standard errors.

32. In most experimental studies in which tumours are seen in various organs of the same animals, it is usually assumed that such tumours occur independently of each other. However, Storer has shown [S53] that this is not necessarily so. In irradiated female BALB/c mice, 21 out of the 66 pairs of tumours tested showed significant positive or negative correlations. Some of the negative associations were due to rapid lethality caused by one of the tumours, and this could be corrected for by appropriate methods allowing for intercurrent mortality. Of the remaining 13 significant correlations, 6 involved tumours known to be endocrine-related, and 7 applied to tumours of other organs. Alterations in host factors were believed to be responsible for the observed associations. These possible complications should be borne in mind in the analysis of dose-response relationships on the assumption of random, i.e., independent, tumour occurrence.

33. The logrank test, the Breslow test, or the wider class of non-parametric generalized rank-sum tests are suitable for the comparison of tumour rates in two or more groups in the case of manifest tumours [K37]. Analogous tests do not exist for double censored data from survival experiments, i.e., for tumours found incidentally. With such data, one must use tests based on the assumption of the equality of competing risks in the two groups under comparison, or one requires knowledge of the degree of difference of competing risks. For experiments with serial killing, suitable standard tests exist.

34. The quantities discussed in paragraphs 28-29 are not based on specific models. In experiments where various groups, exposed to different doses, are compared, estimates may be used that are also non-parametric but are based on models. Most frequently, the proportional hazards model is used. This model is based on the assumption that the tumour rate or the integral tumour rate in non-irradiated animals is increased by a dose-dependent factor:

$$r(t,D) = \lambda(D) r_0(t) \qquad \text{or} \qquad R(t,D) = \lambda(D) R_0(t)$$
$$(1.8)$$

where $r_0(t)$ and $R_0(t)$ are the tumour rates and integral tumour rates for the non-irradiated animals, and $r(t,D)$ and $R(t,D)$ are the tumour rates for the individuals exposed to dose D. By equations (1.1) and (1.6) one could express this model in terms of the actuarial incidence, $I(t)$. However, such expression would be more complicated. The reason is that tumour rates and cumulative tumour rates from independent causes are additive, while the incidence is additive only when its value is small. For manifest tumours, there is a relatively straightforward algorithm for calculation of the proportional hazard coefficients, $\lambda(D)$, employing the method of partial likelihood [K37]. For incidentally observed tumours, one must make use of more complex methods, requiring computer algorithms for non-linear optimization, with the constraint of monotonicity [C36, K38]. The analysis can also be based on the model of accelerated failure times by use of the non-linear optimization methods. This model assumes that the competing-risk-corrected incidence, $I(t,D)$, rises earlier in a way that can be described by a dose-dependent acceleration of the incidence $I_0(t)$ for the control groups:

$$I(t,D) = I_0 [a(D)t] \quad \text{and} \quad R(t,D) = R_0[a(D)t]$$
(1.9)

A similar model is that of time shift [C36], which assumes that the tumour rates, the integral tumour rates, or the incidence may attain the same values at earlier times, in a manner that can be described by a forward shift in time:

$$I(t,D) = I_0 [t+s(D)] \quad \text{and} \quad R(t,d) = R_0[t +s(D)]$$
(1.10)

With both the accelerated time or the time shift models, algorithms for non-linear optimization are required for either manifest or incidentally found tumours.

35. As a further step towards the derivation of coherent time and dose dependencies, parametric models have been used. Particularly important among these is the so-called Weibull model [K37], which postulates tumour rates, and integral tumour rates, increasing as a power of time:

$$r(t) = c\, t^p \quad \text{and} \quad R(t) = c\, t^{p+1}/(p + 1) \quad (1.11)$$

The coefficient c is assumed to depend on dose, while the exponent p may or may not be treated as a parameter that varies with dose. The Weibull model is a special case both of the proportional hazards model and of the accelerated time model. Another frequently used model envisages a log-normal distribution of the times to the tumour, i.e., of a competing-risk-corrected incidence that depends on time as a log-normal sum distribution. Various other models, for example the logistic model, have also been utilized.

36. The preceding paragraphs refer only to acute irradiation. In case of continuous or fractionated long-term exposure, additional complexities are introduced. Under such conditions, the dose increases with time and it may be difficult to identify the relevant value of the accumulated dose. The process of cancer induction is followed by a period of growth until the tumour becomes observable. The dose absorbed during this period is not relevant to the appearance of the tumour. Corrections may therefore be applied by subtracting from the total dose the portion received after the presumed onset of neoplastic growth.

C. THE DEPENDENT VARIABLES IN EPIDEMIOLOGICAL STUDIES

37. Whereas experimental studies use inbred animals that are uniform as regards sex, age at exposure and other conditions, no comparable uniformity is ever encountered in epidemiological human studies. Moreover, various human populations are often subject to a spectrum of influences, of which only some are known or accounted for. In an ideal case, a multivariate analysis should be used to assess the relative importance of factors other than radiation. As this is seldom possible, less rigorous analyses must frequently be accepted which, in addition to the basic quantities previously discussed, use other, somewhat cruder ones. In epidemiological investigations, the follow-up may start shortly after irradiation (prospective studies) or at later times when some or all of the expected tumours may have occurred (retrospective studies). Reliable data collection is more easily achieved in the first case, but the majority of epidemiological studies are based on retrospective analyses.

38. It is not the objective of this annex to deal in detail with all factors and variables affecting the accuracy of risk assessment of radiogenic cancers. However, for the understanding of the following text it is necessary to discuss briefly the expression of the response in absolute and relative terms. The question of risk projection beyond the period of direct observation is intimately linked to the use of so-called absolute and relative risk projection models. These will not be discussed in detail in this annex.

39. As mentioned above, the occurrence of radiation-induced neoplasms may depend on time after irradiation and on the absorbed dose in a variety of ways. In epidemiological investigations it is possible, ideally, to envisage two different situations frequently referred to as the absolute or the relative risk model.

(a) The radiation-induced excess tumour rate—or the incidence rate, as more frequently determined in epidemiological studies—after a latent period increases independently of the spontaneous incidence but as a function of absorbed dose, i.e., the spontaneous and induced rates are additive. Panel (a) of Figure II illustrates this case schematically;

(b) The excess tumour rate, or the net incidence rate, is proportional to the spontaneous age-specific incidence rate, i.e., the dose results in a multiplicative effect of the spontaneous tumour rate over the life span. This relative risk model, corresponding to the proportional hazards model described in paragraph 34, is shown in panel (b) of Figure II [C29].

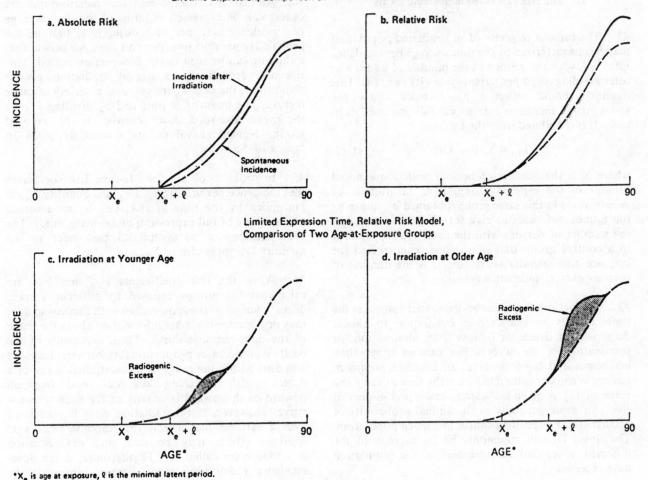

Figure II.   Radiation-induced cancer incidence superimposed on spontaneous cancer incidence, by age. Relative and absolute risk models.
[C29]

40.   For most human tumours, the spontaneous tumour rate is a steep function of age, but quantitatively this dependence varies. For radiation-induced tumours with relatively short latent periods and full expression within a short interval (leukaemia and bone sarcoma) one may distinguish between absolute or relative risk models. A simple absolute model will apply when irradiation at any age is followed by a temporary increase of the tumour rate that does not depend on the magnitude of the spontaneous age-specific rate. A relative model will be preferable when the temporary increase of the tumour rate becomes larger with increasing age at exposure. The latter case is illustrated in panels (c) and (d) of Figure II.

41.   The relative risk projection model implies that the absolute (attributable) risk increases with age; on the other hand, the absolute risk model implies that the excess risk when related to the spontaneous incidence rate, decreases with age. Actually, epidemiological data often show an intermediate pattern, and a decision as to which model is most appropriate for risk estimation is not always possible [C29, T12]. However, recent evaluations of cancer incidences in atomic bomb survivors lend rather strong support to

the relative model. This is so because, for the same age cohort, excess deaths from cancer other than leukaemia increase with age at death in proportion to the age-specific death rate from these cancers in the population of Japan [K39, S59]. A similar conclusion was reached when the time pattern of appearance of second cancers, presumably radiation-induced, was studied in women treated by radiation for carcinoma of the cervix [B93]. Constancy of the relative risk of lung cancer with time after irradiation was also noted in Swedish iron-ore miners [R41] and in United States of America and Czechoslovak uranium miners [I5]. The two projection models have been used for prediction of the numbers of various tumour types in a population having an age distribution similar to the one in the United States, assuming a series of dose-response relationships and applying the appropriate corrections for intercurrent mortality by the life-table technique [C29]. When considering the risk of radiation-induced cancer, whatever the model applied, it is being currently assumed that the distribution of the sensitivity in human population is unimodal, although the character of the distribution is virtually unknown. The question of the possible exceptionally elevated susceptibility of some individuals is discussed in paragraphs 93-97.

173

1. The risk expressed in absolute terms

42. The tumour response of an irradiated population may be characterized by the time average net incidence rate, $\dot{I}_{TA}$, which is defined as the number of additional tumours diagnosed per person-year (PY) at risk. This quantity should reflect a net increase above the spontaneous incidence rate in suitably matched controls. It is calculated from the formula

$$\dot{I}_{TA} = X/P - J/Q \qquad (1.12)$$

where X is the number of persons with a diagnosed tumour in the exposed group; P is the number of person-years in this same group, obtained by summing the number of years at risk for all individuals; J is the number of persons with the same type of tumour in a control group that is matched or corrected for sex, age and calendar years; and Q is the number of person-years in the control group.

43. The period at risk for an irradiated subject is the time, usually in years, from irradiation to cancer diagnosis, or death, or to loss from observation, or termination of the survey. For cancers other than leukaemia and bone sarcoma, an assumed minimum latency is usually subtracted from the time at risk. The value of $\dot{I}_{TA}$ is given as "cancer cases/person-year at risk", or more generally as the annual probability of occurrence of a specified cancer in a given population. The dose, D, will commonly be an average of the different doses that the members of the population have received.

44. If a suitable control group is not available, age- and sex-specific incidence rates of tumours in the general population may be used. Under these conditions, however, tumour ascertainment in the groups may not be fully comparable, and possible selection by conditions that prompted irradiation, or by other co-variates, may result in gross errors.

45. In order to obtain the time average net incidence, I_{TA}, the value obtained from equation (1.12) is multiplied by the average time at risk, i.e., by the average period of observation or, for predictions beyond follow-up, by an assumed time for full expression of the malignancy. For leukaemia and bone sarcoma, this time is known not to exceed significantly 30 years (see chapter V). For other radiation-induced tumours, the period of expression is unknown. In order to derive meaningful projections, a correction for intercurrent mortality becomes necessary, i.e., average life expectancies have to be used. When the distribution of the population by age and sex is known, life tables can be used to this purpose, as in [C29]. As the quantities $\dot{I}_{TA}$ and I_{TA} can be affected by significant errors, due to several circumstances, they must be used with caution. First, as the latent period is not known precisely, the correction for it can only be, at best, an approximation. Secondly (and apart from the above correction) it is unrealistic to assume constancy of the incidence rate over time; if the observation periods for two collectives exposed to different doses do not coincide, then the observations cannot be strictly comparable.

46. Annual risk coefficients for radiation-induced cancer can be expressed in terms of the time average net incidence rate per unit dose, $\dot{F}_{TA}$, that is, the probability per unit time per unit dose per person that a tumour can be seen in the observation period. This risk may depend on sex, age at irradiation, genetic disposition, the organ exposed, and a variety of other factors. The quantity is obtained by dividing $\dot{I}_{TA}$ by the mean absorbed dose received in the exposed group. Numerical values are commonly given in "cases $10^{-6}\,a^{-1}\,Gy^{-1}$".

47. In order to obtain the life-time risk coefficient (net incidence per unit dose), F_{TA}, the quantity $\dot{F}_{TA}$ is multiplied by the time at risk, i.e., by an assumed average time of full expression of the malignancy. The considerations in paragraph 45 that refer to the quantity I_{TA} apply also to F_{TA}.

48. When the risk coefficients F_{TA} and $\dot{F}_{TA}$ are calculated for groups exposed to different average doses, changes of these quantities with increasing dose may provide approximate information about the shape of the dose-response curve. Thus, constancy of the coefficient indicates proportionality between response and dose within the range of doses studied; a rise or a decrease with increasing dose may result from an upward or downward concavity of the dose-response curve. However, if the radiation dose is correlated with a variable that affects the response (e.g., age) spurious effects may be seen and normalization procedures are called for. Furthermore, if the dose-incidence relationship is not linear, expressing the observations in terms of a probability per unit dose distorts the data and introduces additional inaccuracies if individual doses within the exposed population deviate substantially from the average dose to the population. For instance, if the dose relationship contains a dose-squared component, the contribution to the response by individuals with high doses is greater than if linearity applies.

2. The risk expressed in relative terms

49. When the risk is expressed in relative terms, the response is related to the risk of spontaneous cancers (incidence or mortality) in an unirradiated control population. The response variables used are the standardized mortality ratio (SMR), defined as the ratio of mortalities in the exposed group to the mortality in a control group multiplied by 100; and/or the relative risk (RR), which is the ratio of risks observed over expected (each expressed, for instance, per 10^{-6} person and over a given follow-up time). The latter quantity may be applied both to the incidence and mortality indices. The proportional hazard model specifies that if λ_i is the incidence rate of a disease, or the mortality rate for a specific cause of death among subjects in dose group i, it can be expressed as $\lambda_i = \lambda_{i0}\,(RR_i)$, where λ_{i0} is the background or spontaneous rate of mortality or incidence (i.e., the rate experienced by subjects in the absence of exposure to radiation) while RR_i is the relative risk associated with dose group i. The starting point for investigation of a radiation dose-response is the function

$RR_i = 1 + \gamma D_i$, where γ represents the excess relative risk coefficient ($(RR - 1)$ per unit dose). Variation of γ with dose provides information as to the form of the RR-dose relationship.

50. Various statistical methods, including multiple regression analysis, have been used to obtain dose-response relationships, and are presented and discussed in detail in numerous publications, e.g., [G36, J8, K42, S60, W17]. Careful corrections for sex, age at irradiation, attained age at observation and other confounding variables (e.g., ethnicity, exposure to other carcinogens and promoters) are necessary when the shape of the dose-response curve is the object of the study.

D. TEMPORAL RELATIONSHIPS

51. As pointed out in preceding paragraphs, the tumour rate, the cumulative tumour rate and the actuarial incidence depend on time after irradiation and on other factors, such as age at exposure or absorbed dose. It has already been mentioned that the absorbed dose may change the time dependence in a variety of ways. It is necessary, therefore, to consider temporal relations in somewhat more detail.

1. Latent period

52. The latent period is the time between irradiation (e.g., single acute exposure) and manifestation of a tumour. It may be divided conceptually into true latency (the time required from initiation to the beginning of unrestrained growth) and tumour growth (time until the neoplasm can be diagnosed). Reported data are usually latent periods, i.e., the sum of the above times. The length of true latency may be obtained by subtracting an estimated time of tumour growth from the observed latent periods. There are considerable differences between the latent periods of various tumours. Two malignancies in man, leukaemia and bone sarcoma, appear to have relatively short latencies and show an upper limit of the latent periods, so that their full distribution in a population having a normal age structure can be observed. For other tumours the distribution of the latent periods is unknown, because it extends to very long times; the distributions are then usually truncated by the length of the observation period. Median times recorded so far are of the order of 20 to 30 years, but they should increase with extension of the follow-up of the respective groups.

53. If the follow-up is shorter than the minimum latent period, radiation-induced tumours cannot be expected. For more extended studies an inferred minimum latent period is frequently subtracted from the total time at risk, as mentioned before. The minimum latent period is often identified with the time after irradiation at which the incidence rate becomes statistically significant at a given level of confidence above the control values. Figure III shows, however, that, for statistical reasons, the minimum latent period so estimated must vary with dose even

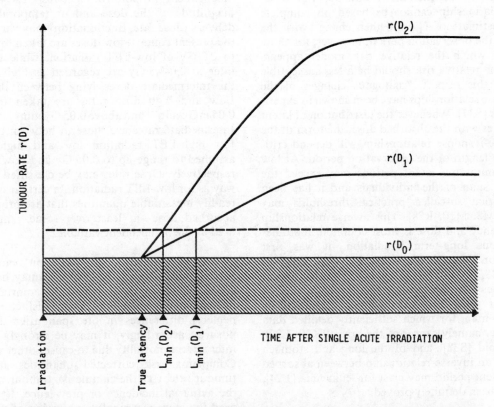

Figure III. Presumed effect of the magnitude of dose upon estimate of minimum latent period. Two doses ($D_1 < D_2$) produce different absolute effects, which have similar time distributions of the latent periods. Shaded area: spontaneous (control) incidence rate; Broken line: upper confidence limit of the spontaneous incidence rate.

under the assumption of the proportional hazard model, i.e., when the tumour rate is increased by a constant factor without change of the underlying temporal dependence. Similarly, shorter minimum latent periods are estimated if the number of individuals in the observed population is larger, because predetermined levels of statistical significance are reached earlier in a larger sample. Other statistical procedures have been developed to analyse the dependence of the latent period on dose [L32].

54. For some cancers, the minimum observable latend periods may change with age at irradiation, as suggested, for example, by studies of human breast carcinoma [B26, M17, S16, T12, T23] and lung cancer incidence in Japanese atomic bomb survivors [K39]. These radiation-induced tumours appear with high frequency at ages when the spontaneous incidence is also relatively high. It follows, therefore, that latency is longer for cohorts irradiated in childhood and adolescence than for individuals exposed in their twenties or thirties. If so, the follow-up to include a complete (i.e., life-time) expression of the effect must vary with age at exposure for different cohorts. It is not known whether this observation can be applied in a general sense to all forms of radiation-induced tumours with long latent periods.

55. In cohorts of advanced age, the life expectancy may be shorter than the average latent periods, and only a fraction of induced neoplasms will be seen. The younger the age at irradiation, the fuller the expression of induced tumours. In the common case of neoplasms with a distribution of latent periods extending significantly beyond the follow-up, the dose-response relationship cannot be based on complete data. The estimate of I_{TA} will then change with the duration of the observation period; however, for those cancers for which the relative risk model appears adequate, the relative risk should be a less susceptible quantity in this respect. Analogous changes of the dose-response relationships have been shown in experimental work [S37]. Whenever the distribution of latent periods varies with the absorbed dose, the form of the derived dose-response relationships will depend critically on the length of the observation period. At low doses, the minimum latent periods may exceed the average life span of the individuals and it has been postulated that so-called practical thresholds may result [E3, M8, M10, R28]. This inverse relationship between latency and dose is most common in studies of continuous long-term irradiation. It was first described for bone sarcoma induced by long-lived isotopes [B48, E3, E4, F8, M4, R18-R20]. The present evidence does not substantiate the existence of such relations for other tumours commonly induced by radiation in man, for which sufficiently detailed data are available, namely cancer of the breast [K39, L22], of the thyroid [S38], and of the lung and stomach [K39, L32]; an inverse relationship between absorbed dose and latent period may exist for leukaemia [L24], but has not been definitely proved.

56. All the above factors must be borne in mind in any discussion of the accuracy and reproducibility of dose-response relationships. Except for tumours with short latencies, such as leukaemia and osteosarcoma, there is generally a lack of data extending to follow-up periods long enough for the dose-response relationship to be assessed with reasonable completeness.

2. Relationships between dose and tumour-free lifetime lost as a result of induced cancers

57. As mentioned above, various malignancies may be characterized by different latent periods. For some malignancies and modes of irradiation the latent periods (mean, median) may vary with dose, the mean values normally increasing with decreasing dose. A quantity that may provide a first approximation to a common denominator for assessment of the harm per induced neoplasm is the tumour-free lifetime lost [I6]. The relationship between this quantity and dose is therefore of interest. Very few papers provide information on the subject, but this will be reviewed, when it is available, in relation to different types of tumour.

E. SUMMARY AND CONCLUSIONS

58. Cancer, as a stochastic radiation effect, can be studied for its dependence on dose and time after irradiation. Different degrees of precision are attainable in experimental and epidemiological studies of radiation-induced tumours. The methods for the estimation of dose-response relationships reflect these differences.

59. The absorbed dose in the relevant tissue is the independent variable for dose-response studies. The magnitude of the dose and its temporal pattern of delivery (dose rate, fractionation) may vary greatly. In the present context, low doses are taken to be those up to 0.2 Gy of low-LET radiation, while those in the interval 2.0-3.5 Gy are regarded as high doses, with the intermediate doses lying between these ranges. Low and high dose rates are taken to be below $0.05 \text{ mGy min}^{-1}$ and above 0.05 Gy min^{-1}, respectively. Intermediate rates are those in between these values. For high-LET radiation low and high doses are assumed to range up to 0.05 Gy and down to 0.5 Gy, respectively. Dose rates may be classified in the same way as for low-LET radiation. In certain studies, more readily measurable quantities that are proportional to absorbed dose—at least over some range—may be used as the independent variable.

60. In experiments on radiation carcinogenesis, various measures of the response may be used. The crude incidence, uncorrected for mortality, is not infrequently applied, but it is unsatisfactory because it neglects differences in life span after different exposures; accordingly, it may be strongly affected by intercurrent mortality due to causes other than cancer. Competing risk corrected quantities such as the tumour rate, $r(t)$, the cumulative tumour rate, $R(t)$, or the actuarial incidence or prevalence, $I(t,D)$, can be used for more meaningful expression of the response. These quantities are always dependent on the post-irradiation time, and must be reported accordingly. They are obtained from the observed time sequence of

tumour appearance and from the variable number of individuals at risk during the observation period. They may be calculated by appropriate algorithms that are different for manifest tumours, i.e., rapidly lethal or readily discovered tumours, and for incidentally observed tumours, i.e., tumours that do not contribute to lethality and that are found only at necropsy. Only a few experiments have so far been analysed according to the requirements of the competing risk theory, and this circumstance has often reduced the potentially useful information from numerous studies.

61. In epidemiological surveys, the response is, in most cases, assessed retrospectively, but less accuracy can be achieved than in well-designed controlled experiments. The genetic composition, the distributions of ages and sex, the forces of selection, and the follow-up periods are often different in irradiated and control groups and require appropriate adjustments. Furthermore, the doses to individual members of a cohort are usually subject to substantial variation, making it necessary to group exposed individuals over broad dose intervals. Also, the less rigorous quantities used in epidemiological studies, I_{TA}, F_{TA}, and their rates, are complex functions of time post-irradiation. The scoring of radiation-induced tumours depends therefore, in a complex way, on the age at irradiation, duration and completeness of follow-up, latent period, and life expectancy of the population. The duration of follow-up may especially influence the magnitude of the response and the shape of the derived dose-response relationship in terms of the absolute (attributable) risk. If the tumours of interest show an increment of the relative risk per unit dose that is not strongly dependent on age at irradiation, the shape of the observed dose-response relationship is less susceptible to duration of the follow-up, provided the minimum latent period has been exceeded, the number of tumours is sufficient for verification of the postulated models, and other relevant co-variables have been corrected for.

62. Human tumours with relatively short latent periods, e.g., leukaemia and bone sarcoma, are not expected to appear after about 30 years. For these tumours, the dose-response relationships in young cohorts can be based on complete manifestation of the effect. For other tumours, of longer and unknown latency, dose-response relationships must be based on the incomplete information resulting from truncation of the response by the short follow-up. A possible dependence of latent periods on dose is of critical importance in determining the shape of the dose-response curve. When mean latent periods decrease with increasing dose, the shape of the relation depends on the observation time and, in some cases, practical thresholds may apply. However, except for ^{226}Ra-induced bone sarcoma, little information of this nature is available from data on man.

63. Projection of tumour incidence or incidence rate beyond the period of follow-up for tumours with long latent periods may be achieved by two alternative models: the absolute and the relative risk projection model. In its simple version, the first is based on the assumption that the rates of spontaneous and of radiation-induced tumours are independent, so that the rate of radiation-induced tumours does not increase proportionally to the age-dependent rate of spontaneous incidence. The second model in its simplest form assumes that irradiation has a multiplicative effect on the spontaneous tumour rate and that the rate of induced tumours is a dose-related multiple of the spontaneous rate. Recent data from several epidemiological studies have shown that, in many cases, the relative risk projection model provides a better fit to the data than the simple absolute risk model. For numerous tumours, however, no firm conclusions can be drawn as yet.

II. ASSUMPTIONS AND LIMITATIONS OF EXISTING MODELS

A. BASIC PHENOMENA AND INFLUENCE OF MODIFYING FACTORS

64. Common features of malignant cells are the unrestrained growth, the ability to infiltrate neighbouring tissues, and often the capacity to give rise to metastases. In a general sense, cancerous cells transmit their malignant characteristics from one generation of cells to another, and therefore somatic mutation could be one of the mechanisms involved as an underlying factor [B71, C32, F14, K20, K29, M50, R31, S43]. On the other hand, epigenetic factors such as dis-differentiation, expression of previously suppressed genes, activation of oncogenes (see annex A to this report) or others [B71, K26, S43, R31, S55] may be envisaged, alternatively or in parallel. Continuous growth through cellular divisions might result either from inactivation of operating or regulatory genes, or from the inability of malignant cells to receive or recognize division-restraining signals, whatever their nature might be.

65. Owing to poor understanding of the origin of cancer, quantitative predictions regarding the effects of ionizing radiation (dependence on dose, dose rate, quality of radiation) cannot be developed from basic principles. Formulation of simplified hypotheses under the form of models is at present a practical step towards understanding basic issues. To this end, detailed knowledge of mechanisms of cancer initiation and promotion would be valuable, but even this cannot be secured at present in a comprehensive form. Quantitative models of cancer induction have been reviewed recently by Whittemore [W8] and Parfenov [P2].

66. Before reviewing selected models, it is necessary to discuss the concept of multi-stage development of cancer. Since the classical studies of Berenblum et al. on chemically induced skin cancer in mice (discussed recently with regard to in vitro oncogenic transformation by Borek [B76]) this concept has gained wide acceptance. The subject has been repeatedly reviewed [B71, C32, D18, F13, F16, F20, M50, R31, R42, S43]. It is commonly assumed that cancer induction is started by a phenomenon of initiation, occurring most likely in one cell, although participation or modifying influences from neighbouring cells cannot be excluded. Further development into a cancerous clone probably

requires several stages, covered under the concepts of promotion and progression, which result eventually in an overt malignancy. These concepts have been reviewed by the Committee in annex I of the 1977 report [U6].

67. Cellular phenomena that take place during development of a cancerous clone are not well understood. Direct involvement of DNA in oncogenic cell transformation has been demonstrated [B14, L33, L34]. Lesions affecting its structure and function must therefore be relevant. Somatic mutation(s)—such as changes of the DNA base sequence; transposition, deletion, translocation and transfection (from one cell to another) of genetic material; enhanced instability of DNA, leading to facilitation of non-repairable DNA damage; induction of recombination between nuclear and mitocondrial DNA; disturbances of DNA methylation; activation of oncogenes—may be involved. But some of these mechanisms are largely hypothetical [B71, B83, F21, G33, R31, S43, S45, S55, V2, V3]. Initiation is followed by a long latent period, during which secondary influences (systemic, exogenous) may influence the final outcome of the process. During this period, the action of secondary factors may accelerate and stimulate (promote) or inhibit, or even reverse the process (anti-promoters, suppressors of malignant transformation). Arguments have recently been presented which show rather convincingly that not all initiated cells, or their clones, will eventually give rise to diagnosable tumours [F22].

68. Whatever the nature of initiation, be it radiation-induced somatic mutation in the classic sense (induction coefficient of 10^{-5} to 10^{-6} Gy^{-1} of low-LET radiation per locus at risk), or any other phenomenon similar to in vitro cell transformation (induction coefficient of 10^{-2} to 10^{-4} Gy^{-1}), the yield of recovered malignant tumours per irradiated cell in vivo is lower by many orders of magnitude. The possibility of a symmetrical "tumour-specific" chromosomal translocation was advocated [F21] as a very rare event that would remove part of this difficulty. However, recent studies in vitro and in vivo (chapter IV) suggest that initiation may not be a rare event when expressed per cell at risk. Therefore, if it is assumed that these processes operate in vivo with comparable efficiency, even for a small fraction of the susceptible cells (10^{-4} to 10^{-6}), a significant number of cells would be transformed every day because of background irradiation alone [M31].

69. The theory of sequential development of cancer may help to explain the discrepancy between data in vitro and in vivo, and the rarity of radiation-induced cancer. If a series of consecutive rare events is required for the initiated cell to become malignant, the final probability of emergence of the malignant clone will be the product of the probabilities of each event. Assuming that only the first event (initiation) is radiation-induced, and that the subsequent ones are rare phenomena, perhaps independent of irradiation, clinical cancer could be many orders of magnitude less likely than initiation itself. Yet, clinical cancer could show a relationship with dose similar to that of initiation, even though (owing to the multi-stage

nature of the process and possible systemic interferences) less regularity would be expected than that observed for stochastic radiation-induced phenomena in single cells under controlled conditions. That this may actually be the case is suggested by the reproducibility of dose-response relationships for some cancers in animals of selected strains. Also, supporting this contention is the fact that the absolute risk coefficient for cancer of the same organs derived from epidemiological observations of different populations (see chapter V) are often similar, although there are exceptions to this rule (see, for example, Figure XXVIII). This may imply that the modifying influence of secondary factors may not greatly change the final probability of induction and the reproducibility of the dose-response relationships. It has been postulated that for some forms of malignancy, such as leukaemias, radiation may be the causal factor, not for the first, but for the last event in a series of rare phenomena [L24, K39]. In any case, initiation is a necessary step, although only a small fraction of initiated cells may develop into a viable clone and into a clinical tumour.

70. The principal aim of a model is to predict the shape of the incidence curves as a function of dose, dose rate, quality of radiation and possibly other factors. Ideally, a model for radiation-induced cancer could provide some basis for the evaluation of risk at low doses [D9, F12, T15] if it could characterize the following processes:

(a) Probability of malignant transformation of a defined target cell. This will most likely vary with the organ, dose, quality of radiation, and temporal pattern of dose distribution. In this respect, the model should include theoretical concepts concerning the nature of the initiating event(s) and not be purely empirical. Mathematical formulations should be compatible with general knowledge of radiation and cancer biology;

(b) Probability of interaction at the systemic level between transformed cells or between developing clones;

(c) Probability of cell killing with dose, as non-viable cells cannot give rise to cancerous clones. This factor, as discussed in chapter III, depends certainly upon the tissues concerned, some of which are particularly susceptible, and upon dose, dose rate and quality of radiation and on other irradiation conditions (in vitro, in situ) [D7, G14, G16, H8, H10, M31, M52, R2, S26, S27, U6, U7, U17];

(d) Effect of numerous host factors, discussed in annex I of the 1977 UNSCEAR report [U6]. Among promoting factors, cell division is perhaps a good example [B36, B85, M6, N6, P22]. Enhanced proliferation can be induced by various mechanisms, including radiation-induced cell death, a phenomenon which is likely to produce a threshold-type dose response. Other factors could be the differentiation of initiated cells, immunological surveillance that suppresses development of malignant clones with antigenic characteristics foreign to the host-system, and hormonal influences;

(e) Effect of exogenous promoting agents leading to more rapid appearance of tumours, to an increase in tumour yield, and perhaps also to changes in the shape of dose-response curves, as shown by several experiments [F21, L26] including those on in vitro oncogenic transformation [H22, L26].

71. Immunological surveillance may be impaired by numerous factors, including ionizing radiation. The degree of impairment would certainly depend on dose, on whether the whole body or only part of it is irradiated, and then on what part and what proportion. It may be postulated that a reduction of immunological capacity of the organism follows a threshold-type response to irradiation. The importance of the immunological suppression in the low and intermediate dose range remains to be established although recent evidence points to a limited role of the immune system. Studies of Mole et al. [M52] on induction of acute myelogenous leukaemia in CBA/H mice, suggest that, at least in this tumour-host system, impairment of immunological surveillance is not very important. Similar conclusions were also reached by Nolibé et al. in respect to lung cancers induced by $^{239}PuO_2$ in rats [N9].

72. Hormonal dependence is well known for some cancers [U6]. By partly or totally inactivating endocrine organs and creating a hormonal imbalance, radiation may accelerate or impair malignant growth in other organs (e.g., breast, thyroid, ovary). Again, it is likely that this type of response would show pronounced dose thresholds. Hormonal influences could also be responsible for the association of various tumours, as observed in experimental animals [S53].

73. In summary, the action of modifying factors might change the resulting dose-response relationships. It is a basic weakness of the models discussed in chapter III that mathematical functions relating cancer incidence to dose reflect only initiation and sterilization of the initiated cells. This is because the precise effect of other modifying factors on tumour induction—as a function of dose—cannot yet be described with reasonable credibility, even if some attempts have been made [M4, P22]. Models, therefore, provide greatly simplified concepts, based on plausible assumptions and hypotheses, which may help in understanding the role of dose, dose rate and radiation quality. The relative importance of the parameters reflecting these quantities in a model can be deduced by comparing data with predictions. However, some of the parameters are the compounded expression of several elementary phenomena that cannot be resolved at present.

74. From available models, risk coefficients for man in the range from about 1 mGy up to about 0.1 Gy can only be obtained by extrapolation from the recorded values (in most cases above 1 Gy) to zero dose. Effects of the host factors discussed above (cell renewal, immunological surveillance, hormonal balance) and exogenous modifying factors upon dose-response relationships are uncertain, and only approximate evaluations may be given. For the purposes of the present annex, the levels of acute doses of low-LET radiation can be broadly separated as follows:

(a) < 0.2 Gy. At this level, data for most tissues are not directly available, but the damage to tissue functions is considered negligible. Therefore, dose-response relationships could be very close to those postulated by models that disregard host factors;

(b) 0.2-2.0 Gy. Damage to tissues, cell proliferation and influence of other host factors would not be expected to play a dominant role. Distortions in the dose-response relations should be relatively minor, and would not grossly bias the extrapolations;

(c) 2.0-10 Gy. Damage to tissues, to immunological functions (for irradiation of the whole or most of the body) and to hormonal feed-back systems may play a significant role. Extrapolations to low doses must therefore become more complex, particularly from the upper end of this range. Great caution is needed to avoid extrapolating from data that are already strongly affected by killing of initiated cells, as this might result in a substantial under-estimate of the risk at low doses;

(d) > 10 Gy. Severe damage to tissues and organs will dominate the response. Data in this dose region are most difficult to evaluate and so complex that extrapolation to low doses could be meaningless. Induced cell repopulation may also become a complicating factor for irradiation times longer than a few days.

A corresponding approximate classification of fast neutron doses would include the ranges: (a) < 0.05 Gy; (b) 0.05-0.2 Gy; (c) 0.2-2.0 Gy; and (d) > 2.0 Gy. It should be noted that the relation between these ranges of low- and high-LET radiation may not be interpreted in terms of RBE.

B. THE THRESHOLD DOSE FOR CANCER INDUCTION

75. It has already been mentioned that for many types of cancer the epidemiological and experimental information available does not suggest the presence of a threshold dose. If initiation is at least partly autonomous, i.e., if it affects a single or very few cells, present understanding of the mechanisms involved suggests that:

(a) The nature of radiation interaction with the cellular target for cancer initiation is stochastic, in the sense that each increment of dose carries a given probability of effective interaction;

(b) The error-free repair of the DNA, which is the most likely target involved, leaves some fraction of the damage unrepaired and the error-prone repair may produce misrepaired sequences in the DNA structure.

As the product of two probabilities greater than zero cannot equal zero, the presence of a threshold cannot be assumed.

179

76. A different situation obtains when the lifetime lost per cancer case (instead of the incidence) is related to dose or dose rate. Few malignancies show a definite inverse relationship between dose rate and latent period (see III.B.2), particularly at chronic exposure. In such cases (e.g., bone sarcomas induced by ^{90}Sr or long-lived radium isotopes) practical thresholds may exist below which no life shortening occurs and a very low probability of tumour appearance applies.

C. UNICELLULAR VERSUS MULTICELLULAR ORIGIN OF NEOPLASTIC GROWTH

77. Under the simplifying assumption that dose-response relationships for radiation-induced cancer reflect mainly the kinetics of initiation, they should include both the dose-dependence of the relevant intracellular phenomena and the interactions of individual (contiguous) cells, if indeed the latter play any role in the process [G30]. Therefore, the question whether a malignant clone arises from transformation of a single cell or of several contiguous cells is of critical importance for the formulation of models. Because understanding of the biological process of carcinogenesis is limited, this question cannot be resolved unequivocally at present. However, most experimental and human observations tend to support—even if indirectly—the monocellular origin of neoplasms. Furthermore, the alternative multicellular hypothesis allows the development of models resulting in such a variety of dose-response relationships as to render the exercise of model-fitting totally meaningless.

78. All these problems were reviewed in depth by Fialkow [F3, F4, F6], Nowell [N5] and others [B60, F13, F14]. It appears from their work that the monocellular alternative is gaining increasing acceptance, except for some rare hereditary tumours in subjects with inborn predispositions (e.g., multiple neuro-fibromatosis [F5]) and other rare tumours, such as condylomata acuminata [F10]. Three main lines of evidence support the unicellular hypothesis [F3, F6, N5]:

(a) The isoenzyme pattern of glucose-6-phosphate dehydrogenase in cancerous cells derived from tumours of heterozygous women, in accordance with the hypothesis that the same X-chromosome of the homologous pair is functioning in all cells of a given neoplasm. A similar pattern was observed recently in 3-methylcholantrene-induced fibrosarcomas in Pgk-1^a/Pgk-1^b mice carrying X-chromosome inactivation mosaicism for the phosphoglycerate kinase (PGK-1) gene [T17];

(b) The homogeneity of immunoglobulins produced by almost every case of myeloma;

(c) The common cytogenetic markers frequently detected in the cells of a single tumour.

This evidence is limited, indirect and compatible with the alternative hypothesis that selection of one clone from among several initially transformed cells might lead to an apparently monoclonal composition of the tumour. So far, however, this possibility has not been widely supported.

D. AUTONOMY OF TARGET CELLS FOR TUMOUR INDUCTION

79. Conceptually, even if initiation is taking place in one cell, the multi-stage nature of cancer development and possible influences of tissue and systemic origin could introduce random fluctuations into the expression of cancers in vivo. For radiation-induced cancer, therefore, such regularity and reproducibility of dose-response relationships as that seen for stochastic radiobiological phenomena in cultured cells would not be expected. Much of the information from animal experiments shows nevertheless that dose-response relationships are reasonably reproducible. Proportionality between initiation frequency and expression may therefore be assumed as a plausible hypothesis.

80. On the basis of microdosimetric considerations Rossi and Kellerer [R17], Rossi [R15, R16] and Rossi and Hall [R43] have pointed out that the observed curvilinear dose-response relationships for neutron-induced mammary tumours in rats and other tumours in mice are inconsistent with autonomous response because at low and intermediate doses there should be a direct proportionality (linearity) between dose and tumour incidence. Therefore, if the dose response is in fact non-linear, this must mean that either initiation or expression are modified by dose-dependent factors, implying a lack of "cell autonomy". If such a conclusion should generally apply, theories concerned with the response of single cells may not be relevant to dose-response relationships for cancer induction.

81. In the original experimental data of Shellabarger on Sprague-Dawley rats [S15], 14 months after an acute x-ray exposure, the incidence of all mammary tumours (adenomas plus carcinomas) per rat showed an approximately linear relationship with dose, up to 0.84 Gy, whereas 0.43 MeV neutron irradiation, with doses from 0.001 to 0.064 Gy, resulted in a tumour incidence roughly proportional to the square root of the dose [S15]. Rossi and Kellerer argued [R17] that, since cell killing would be negligible at such low neutron doses, the form of the observed relationship required the interplay of radiation effects in several cells. For mammary fibroadenomas, such an interaction leads, apparently, to a reduction of the tumour rate per unit dose even at neutron doses of a few tens of mGy.

82. Earlier data by Shellabarger et al. [S15] were later extended, with follow-up of the animals to about 1000 days [S37]. Tumours scored included fibroadenomas and adenocarcinomas, the latter malignant forms being 9-16% of the total. The data expressed as crude incidence or mortality-corrected indices, r(t,D), R(t,D), at various post-irradiation times, essentially confirmed the previous findings. A very high RBE was seen at low neutron doses for both tumour types (about 100 at 0.1 mGy) and the dose-response for the combined tumours was concave downwards for neutrons and approximately linear for x rays. There was also a significant shift of the age-specific r(t) curve in the irradiated animals (acceleration).

83. When the net R(t) values at 800 days (the latest follow-up time for all but one dose groups) were considered separately for fibroadenomas and adenocarcinomas, the following conclusions could be drawn:

(a) For all tumours combined the downward concavity of the curve after irradiation with neutrons results essentially from a low point for the fibroadenomas at 0.064 Gy. Such an effect is not seen for the adenocarcinomas, where the relation is approximately linear, although the experimental scatter precludes accurate assessments in this case;

(b) At 800 days, the departure from linearity of R(t) for the fibroadenomas is much less pronounced than at 400 days [S15] or than that for the incidence of adenocarcinoma [S37];

(c) No account was taken of cell killing in these experiments, although this may have not been negligible already at 0.064 Gy.

84. In view of their high spontaneous incidence (80% throughout the lifetime in females), the mammary tumours in Sprague-Dawley rats must be regarded as an unusual model. This view is confirmed by the facts that only a minor part of these tumours is histologically malignant [S12, S13, S14, S15, U17, V4, V5] and that the very high sensitivity of the Sprague-Dawley rat to the induction of mammary tumours is not seen in other rat strains [B43, B92, C15, S7, S11, V10].

85. In summary, the shape of the dose-response relationship reported for neutron- and x-ray-induced fibroadenomas at low doses in the mammary gland of Sprague-Dawley rats in one study is rather exceptional among all data on radiation-induced tumours. The low yield of adenomas per unit dose at 0.064 Gy, which has been interpreted to show an inhibitory influence by the neighbouring cells, may also be explained in terms of cell killing. Therefore, the observations discussed do not necessarily imply that malignant tumours arise from more than one initially transformed cell, or from interaction of several cells.

86. Other data on benign lung adenomas in RFM mice [U21, U22] may be discussed in this context. Pathogen-free animals were irradiated locally over the thorax with graded doses of fission neutrons (0.05 to 1.5 Gy) and the number of tumours in dissected lungs was counted 9 months after exposure. The effect was fully manifest at 6 months after 0.5 Gy, and intercurrent mortality was negligible. A peaked response, with a maximum around 0.25 Gy, was seen following single neutron doses. Splitting of the dose into two equal fractions, given at 24-hour or 30-day intervals, resulted in no sparing effect of fractionation. Plotting the mean number of adenomas per animal at 9 months against dose gives a slightly upward concave curve in the range of 0 to 0.25 Gy. A quadratic model fits the data very well (P > 0.99) but non-threshold linearity is not excluded (P > 0.8); also, a threshold of 0.05 Gy cannot be rejected, particularly since the gamma-ray curve suggests such a possibility. It is also possible that increasing doses of neutrons up to 0.25 Gy may have an enhancing effect, interpreted either as acceleration or promotion. Such an effect, however, is the opposite of that seen for mammary fibroadenomas in Sprague-Dawley rats. Results of other experiments with neutron induction of various tumours in BALB/c mice [U23] were also advocated as evidence that induction cannot be treated as a phenomenon related to autonomous cells. However, a correction for sterilization of initiated cells could result in approximately linear dose-response curves up to 0.2 Gy.

87. There is yet another explanation for the above data, i.e., that single-cell initiation is modified by enhancing or inhibiting dose-related effects. The nature of these effects (direct or abscopal, cellular or humoral) cannot be specified at present. Tumours requiring hormonal stimulation for their development (as in the case of the ovary) often have threshold dose-responses. In essence, therefore, none of the data discussed are incompatible with the hypothesis that tumour initiation by radiation may take place in a single cell, which from this stand-point must be considered relatively autonomous.

88. It has been pointed out [G15] that the simultaneous initiation of cancerous growth in several interacting cells would be equivalent to a multi-target event. If so, the sigmoid shape of the curve should become more pronounced with an increasing number of participating cells. There is, however, little data to support such a possibility and no known experimental system to test such hypotheses.

89. It may be concluded that if the curve is not obviously sigmoid or threshold-like upon visual inspection, the idea of a monocellular origin of the tumour may be accepted. The argument of a mono- versus a pluri-cellular theory, as well as the question of the degree of cellular autonomy in the origin of cancer, will not be finally resolved as long as the understanding of tumour pathogenesis remains unsatisfactory. As a rule, however, there appears to be no solid biological evidence against the monocellular origin of neoplasms. The assumptions that malignancy is initiated in a single cell, and that there is a reasonable proportionality between tumour induction and expression, have been incorporated—explicitly or implicitly—into most models of cancer induction by radiation. This view is explicitly accepted here as a working hypothesis, even though it is recognized that different opinions have been expressed [B83, M52, R43].

E. NUMBER OF CELLS AT RISK

90. The number of cells at risk of cancer induction in any organ is not known. When discussing this subject, most authors argue that the number of cells in which initiation takes place must be proportional to the number of cells at risk in a given tissue, and that the latter is proportional to the fraction of tissue irradiated. Most models or theories of cancer induction by radiation have accepted this assumption. It does not follow from it that tumour incidence, spontaneous or radiation-induced, is proportional to the total number of cells in any organ, or in the body of various animal

species [B49, M9], because there is no obvious correlation between body size in various species and incidence of tumours.

91. Epidemiological data on leukaemia in man, after irradiation of various fractions of the total active bone marrow, are broadly consistent with the notion that the probability of induction is proportional to the number of irradiated cells at risk, on the assumption that these are uniformly distributed throughout the marrow. Absolute annual risk coefficients derived from various studies fall within a range which is narrower than the variation of the fraction of the irradiated tissue (annex G in the 1977 UNSCEAR report [U6]). The same conclusion may be derived from experiments on cancer induction by total and partial irradiation of the mammary tissue in rats [B28, S10, S12] and by various areas of skin in mice [H11, H12, H13].

92. An important and related question is the effect on tumour incidence of a non-uniform tissue dose distribution. The extreme case is that of the so-called hot particles, i.e., particles with very high concentrations of radionuclides that are deposited in an organ such as the respiratory tract or the liver. Under such circumstances, the dose averaged over the entire organ would be much lower than that in the immediate vicinity of any such particle. Several authors addressed this question by studying carcinogenesis in the lung [I3, L35, S54]. In all cases, as expected from theoretical predictions [M9, M10], hot particles were found to be less effective than similar doses of the same radiation quality distributed in a more uniform manner.

F. POPULATION HETEROGENEITY AND SUSCEPTIBILITY TO CANCER INDUCTION

93. Baum [B16] raised the question of whether linear extrapolation of the risk from the high dose and dose-rate region of low-LET radiation to the low-dose domain is always conservative, in view of a possible difference in susceptibility to cancer induction between groups in the general population. To exemplify the situation, Baum [B16] constructed a model in which three population sub-groups, represented to 1, 10 and 89%, varied in susceptibility (expressed as D_0 values) in the ratio of 100 : 1 : 0, respectively. For each of the sub-groups he postulated a dose-response relationship of the form

$$I_i(D_0) = 1 - e^{-(D/D_{0i})} \qquad (2.1)$$

94. For the most sensitive sub-group (1%) he assumed that cancer induction might be a single-target effect (n = 1) with D_0 of 0.01 Gy; 10% would exhibit a lower sensitivity ($D_0 = 1$ Gy); and for the rest of the population $D_0 = \infty$. According to Baum, the composite response of the total population is dominated in the low-dose region by the highest sensitivity of the 1% sub-group. In the range from about 0.01 Gy to a few Gy, the relationship would be a curve, concave downwards, with response roughly proportional to $D^{0.5}$. The risk per unit dose above 1 Gy would be less than below 0.01 Gy.

95. It is not easy to envisage why susceptibility between groups should be reflected only by D_0, and, if so, why by a factor as large as 100. Moreover, the assumption that the bulk of the population should be totally non-susceptible to induction of malignant disease(s) lacks justification in Baum's paper [B16]. No epidemiological evidence supports this contention, even though it is known that incidence of radiation-induced cancer in man is generally low. Examples of dose-response relationships advocated by Baum to support his argument do not stand up in the face of criticism. The author presented data for acute leukaemia at Nagasaki, and for all cancers, all leukaemias, stomach, lung, and breast cancer at Hiroshima, where incidences rise with a power of dose between 0.1 and 0.8. At present, dosimetric uncertainties preclude a more detailed discussion of atomic bomb survivor data, but preliminary evaluations [K39, S46] of the dose-response relationships for leukaemia, breast cancer and total malignancies for the period up to 1978, using new dose estimates [L27], do not support the above conclusions (this information is still tentative). Therefore, Baum's hypothesis is neither satisfactory on theoretical grounds nor supported by epidemiological observations. The subject itself, however, is obviously important and warrants some exploration.

96. Progress in cancer genetics has shed some light on possible mechanisms of differential susceptibility to cancer development in individuals with various inherited traits [G12, M35]. The relevance of these phenomena to radiation-induced cancer requires attention. The relationship between genetic heterogeneity and incidence of spontaneous cancer, and cancer induced by radiation or other carcinogens, was discussed in detail in annex I of the 1982 UNSCEAR report [U24]. It is again reviewed in annex A to this report. The homozygotes for some genes (ataxia telangiectasia, Fanconi's anaemia and several others) have a significantly increased natural incidence of some forms of cancer and an enhanced sensitivity to other cellular and subcellular radiation effects. Various forms of impaired DNA repair are seen in most of these conditions. In view of their rarity, the affected subjects do not pose a public health problem, but the heterozygous carriers of these genes could also have an increased risk of developing spontaneous cancer. Calculations have shown [V6] that a few percent of individuals in the general population should carry such genes in a heterozygous state. If their capability for DNA repair should be reduced, this might result in an increased proneness to cancer development. Although it is not known at present whether these heterozygous subjects may also be more prone to radiation-induced cancer, this possibility should not be overlooked.

97. If risk coefficients at low doses were higher than those reported in most studies at about 1 Gy, then perhaps such evidence could be interpreted to suggest the presence of population groups particularly susceptible to cancer development. A higher effectiveness of low doses was claimed by Mancuso et al. [M3, K17, K32], who studied the mortality of workers employed in the Hanford works, Richland, United States, dying

with cancer from 1944, for whom death certificates and data on personal radiation dosimetry were available. This information was reviewed by several authors [A7, D14, G5, G25, H20, M30, R3, S2] who pointed to the low statistical power of the original data and to numerous other difficulties in their interpretation. From careful examination of all the evidence, it appears that these data are at present inadequate to prove or disprove that the risk of radiation-induced cancer at low doses is higher than estimated by UNSCEAR in its 1977 report [U6]. This matter will, however, be kept under review.

G. SUMMARY AND CONCLUSIONS

98. The pathogenesis of tumours, both spontaneous and radiation-induced, is at present poorly understood. The probability of cancer induction cannot therefore be derived from general principles. The data available indicate that carcinogenesis is likely to be a complex, multi-stage process. Initiation at the cellular level is followed by a long period of latency, during which numerous changes take place until the tumour becomes clinically manifest. The probability of some of these changes is very low, and during the intermediate stages numerous exogenous factors could accelerate or inhibit the development of potentially cancerous cell clones.

99. There is considerable variation between organs and tissues in the process of cancer development, presumably related to numerous endogenous factors. Among these, the hormonal and the immunological factors are known to be of importance, at least for some forms of cancer. Significant cell killing in tissues may stimulate compensatory cell proliferation and therefore increase the probability of cancer development. The ways in which, and degrees to which, radiation could modify such mechanisms, particularly in relation to dose, are not well understood. It appears likely, however, that dose thresholds such as those operating for non-stochastic effects might apply. This would imply that low or intermediate doses (below approximately 2.0 Gy of gamma rays and 0.3-0.5 Gy of neutrons) delivered acutely might have little or no modifying effect.

100. Under the circumstances described, for predictive purposes the use of simplified models of tumour induction becomes one of the possible choices, even though the degree of simplification is usually such as to exclude consideration of the above modifying factors. This important limitation of the models should be kept in mind.

101. In view of the multi-stage nature of the phenomena described, and of the small probability of occurrence of each step, the proportion of initially transformed cells giving rise to an overt tumour must be extremely small. It may be postulated that at low doses and dose rates, where the host factors mentioned above are not expected to modify primary events appreciably, there is a broad similarity of relationships between dose and tumour incidence, on the one hand, and between dose and probability of cell initiation and survival, on the other. Exogenous modifying factors (e.g., promoters and inhibitors) could alter the slope, and perhaps the shape, of the dose-response curve in some instances; in man very little is known in this respect, apart from the effects of tobacco smoke on lung cancer induction.

102. Monocellular and monoclonal hypotheses are usually assumed in models of radiation carcinogenesis. Most biological data support the notion that cancer, as a rule, starts from a single cell, but unequivocal, direct evidence to support this point is lacking, and alternative interpretations are possible. The monocellular hypothesis is critical in extrapolating the risk from high to low doses. The alternative hypothesis, that concomitant initiation or interaction of several cells is required, lacks sufficient experimental support and makes extrapolation from intermediate to low doses difficult or impossible at present. The postulate of monocellular origin of cancer must be treated, for the time being, as a working hypothesis.

103. The number of cells at risk of radiation-induced malignant transformation is usually assumed to be proportional to the fraction of an organ or tissue irradiated. The experimental evidence in favour of such an assumption is very strong, but, again, it must be regarded simply as a plausible working hypothesis. Gross non-uniformities of the tissue doses, such as those resulting from deposition of the so-called hot particles, normally result in a lower tumour incidence than for comparable doses distributed uniformly.

104. It has been proposed that sensitive sub-groups in the general population might invalidate any linear extrapolation of cancer risk to low doses of radiation, a procedure hitherto believed to provide upper values of the risk. It is known that the very rare homozygous carriers of particular genes (e.g., ataxia telangiectasia, Fanconi's anaemia) are more prone to cancer and that their cells are particularly sensitive to other effects of radiation, such as cell killing. It is also true that the healthy carriers of these same genes in the heterozygous form (a few percent of the general population) are at greater risk of developing spontaneous tumours and also have a slightly enhanced sensitivity to other radiobiological effects. Whether these same individuals may also be at a higher risk of radiation-induced cancer cannot be proved at present and this question requires further study. The epidemiological evidence in favour of the notion that higher risk coefficients per unit dose of low-LET radiation may apply at low, rather than at high, doses appears at present unconvincing.

III. DOSE-RESPONSE MODELS OF RADIATION-INDUCED CANCER

105. Although in principle a large variety of mathematical expressions and models could be fitted to experimental and epidemiological data on radiation-induced tumours, for the purpose of this annex the Committee decided to limit the analysis only to those models that appear to be supported by general knowledge of cellular and subcellular radiobiology.

A. INTRODUCTION

106. When either the crude or the actuarial incidence of various radiation-induced experimental tumours is plotted against a wide range of doses, then, for low-LET radiation, a peak incidence is normally seen at intermediate doses, followed by a decline at high doses. For high-LET particles, the essentially linear initial slope gradually decreases with dose. In some cases, it even becomes negative. The bulk of data is consistent with this generalization [U6]. Evidence in man is much less certain because only a few series cover a sufficiently wide range of doses. Nevertheless, the incidence per unit dose of bone sarcoma [M29, R18], lung carcinoma [K22, S3] and cancer of the breast [S16] decreases at very high doses. Thus, a model of radiation-induced cancer should allow for two opposing trends: a rise of probability of induction with dose and then a decline, resulting presumably either from killing of irradiated potentially malignant cells [G16, M52, R2], or, in some cases, from increased mortality rate at high doses [I5, J7]. Mathematically, this trend may be simulated by multiplying the induction dose-response function by a term describing the probability of cell (or organism) survival as a function of dose.

107. Conceptually, there are two possible approaches to the formulation of models. The first is based on radiobiological considerations, relating, by analogy, the radiation-induced cancer incidence and the influence of various parameters (dose, dose rate, fractionation) to other effects in single cells. Broad similarities have been observed in numerous cases. The alternative approach is an empirical one, aimed at approximating the data (incidence versus dose) by simple mathematical functions. In practice, the two approaches are often applied in combination.

108. There is no reason why any model might be valid for all radiation-induced malignancies: actually, a more reasonable approach would be to determine separately which model is applicable to which type of cancer, a conclusion supported by the bulk of experimental data. There are examples of radiation-induced cancer with pronounced thresholds (e.g., the thymic lymphoma of the C57BL mouse, ovarian tumours in many mouse strains). Indirect mechanisms (destruction of an overwhelming part of target cells in the thymus; killing of a large fraction of hormonally-active cells in the ovary) may explain such sigmoid relationships. Similar data are exceptional in man (see chapter V). Thus, even if threshold-type relationships cannot absolutely be excluded, the most easily induced human tumours, such as those of breast, thyroid and lung (undifferentiated small cell type), as well as leukaemia, do not indicate the existence of a threshold. Therefore, models used for these malignancies do not postulate a threshold. In principle, the models discussed below have been formulated in terms of the absolute risk, but they seem equally applicable to a relative risk increment.

B. DERIVATION AND CHARACTERISTICS OF DOSE-RESPONSE MODELS

1. The linear model

109. The simplest and oldest linear model was developed for x-ray-induced point mutations in Dro-

sophila [G24, M46]. It was based on the postulate that each energy deposition in a cellular target carries a probability of changes in the genome (mutations) and that these may be either irreparable or the result of misrepair. Since radiation energy is transferred in discrete events, all effects should ultimately be linear with dose at low doses when only few cells absorb some energy and their number is directly proportional to dose. The probabilities of an effect assumed to be an all-or-none phenomenon in relation to each dose increment should be additive, and dose rate or fractionation would not be expected to alter the magnitude of the final effect.

110. In the course of time it became obvious that the linear model must be limited to effects showing single-hit kinetics after low- or high-LET irradiation. However, the postulated additivity of effects and the dose-rate independence does not always apply to single-hit effects [E10, H35], showing that in such cases repair processes must also operate to make an otherwise linear relationship dose-rate sensitive. It appears that when a track passing through the sensitive volume is not 100% effective, then its effects may be subject to repair. In other words, the presence of dose-protraction or dose-fractionation effects may not be incompatible with single-hit kinetics.

111. For high-LET radiation, the linearity of the initial slope, modified by phenomena of saturation or cell inactivation (killing), has been widely accepted [B20, I1, M66, U6, U7, U9, U10]. The dose response is described by the following equation:

$$I(D) = a_1 D \, e^{-\beta_1 D} \qquad (3.1)$$

If cells are sensitive to inactivation, the relationship will depart from linearity, even at low or intermediate doses, owing to cell killing. The lower the mean lethal dose $(1/\beta_1)$, the more downwards concave the relationship will be. Recent experiments on neutron-induced tumours in animals (see chapter IV) suggest that this phenomenon—or others [S37, U23, U25, U26]—does in fact operate, causing departure from linearity, even at a few tens of milligray or a few tenths of a gray. This is explained by the fact that cell killing by high-LET particles is very effective with exponential non-threshold survival curves.

112. If equation (3.1) reflects the kinetics of tumour incidence as a function of the high-LET dose, extrapolation to low doses would tend to under-estimate the risk by a factor of $e^{-\beta_1 D}$. Examples and limitations of this postulate will be discussed in chapter IV, in the light of available experimental data.

113. Alternatively, the data can normally be fitted over some range of doses by an equation of the type:

$$I(D) = a_1 \sqrt{D} \qquad (3.2)$$

Such a purely descriptive model implies no linear slope at low doses, even for very radioresistant cells. This seems unlikely, however, on radiobiological grounds. In this latter model, as in any other model involving a downward concavity of the dose-response curve, dose fractionation would produce an increased incidence of tumours if the intervals between fractions were sufficiently long for the effects of each fraction to be considered independent [R37]. By a similar mechanism, the effects at low dose rate could also be enhanced, in comparison with the high dose rate.

114. An interesting variant of the linear model is that developed by Mayneord and Clarke [M9]. They discussed dose-response curves and their relationship with time, in regard to both dose rate and latency in the appearance of tumours. This is of importance because irradiation time and latency may be comparable with the life span of an exposed individual and could, therefore, affect the manifestation of the response. Their point of departure is that irradiation confers a probability of cancer appearance in the future [B48], following a stochastic process. This probability may be estimated by integrating the response of single cells as a function of dose over the number of cells at risk. A linear relationship between the probability of malignant cell transformation and dose was assumed at low doses where cell killing is irrelevant. Because much experimental evidence from chemically- and radiation-induced tumours [B48, E3, E4, F8] pointed to an increase in latency with decreasing dose rate, this particular feature was also incorporated into the model [M9, M10].

115. The result of the analysis was that in all cases, assuming a linear relationship between each increment of dose and risk (the latter distributed in time), non-linear (concave upwards) dose-response relationships were obtained, often with an apparent threshold. This is due to the inverse relation assumed between time of tumour appearance and the dose. According to this model, therefore, in most situations a linear extrapolation of the risk from high to low doses and dose rates is likely to yield a conservative risk estimate. The dose-response relationships should tend to linearity for: (a) long observation times, compared with the median latent period; (b) very heterogeneous populations, i.e., populations with a wide distribution of the latent period after single irradiation; (c) little variation of the median tumour appearance time with the dose. In general, however, the theoretical analysis of Mayneord and Clarke [M10] does not support an overall linear relationship between dose and cumulative tumour rate over finite time intervals in populations having a standard age distribution.

116. Inverse relationships between the mean latent period (from the start of exposure to tumour diagnosis) and dose (or dose rate) are seen mostly for irradiations of long duration, for instance in dogs and mice injected with ^{226}Ra and ^{99}Sr [M33, R28, R32]; in Chinese hamsters, in which the latent period of liver tumours decreases with increasing activity of injected ^{239}Pu [B87]; in rats injected with thorotrast, which produces tumours of liver and spleen [W15]; or rats exposed over periods of weeks or months to various concentrations of radon resulting in lung carcinomas [C34]. Finally, a negative correlation of latency versus mean dose rate was seen in human dial painters with ^{226}Ra and ^{228}Ra body burdens [E3, E4, M14, P11, R18]. It is interesting to note that the inverse dose-latency relationship was much less pronounced for

induction of bone sarcomas after single injections of short-lived ^{224}Ra in rats [M67]. For brief exposures such as for atomic bomb survivors, there is, at least in the younger cohorts, a suggestion that the mean induction period for leukaemia is negatively correlated with dose [L32], although the reference in question seems to compare mostly radiogenic cases with mostly naturally occurring ones. Such a relationship was not detected for breast, stomach and lung cancer in atomic bomb survivors [B17, L32, M17, K39, T12] and for breast and thyroid cancers resulting from medical irradiation [B26, S16, S38]. Moreover, of all cases showing an inverse relation of the latent period against dose, an unequivocal departure from linearity was found only for ^{90}Sr-induced bone sarcomas. The situation for human osteosarcomas induced by ^{226}Ra and ^{228}Ra is not totally clear, and the dose-response relation for leukaemia in atomic bomb survivors is still not available. In conclusion, the inverse relationship between latency and dose does not apply to many tumours. Thus, an upward concavity of the dose-response relationship as a result of this factor alone cannot be viewed as a general phenomenon.

2. The linear-quadratic model

117. For the bulk of experiments on single-cell systems, and for many end-points, the prevailing form of the dose-response curve after acute low-LET irradiation is concave upward, the response rising with a power of dose of between 1 and 2. Broadly similar shapes were also observed for tumours induced by the same radiation. This form of the response is thought to imply that for the occurrence of the final effect the interaction of two elementary effects, usually referred to as sublesions [K4], is required. Repair phenomena and dose-rate effects are usually accounted for by the interaction of these sublesions in time and space [L4, S39, S40], but other interpretations were also proposed [G29, G32]. For effects showing curvilinear responses to low-LET irradiation, linear dose-responses are frequently observed with densely-ionizing particles.

(a) The microdosimetric approach

118. Microdosimetric considerations are important because the distribution of absorbed energy divided by the mass in the volumes believed to be the primary targets of radiation action (i.e., cells or cell nuclei) is very inhomogeneous at low and intermediate doses [F7]. Thus the distribution of specific energy, z (energy absorbed divided by the mass of these volumes), may be more relevant for the analysis of the effects than the organ or tissue mean dose, D.

119. Many experiments indicate that for a number of effects the probability of occurrence, E, after low-LET radiation, rises with a power of dose close to 2. This may be accounted for by the theory of dual radiation action which assumes that the induction of two non-specified sublesions is necessary for the production of the effect (lesion). In the approximation that was first developed in detail [K4], it was assumed that the probability of sublesion interaction does not depend

on their distance within a certain volume (the site). Consequently, the probability of effect should rise in proportion to the mean of the square of the specific energy, i.e., $\overline{z^2}$, in the site. It was shown also that $\overline{z^2}$ is a function of the absorbed dose, D:

$$\overline{z^2} = \zeta D + D^2 \qquad (3.3)$$

where the ζ is a weighted average of the specific energy deposited by single events (energy depositions in the critical structures by individual charged particles). Thus, the probability of a radiobiological effect, E, should be

$$E = K(\zeta D + D^2) \qquad (3.4)$$

The quantity ζ has the dimension of dose and its value denotes the dose at which the contribution of the linear equals that of the quadratic term. For x and gamma rays, and for sites of 1 μm diameter, the value for ζ falls within the range of 0.3-0.8 Gy; for medium-energy neutrons, it is as large as 16 Gy. For smaller sites, the values of ζ are considerably larger, but the ratio of the values for neutrons and for sparsely ionizing radiation is less dependent on site size.

120. Consideration of the values of ζ for radiations with different values of LET and their comparison with biological data, indicates that intracellular distances at which sublesions can interact must be of the order of 0.1 to 1 μm [K4]. High values of ζ for neutrons and alpha particles (relative to x and gamma rays) account for a bulk of radiobiological observations. They show that the RBE of high-LET radiations varies as an inverse function of the square root of their dose and this can be understood on the basis of microdosimetric concepts. This type of dependence can hold down to doses where the response to both radiations becomes linear and the RBE reaches a plateau.

121. Suitable time functions can be inserted into the basic equation (3.4) to describe the interaction probability during the time interval between the formation of two sublesions [R12]. One of the conclusions is that the linear term for single events in equation (3.4) should be independent of dose rate. Therefore, any effect of time distribution may only result in a modification of the quadratic term. This relationship between irradiation time, T, and mean time between induction of a sublesion and its repair, τ, is reflected by a reduction factor, G, that affects the quadratic term:

$$G = 2(\tau/T)^2 (T/\tau - 1 + e^{-T/\tau}) \qquad (3.5)$$

In the presence of recovery, the curves of RBE versus absorbed dose do not change in shape, but are shifted towards higher doses by a factor depending on the dose distribution in time and the recovery time, τ. For a constant dose rate, if the exposure time is much longer than the recovery time, the yield of elementary lesions becomes simply proportional (linear) to dose.

122. The theory of dual radiation action has been applied by several authors to the interpretation of biological results, for example to cell inactivation by ionizing radiation [B62, F7]. In this model, the slope of the survival curve depends explicitly on radiation quality through the quantity ζ [K4]. The theory has also been used as a theoretical basis for the linear-quadratic model for many effects, including mutations, chromosome aberrations and initiation of oncogenic transformation. However, experiments with ultrasoft x rays [C23, G9, G10, G11] and with spatially correlated ions [B88, G31, G32, K41, R38] indicate a strong dependence of the interaction probability of the sublesions on distance, with a dominance of short-range interactions (much less than 0.1 μm) for densely-ionizing radiation. The applicable version of the theory [K5] is a model of higher complexity that is less easily tested experimentally.

123. Alternative explanations were considered for the commonly observed RBE-dose and dose-response relationships for low- and high-LET radiation. In agreement with earlier ideas of Haynes [H27], Goodhead et al. [G29, G32] put forward the notion that a number of cellular and subcellular radiation effects depend both on the production of the primary lesions and on a dose-dependent inactivation of repair mechanisms. Whereas the probability of the primary lesions is taken to increase linearly with dose, impairment of the repair system would depend on absorbed dose and specific energy. It has been postulated that the degree of impairment of repair should display a pronounced dependence upon dose and/or dose rate of low-LET radiation. For high-LET particles there would normally be no error-free repair, independently of dose. Therefore, basically linear dose-responses would be expected for induction at the cellular level of each of the various effects separately.

124. The above concepts have not been widely tested. A variety of factors have been reported that may influence the expression of potential damage, and thus change linear dose-effect relationships to curvilinear ones, and vice versa [F18, H22, L26].

(b) Characteristics of the linear-quadratic model

125. Upward concave dose-response curves that fit well the cumulative cancer incidence as a function of acute doses of low-LET radiation are in themselves no proof that cancer is actually initiated in accordance with a linear-quadratic relationship. Curvilinearity could well result from an inverse relationship between dose and latent period [M10]. However, when follow-up data show a constant latent period with dose, it may be assumed, as a working hypothesis, that the upward concavity reflects a linear-quadratic kinetics of initiation.

126. A generalized linear-quadratic dose-response relationship for radiation-induced cancer would be as follows:

$$I(D) = (a_0 + a_1 D + a_2 D^2) S(D) \qquad (3.6)$$

where I(D) is the incidence (in an ideal case corrected for intercurrent mortality); D is the dose; a_0 is the spontaneous incidence; a_1 and a_2 are coefficients for the linear and dose-squared terms of cancer initiation;

and S(D) is the probability of survival of transformed cells and may be written as

$$S(D) = e^{-(\beta_1 D + \beta_2 D)} \qquad (3.7)$$

In the equation (3.6), initiation may also be treated as a simplification of a more general expression, which includes some repair at low and intermediate doses and dose rates [B95].

127. To test compatibility of the model with experimental and epidemiological data, the parameters in equation (3.6) must be assigned some value. This can only be done by: (a) reasonable analogy with cellular radiobiological effects; or (b) deduction of the values from empirical studies. As to the parameters for cell survival, these are known for many cell lines (e.g., Barendsen [B5, B6, B9-B12, B45]; Goodhead et al. [C23, G9, G10]; Elkind [E2]; and others [A17, B19, B27, C1, C37, D3, D8, F2, F19, H2, H6, J6, K2, K24, L6, M16, M60, R39, S33, T18, T19, W6, W7]), but are not necessarily applicable to specific tumours.

128. The number of unknown coefficients in equations (3.6) and (3.7) is too large to permit their calculation without some constraints. One of these is that all parameters should be positive or equal to zero [C29]. However, this is often insufficient for reasonably stable estimates of β_1 and β_2, particularly when a_1 and a_2 are estimated at the same time. Attempts were made, therefore [B7, B47], to derive independently the quotient a_1/a_2, which facilitates calculations by lowering the degrees of freedom.

129. Assuming that the theory of dual radiation action [K4] applies to the initiation of cancer, there must be a subcellular structure in which the sublesions appear and an interaction distance below about 1 μm where the final lesion leading to malignant transformation is produced. Kellerer and Rossi [K4-K7, R12] did not specify the relevant structure for cell transformation, but the most likely target of radiation action appears to be the genome. In the light of this assumption, and of available evidence, it is not unexpected that models postulating a linear-quadratic relationship presuppose a direct action of radiation on DNA or make reference to phenomena involving DNA (chromosome aberrations, mutations) for derivation of the relevant parameters.

130. Barendsen [B7] selected the values for a_1 and a_2 on the basis of dose-response relationships for chromosomal aberrations in lymphocytes and the rounded values of a_1/a_2 for x and gamma rays were set at 0.5 and 1.0 Gy, respectively. On a similar principle, Abrahamson [A3] and Brown [B47] assumed that, if human radiation-induced cancers are due to mutations or chromosome aberrations in single cells, then information on the quotient a_1/a_2 could be derived from extensive data available in the literature. However, the large variability of the quotient precluded the use of numbers at their face value (e.g., mean or median). Brown showed also an inverse relationship between the DNA content per haploid genome in cells of various species and the a_1/a_2 quotient, the values extending over ranges of 10^3 and 10^4, respectively.

131. For mammalian cells, a_1/a_2 values for mutations and chromosome aberrations, as reviewed by Brown [B47], clustered around 1 Gy (geometric mean, 1.27 Gy). The values of the β_1/β_2 ratio for cell sterilization were generally much higher, with a geometric mean of 7.76 Gy. The difference is due mainly to higher values of the linear parameter for cell killing, in accordance with conclusions [B9, B11] that at low doses there must be a substantial component in cell killing that cannot be identified with the induction of chromosomal aberrations. Brown concluded that if the initial radiation lesion triggering a human cancer is of mutational or cytogenetic nature, then risk estimates derived at 1-2 Gy of low-LET high-dose-rate exposure would, as a maximum, over-estimate the cancer risk at low doses and dose rates by factors of about 2 and about 4, respectively.

132. Concerning cell survival, it has been pointed out repeatedly [B7, E2, F2, K2, M21, S17] that the low-LET survival curves can be described by various models and, among others, by functions of the "single-target" plus "multi-target-single-hit" type

$$S(D) = e^{-(D/_1 D_0)} [1 - (1 - e^{-D/_n D_0})^n] \qquad (3.8)$$

where $S(D) = S_D/S_0$, $_1 D_0$ and $_n D_0$ are mean inactivation doses for single and multiple targets, respectively, and n is the target multiplicity. Alternatively, the linear-quadratic form may be applied, as in equation (3.6).

133. Whether for each cell type there is an initial slope [β_1 in equation (3.7) and ($e^{-D/_1 D_0}$) in equation (3.8)] is still a matter of debate, but this question is rather immaterial in the present context as both functions describe satisfactorily the experimental data for surviving fractions between 1.0 and 0.1 [B9, B11, F2, M21]. Equation (3.6) has been most commonly used in relation to the linear-quadratic model of cancer induction (see [U6, annex G] and [B7, C29, M31]). For high-LET radiation the contribution of the quadratic term is negligible.

134. As a first approximation, for low and intermediate doses, particularly of low-LET radiation, the killing term S(D) may be neglected. This could be justified under the assumption that repopulation of the target cells after irradiation has a promoting effect on the development of radiation-induced cancer roughly proportional to the degree of cell killing [P22]. If, in addition, some of the terms in equation (3.6) and (3.7) are omitted, a transition is possible from the linear-quadratic model to the pure linear or pure quadratic ones (Figure IV). As can be seen from equation (3.6), the model does not assume the presence of a threshold.

135. There are many methodological and biological factors [B10, C1, D8, H6, K24, L6], which make it difficult to select appropriate survival parameters. In particular, cells irradiated in situ might exhibit higher survival capacity than when irradiated in culture or in suspension [G14, H8, H10, M60] (however, for a contrary view, see [A17]). By using a range of survival parameters suitable to describe the most and least

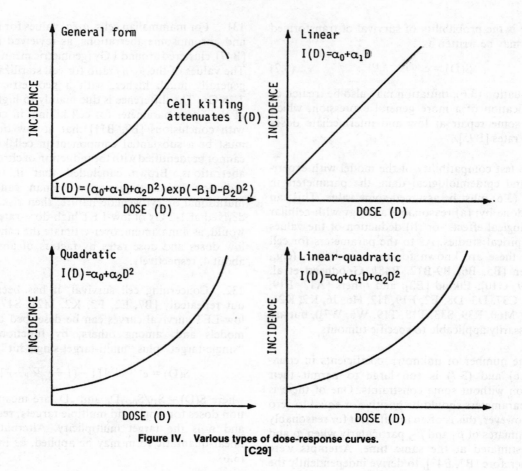

Figure IV. Various types of dose-response curves.
[C29]

sensitive cell lines, one may examine the degree to which cell killing may affect the shape of the tumour incidence data and, hence, the reliability of extrapolation from the intermediate to the low doses. This should provide some indication of the degree of over- or under-estimation of the risk, within the range of values selected for the parameters in question.

136. In an independent analysis, UNSCEAR selected two values of the a_1/a_2 quotient applying to x and gamma rays: 0.5 and 2.0 Gy. For survival, the bone marrow stem cell was selected as the most sensitive. Its survival curve is described by $\beta_1 = 4 \ 10^{-1} \ Gy^{-1}$ and $\beta_2 = 8 \ 10^{-2} \ Gy^{-2}$ [B6]. For the least sensitive cell, a hypothetical line was assumed with survival parameters $\beta_1 = 10^{-1} \ Gy^{-1}$ and $\beta_2 = 8 \ 10^{-2} \ Gy^{-2}$ [B6]. In addition, other survival parameters for radiation-induced human leukaemia cells (Table 1 from [U17]) were used, as follows: $\beta_1 = 3 \ 10^{-1} \ Gy^{-1}$, and $\beta_2 = 10^{-1} \ Gy^{-2}$. To normalize the calculated data, it was further assumed that the lifetime cumulative incidence at 3.0 Gy may be 15,000 cases per 10^6 (5000 $10^{-6} \ Gy^{-1}$). The results in terms of the yield of cases from 10^{-3} to 3 Gy for all combinations are plotted in Figure V.

137. From such an analysis, the following tentative conclusions may be drawn. First, the sensitivity to cell killing has a more pronounced effect on the shape of the dose-response relationships than the a_1/a_2 quotient. (Similar conclusions were reached by Mole [M31].) Secondly, for the cells most sensitive to killing, the

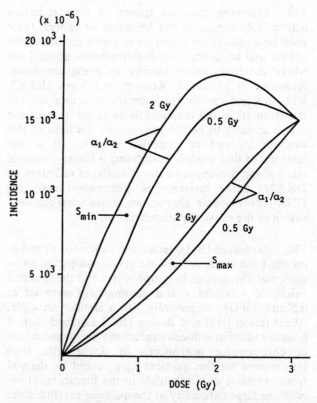

Figure V. Expected cumulative incidences of a radiation-induced cancer according to a linear-quadratic model with a_1/a_2 quotients = 0.5 and 2 Gy and cell survival functions S_{max} and S_{min} as given in paragraph 136. Incidence normalized to 15,000 cases per 10^6 at 3 Gy. For full explanation, see paragraphs 136 and 137.

188

relationship is concave downward, with maxima at 2-2.5 Gy. Since such curves are not observed for human cancers after low-LET irradiation, it is possible that the assumed sensitivity is too high for in vivo irradiation. This would be in accordance with the lower sensitivity of single cells irradiated in situ, which is due mostly to a wider shoulder of the survival curve [D7, G14, H8, H10, M60, S26, S27]. Thirdly, for the cells least susceptible to killing (the carcinomatous cells according to Barendsen [B6, B7]), the over-estimate of the tumour yield per unit dose from 1-2 Gy to 1-10 mGy (relative to linear extrapolation) ranges from 4.0-2.6 at $a_1/a_2 = 0.5$ Gy, to 1.6-1.3 at $a_1/a_2 = 2$ Gy, respectively. The maximum over-estimation of the risk will result from totally neglecting the cell-killing effect. In such a case, extrapolation from 2 and 1 Gy down to about 10 mGy would involve the following over-estimate:

a_1/a_2 (Gy)	Over-estimate by a factor of: from 2 Gy	from 1 Gy
0.50	4	3
2.00	2	1.5

The above differences for a_1/a_2 of 0.5-2 Gy could not be easily—if at all—detected between estimates derived from 1 or 2 Gy and the exceptional estimates available for doses of a few tens of mGy per single dose. The lack of statistically significant difference is therefore compatible with both the linear or the linear-quadratic model.

138. Inspection of equations (3.6) and (3.7) indicates that cell killing may alter significantly the incidence of a given cancer through interaction with the spontaneous incidence, a_0. At very high levels of the latter and with high sensitivity of the cells to sterilization, a dose-related decrease of the incidence would be expected. This in fact was seen in experiments with animals, showing a negative slope of the dose-response relationships for the so-called reticulum cell sarcoma [M19].

139. The slope of the dose-response curve in the complete linear-quadratic model will be described by a differential:

$$d/dD \ \dot{I}(D) = [(a_1 + 2a_2D) - (\beta_1 + 2\beta_2D)(a_0 + a_1D + a_2D^2)] \ e^{-(\beta_1 D + \beta_2 D^2)} \quad (3.9)$$

As D approaches zero this equation simplifies to:

$$d/dD \ \dot{I}(D) = a_1 + 2a_2D - \beta_1 a_0 - D(\beta_1 a_1 + 2\beta_2 a_0) \quad (3.10)$$

To examine the interaction with dose of a_0, a_1 and β_1 and its influence on the curve at low dose, two human cancers were selected: breast carcinoma, with a high spontaneous incidence and moderate sensitivity to cell killing of initiated cells; and leukaemia, with rather low values of a_0 and high sensitivity to sterilization. The notional parameters selected were:

Breast cancer:

$a_0 = 8 \ 10^{-4} \ a^{-1}$ $\beta_1 = 2 \ 10^{-1} \ Gy^{-1}$
$a_1 = 3.2 \ 10^{-4} \ a^{-1} \ Gy^{-1}$ $\beta_2 = 8 \ 10^{-2} \ Gy^{-2}$
$a_2 = 3.7 \ 10^{-4} \ a^{-1} \ Gy^{-2}$

Leukaemia:

$a_0 = 5 \ 10^{-5} \ a^{-1}$ $\beta_1 = 4 \ 10^{-1} \ Gy^{-1}$
$a_1 = 1 \ 10^{-4} \ a^{-1} \ Gy^{-1}$ $\beta_2 = 8 \ 10^{-2} \ Gy^{-2}$
$a_2 = 1 \ 10^{-4} \ a^{-1} \ Gy^{-2}$

When the values of $d/dD \ \dot{I}(D)$ were calculated at 1, 10 and 100 mGy, their ratios to the respective values of a_1 were:

	Dose (Gy)		
	0.001	0.01	0.1
Leukaemia:	0.80	0.82	0.94
Breast cancer:	0.50	0.52	0.64

Thus, at very low doses interaction of cell killing, predominantly with the spontaneous incidence, would introduce some degree of over-estimation of the risk, if this interaction should be neglected in the extrapolation procedure. It appears unlikely, however, that this over-estimation might exceed another factor of 2, over that estimated in paragraph 137.

140. When extrapolation is made from intermediate or high doses of low-LET radiation, delivered at low dose rates or in small fractions (of size much below a_1/a_2), then, due to repair processes, the quadratic terms of equation (3.6) should be reduced. Under these circumstances, dose-response relationships approaching linearity would be expected in which the risk coefficient per unit dose is the same over the range of low and intermediate doses. For high-LET radiation, the contribution of the dose-squared component for most effects in single cells is negligible up to a few tens of Gy. Therefore, the model may be treated as linear, although for some effects the slope of the line may not be dose-rate independent (see III.B.1). Such observations cannot be explained solely on biophysical considerations.

141. It has been pointed out [U17] that the linear-quadratic model of cancer initiation is a simplistic concept and not a pathogenetic theory. The great complexity and the interaction of various phenomena at the cellular level preclude its acceptance as a generalized theory of cancer initiation in all tissues and under all circumstances. The dose dependence of the many modifying mechanisms operating at the tissue and systemic level is still too obscure to allow quantitative predictions over the entire range of doses. However, as discussed in chapter II, it may be postulated that the influence of modifying factors might not be very important in the range of doses up to 1-2 Gy of low-LET radiation (or their high-LET equivalent). Under these circumstances, appropriate extrapolation may be acceptable down from the dose region of 1-2 Gy of x or gamma radiation (or an equivalent dose of neutrons) to obtain risk estimates for the low-dose domain.

142. With all these reservations in mind, the linear-quadratic model has been applied to the results of selected animal tumour experiments where dose, dose rate, dose fractionation, dose protraction and LET were systematically investigated (see chapter IV). In several cases [B7, P22, U2, U3, U25, Y1] the results were in basic agreement with the model's expectations.

3. The quadratic model

143. This model is based on the assumption that for the induction of a given effect two consecutive events are necessary, or two concurrent events separated in space in such a way that their production by a single ionization track is extremely unlikely. Except for irradiation of flattened bone lining cells (see V.E.2.), this assumption is difficult to justify on microdosimetric grounds for low-LET irradiation of normal cells in situ. In tumour radiobiology, this concept may be traced back to the theory of bone sarcoma induction by β emitters [M26, M45, M47]. Proportionality to the square of the dose has been noted for various cancers [H12, H13, M26, M52, R18]: this does not exclude the presence of a linear component, but simply assumes that it may neither be demonstrated nor ruled out on statistical grounds. Therefore, if present, such a component must be relatively small.

144. Recently, Mole et al. [M52] have shown that dose-response relationships for radiation-induced acute leukaemia in CBA/H mice may be characterized by an approximately pure quadratic or linear initiation term for x rays or neutrons, respectively (see IV.B.1). On the basis of microdosimetric considerations the apparent absence of a linear term in the dose-response equation for x rays is difficult to explain when the diameter of a nucleus is of the order of few μm. The proposed hypothesis [M52] was that the interaction of two neighbouring cells is necessary for the initiation of this cancer. Initiation by neutrons is in direct proportion to dose and this was explained by the fact that a single recoil track could cross the nuclei of two neighbouring cells. However, for neutrons of maximum effectiveness (400 keV) the range of the secondary protons is less than most nuclear diameters.

145. The experimental basis of these hypotheses is still debatable, and needs further experimental testing. Moreover, the postulates are difficult to reconcile with the results of transformation experiments of cells in vitro, irradiated at low density (see chapter IV) where it is unlikely that two neighbouring cells may be crossed by a single recoil track or may interact during oncogenic transformation by x rays. Explanations other than the microdosimetric ones must be found to accommodate all these facts.

146. When fitted to the experimental data obtained at intermediate or high doses, the quadratic model will predict effects at low doses to be much less than implied by the linear or the linear-quadratic models within the usual range of a_1 and a_2 values. The influence of the time pattern of dose administration cannot be specified a priori for the quadratic model: if repair is fast and dose-rate-dependent, dose protraction or fractionation could lead to a considerable reduction of the effect, and zero effect could not be excluded.

147. The quadratic model has been used by the Committee on the Biological Effects of Ionizing Radiation (BEIR Committee) [C29] to obtain the lower boundary of likely linear-square dose responses at low doses. Three special models have recently been proposed which assume, or derive from experiments, the basic postulate of the dose-squared concept. They refer to leukaemia in CBA mice [M52], skin cancer in rats [V1] and bone sarcoma in man [M4]. They are reviewed in chapters IV and V, respectively.

C. SUMMARY AND CONCLUSIONS

148. Quantitative models of radiation-induced cancer must allow for two facts: first, that tumour incidence rises with dose at low doses; and, second, that at high doses the effect usually declines (either in absolute terms or per unit dose). This shape of the curve may be modelled by the product of two terms: an initiation term increasing as a function of dose, and a cell-survival term declining with it. The latter term can be neglected at low doses, but this simplification may lead to misinterpretations as the dose increases. There is no reason why any one model should be universally applicable to all radiation-induced types of cancer. Models should be tested in each instance by statistical criteria. In each given tumour system, they should allow for the effect of the main radiobiological variables, such as dose, dose rate, dose fractionation, radiation quality.

149. The linear model implies direct proportionality between dose and the probability of tumour induction. Absence of dose-rate and fractionation effects was thought to be an inherent feature of the linear model, because the biological lesion is assumed to result from a single-track effect. However, examples are known where this is not true, and linear dose-response relationships show shallower slopes with decreasing dose rate. There are few examples of cellular or carcinogenic effects following linear kinetics after low-LET irradiation, while the effects produced by high-LET particles often conform to these characteristics. However, there are examples where dose-rate effects for neutrons are found, in an opposite direction (enhancement) from those normally seen for low-LET exposure. The linear model may be regarded as an upper boundary for the more general linear-quadratic model when the doses at which the linear equals the dose-squared components are high or very high.

150. The model of Mayneord and Clarke assumes linearity between dose and cancer initiation at the cellular level. It also assumes a log-normal distribution of the latent periods for overt tumours and an inverse relationship of latency to dose. Solution of this model for observation times comparable to human life expectancy results in dose-response relationships which are upward concave, sometimes with apparent thresholds. The critical assumption leading to such results is the shortening of the mean latent period with dose. If this were a general rule, then extrapolation of risk from high to low doses would always lead to over-estimates. However, for some radiation-induced tumours in man (thyroid, stomach, breast, lung), the latent period is not obviously dose-dependent; also, curvilinearity is not seen in several cases where there is an inverse relation of the latent period with dose. Thus, it is impossible to generalize the notion that just for this reason curvilinear responses would normally apply.

151. When corrected for cell killing, numerous biological end-points induced by low-LET radiation in single cells show an exponential dependence on dose with exponents of between 1 and 2. On the contrary, the same end-points for high-LET radiation show essentially linear dose-responses. Consequently, the RBE is an inverse function of dose. Low-LET radiation shows pronounced influences of dose rate and fractionation, in contrast with high-LET, for which such phenomena are seldom observed or are observed to a lesser extent. Most of these facts may be accounted for by microdosimetric considerations. They predict that, as a rule, linear-quadratic dose-responses should be expected, where the relative contribution of the two terms is comparable (for low-LET). This prediction is in accordance with numerous experimental data on single cells, and so are the effects of dose rate and dose fractionation that may be deduced from the kinetics of repair of the sublesions postulated in the linear-quadratic model.

152. Recent data on ultra-soft x rays, however, do not conform to the predictions of the theory of dual radiation action in its early approximate formulation. The disagreement could be reconciled in the generalized version of the theory [B98], assuming that some parameters of the biological effect previously taken to be invariable are actually subject to some variability; or that, in case of low-LET radiation, the rate of repair depends on dose and on dose rate. Which of these two alternatives is likely to apply remains to be answered.

153. The linear-quadratic model may be characterized by the quotient of the induction constants (a_1/a_2), which varies with the radiation quality and the specific biological effect. For high-LET particles, this quotient is so high that the contribution of the dose-squared term may normally be neglected. The model then becomes linear. For low-LET radiation (considering chromosomal exchanges, mutations and induction of some malignancies) the a_1/a_2 quotient is between 0.5 and 1.5 Gy. The over-estimation of the probability of effects at about 10 mGy from single-dose data at 1-2 Gy (acutely delivered) by linear (as opposed to linear-quadratic) extrapolation would vary from 1.5 to 3.0 for an assumed reasonable set of parameters.

154. Similar over-estimations would apply to the effects of low-LET radiation delivered at low dose rates, irrespective of the total doses below the level when cell killing becomes important. This would result from the disappearance of the quadratic component of the dose-response curves owing to repair of sublesions.

155. Introducing a cell-killing term into a linear-quadratic model leads, in general, to a lesser degree of risk over-estimation at low doses. The effect of such a term may be analysed by applying a range of experimental cell-survival parameters. Since the killing effect of a given dose might be less in vivo than in vitro, the over-estimation involved in the extrapolation to low doses and dose rates would probably fall between that obtained from typical cell survival parameters in vitro and that obtained by neglecting cell killing entirely.

156. For fission neutrons and alpha particles, the a_1/a_2 quotient is of the order of several tens of Gy and the microdosimetric linear-quadratic model predicts a linear curve, relatively independent of dose rate. At doses where departure from linearity becomes substantial, a significant under-estimation of the risk must result from linear extrapolation to zero doses. Fractionation or protraction of dose may result in enhancement of the effect even at low and intermediate doses, contrary to what is seen at intermediate doses for sparsely-ionizing radiation, where the effect decreases upon fractionation and protraction. These observations, related to high-LET particles, cannot be explained on biophysical grounds.

157. Dose-response curves after low-LET irradiation have been reported for some tumours that suggest either the absence of, or a very small, linear term. In such cases, the curve approaches the purely quadratic, indicating perhaps a very low probability of interaction of lesion in two targets crossed by a single ionizing track, or the presence of highly efficient dose-dependent repair processes. Quadratic models have been proposed for leukaemia in CBA mice and cancer of the skin and bone. They predict a very pronounced reduction of the effect by lowering the dose rate or by dose fractionation. Substantial over-estimation of the risk would derive in these cases from linear extrapolation to low doses and dose rates from high or intermediate single doses.

IV. DOSE-RESPONSE RELATIONSHIPS IN EXPERIMENTAL SYSTEMS

A. PHENOMENA OBSERVED AT THE CELLULAR AND SUBCELLULAR LEVEL

158. In recent years, there has been good progress in understanding the role of oncogenes, and of related phenomena at the macromolecular level, in the causation and development of cancer. The newest data are reviewed in annex A to the present report. This progress, however, has left a considerable gap in the understanding of how these phenomena may be linked to mechanisms of radiation carcinogenesis, and what are the relevant molecular targets [G34]. From qualitative analysis of the available information it appears that a rather wide spectrum of radiation interaction with genetic material should be considered.

159. The present section, therefore, discusses dose-response relationships for radiobiological effects, at the subcellular and cellular level, that might be relevant to the induction of malignancy. Some effects, such as in vitro cell transformation, are probably closely related to in vivo carcinogenesis; the relevance of others is not yet well established, but is not implausible. Among the latter effects are mutations, because there is strong evidence of involvement of the genome in both the process of malignant transformation and of cancerous growth (see II.A). Mutational events that could be linked with carcinogenesis may include point mutations, chromosomal deletions and

translocations, as well as transposition of the genetic material [B71, B72, C32, F14, S43, S56, Y3]. It has been postulated [F21] that "tumour specific" symmetrical chromosomal translocations may be particularly relevant for two reasons: first, there are cancers whose cells consistently show aberrations of this type (e.g., chronic myelogenous leukaemia, Burkitt's lymphoma); second, this chromosomal aberration is compatible with the cell's continuous ability to divide, a pre-condition for a transformed cell to develop into a cancerous clone.

1. Mutations in germ cells

160. The frequency of point mutations as related to dose in germ cells of male and female mice, and of other species, was reviewed in depth in annex H of the 1977 UNSCEAR report [U6] and in annex I of the 1982 UNSCEAR report [U24]. The most recent findings are dealt with in annex A to this report. In summary, there is an unquestionable effect of dose rate and fractionation upon specific locus mutations induced in germ cells of male and female mice by low-LET radiation. Interpretations of these findings differ considerably. Abrahamson and Wolff [A2, A3] postulated that mutational lesions are both one- and two-track events, and tried to fit linear-quadratic equations to the data. The attempt was criticized by Russell [R24, R25, R26] who has long been advocating an alternative hypothesis, namely, that mutations themselves are single-track phenomena, and the apparent multiple-track events reflect damage and saturation of the repair processes at higher doses and dose rates. UNSCEAR reviewed both hypotheses in detail and, in the light of present evidence, accepted that of Russell as a more likely explanation.

2. Mutations in somatic cells

(a) The Tradescantia system

161. The data obtained on plant cells of the species Tradescantia are very valuable because: (a) mutations can be scored down to 3 mGy of x rays (and correspondingly lower doses of neutrons); (b) the amount of data on the effects of dose, dose rate and radiation quality is far better than for any other cellular system; (c) the effect is evidently a somatic mutation (although its molecular mechanism is not clear) and the underlying lesion is most likely chromosomal; and (d) the form of the dose-response curve is similar to that for dicentrics and deletions in mammalian T lymphocytes.

162. Dose-response relationships for somatic mutations in Tradescantia, induced by acute 250-kVp x rays, are plotted on a log-log scale in Figure VI [N2, S20, U19]. Below 0.1 Gy, the curve is linear, but then its slope increases up to 1 Gy, where a dose-squared component sets in, leading to an upward concavity of the curve. Above 1-2 Gy, the curve bends and declines, reflecting, perhaps, preferential killing of the mutated cells (the effect is scored in terms of frequency per surviving cell). The data points below

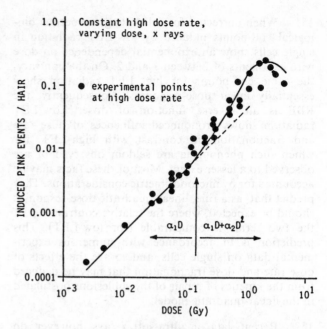

Figure VI. Dose-response curve for induced pink mutations in Tradescantia.
[B99]

1 Gy are well fitted by a non-threshold regression equation of the type $I = a_1D + a_2D^2$, where a_1 and a_2 are constants, presumably for single- and two-track events. Mean values of a_1 and a_2 deduced from three studies [S20, N2, U19] amounted to 5.1 (range 4.6-6.4) $10^{-2} Gy^{-1}$ and 6.5 (5.5-17.3) $10^{-2} Gy^{-2}$, respectively [N1]. In terms of the linear-quadratic model, the a_1/a_2 quotient for x rays varied from 0.33 to 0.83 Gy. For gamma rays, a_1 and a_2 are 2.1 $10^{-2} Gy^{-1}$ and 5.2 $10^{-2} Gy^{-2}$, respectively [N1]. Studies with mono-energetic neutrons (0.065-13.4 MeV) produced a linear dose-response up to 0.05-0.1 Gy [S19, U13] of the form $I = a_1D$. At high and intermediate doses, the RBE of neutrons versus x rays was inversely proportional to the square root of the neutron dose.

163. Reduction of the neutron dose rate had almost no effect upon the yield of mutations [N2, U13]. When the x-ray dose rate was reduced from about 1 Gy min^{-1} to 5-0.5 mGy min^{-1}, the frequency of mutations was an increasingly linear function of the dose, approaching a linear response of the form $I = a_1D$. When the dose rate of x or gamma rays was progressively lowered [M18], and a constant dose of 0.8 Gy delivered over increasing time intervals, lower mutation frequencies were observed approaching asymptotically the limiting value of the respective a_1D for gamma rays. Fractionation of an x-ray dose of 0.6 Gy into two acute fractions of 0.3 Gy each [M18] produced no reduction of the mutation yield up to a 15-minute fractionation interval, but the yield declined with further spacing of the fractions up to 24 hours. Splitting an x-ray dose of 0.05 Gy into two 0.025 Gy fractions given at 5 hours from each other did not reduce the response any further [U27].

164. The influence of fractionation of two x-ray doses (0.7 and 4 Gy) was studied upon induction and repair of two types of somatic mutations (pink and colourless) in this system [W16]. The intervals between

the two fractions varied from 0.5 to 12 hours. Recovery for the two types of mutations differed, in that pink mutations showed recovery at both doses, whereas colourless events showed some recovery at lower doses, but an increased effect at higher doses. Thus, two types of mutations induced by x rays in the same system may have different dose and time kinetics.

165. In summary, the effects of dose, dose rate, fractionation and quality of radiation upon Tradescantia mutations provide, in general, a good example of the linear-quadratic model of radiation action.

(b) Mammalian somatic cells

166. In recent years, significant progress has been made in the methodology of studies of point mutations in somatic cells in culture. Enzyme deficiencies are induced by mutagenic agents, and mutant cells are screened for resistance of developing clones to substances that are toxic to normal cells, e.g., to 8-azaguanine, 6-mercaptopurine or 6-thioguanine in hypoxanthine-guanine-phosphoribosyltransferase (HG-PRT) deficient mutants. Biochemical mechanisms and methods of investigation were reviewed in detail in annex H of the 1977 UNSCEAR report [U6] and in annex I of the 1982 UNSCEAR report [U24] and are discussed again in annex A to the present report.

167. In summary, both linear and curvilinear (concave upwards) relationships have been observed for induction of HG-PRT deficiency in various cell lines by sparsely-ionizing x or gamma rays, and the character of the dose-response curve is evidently related to the genome of the cell studied and not only to the quality of radiation applied [A13, A14, B42, C10, C23, C24, E8, K16]. In cases of curvilinear dose-response relationships, after acute x or gamma irradiation there was also a pronounced reduction of the yield of mutations by dose fractionation. For densely-ionizing radiation (alpha particles, helium, boron and nitrogen ions), the dose-response relationship for induction of HG-RPT deficiency, both in human and hamster cells, was essentially linear [C20, T18]. Induction of forward mutations in Chinese hamster cells by x rays resulted in curvilinear dose-response relationships (concave upwards); moreover pronounced dose-rate effects were observed [S25].

168. Experiments on radiation-induced mutations resulting in HG-PRT deficiency show some correlation between the shape of the survival curve for low-LET radiation and the kinetics of induction of somatic mutations in the same cell lines. This observation has been generalized by Thacker et al. [T10, T9, T8], Munson and Goodhead [M36], Leenhouts and Chadwick [L3, C2] and Goodhead et al. [G29] on different radiations and cells in various stages of the cell cycle, in the sense that there is a relationship of the type $\ln S = -K.M$ where S is the cell survival (S_D/S_0), and M the frequency of induced mutations. This correlation is corroborated by other studies (e.g., [R5]). Thacker [T8] has shown that it applies to exponentially growing cells of several species (man,

hamster and mouse) with the same proportionality constant K. However, the mutation frequency per lethal lesion seems higher for high-LET radiation and lower for ultrasoft x rays [G34].

169. When Thacker et al. studied the same relationship [T19], by irradiating V-79-4 hamster cells grown to plateau phase without re-feeding (most cells in the G_1 phase), they found a similar association of frequency of induced mutations with (log) survival. This was true both after high (1.7 Gy min^{-1}) and low dose rate (down to 3.4 mGy min^{-1}) gamma irradiation. There was considerable repair of sub-lethal and sub-mutational damage with decreasing dose rate. However, when the cells were held for 5 hours after irradiation, before trypsinization and seeding, the potentially lethal damage was effectively repaired, whereas that leading to mutation (HGPRT locus) remained unaffected. Goodhead et al. [G29] interpreted all this to show that the average number of mutagenic lesions in a cell is proportional to the average number of lethal lesions induced by a given radiation. However, results on repair of the potentially lethal damage show that phenomena involved in cell killing and mutation induction can be separated.

170. This conclusion remains to be confirmed. However, if the correlation were generally valid, a linear relationship between frequency of induced mutations and dose of low-LET radiation would be exceptional, because exponential cell-survival curves for x and gamma rays are also exceptional [A17, B63, C9, C21-C23, F2, K21, N8, P7, P15, S33, W6, W7], sigmoid cell survival generally being the rule [B5, B9-B12, B19, B27, B45, C1, C37, D3, D8, E2, F1, F2, F19, H2, H6, K2, K24, L6, M16, M60, S33, T18, W6, W7]. In most cases studied after neutron and alpha-particle irradiation, the survival of diploid mammalian cells is, with few exceptions [H1, C20], a simple exponential function of dose [B5, B9-B12, B29, B45, J6, K2, K3, R39, T18].

3. Chromosome aberrations

(a) Translocations in germinal cells

171. As discussed in annex H of the 1977 UNSCEAR report [U6], the frequency of chromosomal translocations induced by x and gamma rays in spermatogonia, spermatids and oocytes shows a pronounced dose-rate and dose-fractionation effect, and data can be fitted to a linear-quadratic equation. On the other hand, neutrons produce essentially linear dose-reponse relationships without any significant protraction or fractionation effect. These conclusions have been confirmed by more recent data reviewed in annex I of the 1982 UNSCEAR report [U24] and in annex A to the present report.

(b) Somatic cells

172. Studies of chromosomal aberrations in human lymphocytes have been reviewed in the past by UNSCEAR (1969 report, annex C, [U9]), and by others [B15, L13, L12, D4]. In most cases, the yield of

easily identifiable dicentric chromosomes and acentric fragments, induced in G_0 cells, was studied against the dose of various radiations. The asymmetric exchanges are not compatible with cell survival over many generations; however, the yield and kinetics of induction are accepted as representative of symmetrical chromosomal exchanges. The latter may be relevant to present considerations. The subject of dose-response relationships for induction of dicentrics has been thoroughly reviewed by Lloyd and Edwards [L36]. The review included re-calculation of the dose-response functions from original data (62 experiments) using a standardized maximum likelihood method for fitting a linear-quadratic equation. The main conclusions are:

(a) For gamma rays and high-energy electrons, the value of a_1, in the region of 2-2.5 10^{-2} dicentric per cell and gray, appears to be consistent with most observations;

(b) For x rays (180-250 kVp), a representative value of a_1 of about 5 10^{-2} dicentric per cell and gray seems to apply;

(c) The a_2 coefficients for gamma rays, x rays and electrons show less variation than the individual reported values of a_1, and they cluster within the range of 4-8 10^{-2} dicentric per cell and gray square;

(d) For fission neutrons, no significant a_2 term was observed. Typical a_1 values would be 40-90 dicentric per cell and gray. The coefficient tends to increase with lowering of the particle energy, to a peak at about 350 keV (about 160 dicentric per cell and gray);

(e) In several studies [K36, V11, Z1], the yield of chromosome aberrations in human lymphocytes was studied after doses well below 0.5 Gy of x rays. When the data on dicentrics from these studies were pooled [Z1], they fitted a linear function of dose passing through the origin, as would be expected from the values given above. The response for acentric fragments was similar, even though less regular;

(f) At neutron energies above 15 MeV, a significant value of a_2 appears;

(g) For protons with energies > 7.4 MeV, the a_1 coefficients are very similar to those for x rays. The a_2 values are rather lower than for typical low-LET radiation;

(h) For alpha particles, all dose-response relationships (excluding one study with possible methodological complications) are linear, but a_1 values scatter widely, owing probably to systematic dosimetric inaccuracies;

(i) When the value of a_1 is correlated with LET, the coefficient increases with the latter above 5 keV/μm to a maximum at about 70 keV/μm, and then falls off sharply at still higher values of the LET. The a_2 value is roughly constant for low-LET radiation, but virtually absent for high-LET particles.

173. The effects of dose rate and fractionation upon dicentric yield in lymphocytes may be summarized as follows:

(a) For low-LET radiation, the yield decreases with decreasing dose rate (or the extension of irradiation time) and with increasing fractionation intervals. This effect is attributed to the repair of interacting lesions, whose mean life appears to be about 2 hours, although some of the lesions may have a much longer life. Available experimental data and their theoretical interpretation suggest that, for very long irradiation times, the a_2 coefficient would be zero and the a_1 would remain unaffected (linear relationship);

(b) For neutrons, no effects of dose protraction or fractionation were seen.

174. The RBE of neutrons versus x or gamma rays is inversely proportional to the square root of the neutron dose. The limiting value at low dose rates may be obtained from the ratios of the relevant a_1 coefficients.

175. This was also noted when whole blood was irradiated by adding tritiated water prior to initiation of blastic transformation. Doses between 0.2 and 4 Gy β radiation were delivered over 30 minutes or 24 hours. Whereas the dose-response curve for 30-minutes exposures was practically the same as that after acute x rays, the response was close to linearity after longer exposures (the linear component remained unchanged while the quadratic one decreased by a factor of about 3 [P20]).

176. Similar relationships were obtained for dicentrics in the lymphocytes of all mammalian species studied so far (marmoset [B41], Chinese hamster [B41], rabbit [B1, B2, S5], pottoroo [S5], swine [B1, B41, L7], sheep [L7], goat [L7], mouse [B23, B41], rhesus monkey [B61], and other primates [H9, M37]). With protraction or fractionation of x- or gamma-ray doses, the linear term prevails [S4, L9]. With irradiation times exceeding 24 hours the relationships for dicentrics after exposure to gamma rays tend to approach linearity.

177. For acentric fragments, a linear-quadratic relationship is usually observed, but the results are less reproducible [B2, L13]. As these aberrations include both interstitial and terminal deletions, classified together, the relationship does not contradict linearity for single-break aberrations.

178. In conclusion, induction of chromosomal aberrations of the one- and two-break type, in somatic cells in G_0 or G_1, is in broad agreement with the linear-quadratic model for low-LET and with the linear models for high-LET particles. This agreement refers to dose and to the effects of dose rate and fractionation. For single-break aberrations, a linear model should fit the data, but methodological problems make the demonstration difficult.

4. Oncogenic transformation of cells in vitro

(a) General

179. Studies of transformation from the normal to the oncogenic state, on cells in vitro, are very relevant

to the purposes of the present annex. They allow investigation of the mechanisms of cancer initiation without interference of other factors at the tissue and systemic levels. In addition, killing and transformation may be measured in the same target cells, allowing the relative importance of the two effects to be studied at the same time. Morover, in vitro experiments are less expensive and time-consuming than studies on irradiated animals and are easier to analyse, owing to the lack of competing risks and the higher precision of measurements. On the other hand, lack of close intercellular contact and systemic regulation during culture growth is an artifact compared with the situation in situ, and could change—at least quantitatively—the reactions of cells studied. Details of cell handling, such as whether trypsinization has been applied to the cultures, or not, in the course of the experiments, may also substantially modify the results. So far, observations on cell transformation have been limited almost exclusively to fibroblasts, whereas tumours of epithelial origin prevail among radiation-induced cancers in man.

(b) Dose-response relationships

180. Transformed cells are assessed by scoring characteristic colonies recovered in a culture. This directly measures the transformation frequency per surviving cell. Most experiments are reported in this way, but, with some additional effort, information can be obtained on cell survival as a function of dose, and on the plating efficiency. The transformation yield per initial cell at risk may be calculated by correcting the transformation frequencies per surviving cell for the respective survival values and plating efficiency. This latter measure of transformation can seldom be computed from the frequencies per survivors reported in the papers, which often makes it difficult to give a precise description of the dose-response relationships. Many features of the dose-response relationships depend strongly upon the time interval between the establishment of a culture (seeding of cells) and irradiation: new and established cultures should therefore be dealt with separately.

(i) Irradiation of freshly established cultures

181. Borek and Hall [B33] x-irradiated early-passage golden hamster embryo cells in vitro, 24 hours after trypsinization and seeding, with doses from 0.01 to 6.0 Gy (a point at 0.003 Gy x rays was added later [B76]). A dose-response relationship per surviving cell is presented in Figure VII, showing a rise with dose up to 1 Gy, a plateau between 1.5 and 3.0 Gy, and a decline thereafter. The dose-response relationship from the same and subsequent experiments was also expressed per initial cell at risk [B29]. It is impossible to say whether a linear or an upwards concave line would be a better fit of the experimental points along the ascending portion of the curve. A linear fit was assumed by the authors themselves but a linear-quadratic fit was also attempted by Chadwick and Leenhouts [L3]. In a linear plot the line tends to pass through the origin, suggesting no threshold. Below

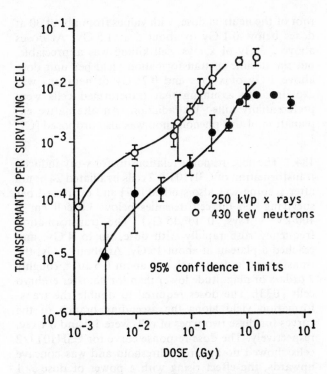

Figure VII.   Dose-response curves for transformation of hamster embryo cells by neutrons and x rays. The curves were obtained by non-parametric least-squares fitting.
[B79]

0.5 Gy of x rays and down to 0.01 Gy the yield of transformants appears to rise with a power of dose < 1. The transformation frequency per Gy of x rays below 1 Gy is of the order of 10^{-2} per cell, which is several orders of magnitude greater than for any somatic mutation [U6] but almost an order of magnitude lower than the total yield of chromosomal aberrations induced by comparable doses of x rays in mammalian lymphocytes [D4]. In a comparison of 300-kVp x and ^{60}Co gamma rays [B76] the RBE of the latter varied from 0.85 at about 1 Gy to 0.5 at a few tens of mGy.

182. Borek, Hall and Rossi [B29] and Borek and Hall [B79] irradiated hamster embryo cells with monoenergetic neutrons (0.43 MeV) and compared the dose-response relationship with that for x rays. The curves representing the relationships, both per surviving cell or per initial cell at risk, were peaked in shape and roughly parallel. A fit to the neutron data similar to that for x rays, but shifted toward lower doses, was obtained (Figure VII) with no suggestion of a threshold. Below 0.1 Gy, the transformation frequency could also be interpreted as rising with a power of dose lower than unity. The RBE of neutrons, at transformation frequencies of 10^{-3} and $5 \cdot 10^{-3}$, was about 12 and about 6, respectively. Measurable transformation was induced even by 1 mGy of neutrons. Accelerated argon ions (429 MeV per atomic mass unit) were roughly as effective as neutrons [B29].

183. Data were also obtained for cell survival [B29]. For x rays a sigmoid survival curve ($D_0 = 1.47$ Gy; $n = 6$), and for 430-keV neutrons a purely exponential curve ($D_0 = 0.5$ Gy), were reported. The RBE of neutrons varied approximately with the inverse square

root of the neutron dose, with values from about 30 at doses below 0.1 Gy to about 5 at 1.5 Gy. At doses above 2-3 Gy of x rays, cell killing was appreciable, but the decline of transformation yield per unit dose above 1 Gy of x rays and 0.25 Gy of neutrons was explained by assuming that transformed cells were preferentially killed by radiation. An alternative explanation of this phenomenon was also proposed [C7, L3].

184. The dose-response relationship for x-ray-induced transformation of C3H10T1/2 cells irradiated 24 hours after seeding was also studied [T7] and expressed per surviving cell (at cell densities below 3.8 cell cm^{-2}; 100-kV x rays, 0 to 15 Gy). The transformation frequency rose rapidly with dose, up to 4 Gy, and reached a plateau at about 15 Gy. At about 1 Gy, the transformation frequency was about $0.5\ 10^{-4}$, roughly 2 orders of magnitude lower than for hamster embryo cells [B33]. The doses required to double the transformation yield along the ascending branch of the curves for these two types of cells were 1.0 and 0.1 Gy, respectively. The dose-response curve for C3H10T1/2 cells showed no apparent threshold and was concave upwards, the effect rising with a power of dose > 1 and close to 2.

185. In a later study, Miller et al. [M23, M41] examined, under a similar experimental protocol in the same C3H10T1/2 cells, the effect of single and split doses of 300-kVp x rays. The single-dose response curve had a complex, curvilinear shape. The transformation frequency was less than proportional to dose between 0.1 and 0.3 Gy, almost flat between 0.3 and about 1 Gy, and then rising with the square, or higher, power of dose. A plot of the data at 0.1-10 Gy on a log-log scale, per surviving cell, is given in Figure VIII. Interpretation of the shape of this dose-

response relationship is very difficult, particularly in the dose range below 1 Gy.

186. Yang, also, studied the transformation of C3H10T1/2 cells by x rays and energetic silicon ions (initial energy 320 MeV per atomic mass unit, residual range in water 4.5 cm, dose average LET = 88 keV/μm) [Y5]. This radiation was more effective than 225 kVp x rays (RBE not given). Cells kept in a highly confluent state for some time after irradiation were able to repair part of the transformation damage induced by x rays, but not that induced by accelerated silicon ions.

187. When C3H10T1/2 cells were irradiated with neutrons (35-MeV $d^+ \rightarrow$ Be), the results were as in Figure IX [B79]. The dose-response curve is shifted towards lower doses with a similar dose-independent plateau as for x rays. The RBE increased with decreasing dose and was similar for both transformation and cell killing.

188. Lloyd et al. [L15] studied transformation in C3H10T1/2 cells by irradiation with 5.6-MeV alpha particles, showing a higher effectiveness as compared with x rays (the relationship of irradiation- and seeding-time is not available). For alpha particles, the dose-response relationship is of a grossly curvilinear (concave upward) character, the effect rising with approximately the cube of the dose. When expressed per surviving cell, the maximum transformation rate was seen at about 2 Gy.

189. C3H10T1/2 cells were transformed by 100-kVp x rays, fast fission neutrons (mean energy 0.5 MeV, 8-20% gamma contribution) and cyclotron neutrons (mean energy 38 MeV, 8% gamma contribution). The dose ranges were: 1.5-11 Gy, 0.5-5 Gy, and 1.5-6 Gy, respectively [B89]. The cells were irradiated 36 hours after seeding. For fission neutrons, the response per survivor was most effective and the initial portion of the curve was only slightly concave upwards. X rays were least effective and 38-MeV neutrons produced curves very similar to those of x rays. For both radiations, the dose-response curves were grossly concave upwards at their ascending portions. A plateau of effect at high doses was reached for all radiations tested. It is worth mentioning that for each radiation the survival curves had pronounced shoulders, which were roughly proportional to the degree of curvilinearity of the dose-transformation curves. The RBE relative to x rays at the transformation frequency of $5\ 10^{-4}$ was 1.2 and 3.8 for 38-MeV and 0.5-MeV neutrons, respectively.

190. Transformation of BALB/3T3 cells by ^{238}Pu alpha particles and x rays was studied by exposure of freshly seeded single cells or confluent cell monolayers [R39]. The dose ranges were 0.5-2.5 Gy and 0.5-5 Gy for alpha particles and x rays, respectively. When calculated per surviving cell the rise of transformation frequency with dose was exponential (steeper than proportional). However, when the results were expressed as transformants per exposed cell, for alpha particles the highest yield was induced already by a dose of 0.5 Gy, with a slight decline thereafter. This

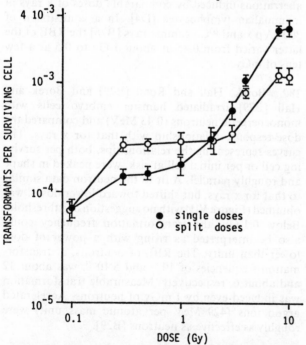

Figure VIII. Dose-response relationships for the number of transformants per surviving C3H10T1/2 cells, following single or split doses of 300-kVp x rays. In the case of split doses, the radiation was delivered in two equal exposures, separated by 5 hours.
[M23]

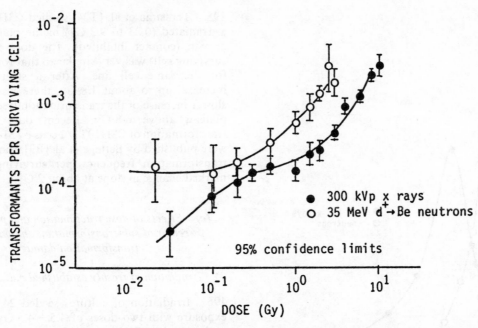

Figure IX. Pooled data obtained for the fraction of transformants per surviving C3H10T1/2 cell following irradiation with x rays or neutrons.
[B79]

may be attributed to highly efficient cell sterilization by alpha rays. A high effectiveness of the alpha particles, relative to x rays, was noted, but the precise shapes of the curves at the lower end of the dose scale cannot be established. Little studied the transformation by x rays of freshly seeded cells (20 hours prior to exposure) of BALB/3T3 mouse [L10]. Although there was some indication of an upward concave curve, the statistical uncertainty of the data does not allow precise conclusions.

191. Golden Syrian hamster embryo fibroblasts, seeded about 12 hours before, were exposed for 17 hours to varying concentrations of methyl ^{3}H-thymidine [L33]. The number of transformants per surviving cell (and mutants at HGPRI locus) showed a proportionality to the concentration of the substance. Tritiated uridine, which is not incorporated into DNA, was ineffective in inducing both oncogenic transformation and mutations.

192. BALB/3T3 embryo fibroblasts, synchronized in the S-phase, were incubated for 16 hours with the DNA precursors ^{3}H-thymidine and ^{125}I-iododeoxy-uridine (^{125}I-dUrd) [L34]. The incorporation of the radionuclides into cellular DNA was proportional to concentration in the culture medium. The transformation frequency per survivor, versus concentration of activity per cell, was linear in both cases—without suggestion of a threshold—up to a frequency of about $5 \cdot 10^{-4}$. The ratio of the initial slopes of ^{125}I-dUrd versus ^{3}H-thymidine dose-response curve was about 25. In the same experimental series, the transformation by x rays was somewhat irregular, with an approximately exponential increase of the transformation frequency with dose over the whole range of doses (0.5-6 Gy). The high effectiveness of ^{125}I-dUrd was explained by the release of a cluster of low energy

Auger electrons (about 25 per decay), leading to a very high energy deposition in the vicinity of the DNA double strand.

(ii) *Late irradiation of cultures*

193. Dose-response relationships for in vitro transformation of cell line C3H10T1/2 by acutely delivered x rays (50-kVp, 0.18 mm Al filtration) and neutrons (fission, mean energy 0.85 MeV) were reported by Han and Elkind [H1]. In contrast with the experiments reviewed above, cells were irradiated 48 hours after seeding. When the transformation rate was expressed per initial cell at risk, the decline of the yield beyond the maximum had the same slope (or D_0) as for the killing of non-transformed cells, suggesting that sterilization by high doses of normal or transformed cells was similar. On linear co-ordinates (Figure X), the ascending portions of the dose-response curves (per initial cell at risk) for x rays was concave upwards (at least above 1.5-2 Gy) but details cannot be established from the graphs. For neutrons, the ascending portion of the curve appears to be close to linearity. The RBE of neutrons increased with declining doses, and the maximum attainable transformation frequency by neutrons was higher by about 50% than that for gamma rays (per initial cell at risk). In contrast with the data of Miller et al. [M23] (Figure VIII) there was a significant flattening of the yield above 4 Gy of x rays, when the data were expressed per surviving cell [H14] (see Figure XI).

194. Watanabe et al. [W18] irradiated golden hamster embryo cells 72 hours after establishing the culture. The exposures varied from 50 to 600 R at exposure rates of 5, 75 and 600 R/min. Additional exposures (1-50 R) were applied at the dose rate of 5 R/min. The

197

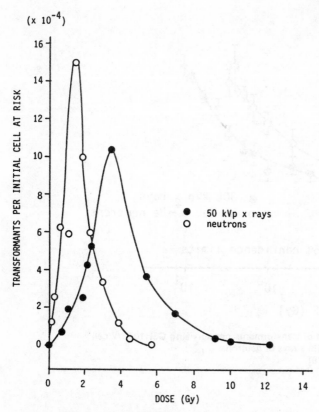

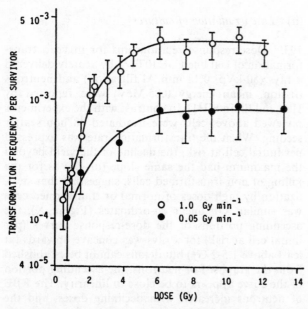

Figure X. Changes in transformation frequency of C3H10T1/2 cells after single exposures to x rays or fission-spectrum neutrons.
[H1]

Figure XI. Frequency of neoplastic transformation of C3H10T1/2 cells expressed per surviving cell as a function of dose of gamma rays delivered at high or at low dose rate. Error bars represent the standard errors of the data pooled from various experiments.
[H14]

logarithm of transformation frequency per survivor was approximately linear up to 100 R, and had a very shallow increase from 200 R onwards (semi-plateau). From the graphical presentation of data, it appears that up to 75 R, at 5 R/min, the dose-response relationship is linear, with no suggestion of a threshold.

195. Terasima et al. [T24] studied C3H10T1/2 cells, x-irradiated (0.23 to 9.3 Gy) in the plateau phase of growth (contact inhibited). The dose response (per surviving cell) was very similar to that found by others for the same cell line. After a steep exponential increase, up to about 1.8 Gy, there was a gradually slower increase of the transformation frequency with a plateau above 6-8 Gy. Recent data on in vitro transformation of C3H10T1/2 cells by 31-MeV protons were published by Bettega et al. [B3], showing that the transformation frequency per surviving cell had a marked change in slope at about 2 Gy.

(c) Effects of dose fractionation and protraction; repair of sub-transformation and potential transformation damage

(i) Irradiation of freshly established cultures

196. Irradiation of cultures seeded 24 hours before exposure with two doses of 4.5 + 4.5 Gy of x rays at various intervals (zero to five hours) showed that survival of C3H10T1/2 fibroblasts nearly doubled when the interval exceeded 2 hours, with no further increase for longer intervals [T4]. For doses of 1.5, 3.0 and 8.0 Gy in two equal fractions at five-hour intervals, the transformation frequency per surviving cell remained unaltered at the lowest dose, but declined significantly (p = 0.005) at the two higher doses.

197. Hamster embryo cells in culture (seeded 24 hours earlier) showed a doubling of the effect after split, as opposed to single, doses of 0.5 or 0.75 Gy [B90]. At the same time, the survival of irradiated cells increased only marginally. When the experiment was extended [B64] by studying the effect on the transformation frequencies of splitting 1.5, 3 and 6 Gy of x rays, no enhancing effect of 2×0.75 Gy, as opposed to 1×1.5 Gy, was noted. Fractionation of 3 and 6 Gy led to a reduction of the total effect.

198. Miller and Hall [M23] studied dose fractionation on C3H10T1/2 fibroblasts, plated 24 hours before x-ray treatments (0.3 to 8.0 Gy). Their results confirmed the sparing effects of splitting the dose above 1.5 Gy (with a possibly incidental deviation of the points at 4 Gy) and an enhancement of transformation below that dose. The experiment was repeated [M41], and the dose range expanded to include 0.1 and 10 Gy. The results are presented in Figure VIII. In addition, a dose of 1 Gy was split into 2, 3 or 4 equal fractions [H21]. An almost proportional (2-, 3- and 4-fold) enhancement of transformation was observed. Also, when a dose of 1 Gy of ^{60}Co gamma rays was delivered at a low dose rate (over 6 hours) the effect was significantly enhanced, by a factor of about 3, by comparison with acute exposure (over 10 min) [H21]. In conclusion, using this experimental protocol, in the range 0.3-1 Gy there is an enhancement of the effect by splitting the dose into two equal fractions within 5 hours or by protracting the dose over a similar interval. At 2 Gy, there is no effect. There is a decline of the yield after fractionation at higher doses. Approximately the same trend is seen when the data are expressed per initial cell at risk.

199. Little [L10] reported dose-fractionation experiments on BALB/3T3 cells seeded 24 hours before the first exposure with essentially identical results. The fractionated doses ranged from 0.1 to 3.5 Gy, and similar observations were also made in still another study by Suzuki et al. [S44]. It may be concluded, therefore, that enhanced transformation (per survivor) below 1.5 Gy of x rays after fractionation within 5 hours is a phenomenon observable in all cell lines studied so far, irradiated in freshly established cultures. Such an effect might be deduced from the curves in Figure VIII [M23]. In fact, if an independent action of the two dose fractions is assumed, the decrease above 2 Gy, where the response rises with D^2 or with a higher exponent, is easily understood. Similarly, below 1 Gy, over the plateau, where the effect is roughly independent of dose, fractionation should increase the yield, as observed.

200. Figures VIII and IX show clearly that a linear extrapolation down from intermediate (1 Gy) and high (2-3 Gy) doses of x rays would lead to an underestimate of the real transformation frequency, particularly with respect to the effect of split doses in the low-dose region. The greatest under-estimate, by a factor of 4-6, would be encountered when the effect of single doses in the range 1-3 Gy is linearly extrapolated to predict effects of split total doses of 0.1-0.3 Gy. The relevance of this finding to tumour induction in vivo has been commented upon by several authors [B76, H21, M41].

(ii) *Late irradiation of cultures*

201. Data on fractionation were reported by Han and Elkind [H1] for x rays (0.75 Gy) and fission neutrons (3.8 Gy) on C3H10T1/2 cells exposed 48 hours after seeding. The transformation rate after doses of this magnitude was on the declining part of the curve when expressed per initial cell at risk. Fractionation of the neutron dose within 0 to 16 hours had little, if any, effect on single-dose survival and caused a slight reduction of the transformation yield, perhaps within the limits of experimental error. With x-ray fractionation times up to 5 and 10 hours, the frequency increased and then declined to the level of the non-fractionated exposure at about 16 hours. The increase was within a factor of 2 and its statistical significance uncertain. When expressed per survivor, the transformation frequency after x irradiation declined steadily to a plateau at 12-16 hours fractionation interval, reflecting essentially an expected and considerable effect upon survival of the non-transformed cells. This observation, therefore, confirmed other findings [M23, M41] that fractionation of high x-ray doses in this cell line reduces the transformation frequency when expressed per surviving cell.

202. Han and Elkind also irradiated C3H10T1/2 cells, 48 hours after plating, with ^{60}Co gamma rays at high (1.0 Gy min^{-1}) and low (0.05 Gy min^{-1}) dose rate [H14]. The range of doses varied between 0.2 and 13 Gy. The transformation frequency per survivor (Figure XI) was consistently reduced at the lower dose rate, as was cell sterilization. The reduction in

transformation yield was by a factor of about 5 above 6 Gy and by a factor of about 3 at 2 Gy, and was still present at doses of 0.5 and 0.2 Gy [E9, H26].

203. Hill et al. [H30] studied the effects of gamma-ray fractionation in the same system. Throughout the dose range tested (0.25-3 Gy), fractionation of the dose into 5 daily fractions resulted in a significant reduction of transformation frequency. Up to 1.5 Gy delivered unfractionated, and up to 3 Gy fractionated regimes, the dose response could be fitted by a straight line passing though the origin (Figure XII). The yield

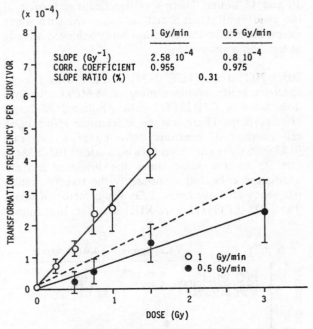

Figure XII. Transformation frequency of C3H10T1/2 cells per surviving cell against dose of gamma rays. Open circles: acute exposure at 1 Gy min^{-1}; Dashed line: continuous exposure at 1 mGy min^{-1}; Closed circles: five fractions at 0.5 Gy min^{-1}, given at 24-hour intervals.
[H30]

of transformants per unit dose was 3 times lower after fractionated than after single doses, and very similar to the dose-response curve for the lower dose-rate exposure referred to above [E9, H26]. Increasing the fractionation intervals beyond 24 hours, and reducing the dose per fraction, led to a further slight reduction of the effect. This suggested that there may be a limit beyond which further dose protraction cannot reduce the transformation frequency. Trypsinization per se, or delivery of the dose within 7 days of growth in culture, did not affect the yield of transformants per unit dose, provided they took place at least 40 hours after seeding. Confluence of the cells was excluded as a possible reason for the observed fractionation effect. These results of dose fractionation and protraction below 1.5 Gy are in striking contrast with those observed when the cells were irradiated 24 hours after seeding [H21, M23]. The difference was attributed to atypical conditions of cellular growth early after plating and to the action of radiation on parasynchronous cells [H30].

204. Watanabe et al. [W18] irradiated golden hamster embryo cells, sub-cultured 72 hours earlier, with x rays

at various exposure rates: 5, 75 and 600 R/min. Throughout the whole range of exposures tested (50-600 R), the lower dose rates produced a reduced yield of transformed cells, even within the 50-100 R range where the dose-response relationship was practically linear. At equal survival levels (which were inversely related to dose rate), the transformation frequency was higher in cells irradiated at higher than at lower dose rates. Terasima et al. [T24] studied the effect of fractionating x-ray doses (0.93, 1.86 and 3.72 Gy) in C3HT101/2 cells irradiated in the plateau phase. Equal fractions were spaced at intervals of 3, 10 and 15 hours. There was significant reduction of the yield at all doses tested, as compared with single doses, the maximum reduction being achieved already at the 3-hour interval.

205. Hill et al. [H26, H34] worked with fission-spectrum neutrons (mean energy 0.85 MeV) at various dose rates in C3H10T1/2 cells irradiated 48 hours after seeding. There was no discernible effect upon cell survival of neutrons delivered at a low rate (0.43-0.86 mGy min^{-1}) versus a high rate (0.103-0.38 Gy min^{-1}). At the same time, the low-rate neutron irradiation enhanced significantly the transformation frequency at doses below 1 Gy (by a factor of about 9 at 0.025-0.1 Gy) (Figure XIII), an effect that cannot

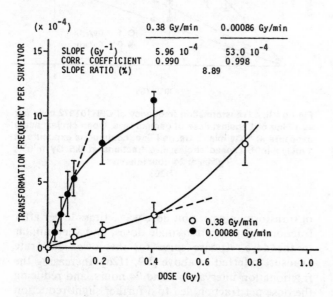

Figure XIII. Oncogenic transformation of C3H10T1/2 cells exposed to fission-spectrum neutrons at high and low dose rate. Dashed lines indicate the linear regressions fitted to the initial portions of the curves.
[H34]

be explained on biophysical grounds. Above doses of 1.5-2.0 Gy, the effect of the dose rate disappeared and dose-response relationships converged to a plateau of 5 10^{-3} transformants per surviving cell.

206. The influence of dose fractionation (5 fractions over 4 days) of fission-spectrum neutrons, delivered at a rate of 0.1 Gy min^{-1}, was studied by the same authors. Over the whole range from 0.103 to 1.12 Gy, an enhancement of effects by fractionation was observed. The ratio of linear slopes of the dose-

response curves at low doses was about 8. The increased effectiveness of the low dose rate and of the fractionated neutron irradiation was explained either by the induction of more efficient error-prone repair or by facilitation of the expression of "sub-effective transformation damage", whatever this means [H37]. A recent study on transformed mammary epithelial cells transplanted in vivo to virgin female BALB/c mice suggests that the effect of fractionated neutron exposures may be analogous to chemical promotion and is due to an enhanced expression of the transformation damage [U28]. The effects of fractionation schemes applied to the cells in an asynchronous growth indicate that x and gamma irradiation—by analogy with sublethal damage—result in error-free, reparable, sub-transformation damage. The transformation damage induced by neutrons either does not undergo repair, or is subject to error-prone repair [E10, H37]; however, why the latter should be more effective at protracted or fractionated low doses is not clear.

207. Terzaghi and Little [T5] found that irradiating C3H10T1/2 cells with x rays in a density-inhibited state, and delaying plating up to 48 hours substantially increased survival rates. Delay for 2 to 4 hours caused marked increase of the transformation rate. Further delay of plating reduced the yield of transformants to very low levels after 48 hours. Terasima et al. [T24], however, did not observe any initial increase of the transformation frequency, as the potential transformation damage fell over the first 3 hours of delayed plating. The rate of potential transformation repair in C3H10T1/2 cells depended strongly on a particular batch of fetal calf serum used in the cell culture medium, both before and after release from confluence [T11]. Lack of serum was accompanied by a high degree of repair (80% over 6 hours) after keeping the irradiated cells (x rays, 3.7 Gy) in the non-proliferating state. Some batches of serum totally prevented the occurrence of repair. No repair of potential transformation could be found after irradiation with alpha particles [R39] and accelerated heavy ions [Y5].

208. When potentially lethal damage was studied by holding these cells in confluence after irradiation for varying lengths of time, a pronounced repair was observed for x rays and none for alpha particles [R39]. Equally, no repair of potential transformation damage was seen for up to 220 hours after alpha particle exposure, whereas the x-ray-induced potential damage was efficiently repaired.

209. The results of other experiments [L23] suggest that two separate processes may be involved in the recovery of damage: first, DNA repair leading to enhanced survival; and, second, a slower error-prone repair process responsible for changes in DNA and leading to mutation and transformation. It should be stressed that the frequencies of transformation reported for most in vitro experiments apply to actively proliferating cell populations and may not be representative of situations where the overwhelming majority of cells is in the resting state, as in most organs in vivo.

(d) Other factors affecting oncogenic transformation in vitro

210. Numerous factors affect the yield of in vitro oncogenic transformation. Among these, a basic role is played by both the time and the density at which cells are seeded.

211. Studies on three cell lines (hamster embryo, C3H10T1/2 mouse embryo and mouse BALB/3T3 cells), have shown [B34, K12, L10, T6] that several post-irradiation cell divisions—4 to 6, depending on the cell line studied—are necessary for expression or fixation of the transformed state. Of these, at least one must take place in the first 24 hours post-irradiation.

212. Terzaghi and Little [T7] investigated the influence of cell density on the transformation frequency per surviving cell. Above 400 viable cells per dish (about 5 cell cm^{-2}), there was a steep decline from plateau values of transformation observed at lower cell densities. The authors suggested that this effect could be the result of an incomplete expression of transformation due to early confluence, which lowers the number of cell divisions during exponential growth below that necessary for full expression of transformation [B71, B72, L26]. Han and Elkind observed, in the same cell line, a similar relationship between the density of seeded cells and the transformation rate after x-ray and neutron irradiation [H1]. Direct cellular contact cannot operate at such cell distances, but a diffusible mediator substance might prevent occurrence or growth of the transformed clones [L15].

213. Lloyd et al. [L16] experimented on co-cultivation of transformed C3H10T1/2 cells with non-transformed ones. When transformed cells were seeded at low densities, together with normal cells, at some ratios of the two cell types (1:50 to 1:500, respectively), expression of the malignant state could be completely prevented. Adding non-transformed cells in greater numbers again elicited this response. The experiment points clearly to a very complex nature of the interaction between transformed and non-transformed cells, even in vitro.

214. The data by Kennedy et al. [K26] are of importance because they throw some light on the complexity of the phenomena leading to oncogenic cell transformation in vitro and could modify substantially the current interpretation of this radiation effect. These authors studied the influence of re-suspending C3H10T1/2 cells after irradiation, once confluence was reached. When dilutions at the time of re-seeding were progressively increased, the number of originally irradiated and inoculated cells per plate decreased to very low values. In spite of that, after a constant dose of 4 Gy of x rays, the number of transformed foci per plate remained practically constant. This indicates that the number of transformed foci per plate is apparently independent of the number of cells initially irradiated. It is interesting to note that similar results were obtained when the effect of inoculum size was studied on the appearance of tumours, after in vitro irradiation of monodispersed thyroid or mammary cells injected into the fat pads of rats [G30]. These observations are in direct conflict with the expectation that—if initiation of a cell is a rare phenomenon—the probability of observing a tumour should rise in proportion to the size of the inoculum.

215. It has been suggested [K26, G30] that exposure to radiation results in some change of the cellular state in many or, after high doses, in all cells. Gould postulates that initiation is not an all-or-none phenomenon, but that its intensity rises with dose up to a saturation level, which is reached in C3H10T1/2 cells at 5-6 Gy after ^{60}Co gamma irradiation or 3 Gy of neutrons. The change is probably transmitted to the whole progeny of surviving cells. The nature of initiation—genetic or epigenetic—is unknown, but the latter would presumably be suggested by these observations. This interpretation is not easily reconciled with the demonstrated direct involvement of DNA in the carcinogenic process [B14, L33]. Only a second rare phenomenon (perhaps mutation), would lead to a phenotypically recognizable transformation at confluence of C3H10T1/2 cells. The probability of this second phenomenon should be in some proportion with the degree of initiation.

216. A report by Hall et al. [H28] challenged the hypothesis that commitment of irradiated cells to the transformed state takes place at confluence. By re-plating cultures at different times after irradiation and testing for distribution of transformed foci among the plates, the authors could show that commitment takes place within 1 week of exposure. This observation is in agreement with a study [B91] on in vitro oncogenic transformation of C3H10T1/2 cells by 7β,8a-dihydroxy,9a,10a-epoxy,7,8,9,10-tetrahydro-benzo(a)-pyrene. The results of this study showed that acquisition of the ability to form transformed foci occurred within 2 days of exposure to a carcinogen. Hall's experiments [H28] also showed that increasing the density of cells in culture probably suppressed expression of the transformed state. These results do not contradict the fact that at 4 Gy of x rays the probability of initiation per cell is close to 1, but they, have been interpreted to challenge the postulated non-stochastic nature of initiation [K26].

217. The presence of thyroxin in the culture medium at a physiological concentration was shown to be a prerequisite for transformation to occur in Syrian hamster embryo and C3H10T1/2 cells [B73, G26, G27]. Thyroxin is required for protein synthesis only within a few hours of irradiation and its action can be reversed by an agent blocking protein synthesis, e.g., cycloheximide.

218. Other factors were shown to enhance transformation in culture during or after irradiation. Extensive investigations were made on a well-known promoter of in vivo carcinogenesis, the active ingredient of croton oil, 12-0-tetradecanoyl-phorbol-13 acetate (TPA). By adding TPA to the cultures within 96 hours of irradiation, Kennedy et al. [K10] showed enhancement of the x-ray transformation frequency (or its expression) in C3H10T1/2 mouse embryo cells.

The effect was particularly marked after doses of 0.5-1.0 Gy. These data indicate that promoting agents can increase the levels of x-ray-induced transformation in vitro, just as they enhance carcinogenesis in vivo. It was also shown [K27] that the most effective period of exposure to TPA is that of exponential growth. However, a delay of TPA application, e.g., addition to cultures re-seeded after confluence, did still lead to a significant enhancement of oncogenic transformation.

219. When TPA was added for six to seven weeks (at 0.1 μg/ml of medium) to cultures of C3H10T1/2 cells irradiated with graded doses of x rays (0.25-4.0 Gy), there was not only an absolute increase of transformation frequency, but also a change in the shape of the dose-response relationship, from curvilinear (upward concave) after x rays alone to linear (Figure XIV). The

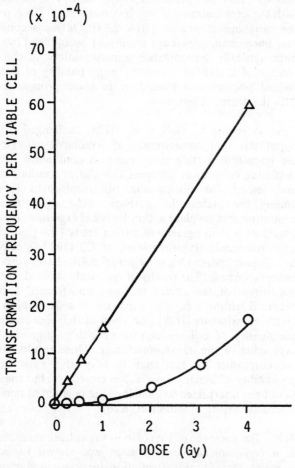

Figure XIV. Influence of post-irradiation incubation with the tumour promoter TPA on x-ray transformation of mouse C3H10T1/2 cells. ○ x-irradiation only; △ TPA (0.1 μg/ml) added for the entire period of expression.
[L26]

action of TPA was especially pronounced at doses in the low and intermediate range [L26]. A very similar effect of TPA on the shape of the dose-response curves for x-ray-induced and neutron-induced transformation of C3H10T1/2 cells was also seen in another study [H22].

220. Numerous mechanisms of action for TPA have been advocated, including inhibition of the cell-to-cell communication [H22, T15]; enhancement of chromosomal rearrangements [K28]; production of short-lived radicals [B76]; and action via mechanism of cellular differentiation [B74, S43]. Increase of cellular proliferation is a phenomenon that often accompanies promotion [F14], but it is doubtful whether it is at all necessary, or sufficient [D13, K27]. The TPA promoting effect is apparently not related to any of the known DNA repair processes [K27].

221. Enhanced transformation of various cell lines was also noted after addition to the medium of the epidermal growth factor, a natural hormone-like polypeptide [F15]; bromodeoxyuridine [R30]; high concentrations of insulin [U29]; cortisone [K30]; and interferone [B46]. The particular batch of fetal calf serum used may also have a profound influence on the transformation frequency eventually observed [T11]. A new promoter, dihydroteleocidin B, an antibiotic derivative recently discovered, has a promoting capacity per unit mass about 100 times higher than that of TPA [H31]. A synergism between x rays and a food pyrolysate product 3-amino-1-methyl-5H-pyrido-(4-3b)indol (Trp-P-2), itself a mutagen and carcinogen isolated from boiled meat and fish, has also been shown [B76] in Syrian hamster embryo cells. Hyperthermia (43°C for 60 minutes or 45°C for 15 minutes before irradiation) caused some increase of the x-ray-induced transformation frequency in C3H10T1/2 cells [C33]. The nature of most enhancing agents mentioned above suggests that the mechanisms of action are epigenetic rather than likely to cause structural changes in the genome itself.

222. There are also suppressing (inhibiting) factors. Kennedy and Little [K35] and Little [L26] described suppression by the protease inhibitors antipain and leupeptin. In other studies [B65, G28] it was shown that antipain added to cultures before irradiation enhanced the yield of transformants, while addition shortly after exposure reduced the transformation frequency, and addition 1 or 2 days later was ineffective. Inhibition of radiation-induced oncogenic transformation was also observed when inhibitors of poly(ADP-ribose) synthesis (benzamide, 3-amino-benzamide) were added to cultures of C3H10T1/2 and golden hamster embryo cells [B96].

223. An inhibition (by a factor of 3) of transformation in C3H10T1/2 cells was observed by adding, 24 hours before exposure, a non-toxic derivative of vitamin A, trimethyl-methoxy-phenyl, analogue of N-ethyl retinamide (Ro-H-1430) and other retinoids [B73]. The retinoids irreversibly suppressed oncogenic transformation when present in culture for only a few days after irradiation. Later addition of TPA to the culture remained ineffective. The retinoids may act by suppressing the carcinogen-induced progression of the neoplastic process [B76].

224. Selenium compounds [B73], actinomycin D [K31] and lymphotoxin [D19, E6, R44] also inhibit radiation-induced transformation. When superoxide dismutase was added to irradiated C3H10T1/2 cultures from irradiation to expression of transformation, the frequency of radiation-induced transformants was

greatly reduced, whether or not the drug was present during x-ray exposure [M49]. Quantitatively, the effects of oxygen and misonidazol upon oncogenic transformation and cell killing of C3H10T1/2 cells are very similar [B97].

(e) Conclusions

225. The oncogenic transformation in vitro of hamster embryo cells and several established mouse fibroblast lines by ionizing radiation shows numerous similarities in respect of dose-response relationships, effects of dose fractionation, and influence of cell density upon transformation frequency.

226. The mechanisms of transformation are still imperfectly understood and several methodological questions are not yet fully resolved. The subject has been thoroughly reviewed [B71, B76, G34, L26, Y3]. Transformation is probably a complex multi-stage phenomenon that includes initiation, progression and final expression of malignant foci. A number of promoting and suppressing factors may affect the frequency of transformation and therefore the shape of the dose-response relationships.

227. For these reasons, analysis of dose-response relationships for low- and high-LET radiation must, for the time being, remain descriptive. After single doses of x rays or neutrons, the dose-response curves have some features in common with those seen in vivo for many experimental tumours. For example, when expressed per initial cell at risk, transformation shows an initial rise of the frequency with dose, then the curve reaches a peak and the yield declines at still higher doses. The lower efficiency of gamma rays at the low, as opposed to high, dose rates in cultures established at least 40 hours before irradiation is also in accordance with most observations in vivo. The same applies to the RBE values of neutrons and alpha particles, which are definitely higher than unity and tend to decline with increasing dose, in agreement with the general understanding of cellular radio-biology [B11, K7]. Neutron dose fractionation upon oncogenic transformation in vitro produces effects that are similar to those seen recently in some—but not all—experiments in vivo. There are, however, differences, particularly when comparisons are made with cells plated shortly before irradiation. The most important is the rise of the transformation frequency with a power of dose less than 1 at intermediate doses (< 1.5 Gy). This shape of the curve may be linked with the enhancing effect of fractionation of x ray doses in the same region, a phenomenon observed in all cell lines tested so far.

228. If enhancement of transformation by fractionation applied in vivo, the complex nature of the low-LET dose-response relationship for single doses might imply an under-estimation of cancer induction when risk coefficients for man are extrapolated from the intermediate down to the lowest doses. Similarly, in the case of fractionated exposure, there might be an even greater under-estimation, owing to the enhancement produced by dose fractionation and protraction in some trans-

formation experiments with low-LET radiation. However, in the light of present knowledge—which is still insufficient—such conclusions are premature, for the following reasons:

(a) No dose-response relationship has been observed for tumours in animals with a plateau below 1 Gy after single acute doses of x or gamma rays. It is also quite clear that no enhancement of tumour induction by fractionation or protraction of external low-LET irradiation has ever been noted at doses below 1 Gy (with one possible exception, see IV.B);

(b) The dependence of the dose-response relationships on the length of the culture period before irradiation shows that the irregular shape of the dose-response curves and the enhancement of fractionation in freshly plated cultures result from irradiation of para-synchronous cells and may therefore be considered an artifact [H37];

(c) The effects of low-LET dose fractionation and protraction on established cell cultures are in general agreement with observations related to other effects at the cellular level (induction of mutations, chromosome aberrations, cell sterilization).

B. TUMOURS IN EXPERIMENTAL ANIMALS

229. In its 1977 report [U6], UNSCEAR reviewed experimental data on radiation-induced tumours, including an examination of the dose-response relationships then available. The essential conclusions were that the peculiarities of each tumour model were such as to prevent large generalizations. There were difficulties in interpreting tumour induction curves on the basis of simple mechanisms of action, in view of the complex interplay of primary and secondary contributing factors. With few exceptions, the data came from observations at doses above 0.5 Gy. Data were insufficient to define, unambiguously, dose-effect relationships in the low and sometimes also in the intermediate dose region.

230. With the exception of the mammary tumour of the Sprague-Dawley rat, dose-incidence curves obtained at high dose rates with low-LET radiation showed a slope that increased with increasing dose, not incompatible with a linear-quadratic trend. With high-LET radiation, on the other hand, dose-effect relationships tended to be more linear and their initial slopes showed relatively little change with dose rate and fractionation. However, with low-LET radiation, a decrease in dose rate led mostly to a decrease of the oncogenic effect, following some inverse function of the exposure time. It appeared difficult to quantify this decrease because the shape of the dose-induction relationships was often altered by the change in dose rate. It was clear, however, that the sparing effect of low dose rate or fractionation was higher for low- than for high-LET radiation. Occasional departures from this general scheme were attributed to the peculiarity of the model systems tested, rather than to real exceptions of established radiobiological mechanisms.

231. The National Council on Radiation Protection and Measurements [N1] evaluated the influence of dose and its distribution in time on the induction curves for tumours, with different radiations and a wide range of dose rates. The ratio of the linear non-threshold curves fitted to the high- or to the low-dose-rate experimental points was taken to be a measure of the "dose-rate effectiveness factor" (DREF). DREF values referring to 10 different experimental tumour systems varied from 1.1 to 6.7, the majority of the values clustering between 3 and 5. This analysis led to the conclusion that in most cases the risk of low-LET radiation would be significantly overestimated if non-threshold linear extrapolation of the data for high-dose-rate were applied to low-dose-rate irradiation. Moskalev et al. [M61, M68] came to the same conclusion when reviewing the available scientific literature. New data that have become available since 1977 are reviewed below.

1. Myeloid leukaemia

232. Robinson and Upton [R7] re-analysed part of the original data on radiation effects in RF mice [U14-U16], correcting for competing risks. About 2000 male mice, irradiated with 250-kV x rays at doses between zero and 4.5 Gy, were selected. Early causes of death (myeloid leukaemia, M, and thymic lymphoma, T) or late causes (reticulum cell sarcoma, L, or others, R) were analysed separately by a non-parametric Kaplan-Meier survival function and its logarithmic transform (the cumulative force of mortality, cum. F.M.). Models were set up for treatment of these two categories, on the assumption of independence between the various causes of death. For causes M and T, there was a significant decrease of the latent period with dose up to 3 Gy. When the effect of dose on the integral tumour rate of M (which corresponds to the cum. F.M.) was studied, the form of the relationship for this cause of death peaked, with a maximum between 2 and 3 Gy and a further decline up to 4.5 Gy, depending on the age at irradiation of the animals (which was 5-6 weeks for group A and 9-10 weeks for group B) (Figure XV). The model for fitting the experimental data was such that the estimate of the ultimate value of the cum. F.M. corresponded to the number of leukaemogenic cells per animal. These were assumed to have a linear-

quadratic dose dependence for induction, and linear-quadratic kinetics for killing. Following Barendsen [B7], the authors took an a_1/a_2 quotient of 0.5 Gy and a β_1/β_2 quotient of 3 Gy. The fit of the data actually produced a β_1/β_2 quotient of 2.4, which is in reasonable agreement, considering the assumptions involved. It was concluded that the data were consistent with the postulated linear-quadratic dose-response model.

233. Petoyan and Filyuskin [P22] tested another model on x-ray- and neutron-induced (high dose rate) leukaemia in RF mice [U16]. The basic assumptions of the model were:

(a) Initiation in the bone marrow stem cells is a two-track phenomenon, perhaps a symmetrical chromosomal translocation;

(b) The sensitivity of initiated and non-initiated stem cells to killing by radiation is the same;

(c) Most of mitotic cell death is due to asymmetric chromosomal exchanges, which have a functional dose dependence basically similar to that of the symmetrical translocations. Therefore, the shape and parameters of the dose-response functions for induction of symmetrical exchanges and cell death should be similar for a given cell line;

(d) The promoting influence of radiation is brought about through an enhancement of mitotic activity and, therefore, the degree of promotion should be inversely proportional to the post-irradiation survival of stem cells;

(e) The probability of scoring an overt malignancy during the remaining life span is a complex function of the "spontaneous" incidence of a given malignancy.

234. The parameters of the model were defined by selecting from independent sources the survival functions of bone marrow stem cells irradiated with x rays and neutrons. The model was fitted to experimental data on the incidence of leukaemia in the RF mouse [U16] by the maximum likelihood method, using a single set of two adjustable parameters; the same set was applied to x rays and neutrons. A good fit was obtained, by visual inspection, and the dose-response curve showed a slight upward concave curvilinearity and linearity of the initial ascending part of the curve for x rays and neutrons, respectively. Linear extrapolation from 1.5 Gy to the low-dose region would lead to a small over-estimate of the risk for x rays, but would be adequate for neutrons. The assumption that the dose-response functions for the initiation and cell killing are similar could be criticized on the basis of available information [B9, B11], but the postulate may be accepted as a first approximation to reality.

235. Mole et al. [M2, M52, M64-M66] studied the induction of acute myeloid leukaemia by x rays, gamma rays and fission neutrons in male CBA/H mice that have almost a zero incidence of this disease. With little intercurrent mortality from competing causes of death, this tumour model is also less sensitive to systematic bias from such causes than that on RF mice [R7].

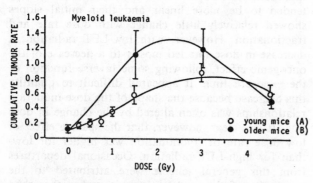

Figure XV. Final cumulative tumour rate ± standard error versus dose for myeloid leukaemia in x-irradiated RF mice.
[R7]

236. Mice were exposed to one of ten doses of x rays (from 0.25 to 6 Gy, delivered at the rate of 0.5 Gy min^{-1}) and then followed until they died [M52, M64]. Median survival in all groups was very similar. There was essentially no association between latency and dose. The results were fitted to a four-term polynomial of the general form $I = (a_1D + a_2D^2) \exp - (\beta_1D + \beta_2D^2)$ as well as to four simplifications with three or two parameters only. All fits were acceptable in a statistical sense (P for goodness of fit = 0.34-0.44), but only two equations had all parameters positive and significantly larger than zero (p < 0.05). These were: $I = a_1D \, e^{-\beta_2D^2}$ and $I = a_2D^2 \, e^{-\beta_1D}$. The former was rejected on the ground that cell survival depending solely on the square of dose is normally not found. The observed incidence could best be fitted by the latter relationship, as shown in Figure XVI. In another recent study of the induction of myeloid leukaemia in CBA male mice by whole-body x irradiation (250 kVp, HVL 1.5 mm Cu) [D3], the age-corrected incidence after doses of 1, 3, 5 and 7 Gy was essentially superimposable on the data by Mole [M52] (see Figure XVI). A purely exponential survival for haemopoetic cells is probably a simplification of reality, but survival curves for bone marrow stem cells usually show only a small shoulder at low doses. For in vivo irradiated bone marrow stem cells McCulloch and Till [M16] found $D_0 = 0.95$ Gy and n = 1.5. Mean values for 17 measurements of D_0 for spleen-colony-forming units in different mouse strains irradiated in vivo with x rays were in the range 0.95-1.61 Gy [H32]. The value of β_1 (0.7-0.11 Gy^{-1}) found by Mole [M52] is compatible with this range.

237. A contribution of a dose-linear term (a_1D) to the dose-response relationship in Figure XVI cannot be excluded on purely statistical grounds. The a_1/a_2 quotient estimated for the complete four parameter model was negative, but the upper 95% confidence limit was 1.29 Gy; and therefore, values of 0.3-0.5 Gy cannot be excluded as very unlikely. Moreover, when the data were tested on three models with a number of

adjustable parameters greater than two, one or two of the parameters were always insignificant. From the simplified two-parameter models, one had to be chosen on the basis of additional information, and this implies a constraint a posteriori even if none had been chosen a priori. In summary, it appears that complete parameters for cell initiation and survival cannot be estimated, independently and simultaneously, solely from the data. However, when a likely shape of the survival function is assumed, the kinetics of initiation for low-LET radiation appears, in this case [M2, M52, M64], to be concave upwards with a pronounced D^2 component.

238. Induction of myeloid leukaemia in CBA/H mice was also studied after brief (0.25 Gy min^{-1}) and protracted exposure to ^{60}Co gamma rays (1.5, 3.0 and 4.5 Gy) [M65]. Protracted exposures were delivered either as daily fractions (0.25 Gy min^{-1}, 5 days per week for 4 weeks) or at a constant rate of 0.004-0.11 mGy min^{-1}. The latter two modes of exposure did not differ in their effectiveness and gave a rather constant response at 5-6% incidence for doses above zero. The shape of the dose-response curve is very similar to that observed for leukaemias induced by fractionated x-ray treatment for ankylosing spondylitis [S49]. The response after acute irradiation was higher by a factor of 2.2, 2.8 and 5 for the three doses, respectively. The most effective gamma-ray dose for leukaemia induction was higher than that of x rays.

239. Irradiation of CBA/H male mice with fission neutrons was performed at high rate (exposure times, 2-20 minutes) with 7 air-midline kerma values in the range from 0.02 through 2 Gy [M66]. The observed incidence of acute myeloid leukaemia was fitted by the equation $I(D) = (4.5 \pm 1.25) \, 10^{-1}D \, e^{-(1.01 \pm 0.28)D}$ (P = 0.25). Neither a purely linear model without correction for cell killing, nor the dose-squared model that fitted the x-ray data, could be satisfactorily interpolated to the neutron data (P for goodness of fit in either case < 10^{-4}).

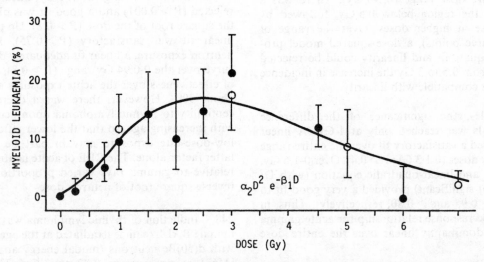

Figure XVI. Dose-response relationship for incidence of myeloid leukaemia after brief exposures of male CBA mice to 250-kVp x rays. Closed circles, data from Mole [M52]; Open circles, data from Di Majo et al. [D3].

240. In experiments by Ullrich and Storer [U20], specific-pathogen-free (SPF) RFM/Un mice of both sexes were irradiated at 10 weeks of age with ^{137}Cs gamma rays at 0.45 Gy min^{-1}, with doses ranging from 0.1 to 3 Gy. Myeloid leukaemia was less frequent in the females, in which the age-corrected incidence reached significance over the control level at 1.5 Gy. Although both a linear and a linear-quadratic model provided a satisfactory fit to the data (P > 0.5 and > 0.8, respectively), the dose-squared component was not significant and linearity predominated between zero and 3 Gy.

241. In male mice, the incidence was significantly higher than control, even at 0.5 Gy, and the form of the relationship was similar to that in females: it could be described either by a linear (P > 0.5) or a linear-quadratic model (P > 0.35), with a very small and non-significant dose-squared term. The ratio of the linear slopes for the two sexes indicated that males were more susceptible by a factor of about 5. Low-dose-rate (0.083 Gy per day) gamma exposure [U3] was very much less effective in inducing myeloid leukaemia in the female mice; no significant increase above controls could be reached even at 2.0 Gy. After acute and chronic neutron irradiation, the incidence of the disease was very low and did not permit any detailed study of dose-response relationships. In either case, the peak incidence was observed at 0.47 Gy, but the results were not significantly different from controls (p > 0.05).

2. Thymic lymphoma

242. Ullrich and Storer [U2, U3, U5, U20] studied the dose-response relationship and dose-rate effects for ^{137}Cs gamma rays and neutrons in SPF 10-week-old RFM/Un mice. The response was assessed as age-corrected incidence, standardized to the distribution of the age at death of control animals. In females, thymic lymphoma was efficiently induced by gamma rays at 0.45 Gy min^{-1}; the incidence was significantly higher than in controls in all groups receiving 0.25 Gy or more. No simple model could describe the response over the entire dose range (0.1-3 Gy). There was a steep rise in the region below 0.5 Gy, followed by a shallow rise at higher doses. Over the range of 0-0.25 Gy (three points), a dose-squared model provided an adequate fit and linearity could be rejected (P < 0.06). From 0.5 to 3 Gy the increase in incidence with dose was compatible with linearity.

243. In males, the significance of the difference above controls was reached only at 1 Gy. A linear model provided a satisfactory fit over the entire range of gamma-ray doses (0.1-3 Gy; P > 0.4). Over 0-1.5 Gy, both a linear and linear-quadratic equation (with D^2 coefficient not significant) provided a very good fit to the data (P > 0.95 and > 0.80, respectively). Thus, in males the dose-response relationship for acute gamma rays was predominantly linear over the entire dose range.

244. Lowering the dose rate to 0.083 Gy per day considerably decreased the incidence of thymic lymphoma in the females and changed the form of the curve from quadratic followed by linear to linear-quadratic with a negative linear component. Simple linearity could be rejected (P < 0.001). It is quite clear that in the RFM mouse, after low-LET exposure, there is no suggestion of the threshold-type response found by Kaplan and Brown [K33] in C57Bl mice. In these older data there was a statistically verified threshold in the dose-response relationship. As may be seen in Figure XVII (kindly provided by G. Walinder), fractionation of the dose into 1, 2, 4 or 8 fractions with one-day spacing, is without effect upon the incidence of the lymphoma. When plotted against exposure (either simple or fractionated) the incidence may be fitted by a linear function of the form I = aD − b where a = 0.112, and b = −21.6 (significantly different from zero); the coefficient of correlation is very high (0.903).

245. In experiments by Maisin et al. [M62], 12-week-old male BALB/c mice were exposed to single or to fractionated doses of ^{137}Cs gamma rays (10 equal doses separated by 1 day) in the dose range from 0.25 to 6 Gy. The dose-response curve for thymic lymphoma was of a threshold type, the actuarial incidence rising above control only at 4 and 6 Gy. Single doses were more effective at 4 than at 6 Gy.

246. Other data on thymic lymphoma induction by x rays in neonatal (C57Bl/6 JNrs × WHT/HC) F$_1$ mice were reported [S48]. Even though the incidence in females and males at three exposure points (200, 400 and 600 R) could be fitted to a linear-quadratic equation with a negative linear term (P > 0.80), the data adequately fit a threshold-type response such as that presented in Figure XVII for the C57Bl mice.

247. Fast neutrons (acutely delivered doses at 0.05 and 0.25 Gy min^{-1} and chronic doses at 0.01 Gy per day, with total doses between 0.1 and 3 Gy) induced thymic lymphoma in female RFM mice [U5]. In the range 0.25-0.5 Gy, the RBE with respect to high-dose-rate ^{137}Cs gamma rays was between 3 and 4. For acute neutron exposures, the dose-response curve was concave downward. In the range 0-0.94 Gy, linearity could be rejected (P > 0.001) and a good fit was obtained with the square root of the dose (P > 0.8). Up to 0.47 Gy, a linear fit was satisfactory (P > 0.75). For chronic neutron exposure, a linear fit adequately described the curve over the 0-0.94 Gy range (P > 0.8); and the loss of effectiveness over the acute exposures amounted to about 30%. However, there was a decrease of susceptibility to thymic lymphoma upon acute exposure with increasing age, so that the lower efficiency of the low-dose-rate exposure may in part be due to this latter factor alone. The RBE of acute neutron exposure relative to gamma rays varied proportionally to the inverse square root of neutron dose.

248. Induction of thymic lymphoma was also studied in male BALB/c mice irradiated at the age of 12 weeks with d(50)Be neutrons (modal energy about 23 MeV) [M63] at doses from 0.02 to 3 Gy. The actuarial incidence of thymic lymphoma fitted the same sigmoidal threshold-type curve found for ^{137}Cs gamma rays [M62].

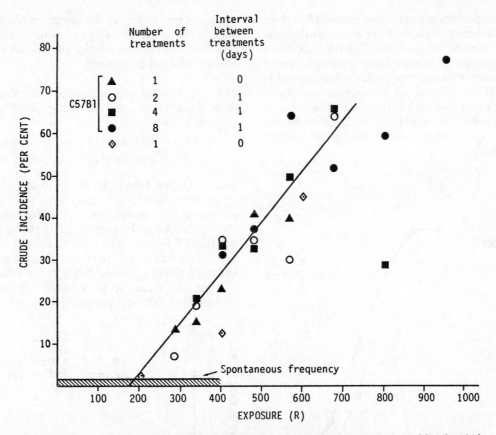

Figure XVII. Crude incidence of thymic lymphoma in C57Bl mice given single and fractionated x-ray doses at 1 day interval [K33]. Rhombard symbols represent the crude incidence of thymic lymphoma in neo-natal (C57B1/6 JNrs × WHT/Ht) F₁ mice [S48].

3. Other reticular tumours

249. The so-called mouse reticulum cell sarcoma is a group of neoplasms showing a decline of the incidence with dose after whole-body x irradiation [C19, K25, U3, U5, U20]. Ullrich and Storer [U3, U5, U20] studied the age-corrected incidence of reticulum cell sarcoma among SPF RFM/Un male and female mice irradiated with gamma rays (0.45 Gy min⁻¹ or 0.083 Gy per day) and in RFM/Un female and BALB/c mice irradiated with fast neutrons (0.05, 0.25 Gy min⁻¹ and 0.01 Gy per day). All treatments produced a decrease of reticulum cell sarcoma with dose, neutrons being more effective than gamma rays, and chronic exposures less effective than acute ones. The difference between acutely and chronically delivered gamma rays was more pronounced than that for neutrons. There was a clear, inverse relationship between the increase of thymic lymphoma and the decrease of reticulum cell sarcoma, suggesting some link between various radiation-induced reticular neoplasms which could greatly affect the observed dose-response curves.

250. Male mice (C57BL/Cne × C3H/Cne)F₁ hybrids received lethal whole-body irradiation (9 Gy) and were rescued from early death due to haematological failure by a homologous bone-marrow graft [C18]. In these mice, the spontaneous incidence of reticulum cell sarcoma of about 50% is reduced in irradiated survivors to a few per cent. Shielding of a part of the marrow during exposure affords a similar protection against early post-irradiation death and effectively depresses the incidence of the tumour. It was suggested that whole-body irradiation sterilizes cells from which these neoplasms originate [C18, C19] and that the D_0 for these cells is similar to that for the bone-marrow stem cells [M20].

251. Further studies [M20] showed that in vivo irradiation of the bone-marrow graft with doses of 2 and 4 Gy of x rays before transplantation into hosts given whole-body irradiation (9 Gy) provides the same protection against early death, but leads to a significantly elevated incidence of reticulum cell sarcoma in animals given irradiated marrow. The incidence expressed per number of injected marrow cells rises with dose, amounting to $1.65 \cdot 10^{-8}$, $1.90 \cdot 10^{-8}$ and $2.38 \cdot 10^{-8}$ tumours per cell irradiated with 0, 2 and 4 Gy. When related to the number of injected surviving stem cells, the incidence rose steeply from $4.3 \cdot 10^{-5}$ through $9.7 \cdot 10^{-4}$ and $6.4 \cdot 10^{-3}$ at 0, 2 and 4 Gy, respectively. It is an unproved assumption that the tumours originated from these cells. If this hypothesis could be accepted, the dose-response would display a pronounced curvilinearity (concave upwards), the effect rising with a power of dose appreciably greater than 1, and even the presence of a threshold dose could not be rejected.

252. In the same animal model, studies [M19] were made on whole-body irradiated mice with shielding of one or two hind legs, from which shielding was removed for a variable fraction of irradiation time, thus exposing some of the protected marrow in situ to graded doses of x rays up to 8 Gy. The observed

incidence of reticulum cell sarcomas increased in these mice to a maximum at about 5 Gy and then declined with further increase of the dose. The final incidence of these neoplasms in all experiments with exogenous and endogenous bone-marrow protection is plotted in Figure XVIII, showing in all instances a curvilinear (upward concave) rise with x-ray dose. The form of these relationships is similar to that observed for many other radiation-induced tumours in animals irradiated in vivo.

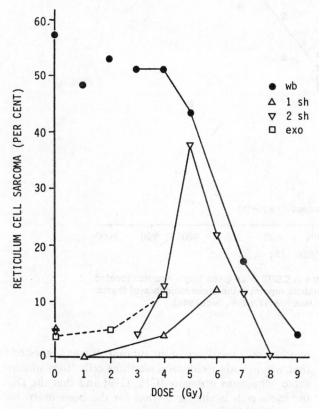

Figure XVIII. Final incidence of reticulum cell sarcoma as a function of dose under three different experimental conditions: (a) whole-body irradiation (wb); (b) shielding of one (1 sh) or two (2 sh) hind legs; (c) syngenic bone marrow transplantation (exo). [M19]

4. Tumours of the thyroid

253. An extensive study of thyroid tumour induction by 250-kVp x rays and ^{131}I in about 3000 6-week-old female Long-Evans rats was reported by Lee et al. [L29]. The study aimed at comparing the effectiveness of the two radiations delivered at different dose rates (2.8 Gy min^{-1} for x rays; the maximum dose rates for ^{131}I in individual groups were estimated at 0.17, 0.69 and 1.6 mGy min^{-1}). Local doses of x rays to the thyroid were 0.94, 4.1 and 10.6 Gy. Total doses delivered by ^{131}I were estimated at 0.8, 3.3 and 8.5 Gy. The role of pituitary irradiation in the induction of thyroid cancer was also explored by delivering doses of 4.1 Gy of x rays to the pituitary alone, or to the thyroid and the pituitary together: findings were negative in this respect.

254. Tumours included were those that appeared later than 6 months in rats dying before the age of 26 months and in animals sacrificed at 24 months. The

results were given as incidence corrected for the slightly enhanced mortality of irradiated versus control rats. Data on tumour multiplicity and on tumours per animal were not presented.

255. A least square fit yielded the following functions describing the dose-response relationships (Figure XIX):

$$I(D) = 7.47 \ 10^{-4} \ (D + 10)^{0.6838} \text{ for x rays}$$
$$I(D) = 1.78 \ 10^{-3} \ (D + 10)^{0.5348} \text{ for } ^{131}I$$

where D is the dose given in rad (0.01 Gy). The exponents were significantly lower than unity (p < 0.001), indicating that the incidence of thyroid carcinomas in these rats rose with approximately the square root of the low-LET dose. Thus, there was no difference in the effectiveness of the two radiations over the observed range of doses, but a lower effectiveness of ^{131}I per unit dose (up to a factor $\simeq$ 3) could not be excluded on statistical grounds [N10].

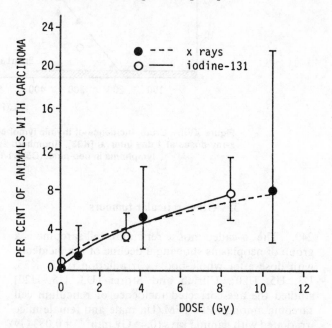

Figure XIX. Incidence of thyroid carcinoma as a function of mean thyroid dose from injected iodine-131 and localized x irradiation. Error bars are estimates of the 95% confidence limits. [L29]

256. For adenomas, the two dose-response relationships were slightly different (p < 0.01) and when fitted by exponential equations they assumed the following forms:

$$I(D) = 0.0245 \exp (0.00207 \ D) \text{ for x rays}$$
$$I(D) = 0.0240 \exp (0.00123 \ D) \text{ for } ^{131}I,$$

where D is the dose in rad (0.01 Gy). At no dose point was there a significant difference between the effect of the two radiations. However, due to the large variability of the observations, some difference in the effectiveness could not be excluded. Control incidence of medullary tumours was not affected by either radiation.

257. The downward concavity of the dose-incidence curve for carcinomas was attributed to killing of initiated cells. If an in vivo survival curve of thyroid

follicular cells with $D_q = 4.9$ Gy and $D_0 = 4.5$ Gy is assumed [D15, M51], then the dose-response curve for initiation of carcinomas or adenomas in this experiment may be expected to rise with a power of dose either close to or greater than unity. The slope of the initial portion of the dose-incidence curve for carcinomas was estimated at $1.9 \cdot 10^{-2}$ Gy^{-1}, which is close to the estimate for humans [S60].

258. The presence of a strong linear component in the relationships is suggested by the absence of a clear dose-rate effect, at least in young animals. This observation contradicts previous findings (reviewed in [D16, W12]) that, per unit dose, x rays are more efficient for thyroid tumour induction than ^{131}I. The study reviewed here [L29] differs from the older ones in two important aspects: first, the range of doses is below 10 Gy, and thus cell killing and other non-stochastic effects would not be expected to prevail; second, the number of animals used is large and gives the study good statistical credibility. Nevertheless, the findings refer only to one sex of one particular strain of rats. These experiments do not support the suggestion [R29] that irradiation of the pituitary gland may give rise to increased incidence of thyroid cancers in children irradiated for treatment of tinea capitis.

5. Mammary tumours

259. The age-corrected incidence of mammary adenocarcinomas was studied in SPF female BALB/c mice after high- and low-dose-rate exposure to gamma rays [U3, U25] as well as to high-dose-rate, low-dose-rate and fractionated exposures to fission neutrons [U4, U25, U26]. After acute gamma-ray exposure (doses 0.1-2 Gy) the incidence increased rapidly over the range 0-0.25 Gy, with a rather irregular plateau appearing at higher doses. The irregular response was consistent with the models $I(D) = 7.7 + 35 D + 150 D^2$ $(P > 0.4)$ for the high dose rate and with $I(D) = 7.7 + 35 D$ $(P > 0.4)$ for the low dose rate, in accordance with the linear-quadratic model. Ramzaev et al. [R1] described a "supra-linear" response for induction of mammary adenocarcinoma in mice irradiated over ten generations through constant feeding of ^{137}Cs and ^{90}Sr.

260. Acute irradiation of BALB/c mice with fission neutrons (0.05-0.25 Gy min^{-1}) [U25] yielded a dose-response that was downward concave over the range 0-0.5 Gy (the lowest dose being 0.025 Gy) and would be poorly described by a linear model. A good fit was obtained by a model $I(D) = 7.9 + 27 \sqrt{D}$ $(P > 0.85)$. In the range 0-0.1 Gy, the response could be well fitted by a linear model $I(D) = 7.9 + 114 D$.

261. When fission neutron exposures were split into two equal fractions delivered 24 hours and 30 days apart [U26], there was no difference with respect to the single dose-response for the 24-hour interval, but for the 30-day interval there was an increase of about 30-40% only for the highest dose tested (0.5 Gy). In the latter case, the curve was still bending over in the range 0-0.2 Gy. Protracted irradiation (0.01-0.1 Gy per day) led to a significant enhancement of the effect

relative to the acute exposure, and over the whole range of doses. This was interpreted either as a promoting effect or as stimulation of progression of the growth of malignant clones. The maximum RBE of neutrons was 33; this was calculated as a ratio of the linear slope for the gamma and neutron curves (for single irradiation at low dose rates).

262. Two-month-old female, Sprague-Dawley rats were followed by Shellabarger et al. [S37] for their entire life span after single exposures to 250-kVp x rays (0.28, 0.56 and 0.85 Gy) and 430-keV neutrons (0.001, 0.004, 0.016 and 0.064 Gy). The animals were observed for appearance of adenocarcinomas and fibroadenomas. In all irradiated groups the tumour rate increased steeply with age and the effect of irradiation could be described as a forward shift in time of the spontaneous age-specific tumour rate.

263. The response was expressed separately for carcinomas and adenomas as mortality-corrected prevalence and cumulative tumour rate [R(t,D)]. The fibroadenoma and total mammary tumour responses were approximately proportional to x-ray dose over all times, while neutrons produced a downward concave relationship, rising with a power of neutron dose less than unity. The increase in R(t,D) was significant even at 1 mGy of neutrons and the forward shift of the prevalence, corrected for age-specific mortality, caused by this dose was equivalent to 35 days. The R(t,D) for fibroadenomas at 800 days was less curvilinear than at 1 year after exposure. The distribution of tumours was non-random among the animals (over-dispersion was noted relative to Poisson distribution). The response for adenocarcinomas was statistically uncertain, owing to the small number of tumours involved, but linearity is the best approximation to the dose-response relationship.

264. In this study [S37], the RBE varied roughly with the inverse square root of the neutron dose. At the highest doses studied it exceeded 10; at the lower end of the dose scale, it approached a value of 100. The implications of these observations were already discussed in chapter II.

265. In other experiments [V9], female Sprague-Dawley rats were acutely exposed whole-body to fission neutrons, or to protracted doses of 0.02, 0.06 and 0.5 Gy (over 242 hours in one month). The prevalence of mammary tumours at 10 months after exposure increased, relative to single irradiation, at all doses tested. Protraction of gamma-ray exposures (150, 300, 450 R) in a similar pattern reduced significantly the prevalence seen after corresponding single exposures. The RBE values for neutrons, measured at 20% prevalence, were 16 and 68 for acute and chronic irradiation, respectively.

266. Breast tumours (histology not specified) in young female Sprague-Dawley rats were studied [G35] after acute (over one hour) and chronic (over 10 days) x irradiation, as well as after internal irradiation by tritium, administered as tritiated water (75 and 90% of total dose delivered over 10 and 20 days, respectively). The doses of 200-kVp x rays varied from 0.29 to 2 Gy,

and those of tritium from 0.5 to 4 Gy. The competitive-risk-corrected tumour rate was calculated up to 450 days after the start of exposure and the integral values were linearly related to dose for all three irradiation modes. The effectiveness of tritium per unit dose did not differ from that for the chronic x-ray exposure. The latter produced effects similar to those of acute exposure at 0.6 Gy, but was 25-30% less effective at about 1.8 Gy.

267. X-ray-induced and neutron-induced (0.43 MeV) mammary tumours were studied in weanling, virgin female ACI rats [S52], irradiated at 88-89 days. The doses for x rays ranged from 0.17 to 3 Gy and for neutrons from 0.01 to 0.36 Gy. The animals were irradiated either 2 days after implantation of a pellet containing 5 mg of diethylstilbestrol (DES) or without prior hormonal treatment. Fibroadenomas and adeno-carcinomas were diagnosed histologically and recorded separately. DES greatly increased the incidence of spontaneous and radiation-induced adenocarcinomas in this strain, which has a low spontaneous incidence of mammary neoplasms. Significant excess prevalence was detected in DES-treated rats even at the lowest neutron dose; for x rays, the significance occurred at 0.17 Gy. The RBE varied inversely with the square root of the dose and approached a value of 100 at the lowest end of the range.

268. Appearance of tumours in rats not treated with DES was followed, on the average, to about 750 days after irradiation. For x rays, the cumulative tumour rate at 600 days (for the sum or for each type of tumour separately) rose almost linearly with the dose. The same applied to adenocarcinomas after neutron irradiation, but for fibroadenomas a downward con-cave relationship could not be excluded. The RBE of neutrons for the sum of tumours tended to decrease with dose over the range of doses tested, but did not vary much from an average value of 10. The length of tumour-free life lost due to the sum of benign and malignant tumours was a linear function of dose, for both x rays and neutrons, and for the whole range of doses tested.

269. When non-inbred female rats were irradiated externally, with single, increasing doses of β rays from a ^{90}Sr + ^{90}Y source, the rise of the crude incidence of mammary carcinoma was linear with dose, up to 4 Gy [M68, M71]. These animals were also irradiated, starting at the age of 8 weeks, singly, with doses of 16 Gy (from the published text it appears likely that the doses refer to the surface of the body); daily (5 days a week) at 0.8 Gy per day for 4 weeks; or once every two weeks with 0.8 Gy over a period of 39 weeks. The observed life shortening differed signi-ficantly from the control value, but not between groups with various irradiation schemes. There was an obvious acceleration of the appearance of mammary tumours after irradiation, and the fractionated schemes were slightly less effective, although this difference could be accounted for by the fact that, on average, the fractionated exposures were delivered somewhat later in life. The crude incidence over lifetime was elevated in all irradiated groups to 100% from 40% in controls. This experiment [M71] supports the notion

that fractionation of low-LET radiation has little effect upon the incidence of mammary tumours in rats.

270. Other authors reported that mammary tumours were also induced in female Sprague-Dawley and in WAG/Rij rats by x rays, and by monoenergetic 0.5-MeV and 15-MeV neutrons [B86, B92]. There was no evidence that a virus played any role in mammary carcinogenesis in these animals. The rats were 8 weeks old when irradiation was started with fractionated doses or given as single doses (absorbed doses in the glands). They were kept until their death, and the frequency of fibroadenomas and carcinomas was based on histological examination.

271. The probability of animals surviving without evidence of a tumour was calculated according to the Kaplan and Meier life-table analysis. Weibull func-tions were fitted to these data and showed that irradiation caused an acceleration in the appearance of fibroadenomas and carcinomas in both strains of rats. X-ray fractionation (10×0.2 Gy at one-month intervals) in WAG/Rij rats was marginally less effec-tive, in respect of the appearance time of mammary carcinomas, than a single dose of 2 Gy. Fractionation of 0.25 Gy of neutron into 10 equal fractions at one-month intervals was also without a significant effect relative to 1×0.25 Gy.

272. When dose-response relationships were calcu-lated from actuarial incidence data at 95 weeks of age, the results for carcinomas in WAG/Rij rats for x rays and 0.5 MeV neutrons showed such a wide scatter as to preclude unequivocal inferences about the character of dose-response relationship. For fibroadenomas (Figure XX) the response for x rays (0.25-4 Gy) was proportional to dose. The response for 0.5 and 15 MeV neutrons (0.025-0.8 or 1.6 Gy, respectively) showed a saturation effect. In Sprague Dawley rats, the actuarial incidence of fibroadenomas showed

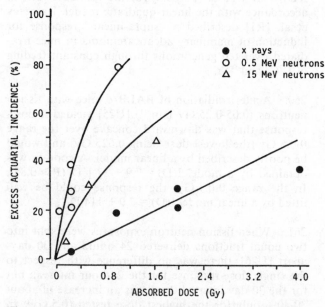

Figure XX. Actuarial incidence at 92 weeks of age of mammary adenomas in WAG/Rij rats as a function of dose for various types of radiation.
[B92]

saturation effects at high doses of all radiations. The RBE of neutrons was much lower than that observed in other studies on the same strain [S37, S52]. Carcinomas were so rare that no dose-response relationship could be established.

273. When the prevalence of mammary adenocarcinomas was studied at 10 months after x-ray exposure (200 R) in female Sprague-Dawley rats irradiated as young virgins or as pregnant, lactating or post-lactating animals [H23], no effect of the physiological state upon the incidence could be found. This result is at variance with the age-effect seen in women (see chapter V).

274. Numerous studies show that several factors may influence the development of radiation-induced mammary tumours in various strains of rats. Some of these studies were considered in annex L of the 1982 UNSCEAR report [U24]. A strong influence of genetic factors on neutron-induced mammary carcinogenesis was reported by Vogel et al. [V10]. After a single dose of 0.5 Gy from fission neutrons, the highest (56%) prevalence at 1 year after exposure was seen in Sprague-Dawley and Long-Evans females; the lowest (5%) was observed in Wistar, and an intermediate one (25-29%) in Buffalo and Fischer-344 rats. Wide variation in susceptibility to mammary tumour induction was also found by Broerse et al. [B86, B92] for Sprague-Dawley, WAG/Rij and BN/BiRij rats.

6. Lung cancer

275. Lung adenocarcinomas were induced in BALB/c female mice by gamma irradiation at 0.45 Gy min^{-1} and at 0.083 Gy per day in the dose range 0.1-2 Gy [U2, U3, U25]. After acute exposure, the age-corrected incidence could be related to dose by a linear [I(D) = 10.9 + 11 D; (P > 0.7)] or a linear-quadratic model [I(D) = 11.9 + 4.1 D + 4.3 D^2 (P > 0.7)]. At low dose rate, the dose-response relationship was linear with the same slope [I(D) = 12.5 + 4.3 D (P > 8)] as at high dose rate in the linear-quadratic model. This model, therefore, seems to describe adequately the response in question.

276. After single acute exposure to fission neutrons (doses 0.025-2 Gy; 0.05-0.25 Gy min^{-1}), the relationship was downward concave with a maximum at 0.5 Gy [U25]. Over the range 0-0.5 Gy the data were consistent with a square-root model [(D) = 13.6 + 29 $\sqrt{D}$ (P > 0.7)]. A linear model could not be rejected but was obviously unlikely. In the ranges 0-0.2 Gy, the data were fitted by a linear model [I(D) = 14.7 + 76 D (P > 0.7)]. When the doses were split into two equal fractions, no difference was seen for 24-hour fractionation [U26]. A slight increase of the incidences was noted for 30-day fractionation, but only at the highest dose of 0.5 Gy. For this irradiation mode the dose-response became practically linear up to 0.5 Gy.

277. Protracted neutron irradiation (8.3 10^{-5} Gy per day and 8.3 10^{-6} Gy per day) was more effective than the high-dose-rate exposure and, as in the case of 30-day fractionation more nearly linear over the

entire dose range [U26]. Higher effectiveness for 0.5 Gy at chronic and at 30-day fractionated exposure is unlikely to result from repair of sub-transformation damage, as no repair was seen for fractionation over 24 hours. The effect was attributed to repopulation of alveolar target cells. The maximum RBE of neutrons from the ratio of the linear slopes at low doses was 18.5. When derived from the square root of the dose model, it equalled 70.7/$\sqrt{D_n}$.

278. Chmelevsky et al. [C34] analysed the induction of lung carcinoma in male Sprague-Dawley rats which were 90-days old at the start of an exposure to radon in equilibrium with its short-lived daughter products. The radon concentrations and the duration of daily or weekly exposure were varied. The total duration of the inhalation period was kept within one to six months. The dose was defined as a product of potential alpha energy concentration and exposure time, and expressed in working level months (WLM^c); the range of dose covered zero to 14,000 WLM delivered at various rates.

279. Animals were studied at death for the presence and histology of lung neoplasms. In this species, lung cancer is almost never a cause of death; therefore independence between disease and death could be assumed and the data could be treated as fully censored. The prevalence of neoplasms as a function of time was estimated for each exposure group by non-parametric methods in the form of a monotonically increasing function (by a most-likelihood fit). Three models were selected for fitting prevalence to dose: a time shift, an acceleration, and a proportional hazard model. The fit of the data to all three models was equally good; none could be discarded on statistical grounds.

280. The crude and mortality-corrected incidence of lung carcinomas was calculated from the prevalence function up to 900 days. The results of the actuarial incidence are shown in Figure XXI. The initial slope (below 1000 WLM) is practically linear in both cases. When the incidence was fitted to a function of cumulative exposure E of the type I(t;E) = K E^p, the parameters obtained at t = 850 days were: K = (3.4 ± 1.4) 10^{-4} and p = 0.92 ± 0.07. When linearity was assumed to apply over this range of exposures, the proportionality coefficient was (2 ± 0.5) 10^{-4} per WLM. Perhaps by accident, these values are very similar to those found for man (chapter V). At doses above 3 10^3 WLM, the response flattens off. At doses above 4 10^3 WLM, the exposures at high dose rate (> 1600 WLM per month) are less effective in inducing tumours than those delivered at lower rates. The data do not suggest a threshold, which, if present, would have to be much lower than 65 WLM. The character of the dose-response relationship is basically similar to that seen

---

^{c}The concentration of potential alpha energy of short-lived radon-222 daughters is sometimes expressed in units of Working Level (WL). This level corresponds to any mixture of these daughters which, upon complete decay, will emit alpha particles with total energy of 1.3 10^5 MeV per litre of air (2.08 10^{-5} J m^{-3}). The Working Level Month (WLM) corresponds to exposure to a mean concentration of 1 WL for the reference period of 170 hours. 1 WLM = 170 WL hours = 2.2 10^4 MeV h m^{-3} = 3.5 10^{-3} J h m^{-3}.

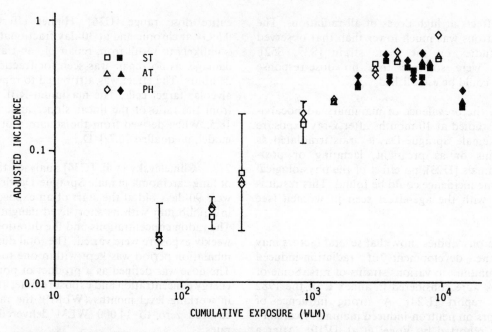

Figure XXI. Adjusted incidence of lung carcinoma in rats as a function of the cumulative exposure (WLM), calculated on the basis of three models: ST, time shift model; AT, accelerated time model; PH, proportional hazard model. Open symbols: exposure rate < 1600 WLM per month; Solid symbols: exposure rate > 1600 WLM per month.
[C34]

in uranium miners (chapter V). The loss of tumour-free life (the so-called "effect period" [U6]) was also studied in these rats as a function of cumulative exposure. Agreement between the models is less close than for the mortality-corrected incidence; however, linearity seems to prevail up to 1-2 10^3 WLM.

281. The actuarial incidence of lung carcinomas was studied [C38] in Sprague-Dawley rats, after whole-body irradiation with fission neutrons, and evaluated by methods of analysis similar to those described for radon-induced cancers [C34]. The neutron doses ranged from 0.012 to 8 Gy. The doses up to 2.3 Gy were delivered within 1 day and the higher doses were protracted over periods from 14 to 42 days to secure early survival of the animals. The time-related prevalence of pulmonary cancers was fitted to shifted-time and accelerated-time models and an actuarial incidence was calculated which did not depend upon the model chosen (Figure XXII). The dose-response

relationship could be linear up to about 0.5 Gy. At higher doses, the curve does flatten, but does not decrease (actually, the absence of a decrease is due to correction for life shortening). In the low-dose range, the efficiency of neutrons versus radon in inducing pulmonary carcinomas exceeded 3 WLM/mGy. At higher doses, it was lower. Recalculation of this ratio in terms of lung doses, rather than exposures, indicates that the efficiency of neutrons, relative to alpha particles, is about 14 when expressed in terms of the bronchial dose and about 2 in terms of dose to the **pulmonary parenchima [T3]**.

282. An exhaustive review of lung cancer induction by inhalation of various radionuclides in different animal species was compiled by an ICRP Task Group and published as ICRP Publication 31 [I3]. When the data from various experimental series were combined for an analysis of dose-response relationships a very wide scatter was apparent. Whereas for various alpha-emitting transuranic nuclides a linear fit to the data did not appear unreasonable, a linear dose-response relationship did not adequately describe the experimental points obtained for beta and gamma emitters. For these an upward concave dose-response relationship was typical.

7. Lung adenomas

283. Induction of benign lung adenomas in RF mice was studied [Y1] by locally-delivered, acute doses of x rays of between 2.5 and 15 Gy. The dose-response curve for tumours recorded 12 months thereafter, when plotted on a log-log scale, had a slope of 1 below 7.5 Gy and a steeper increase of the tumour yield at higher doses. In terms of a linear-quadratic model, this would imply induction of tumours by single-track kinetics in the lower portion of the curve

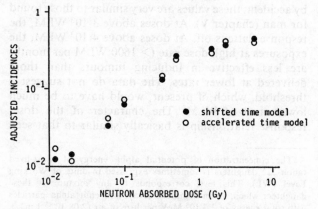

Figure XXII. Adjusted incidence of lung carcinomas in neutron-irradiated male Sprague-Dawley rats.
[C38]

and two-track kinetics in the steeper region of the relationship. A split-dose experiment with fractionation intervals of 24 hours confirmed that the number of adenomas per animal was lowered by fractionation, but only above 7.5 Gy, where repair of interacting lesions would, theoretically, be expected.

284. Induction of lung adenomas by localized irradiation of the thorax with 300-kVp x rays and fast neutrons was also studied in 10-12-week-old female SPF RFM/Un mice [U21]. After 0.5 Gy of neutrons, the number of tumours per mouse at 6 months did not increase further and it was assumed that by 9 months it should have been complete. The doses of x rays ranged from 1 to 9 Gy and of neutrons from 0.05 to 1.5 Gy. The level of mortality did not influence the results substantially. For acute x irradiation, linearity could be excluded and the dose-response curve could be described by: (a) a linear-quadratic model with an initial negative linear slope (P > 0.90); and (b) a threshold model of the form $P(t;D) = c + a (D - D^*)^2$ (P > 0.99), where D^* is the threshold dose, estimated to be 2.47 Gy. For neutrons, the average number of adenomas per mouse rose about linearly to 0.25 Gy, peaked at 1 Gy, and then declined by a factor of about 2 toward 1.5 Gy. Over the range 0-0.25 Gy, the rise was approximately linear (P > 0.50). A proportionality to $\sqrt{D}$ could be rejected over this range (P < 0.05). Also a linear threshold model with threshold dose at about 0.07 Gy described the response within the range 0-0.25 Gy very well (P > 0.99). For the linear model, the RBE of neutrons increased from a value of 25 at 0.15 Gy neutrons to one of 40 at 0.01 Gy.

285. Splitting of the dose of either radiation into two equal fractions separated by 24 hours or 30 days was also tested [U22]. Under these conditions, there was a reduction in tumour yield for x-ray doses above 4.0 Gy, and the response tended to become more nearly linear. There was no difference between responses with doses split by 24 hours or 30 days. Recovery was complete by 24 hours, and amounted to 50% of the initial effect. After split neutron irradiation, no recovery could be seen. Linearity for all data combined over the range 0-0.25 Gy could not be rejected (P > 0.8), but better fits were obtained with a dose-squared model (P > 0.99) or with a model using a threshold dose at about 0.054 Gy. If it is accepted that decline of the tumour yield at high doses reflects killing of potentially transformed cells, then linearity over the range 0-0.25 Gy becomes rather improbable, as already discussed in chapter II. However, an alternative explanation of the slight upwards concave curvilinearity in the 0-0.25 Gy range could be a possible inverse relationship between latency and dose.

8. Ovarian tumours

286. Induction of ovarian tumours by x rays and neutrons was studied by Ullrich et al. [U2] using SPF RFM mice. An acute gamma-ray exposure (0.4 Gy min^{-1}) induced various types of ovarian tumours, and their age-corrected incidence increased rapidly over the dose range 0-0.5 Gy. At higher doses, there was a plateau of the response with a marginal rise of tumour incidence with increasing doses. Over the range 0-0.5 Gy linear and dose-squared non-threshold models could be rejected (P < 0.01) while a linear-quadratic model with a negative linear component adequately described the relationship (P > 0.25). Since, according to the authors, no biological meaning could be attributed to such a model, threshold models were tested and a linear one was again rejected (P < 0.01). However, a threshold dose-squared model (threshold estimated to be 0.12 Gy) provided a satisfactory fit (P > 0.75) over the dose range up to 0.5 Gy. At 0.08 Gy per day, a significant incidence was seen at 1 Gy, where it corresponded to that seen after 0.25 Gy acute exposure. Again, non-threshold linear and dose-squared models could be rejected (P < 0.01) as well as the threshold dose-squared one. An adequate fit was obtained for a threshold linear model with a threshold dose of 0.7 Gy and a linear-quadratic model with an initial negative linear slope (significantly negative at the 5% level).

287. After neutron irradiation [U5], the ovarian tumour incidence in RFM mice was lower at 0.01 Gy per day than at 0.05 and 0.25 Gy min^{-1} for all dose levels. The decline was attributed partly to the reduction of the dose rate and partly to an age-related decrease of susceptibility. This suggests that a true dose-rate effect was perhaps observed in this tumour system after high-LET irradiation.

288. Ullrich [U23, U25, U26] studied the age-corrected incidence of all ovarian tumours (granulosa cell tumours, luteomas, tubular adenomas) in BALB/c female mice, induced by gamma radiation and fission neutrons. High-dose-rate gamma irradiation (in the range 0.1-2 Gy) increased the incidence steeply from control levels (about 2.5%) at 0.1 Gy to 77% at 0.5 Gy, with a plateau at higher doses. As previously observed for RFM mice, the dose-response relationship was consistent with a threshold model, and the linear, dose-squared and linear-quadratic models could be rejected (P < 0.01). Irradiation of BALB/c mice with fission neutrons (0.025-2 Gy) led to a steep increase in the incidence of ovarian tumours from control level at 0.025 up to 76% at 0.5 Gy, with a slight decline towards 2 Gy. Over the dose range 0-0.5 Gy, a variety of dose-response models could describe the data, including the non-threshold models (linear-quadratic, dose-squared) and a threshold-type model. The linear non-threshold model could, however, be rejected (P < 0.01). A threshold model would be consistent with both the postulated role of non-stochastic mechanisms involved and the data for gamma radiation. Because of the apparent threshold, at low doses any estimate of RBE is meaningless. From 0.2 Gy upwards the RBE is close to unity [U25]. Splitting the neutron dose at 24-hour and 30-day intervals was ineffective, the data being practically indistinguishable from the single-dose series. At protracted exposures, the neutrons were less effective than when delivered acutely but, for instance, 0.4 Gy yielded the same result whether delivered over 4 or 40 days. This indicates that the difference with regard to acute exposure is a true dose-rate effect and not a change of susceptibility to tumour induction with age. The observation is similar to that for the RFM mouse, but no explanation is available.

289. In other experiments [Y2], mice received a series of x-ray doses over a variable time T and the animals were followed for incidence of ovarian tumours. The results were later re-analysed [K8] on the assumption that the cumulative net incidence (prevalence) is described by the equation

$$F(t) = f[a_1 D + q(T)D^2] \qquad (4.1)$$

where the form of the function is left undecided and $q(T)$ is a reduction factor for recovery of the damage with protraction of irradiation. The optimal fit to the data was obtained for an assumed exponential decay of the sublesions $T = 15$ h. The optimum value for a_1 for the linear term was zero, and a_1/a_2 quotients greater than 0.04 Gy in terms of the linear-quadratic model could be excluded when data were corrected for time-dependent repair using non-linear optimization. In essence, no linear component could be found, and incidence was proportional to the square of the dose over a wide dose range.

9. Pituitary gland tumours

290. In female RFM mice, pituitary tumours increased irregularly with gamma-ray dose over the range 0.05 to 3 Gy (0.45 Gy min^{-1}) and the age-corrected incidence was not significantly different from control. A linear-quadratic response adequately described the data ($P > 0.6$), but a linear response could not be excluded ($P > 0.2$) [U2]. In male mice, the effect was so slight that the dose-response could not be investigated. Lowering the dose rate (0.083 Gy per day) caused a less efficient induction of pituitary tumours in the same mice [U3]. If a linear-quadratic response was assumed at high dose rate, the linear component was very similar under both conditions and the lower dose rate eliminated the contribution of the dose-squared component. Neutrons induced a large number of pituitary tumours with an RBE greater than 5. A dose rate of 0.01 Gy per day appeared as effective as 0.05 and 0.25 Gy min^{-1} up to 0.2 Gy, but rather less effective at 0.47 and 2 Gy.

10. Harderian gland tumours

291. These tumours were induced by gamma rays in both male and female RFM mice, and the response in the two sexes was very similar. The data on age-adjusted incidence appeared to fit best a linear-quadratic model ($P > 0.25$ and > 0.99 for females and males, respectively), but linearity could be excluded only for females ($P > 0.05$). The low-dose-rate gamma irradiation substantially reduced the incidence of tumours, and a good fit ($P > 0.90$) to the equation was obtained with the same linear coefficient as for high dose rate but without a dose-squared term [U2, U3]. The same tumours showed a marked sensitivity to induction by neutrons, with an approximately linear increase in age-adjusted incidence as a function of dose up to about 0.5 Gy, with a plateau at 1 Gy and a decline at 2 Gy. No significant effect of the dose rate was observed [U5]. When the age-adjusted incidence of harderian gland tumours was studied in whole-body x-irradiated CBA mice [D3] it was found

that the dose-response curve rose as a function of dose up to 3 Gy (there were, however, only 3 points) and then became flat. Correction of these data for cell killing (a survival curve was determined independently) resulted in a dose-response curve per surviving cell which rose with the square of the dose between 1 and 7 Gy.

11. Skin tumours

292. Skin cancer can be induced in experimental animals, mostly CBA mice and CD rats, by both densely- and sparsely-ionizing radiation, and relevant experiments were reviewed in the 1972 and 1977 UNSCEAR reports [U6, U7]. For both species, highly curvilinear dose-response relationships were reported for β particles and high-energy electrons [B59, H12, H13] as well as for accelerated (40 MeV) helium nuclei, which also produced a curvilinear response in CD rats [B59]. From detailed considerations of depth-dose distribution versus efficiency of cancer induction, and from the association of the latter with damage to the hair follicles, it was concluded that radiation-induced skin cancer in this latter strain is likely to originate from cells located in the follicles.

293. The induction of epidermal and dermal skin tumours was again studied in 3-month-old female CBA/CaH mice (3125 exposed, 612 controls), irradiated locally over one-third of their skin surface (mid-torso) by β particles emitted from a ^{204}Tl source [H33]. The radiation neither penetrated the abdominal wall nor reached the bone marrow. Tumorigenic doses were taken to be 75% of the nominal dose at the body surface for epidermal tumours, and 65% for dermal ones. The nominal doses ranged from 5.4 to 260 Gy, and the dose rate varied from 2 to 0.017 Gy min^{-1}. Most tumours arose well within the irradiated area and only a few at the edge. Over 70% of all tumours were dermal (fibromas and fibrosarcomas), and about 60% of the dermal and epidermal ones were malignant. It was confirmed histologically that fibromas could become malignant, and multiple tumours were noted in 12-15% of tumour-bearing mice irradiated at the highest rates. The incidence of tumours was expressed per unit area of skin. Reduction of dose rate from 1-2 to 0.11-0.22 Gy min^{-1} did not alter the incidence appreciably; at 0.05-0.08 Gy min^{-1}, the incidence of epidermal tumours was reduced at all except the highest doses (120 Gy).

294. The incidence of dermal tumours began to increase significantly with doses to the dermis of about 16 Gy and rose steeply into a plateau above 60 Gy. The incidence of epidermal tumours increased significantly and then rose steeply when the dose in the epidermis exceeded 21 Gy. The peak incidence was reached at 60 or 100-120 Gy and fell at still higher doses. At exposure rates of 0.017-0.024 Gy min^{-1}, no epidermal tumours occurred and the incidence of dermal tumours was very much reduced. At lower rates, therefore, a range of high doses was ineffective in producing skin tumours. The dose-response curve resembled those typical of non-stochastic effects, with an apparent threshold at about 10 Gy.

295. The series irradiated at the highest dose rate (1.1-2.2 Gy min^{-1}) had sufficient statistical power to distinguish between various dose-response models. The observed incidence was fitted to a series of models incorporating both initiation and cell-killing terms at various powers of dose, as well as threshold doses [P21]. From a rather elaborate analysis it was concluded that only one non-threshold model could not be discarded, and this was for induction of epidermal tumours with a very high exponent of dose (about 4) in the induction term. The incidence above apparent thresholds usually rose very steeply with dose. The authors suggested that the apparent thresholds may be due to some relatively radioresistant factor in the skin that restrains potential tumour cells, and that this factor can be overcome by very high doses, and also perhaps by aging.

296. In CD rats, the incidence of tumours over the ascending part of the curve rose roughly with the fourth power of the electron dose [B59, H12, H13] and with the square of the dose of alpha particles [B59]. However, these conclusions are only approximate, because the data were insufficient for more detailed analysis. The value of the RBE of alpha particles at about 1 tumour per animal, relative to high energy electrons, was roughly 3. The peak incidence of skin tumours always occurred at several tens of Gy of sparsely-ionizing radiation.

297. Fractionation of the electron dose [B57, B58] showed that suboncogenic damage was repaired with a half-time of about 4 hours. This observation suggested that the repair process was operating at the cellular level, as for sublethal damage. Experiments on the influence of dose fractionation were also made with 10-MeV protons [B56]: when fractions were separated by 24 hours, a reduction of the effect was interpreted as showing complete repair of recoverable damage. It was concluded, therefore, that for skin tumour in CD rats 10-MeV protons have the usual characteristics of both high- and low-LET radiation: an RBE of about 3, typical for the former, but recovery at fractionation and yield of the effect proportional to a power of dose greater than one, typical for sparsely-ionizing radiation.

298. It is difficult to say to what extent skin cancer induction in rats is an adequate model—qualitatively or quantitatively—for man. A relatively low sensitivity of human skin to cancer induction by radiation was noted in annex G of the 1977 UNSCEAR report [U6] and in the BEIR III Report [C29]. On the other hand, histogenesis of most skin cancers in rodents is different from those of the human skin [L8]. Albert, Burns and Shore [A4] suggested that radiation-induced cancers in CD rats, and in children irradiated for tinea capitis, show similarities in the distribution of the latent periods when time is normalized for both species to their mean life spans. However, the fractions of total skin surface irradiated were different in animals and in children, so that any similarity could be fortuitous.

299. On the basis of data in CD rats, Vanderlaan et al. [V1] proposed a mathematical model of skin cancer induction by ionizing radiation. The model is based on the hypothesis that radiation can initiate a cancer by converting normal cells (S_1) to potentially malignant cells by one of two routes: a reversible route involving two steps ($S_1 \rightarrow S_2 \rightarrow S_3$, the reversible stage being S_2) and an irreversible single-step process ($S_1 \rightarrow S_3$). It was assumed that the initiation process takes place in single cells but its nature was not specified. Cells in the intermediate stage S_2 can revert to the normal state S_1 at a rate λ assumed to be constant and independent of dose. The probability of developing carcinoma of the skin was assumed to be proportional to the number of irreversibly transformed cells S_3. Expression of the latter as a function of time after irradiation was obtained from solution of a pair of differential equations. The solution showed that the relationship of cumulative incidence versus dose was dominated by the dose-squared component. In this model, the relative values of the linear and squared components are not predicted by LET or any other microdosimetric consideration. From experimental observations, Vanderlaan et al. [V1] concluded that, after a dose-independent tumour-free interval, throughout the remaining life span the tumours appear at an approximately constant rate, directly proportional to the dose. However, the experimental data show a considerable scatter for all radiations used.

300. From fractionation experiments, a decrease of unrepaired damage with time was deduced, with a half-life of about 4 hours. For estimation of the dose-rate effect on the yield of tumours, a dose-rate factor DRF (the ratio of acute to protracted dose for the same yield of S_3 cells) was calculated, and it was predicted that the reduction of the carcinogenic response at low dose rate would be very pronounced. This was confirmed in fractionation experiments with 0.8-MeV electrons [A18], showing that weekly exposure to fractions of 2 Gy per week (130 Gy in 65 weeks) yielded the same incidence as a single exposure to 15 Gy.

301. In conclusion, all the data discussed above suggest that linear extrapolation of skin cancer risk from the rates observed at high acute doses to the low-dose range would greatly over-estimate the risk. To what extent these conclusions might apply to man is still, however, an open question.

12. Bone tumours (internal irradiation)

302. Although the data discussed in the following paragraphs are often referred to in terms of the average skeletal dose, it should be borne in mind that the relevant dose for the effects in question is that delivered to the bone-lining cells. The crude incidence of bone sarcoma induced by ^{239}Pu, ^{249}Cf, ^{252}Cf, ^{241}Am, and ^{226}Ra was compared in C57Bl/Do mice and albino mice [T22]; the data seemed compatible with linearity of the dose-response relationships for all radionuclides. However, the scarcity of data points for each series makes this conclusion at best tentative. It will be recalled that linearity of the dose-response was also seen earlier for bone sarcoma induction by ^{226}Ra in CF1 mice [M69].

303. The question of a practical threshold in bone sarcoma induction following internal irradiation by bone-seeking radionuclides was raised originally by Evans [E4]. This issue was addressed again by a study of Raabe et al. [R32, R40] who tested the hypothesis on the basis of results on beagle dogs. Two groups of animals were given: (a) ^{226}Ra in 8 fortnightly injections of graded activities, the median age during the injection period being about 14.5 months, to simulate the human experience with radium; and (b) ^{90}Sr by continuous feeding at various levels of ^{90}Sr/Ca ratio from mid-gestation through 540 days of extra-uterine life, to simulate the human contamination from the environment.

304. On inspection, the mortality data showed that at higher dose levels survival declined as the dose rate to the skeleton increased. The mean latent period of osteosarcomas varied inversely with the time-averaged dose rate calculated for individual animals from periodic measurements of whole-body activity (Figure XXIII). When the survival period t was plotted against the mean dose rate to the skeleton, the data could be fitted to the relationship $t = K D^{-S}$, where K and S were parameters determined by a least-squares procedure. When a log-normal distribution of times to death from osteosarcoma for a given dose rate was assumed (on the basis of empirically tested distributions), K and its geometric deviation ($\pm \sigma_g$) for radium and strontium-90 were 2500 ($\pm$ 1.24) and 8400 ($\pm$ 1.72), respectively. The corresponding values for $S \pm S.E.$ were 0.29 ± 0.01 and 0.77 ± 0.05. For 116 and 27 dogs dying with malignant bone tumours in groups given radium-226 and strontium-90, respectively, the fit to the function was good, with correlation coefficients of 0.92 and 0.95.

305. From inspection of the regression lines, it appeared that, if the relationship held down to the lowest dose rates, there must be latent periods in the low-dose range exceeding the normal life span. A practical threshold was therefore defined as the dose rate corresponding to the intersection of the regression line log(t) versus log(D) (Figure XXIII) minus three geometric standard deviations of the mean survival time t for control dogs. For dogs injected with ^{226}Ra, the threshold dose rate so defined was 0.11 mGy per day, corresponding to a lifetime dose of 0.5 Gy and a probability of about 0.7% of incurring a sarcoma towards the end of life. Corresponding values were not given for ^{90}Sr-contaminated animals but they would be expected to exceed the values for radium by one or two orders of magnitude.

306. The S values derived from dogs injected with radium were used to fit the data on latency and skeletal dose rate in women dial painters and in RFM mice. There was a high degree of correlation between the species' average life span L (years) and K values calculated for each species according to the relationship

$$K_m = [655 \pm 57 \,(S.E.)] + [119 + 1 \,(S.E.)] \, L \quad (4.2)$$

It could be concluded that a practical threshold for ^{226}Ra in man is 0.039 mGy per day and a total dose of 0.8 Gy. The relative effectiveness of ^{90}Sr and radium, in terms of doses inducing equal effects in dogs, was also estimated; it varied in some proportion to the average dose from ^{90}Sr to the skeleton. If this relation holds down to the lowest doses, a practical threshold of dose rate and cumulative dose for ^{90}Sr would be at least one or two orders of magnitude greater than those for ^{226}Ra.

307. The same methodology was applied [R40] to a study of relative effectiveness for the induction of bone sarcoma in young beagles injected with nine α-emitting bone-seeking nuclides. All nine studies showed, with relatively good precision, a three-dimensional, log-normal, response relationship represented in two dimensions by the equation $t = KD^{-S}$. S was found to be, on average, 0.29 ($\pm$ 0.01 S.E.) for all radionuclides.

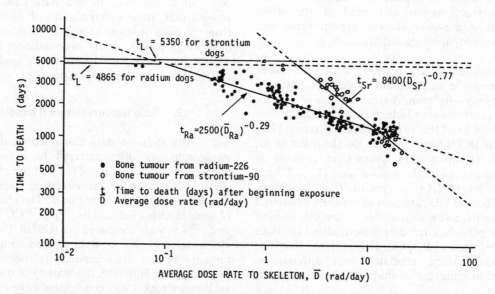

Figure XXIII. Comparison of the dose-response relationships for radium-226 and strontium-90 in beagle dogs that died of primary bone cancer. The data show the median time, t_L, of spontaneous deaths among unexposed controls and the fitted functions in irradiated animals.
[R32]

A practical threshold dose or dose rate, below which bone sarcoma deaths are very unlikely, is suggested at low dose rates for all these radionuclides, just as it was reported for ^{226}Ra [R32]. Mean skeletal doses at which the defined practical threshold was reached were lower than for ^{226}Ra (0.5 Gy) by the following factors: ^{228}Ra, 3.0; ^{241}Am, 6.4; ^{249}Cf, ^{252}Cf, ^{253}Es, 6.6; ^{239}Pu, 9.0; ^{228}Th, 10.7; ^{238}Pu, 15.5. If these factors were expressed in terms of the doses to the bone-lining cells, their spread would be considerably reduced.

308. The reasoning of Raabe et al. [R32] is based on an empirical linear regression of survival times versus mean skeletal dose rate in animals dying with, or due to, malignant bone tumour. However, in the low-dose-rate groups and among the controls a majority of animals were still alive at the time when the experiments were evaluated. There is some uncertainty in the data as to the mean survival values and their distribution among control animals. The data could also change somewhat as a result of further follow-up. The derived practical thresholds must therefore be treated as tentative at best and any final assessment must be deferred. Moreover, any hypothesis regarding species-related interpolation of the risk neglects differences in susceptibility to the induction of bone sarcoma among various strains of mice and breeds of dogs. Alternative interpretations of the data were presented by Mays [M69]. However, the concept of a practical threshold for bone sarcoma is important for risk assessment, because, if extrapolation of the basic relationships is correct, there must be values of the dose and activity at which no radiation-induced life shortening occurs, and therefore the somatic component of the index of harm [I6] can be taken to be zero.

309. Osteosarcoma induced by ^{239}Pu in 294 beagle dogs of both sexes was studied following single injections at ages between 400 and 800 days [W14]. The activity injected ranged up to about 0.11 MBq/kg body weight, in 7 groups of animals [M11]. Times at death due to osteosarcomas were fitted to the Weibull distribution function and described in terms of cumulative hazard or hazard rate, in both cases as a function of time after injection. The power functions of time for cumulative hazard or hazard rate corresponding to R(t,D) and r(t,D) for tumours detected at death in individual injection groups were fitted to the data by a most likelihood method. The plots on a log-log scale were virtually parallel for all groups, and therefore the proportionality constants of the lines could be analysed as a function of the injected activity of ^{239}Pu. Below 37 kBq/kg, there was a strong inverse relationship between the injected activity of plutonium and the time at which a given value of R(t,D) was reached. At the highest injection level the hazard was lower than in the preceding group, probably due to cell killing or some other non-stochastic effect. When the highest activity level (0.095 MBq/kg) was discarded, the data for R(t,D) (below 37 kBq/kg) gave an acceptable fit to a pure quadratic model (P = 0.19) and linearity could be rejected (P < 0.001). A model containing both a linear and a quadratic component did not fit the data better than the quadratic one, where R(t,D) depended also on time after injection to the power of 5.9.

310. The same data were studied in parallel [W14] by the generalized Marshall-Groer model for bone sarcoma induction [M4] (see V.E.2 for details). The solution of the model showed lack of a linear component in the relationship between effect and cumulative dose. The best fit was obtained for a quadratic relationship between dose and R(t,D) for osteosarcoma. Since many animals injected with the lower activities are still alive, a linear contribution to the dose-incidence relationship might still appear after further follow-up. When the same data [P17] were treated in terms of a non-parametric proportional hazard relative risk model, both a linear and a quadratic function could be fitted to the data and neither could be excluded. However, if—as was legitimately done by Whittemore [W14]—the data for the highest injection level are omitted, the results again support a roughly quadratic rise of the relative risk with injection level.

311. An experiment has been completed [W19] on 160 young beagle dogs, injected at the age of 17 ± 2 months with saline (controls, 44 dogs) or with increasing amounts of ^{226}Ra (8 levels from about 260 Bq to 370 kBq/kg). The average α-particle dose to the skeleton varied from 0.35 to 190 Gy. Most of the primary bone tumours were osteosarcomas. Bone sarcoma incidence was a monotonically increasing function of the dose up to 70 Gy. The dose-response fits well a linear non-threshold model over the six lowest dose ranges with a slope of 3.3% per Gy. No tumours were found in the controls or in the 0.35 Gy group, but 1 tumour over 25 dogs was found in the next group with a mean skeletal dose of 0.85 Gy. No significant change in bone tumour incidence was seen among the three highest dose levels at which the incidence exceeded 90%, and the life span was considerably shortened. There was very little, if any, life shortening at the five lowest levels up to 9.5 Gy.

13. Liver

312. Liver tumours were induced in Chinese hamsters by ^{239}Pu citrate injection, and the crude incidence for the few dose points available suggested an initial approximately linear rise up to 2.7 Gy at the time of 50% survival. At the highest dose of 14 Gy, the effectiveness per unit dose was much lower [B87].

313. The dose-response relationship of injected thorotrast was studied in female Wistar rats for the sum of liver and spleen tumours [W15]. In some of the experimental groups, the preparation was enriched with ^{230}Th in order to study the influence of the mass of injected colloidal thorium dioxide. For a constant dose rate (activity), an increase in mass by a factor of 10 proved more effective in respect of life shortening. When the crude percent incidence (I) of all benign and malignant liver tumours was plotted against the relative dose rate ($\dot{D}$), a linear dose-response relationship was observed: $I(\dot{D}) = 3.3 \pm 0.79\,\dot{D}$ with a correlation coefficient of 0.97. The I value at $\dot{D} = 0$ does not differ essentially from the observed control incidence of 2.7%.

14. Combined tumour data and indirect inferences

314. Life shortening by radiation was reviewed in depth in the 1982 UNSCEAR report [U24]. It was concluded that, in the intermediate- and low-dose region, life shortening is due essentially to a higher tumour mortality. This does not mean, of course, that dose-response relationships for both endpoints are directly comparable, because, even for the same radiation, the mean latent period of some tumours varies with dose, dose rate, age at exposure, etc. However, if life shortening is the major consideration, then comparison of results from various dosage schedules for the same radiation and in the same strain of animals could provide some indication as to what the comparative incidences and/or latent periods might be. This seems particularly interesting for neutrons, for which no human data are available.

315. Life shortening and incidence of various diseases, including leukaemias and malignant tumours, were studied in male BALB/c mice [M62] after single and fractionated doses of gamma rays split into 10 equal fractions delivered at intervals of 1 day. The doses ranged from 0.25 to 6 Gy. The causes of death were ascertained by autopsy and histological examination, and actuarial incidences were calculated, with correction for competing risks. In general, single exposures were more effective than fractionated ones with regard to life shortening. Over the whole range of doses, the incidence of all leukaemias and cancers combined appeared significantly higher after fractionation. However, the dose-responses were very flat and included more than 70% of spontaneous cancers. For all carcinomas and sarcomas, except lung carcinomas (for which the spontaneous incidence in BALB/c males is very high), a higher effectiveness of fractionated doses was seen only after doses above 1 Gy.

316. These observations must be taken with some caution, due to the very high spontaneous tumour incidence; to the lack of statistically significant differences between incidences of individual tumours after two modes of irradiation; to the generally flat dose-response relationships; and to the fact that, as shown by Storer [S53], this strain has a number of significant associations between various tumours. Finally, the effect of single and fractionated gamma-ray doses upon life span was opposite to that seen for combined cancer incidence, showing, perhaps, that in this case a specific combination of induction and acceleration of some tumours could have played a significant role.

317. Whereas incidence of all carcinomas and sarcomas combined (except lung carcinomas) showed a negative trend after single doses of gamma rays on the same strain [M63], an almost linear increase was seen after single doses of d(50)-Be neutrons in the range from 0.02 through 3 Gy.

318. Life shortening of B6CF1 mice was studied by single, fractionated (short- and long-term), and life-long exposures to gamma rays and fission (0.85 MeV) neutrons [T20, T21, T25]. When survival data were compared for doses given in 24 weekly fractions or as single exposures, the effectiveness of gamma radiation was consistently decreased by fractionation. However, for neutrons the same fractionation scheme increased the effect throughout the whole range of doses, down to 0.05 Gy. It was argued, therefore, that neutron fractionation in the intermediate- and high-dose range led to an increased incidence of tumours, or their earlier appearance, or both.

319. Thompson et al. [T26] recently published new additional data on life shortening induced by single exposures of B6CF1 female mice to fission neutrons in doses down to 0.01 Gy. They concluded that the assumption of a response proportional to $D_n^{0.5}$ grossly overestimated the life shortening induced by 0.01-0.03 Gy of neutrons and that the data up to 0.1 Gy of neutrons were best fitted by a linear dose-response relationship. The limiting value for the RBE fission neutrons compared with gamma rays was in the region of 12 to 16, depending upon the method used to analyse the data. No consideration was given in any of these publications to RBE values at low doses for fast neutrons as compared with the standard reference radiation, i.e., x rays of about 200 kVp.

320. In another experiment [S57], life shortening was studied in female BALB/c mice exposed to single doses of fission neutrons (mean energy 1.3 MeV) or given into two equal fractions at either 1- or 30-day intervals (whole-body doses from 0.02 to 2 Gy). Protracted exposures from a ^{252}Cf source were also used at rates from 1 to 100 mGy per day (total 0.025 to 0.4 Gy). Life span was considerably shortened between zero and 0.5 Gy for both single and fractionated exposures, and then a plateau ensued. The data were fitted by a linear and a square-root model. Both models adequately described the results below 0.4-0.5 Gy for single, fractionated and protracted exposures, with the exception of a 30-day protraction scheme where the square-root model could be rejected and the linear one still provided a good fit. In contrast with the observations in B6CF$_1$ mice, no increase in effectiveness on life shortening was observed for fractionation and protracted exposures to neutrons below 0.5 Gy. Only at 0.5 and 2.0 Gy was a significantly increased effect of fractionated doses observed.

321. Storer and Mitchell [S62] analysed published data from the Oak Ridge and Argonne laboratories on the shape of the dose-response curves for life shortening induced by single exposures to fission neutrons at doses from 0.025 to 0.2 Gy and by fractionated exposures resulting in total doses up to 0.8 Gy. The response was found to be proportional to $D_n^{0.9}$ to $D_n^{1.0}$, and not to the function $D_n^{0.5}$, which does provide a reasonable description of the dose-response curve at higher neutron doses. The limiting RBE of fission neutrons compared to gamma rays was found to be 18-29 if the response were proportional to $D_n^{0.9}$ and to be 13-22 in the equally likely event that the response were proportional to $D_n^{1.0}$. The range of RBE in both cases was determined by the strain and sex of the mice. Thus, the most recent publications [S62, T26] suggest that a linear dose-response model rather than a square-root model is appropriate at low neutron doses.

C. SUMMARY AND CONCLUSIONS

322. On the assumption that cancer is initiated by lesions in the genome of a single and relatively autonomous cell, the kinetics of induction of point mutations and chromosomal aberrations, mostly symmetrical translocations, could perhaps throw some light on the form of the dose-response relationship for cancer initiation. Studies of cell transformation in vitro could also provide some information in this respect. These end-points cannot, however, provide insight into other factors affecting tumour development at the tissue and systemic level: thus, the relevant conclusions must be regarded as over-simplifications of the real situation.

323. The dose-response relationship for point mutations induced by low-LET radiation in mouse male and female mouse germ cells appears to be curvilinear (upward concave). It also appears to be greatly dependent on dose fractionation and protraction as a result, at least in part, of repair of primary damage at the cellular level. At very low dose rates, linearity and independence of dose rate have been observed. For high-LET radiation the usual form of the curve is linear for all dose rates; fractionation and protraction effects are marginal or absent. Under these conditions, linear extrapolation from high and intermediate doses delivered at high dose rates, down to low doses and dose rates, would over-estimate the mutation rate by sparsely-ionizing radiation. For high-LET radiation, a linear extrapolation provides an adequate estimate of the risk.

324. The induction of somatic mutations in the stamen hair of the plant Tradescantia was studied over a wide range of doses, dose rates and radiation qualities. This system provides direct and extensive information at very low doses of x and gamma rays and of neutrons. The relevant dose-response relationships fit very well a linear-quadratic model for low-LET radiation and a linear model for neutrons.

325. Data on various other types of somatic mutations are also available in several established and early-passage mammalian cell lines. For x- or gamma-ray doses delivered acutely, the observed dose-response relationships are mostly curvilinear, with pronounced fractionation effects in the few instances tested. Exceptions showing linear responses (e.g., human fibroblasts) are also found, showing that the shape of the curves depends on the biological characteristics of the cells. High-LET particles induce mutations in a linear proportion to dose. Sub-mutational damage is readily reparable after low-LET radiation but not after high-LET particles. Studies in several cell lines show a simple inverse relationship between the induction of somatic mutations by low-LET radiation and the logarithm of cell survival. This must imply that linearity of the observed response is accompanied by simple exponential cell survival. Since for low-LET radiation this is an exceptional finding in mammalian cells, the inverse relationship between survival and mutation must, as a rule, imply an upward concave dose-response for induction of somatic mutations, similar to that described for Tradescantia.

326. For low-LET radiation, data on chromosomal exchanges in germinal and somatic cells are, almost without exception, in agreement with a linear-quadratic model, both in respect of dose and of time-dose relationships. For terminal deletions, linearity would, in theory, be expected for all types and dose rates of radiation, but curvilinearity is often seen in some cells (e.g., lymphocytes). This is attributed to the difficulty in distinguishing between terminal and interstitial deletions that have linear and quadratic relationships, respectively, with resulting curvilinearity of the response for both types combined. For high-LET radiation the response is linear and practically unaffected by dose protraction or fractionation.

327. Much work has been done over the last few years on radiation-induced oncogenic transformation in vitro of several established and some early-passage mammalian cells. Numerous factors affect the observed transformation frequency. These include: cell density at irradiation and post-irradiation; cell-cycle stage; time between seeding and exposure; phase of growth at exposure; mitotic delay; and promoting and inhibiting agents. The experimental model appears to be much more complex than originally envisaged for cells in culture, and cell-to-cell influences are found to be present.

328. Cells irradiated with a wide range of doses and types of radiation show dose-response curves that have some features in common with those reported for tumour induction in animals. These are: an initial rise of the transformation frequency with dose up to a maximum and an ensuing decline or plateau; a higher transformation efficiency by high-LET radiation; and a decline of the transformation yield by low, as opposed to high, dose rate of gamma rays in cells irradiated in culture 40 hours or later after seeding. An enhancement of the oncogenic transformation in vitro by a reduction of dose rate of fission neutrons at low and intermediate doses is similar to that which has been described in some, but not all, experiments on tumour induction (or life shortening) in animals.

329. However, several features of the single-cell studies are at variance with animal studies. These are mostly for cells irradiated shortly after seeding: a shallow rise of the transformation rate over the range of intermediate doses, with a power of dose less than unity; an enhancing effect of low dose rate and dose fractionation for low-LET radiation for a fractionation interval of about 5 hours at doses below 1.5 to 2.0 Gy, with reduced transformation at higher total doses. These results most probably indicate a non-homogeneous sensitivity to transformation of the irradiated cells, due to the non-random distribution of cell-cycle stages in freshly seeded cells. If so, they would not be representative of most situations in vivo.

330. The above results were sometimes interpreted to imply that linear extrapolation to zero dose from the transformation frequency at high doses could lead to an under-estimation of the effect at doses below 0.5 Gy, particularly for fractionated and protracted exposures. For the time being, however, while taking note of the complexities referred to above and of the

enhancing effect of fractionation, UNSCEAR does not encourage a direct projection of the in vitro data to the situation in vivo, particularly when irradiation is performed early after seeding. Further analysis of various culture conditions, and a better understanding of the mechanisms of initiation, oncogenic transformation and progression in vitro, is required for meaningful extrapolations to tumour induction in vivo. It appears likely that results obtained from asynchronous cell cultures (i.e., those irradiated later than about 40 hours after seeding) and those irradiated in density-inhibited state may more adequately represent the situation in vivo.

331. New dose-response relationships for a variety of tumours generally support the conclusions reached in the 1977 UNSCEAR report, the most important being the specificity of the response for each tumour-host system. The new experiments enlarge the data base, particularly at the lower end of the dose scale, down to 150 mGy of gamma rays and to a few tens of mGy for neutrons. They justify more specific statements than hitherto possible about the form of some dose-induction relationships.

332. For sparsely-ionizing radiation, most curves are upward concave and may be fitted by linear-quadratic or quadratic (leukaemia in CBA/H mice) models, but in some cases approximate linearity may apply. This is so with mammary fibroadenoma and carcinoma in Sprague-Dawley, adenomas in WAG/Rij and carcinomas in AC rats, thymic lymphoma in RFM mice, and lung adenocarcinoma in BALB/c mice. Thymic lymphomas in most mouse strains and tumours with a pronounced hormonal dependence (e.g., ovarian tumours), show curves with pronounced thresholds. They may reflect the role of non-stochastic mechanisms in the development of these tumours, such as the need to inactivate a large proportion of hormonally-active cells in the ovary, or to kill a large proportion of cells in the thymus.

333. The incidence of the so-called reticulum cell sarcoma after whole-body irradiation usually declines with increasing dose in several mouse strains. Animals protected from early radiation death, by either bone-marrow transplantation or partial marrow shielding, show a very low incidence of this neoplasia. It has been suggested that by relating the number of induced tumours in these animals to the number of irradiated marrow stem cells at risk (assumed to be the targets for tumour induction) it may be possible to estimate in vivo the incidence of tumours per cell at risk. The x-ray dose-response curves obtained under these assumptions are curvilinear (upward concave).

334. Induction of skin cancer in rats and mice by local low-LET irradiation requires high doses. The dose-response relationships are therefore grossly curvilinear (upwards concave) and apparent or real thresholds cannot be excluded. Fractionation and protraction of doses greatly reduces the carcinogenic action of radiation in the skin of rodents.

335. Dose-rate studies with sparsely-ionizing radiation almost invariably show a decreased incidence with decreasing dose rate. In some instances (lung adenoma in RFM and BALB/c mice and harderian or pituitary tumours in RFM female mice), lowering the dose rate results in a more nearly linear dose-response relationship in which the dose-squared component is substantially reduced or abolished.

336. For neutrons, the ascending slopes of the dose-response curves are closer to linearity than for gamma rays. However, in some cases (lung adenoma in RFM mice), curvilinearity is suggested at low doses, even though linearity cannot be excluded. Factors such as a dose-related latency may perhaps contribute to this curvilinearity. In other cases, neutron-induced tumours rising with a power of dose less than unity have been confirmed at low doses. The downward concave shape may be accounted for by killing of potentially neoplastic cells.

337. For most tumours, either no effect, or an enhancement of the tumour yield by a lower neutron dose-rate or fractionation, has been documented. At low and intermediate neutron doses, such effects are less pronounced than for x rays. At high doses, an enhancement of tumour incidence by fractionation or protraction is often observed, but the overall picture is not as simple as cellular data might imply. Factors operating at the tissue level, or perhaps systemic influences, could modify the final tumour appearance to some extent.

338. Pulmonary carcinomas induced by low doses of inhaled radon and of neutron irradiation show an essentially linear non-threshold relationship with cumulative exposure or dose, respectively. High exposure rates of radon daughters at high total exposures are, however, less efficient than low rates. For neutrons also, the effectiveness per unit dose decreases at high doses. These observations are in line with results of epidemiological studies in miners exposed to radon daughter products.

339. Analyses of the latent period of bone sarcoma after incorporation of ^{226}Ra and ^{90}Sr in dogs and mice show an inverse relationship between mean latent period and mean dose rate to the skeleton. According to these observations, there may be a practical threshold for these tumours. Under these circumstances a linear extrapolation of the incidence rate and of the length of life lost per induced bone sarcoma down to zero, from values recorded at high doses, would surely overestimate the risk at low doses. This also applies to tumours induced by β-emitting bone seekers.

340. Studies of bone sarcoma induced by alpha-emitting bone-seeking radionuclides, particularly ^{226}Ra, support a linear activity-response relationship for crude incidence. However, for ^{239}Pu, more refined statistical analyses of data from dogs injected with this nuclide, and observed for longer times, have shown that a purely linear dose-response relationship between integral tumour rate (cumulative hazard) and administered activity is highly unlikely. The same seems to apply to the relationship between dose rate to cells at risk and tumour rate (hazard rate). The appearance of a linear component in the curves cannot be excluded

in the follow-up of animals that are still alive but at present the dose-squared component is dominating.

341. The most recent data on radiation-induced life shortening in mice suggest that a linear dose-response model applies at low neutron doses, while at intermediate and high doses the response follows a square-root function of the dose. Fractionation and protraction of the neutron dose increases the effect of life shortening in some experiments, but not in others; fractionation of low-LET radiation reduces the effect. To the extent that life span shortening in irradiated mice can be attributed to the induction of new tumours, these conclusions may also be applicable to radiation carcinogenesis.

V. DOSE-RESPONSE RELATIONSHIPS FOR TUMOURS IN MAN

342. Data on the incidence of radiation-induced human cancer, at different levels of dose, may be tested for consistency with various models in two ways: directly or indirectly.

343. Indirect inferences may be drawn from limited comparisons in the few instances where risk coefficents (F_{TA} or $\dot{F}_{TA}$) are available at two ends of the scale: high and low doses (total or per fraction). Risk coefficient which are not substantially different under such circumstances will be taken to be consistent with a linear-quadratic or a linear model, because in most cases the variability of data precludes a clear distinction between the two models. Theoretically, for a dose-squared model, an appreciable difference would be expected between F_{TA} or $\dot{F}_{TA}$ at low and intermediate doses, but examples of this kind have not been found for the types of cancers reviewed.

344. In direct studies, attempts may be made to fit various models to the epidemiological data over a wide range of doses. There are often shortcomings to these data (dosimetric uncertainties, a narrow range of doses, pre-selection of groups, ill-defined controls, possible influence of confounding variables, errors of sampling) and consistency with a model rarely, if ever, excludes a fit to alternative models. Thus, consistency of a set of data with a given model should not be taken as evidence that only that model provides an adequate description.

345. Much information on dose-response relationships for radiation-induced malignancies (e.g., leukaemia, cancer of the breast) has been derived in the past from the follow-up of atomic bomb survivors at Hiroshima and Nagasaki. These cohorts represent the statistically most powerful set of data available for dose-response studies, because of the great number of person-years at risk, the wide range of doses, and the relative lack of selection of the samples.

346. The dose-response data in these groups were based on the so-called T65 dosimetry. Since 1980 this dosimetry has been under revision [K34, L27, L30, R4, R6] and a new dosimetry system (DS86) is being installed at the Radiation Effects Research Foundation in Hiroshima as of March 1986. Preliminary estimates based on somewhat more detailed analyses and the current state of knowledge (for a preliminary review see [B77]) differ substantially from those of T65 dosimetry. It appears now that the gamma-ray component had been under-estimated in Hiroshima by a factor of 1.5 to more than 2, and the neutron component had been over-estimated by a factor of about 10 in Hiroshima and of about 2.5 in Nagasaki. As a result, much of the information based on T65 dosimetry will have to be re-assessed upon completion of the ongoing dosimetric revision and will be reviewed by UNSCEAR in the future. However, there is no question as to the qualitative validity of the previously accumulated information about the effects of age and sex upon the incidence of various neoplasms in atomic bomb survivors. The same applies to the clinical and pathological forms of diseases and to the distribution of their latent periods, which are discussed here.

A. LEUKAEMIA

1. Direct studies

(a) Leukaemia in atomic bomb survivors

347. From the information collected in the Life Span Study Sample it appears that the age at time of irradiation had a pronounced effect on the magnitude of the risk when expressed in absolute and relative terms. The effects of sex differences were also discussed in the 1977 UNSCEAR report [U6]. The age-adjusted leukaemia mortality rates reveal that the risk of leukaemia (all types) in males is significantly higher than in females. For both cities combined, the male : female ratio is 1.36, 2.86 and 1.56 for the TD65 kerma categories of 0-0.09, 0.1-0.99 and > 1 Gy, respectively. The distribution of cases in time varied with the type of leukaemia and with age, as shown schematically in Figure XXIV [O1].

(b) Leukaemia in x-ray treated spondylitics

348. Smith and Doll [S49] studied mortality through 1970 in 14,111 ankylosing spondilitis patients given a single course of irradiation during the period 1935-1954. Of these patients, 98.5% were traced to their death, to the date of emigration from the United Kingdom, to the closing date of follow-up (1 January 1970) or to the end of a year after a second treatment, whichever was the earliest. The average period of follow-up of those with one course of treatment was 16.2 years. Causes of death were obtained from death certificates.

349. The number of expected deaths in the cohorts were calculated from age- and sex-specific mortality rates for England and Wales in the respective calendar five-year intervals. An analysis of mortality revealed that the number of deaths was 66% more than

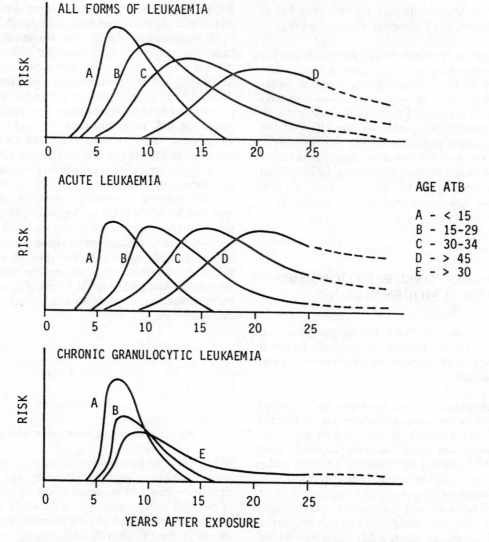

ALL FORMS OF LEUKAEMIA

RISK

0   5   10   15   20   25

ACUTE LEUKAEMIA

RISK

0   5   10   15   20   25

CHRONIC GRANULOCYTIC LEUKAEMIA

RISK

0   5   10   15   20   25
YEARS AFTER EXPOSURE

AGE ATB

A – < 15
B – 15-29
C – 30-34
D – > 45
E – > 30

Figure XXIV. Schematic model of the influence of age at the time of the bombing (ATB) and calendar time on the leukaemogenic effect of radiation (heavily exposed survivors).
[O1]

expected in the patients (1759 versus 1062 expected). The total excess of leukaemia, as well as that for neoplasms, was highly significant (p < 0.001), and did not differ among males and females (the latter made up only one-sixth of the population).

350. The only malignancies for which the dose-response relationship has been studied were leukaemias. The excess death rate was high, the overall observed/expected (O/E) ratio being 4.79 (3.06 and 5.10 in women and men, respectively). The time trends were characteristic, with the death rate rising even at 2 years after the first irradiation, peaking at 3 to 5 years, and declining to the control level more than 20 years after treatment. Chronic lymphatic leukaemia was apparently not increased by the treatment. The relative risk of leukaemia (O/E ratios) was equally increased in all age groups (age at first treatment). The excess risk coefficient per 10^5 person-years rose from 251, in those younger than 25 years, to 1366 in patients treated at more than 55 years of age. In this instance the radiation-induced leukaemia incidence increased temporarily in proportion to the age-specific spontaneous incidence (at age of exposure), as represented schematically in Figure II, c and d.

351. As the distribution of local absorbed and mean doses to the bone marrow among all patients is unknown, it had to be reconstructed through an extensive phantom study in all patients who died with leukaemia and in a sample of all followed-up patients. The doses ranged from 0.5 to 7 Gy, with a rather uniform distribution of frequency, involving 90% of cases below 5 Gy. The proportion of cases above 6.5 Gy did not exceed 2%. The mean marrow dose was 2.49 Gy.

352. The excess leukaemia mortality rate, plotted versus the mean dose to the marrow is very erratic, and a zero response (independence of mortality rate on dose) may not be excluded on purely statistical grounds. However, due to the time characteristics of the mortality, and to the fact that no increase of leukaemia mortality was seen in non-irradiated spondylitics [R33], the non-zero effect at zero dose was discarded as very unlikely. Three models, a linear, a linear with cell killing, and a quadratic with cell killing were fitted to the data by the method of maximum likelihood. Such a method is not formally correct for the last model because simple averaging of organ doses when a large fraction of marrow was unexposed,

must lead to erroneous results when a dose-squared dependence of initiation of the cells is assumed. The first model could be discarded ($P < 0.03$), and the fit obtained for the second was satisfactory ($P = 0.28$).

353. The coefficient of the linear slope in the second model gave a risk coefficient in accordance with most other estimates of leukaemia risk. However, owing to the erratic character of the dose-response, this value must be taken with caution. The cell-killing term cannot be taken in its usual meaning of mean lethal dose, because absorbed doses to the irradiated fraction of the marrow were 2.5 times higher than the mean. Moreover, the fractionated treatment allowed sublethal repair and cellular repopulation to occur.

2. Indirect evidence

354. The risk of leukaemia was studied in radiologists exposed to x and gamma rays either at low dose rates or at higher rates, but in small fractions, accumulated over decades [M7, S8]. The risk was significantly elevated. The records of mortality of the 1920-1927 cohort followed for 50 years showed excesses of 390 and 170 deaths per 10^6 person-years at risk due to leukaemia and to aplastic anaemia, respectively. Calculation of risk per unit dose to the marrow is affected by great uncertainty about the doses accumulated. The diagnoses are also very uncertain. The BEIR Committee [B20] estimated the likely average value to be about 6 Gy, with a resulting annual risk coefficient of 70 leukaemia deaths per 10^6 Gy^{-1} a^{-1}. This value is not significantly different from estimates for low dose and dose rate derived by UNSCEAR in annex G of its 1977 report [U6] from studies on other acutely-irradiated groups (spondylitics, females irradiated for induction of menopause, or other benign conditions) given doses and/or fractions above 1 Gy. If the above estimates of dose were in error in either direction by a factor of 2-3, the derived risk would still appear similar to that deduced from studies on acute irradiation, and therefore consistent with the linear or linear-quadratic model of induction of leukaemia.

355. In conclusion, therefore, it may be assumed, on the basis of the present fragmentary information, that the dose-response relationship for leukaemia after acute low-LET irradiation is likely to follow a linear-quadratic model.

B. CANCER OF THE BREAST

356. The female breast is one of the most sensitive organs for cancer induction by ionizing radiation [B20, I1, M28, U6]. The data reviewed in annex G of the 1977 UNSCEAR report [U6] have been given either in terms of mortality or morbidity, but the latter category will preferentially be discussed here. Epidemiological data relate to three categories of exposure: atomic bomb explosions, therapeutic irradiation for benign conditions (e.g., mastitis), and tuberculosis patients undergoing multiple fluoroscopies for pneumothorax or pneumoperitoneum. Since the 1977 UNSCEAR report [U6] new information has become available [T12, T23] and several attempts have been made to fit cancer induction models to the relevant epidemiological observations [B24, B25, L1, L22].

357. Dosimetric estimates were retrospective in all studies. The uncertainties were particularly great in the Nova Scotia Fluoroscopy Study [M39, M40], where subjective judgement made assessment of the likely confidence limits unfeasible [B20, B25]. This study, therefore, should not be used for discussion of consistency with dose-response models. The Swedish radiotherapy study [B4] is also limited by the absence of an appropriate control group and by a possible association between fibroadenomatosis or chronic mastitis and increased cancer risk. The following discussion, therefore, is based principally on studies of three series: atomic bomb survivors (tentative), the Massachusetts fluoroscopy study, and the Rochester mastitis patients.

358. Several factors could affect the results of such studies, if not appropriately accounted for. These would mostly be age at irradiation, age at manifestation of the effect, length of the latent period, duration of the period at risk, and relationship between latency and dose.

359. Age at exposure is a major determinant of the breast cancer risk. The three studies cited provide strong evidence of cancer induction in females exposed below age 30, with girls of 10-19 years having the greatest absolute risk. The coefficient of the relative risk increment was already highest in the lowest age bracket (0-9 years) at the time of the bombing, but the absolute attributable risk coefficient for this age was lower by a factor of 2 when compared with that for the next age bracket, i.e., 10-19 years. The absolute and relative risk coefficients for ages 20-39 years remain approximately constant [T23]. The fluoroscopy data are scarce for ages 40-49 years, and absent for older ages at irradiation. The atomic bomb survivors showed no significantly elevated cancer incidence when exposed at ages higher than 40. On the other hand, the Swedish radiotherapy data [B4] imply a radiation risk at all age groups, including 40-49 and greater than 50 years, but statistically the estimates at older ages are uncertain. The possibility that concomitant ovary irradiation in atomic bomb survivors at, or close to, menopause might have been responsible for this protective effect (due to sterilization) was suggested by Boice et al. [B25] and Kato and Schull [K39], but this explanation must remain hypothetical. It has more recently been suggested [T23] that differences in the distribution of the risk at ages above 40 parallel the age-specific incidence of mammary cancer in the various countries (Japan, United States of America, Sweden). Taken together, the data show that the risk is highest when the hormonal action affecting the gland is most intense [T23]. It should be mentioned, however, that the follow-up of the younger age cohorts is still incomplete.

360. The increased incidence becomes manifest in all groups at ages above 30 and particularly at the ages of highest natural incidence rate of the disease. This

observation calls for the use of age-corrected incidences in the exposed and control groups. The so-called minimum latent period can be estimated approximately from all observations [B25], but pitfalls of such estimates have been discussed in chapter I. In the Massachusetts, Nova Scotia and Canadian fluoroscopy series, no excess of breast cancer could be seen for the first 10 years after exposure. In atomic bomb survivors, and in the Swedish radiotherapy patients, the increased risk—particularly in those irradiated at ages above 30 years—could be seen even at 5-9 years after irradiation. Thus, it appears that in younger women (under 30 years) the minimum latent period is perhaps close to 10-15 years, and still longer in irradiated children, whereas in the older women it may be shorter (about 5 years). This observation is important for the selection of a period at risk in calculations of the excess incidence. All studies [B26, S16, T12, T23] show a continuing excess cancer incidence up to follow-up times of 30-45 years in women older than 30 years at exposure. There is, as yet, no indication of a decreasing risk even at the longest follow-up of 45 years. There also appears to be no relationship of latency to dose [L32].

1. Radiotherapy for mastitis

361. The Rochester study on women treated for mastitis [S16] was reviewed in detail in annex G of the 1977 UNSCEAR report [U6]. Only those aspects dealing with the shape of the dose-response relationship are discussed here. By dividing the irradiated group into five dose sub-groups, a dose-response relationship was obtained which was controlled for age and for interval since entry into the study, by means of the Mantel combination χ^2 technique, and by test of linear and quadratic trend. The interval at risk for the irradiated group was from 10 to 34 years after exposure. In a first analysis, the average dose to both breasts was used as the independent variable: the data are presented in Figure XXV. The difference between controls and irradiated women was significant ($p = 0.01$) and the linear trend χ^2 test for association with dose was highly significant ($P = 0.0006$). The incidence increased linearly up to about 4 Gy, and then dropped at higher doses. No significant quadratic trend with a coefficient greater than zero occurred. The second analysis was based on doses to single breasts. The relative risk for the period 10-34 years after irradiation was highly significant ($P < 0.0001$), and amounted to 3.3 when controlled for age and interval since entry into the study. The results in terms of relative risk are presented in Table 1, together with results of the first analysis. Significance was obtained for the linear gradient ($P < 0.0001$) and for a quadratic effect with a negative coefficient ($P = 0.0003$). The latter reflects a decreased carcinogenic effect above 4 Gy, owing perhaps to cell killing or other influences.

362. The possible effects of fractionating the dose were analysed within a range of total doses below 3.5 Gy. The analysis compared breasts receiving one or two treatments (mean dose = 1.9 Gy) with three or more treatments (mostly 3-4, mean dose = 2.86 Gy).

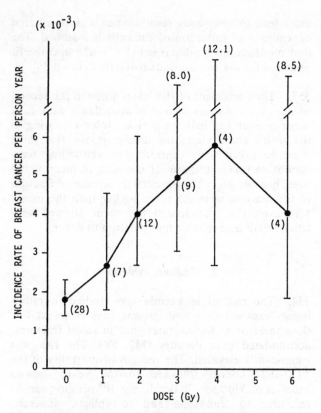

Figure XXV. Breast cancer incidence rate as a function of the average dose to both breasts in mastitis patients for the interval 10-34 years after irradiation. Error bars represent 80% confidence intervals. Numbers in parentheses are breast cancer cases in each dose group.
[S16]

Single, non-irradiated breasts served as controls. For a risk interval of 10-34 years post-irradiation, the adjusted coefficient of the absolute (attributable) risk of breast cancer was 910 10^{-6} Gy^{-1} a^{-1} per breast in the 1-2 fraction group, as compared with 1120 10^{-6} Gy^{-1} a^{-1} per breast in the 3-4 fraction group. Thus, fractionation did not appear to reduce the carcinogenic effect, although the validity of the comparison is limited by the difference between mean doses in the two subgroups.

363. The annual absolute risk coefficient during the period, using the average dose to both breasts, and age- and interval-adjusted incidence rates (irradiated adjusted to controls), was calculated as 830 10^{-6} Gy^{-1} a^{-1}. For irradiation of a single breast, the age- and interval-adjusted estimate of the coefficient amounted to 496 10^{-6} Gy^{-1} a^{-1}. If this figure is doubled for the two breasts, it is consistent with the average for two breasts given above.

2. Pneumotherapy patients

364. The Nova Scotia series on breast cancer induction by repeated fluoroscopies [M1, M39, M40] showed that repeated low doses of diagnostic x rays, when delivered to the gland in sufficient amounts, led to an increased risk of tumours. The doses were

estimated retrospectively, but the margin of uncertainty was so large [B20, B25] that detailed discussion of the likely shape of the dose-response relationship is difficult. However, the fact that the risk estimate was similar to that derived from other studies suggests additivity of the effect and thus approximate linearity of the dose-response relationships.

365. A follow-up study of Boice and Manson [B26] on female tuberculosis patients has been discussed already in annex G of the 1977 UNSCEAR report [U6]. The methodology of estimating the radiation dose to the breasts was described in detail in a separate report [B24] and warrants some discussion because it is critical for the assessment of the dose-response relationship. The data on the number of fluoroscopies were abstracted from the medical records and checked by interview. It was estimated that 63% of the patients faced the physician during the fluoroscopic examination, 16% faced the x-ray tube, 21% had variable positions, and 12% reported being rotated during examination.

366. Out of the 15 former tuberculosis physicians interviewed, 29% reported that they examined their patients with breasts directed to the x ray tube. Sixty-nine per cent conducted the fluoroscopy with the beam-shutters wide open and 81% always scanned the opposite lung. The average time of examination was given as 15 s (3 to 60); 70-80 kVp and 5 mA were the usual parameters of x-ray machines employed; and 1 mm Al filtration was added in 1948.

367. Exposure measurements were made on three representative types of fluoroscopy units, and exposure rates were determined at the fluoroscope panel. Half-value layers for a range of tube voltages and added filtrations were also checked. The exposure measurements were translated into average conditions before and after 1948. Based on these data, estimates were made of absorbed dose in the breast, by means of a Monte Carlo radiation transport method in relation to an anthropomorphic phantom. The shape of the breast was geometrically simulated, separately for an adult and for an adolescent breast. A typical elementary composition of the gland was assumed. The absorbed dose in the breast per 1 R skin exposure (free in air) was calculated for selected exposure conditions: 2 beam qualities, 2 patient orientations, 2 breast sizes and 4 field sizes. These calculations were approximately in agreement with TL dosimetry in a phantom.

368. Cumulative breast doses of all fluoroscoped patients were calculated from all the above information (medical records, physician interviews, patient contacts, exposure measurements and absorbed dose calculations). Females under 17 years of age were assigned doses for the adolescent breasts and the older ones doses for adult breasts. Individual orientations could not be determined and it was assumed that 25% of all examinations were performed in the antero-posterior position, and both breasts were assumed to be in the unshuttered beam 81% of the time while fluoroscoping a unilateral lung collapse, and 19% of exposure time was assigned to the ipsi-lateral breast. Average doses were computed by adding the dose received by the directly exposed breast and the scatter dose received by the opposite breast, and dividing by 2. In a few cases of bilateral lung collapse, both breasts were assumed to be in the beam for 100% of the time.

369. Uncertainties affecting dose estimates based on so many variables, sometimes estimated from memory of 20 to 45 years previously, must be affected by considerable errors and should therefore be taken with great caution. It is very difficult to say whether average breast doses calculated by Boice et al. [B24, B26] are representative of the the real situation and what might be the systematic errors involved. However, the shape of the dose-response relationship should perhaps not be affected by a systematic over- or under-estimate of the real dose.

370. For the exposed women, the onset of the period of risk for breast cancer development was assumed to be the date of the first fluoroscopic examination, and, for the non-irradiated controls, the date of admission to the sanatorium. Expected breast cancer cases were determined with the use of the age- and calendar-specific incidence rate for the neighbouring state of Connecticut, where a cancer registry has been in existence since 1935. The number of expected breast cancers in the exposed group was calculated by multiplying the age- and calendar-specific women years (WY) at risk by the corresponding incidence rates in Connecticut. Standard morbidity ratios and absolute risk coefficients were calculated. The end of the period at risk was regarded as: the date of cancer diagnosis; or the date of death from another cause; or 1 July 1975 for those found alive; or the last date at which the woman was known to be alive, for those lost from the follow-up.

371. The number of breast cancers found among the irradiated women was 41, as against 23.3 expected (excess significant: $p = 0.0006$). Among the controls, 15 cancers were found, against 14.1 expected. The observed/expected ratios were, correspondingly, 1.76 and 1.06. The absolute excess risk increased with increasing numbers of fluoroscopies up to 100-149: a decrease after a greater number was suggested. Nevertheless, a linear increase could not be excluded [χ^2 (trend) = 4.1, $P = 0.04$; χ^2 (departure from linearity) = 6.9, $P = 0.14$].

372. When the incidence rate was calculated as a function of the average dose to the breast, the results were as shown in Figure XXVI. The average dose to the breast per examination was estimated to be 0.015 Gy, and the mean cumulative dose to the breast amounted to 1.5 Gy [B24]. No decrease in the excess incidence per unit dose was apparent at doses above 4 Gy (the highest average was 5.74 Gy) and the dose-response was consistent with linearity down to the lowest dose group (0.32 Gy average) [χ^2 (trend) = 9.4, $P = 0.220$; χ^2 (departure from linearity) = 1.6, $P = 0.8$]. Some differences between the relationships for dose and for number of fluoroscopies resulted from fluoroscopic examinations in different positions of the patients, in different periods, at various ages and for different sizes of the breast.

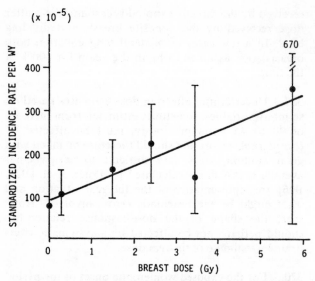

Figure XXVI. Standardized incidence rate of breast cancer in fluoroscoped pneumothorax patients per 100,000 women-years (WY) at risk, as a function of estimated cumulative breast doses. Error bars represent 80% confidence limits.
[B24]

373. The breast cancer risk appeared after 15 years, and the excess risk was present for at least 40 years after initial exposure. The average age at cancer diagnosis was 48.4 years (the greatest risk appeared among women aged 40-49 years at diagnosis) and the mean latent period from exposure to diagnosis was 24.4 years. The radiation risk coefficient derived from subjects of this study living 10 or more years after the first exposure was 620 excess cases per 10^6 women-year and Gy (280-1070 are the 90% Poisson confidence limits).

374. In 1980 Land et al. [L22] reported a comparative study fitting the same set of models to mammary cancer incidence data from 3 main studies: atomic bomb survivors, Rochester mastitis and Massachusetts fluoroscopy series. They assumed that the level of breast cancer response to irradiation may depend on age at exposure. To avoid confounding of dose and age, the dose-specific data were age-standardized using the overall age distribution of each series as an internal standard. It was assumed that the shape of the dose-response curve was not dependent on age. Linear, linear-quadratic and quadratic models, with or without a cell-killing term, were fitted to the data. The linear component was omitted from the killing term as it did not improve the statistical fit, but increased the statistical uncertainty in other parameters. This procedure is, however, biologically implausible. Another constraint was that no parameters should be negative.

375. The model assumed that the control incidence rate, a_0, was equally affected by presumptive cell sterilization, implying that all transformed or potentially transformed cells from which cancers would later develop were already present at the time of exposure. This unproved assumption requires that latent periods for spontaneous and radiation-induced breast cancers should be the same, or longer for the former, and is in fact supported by the apparent lack of dependence of the latent period on dose, as shown by Land et al. [L32].

376. The results of the above fits are presented in Tables 2 and 3, according to the notation in equations (3.6) and (3.7). For the Massachusetts series, parametric constraints reduced the linear + killing model to linear, and the linear-quadratic + killing model to linear-quadratic. For the Rochester series, the linear-quadratic model was reduced to linear. For the mastitis series, accounting for cell killing improved the fit significantly (Table 3). Better results were obtained in this respect when single-breast data were used from the mastitis series, where the linear + killing model gave a substantially improved fit (P = 0.27) over the linear model (P = 0.012). This suggests that cell killing at 4-14 Gy may be a real effect in unfractionated or relatively unfractionated exposures. The quadratic and quadratic + killing models did not fit the age-standardized data as well as did the models with the linear term $a_1 D$. The results show that low-dose risk estimates for breast cancer induction should be based on models with a pronounced linear term. The values for the a_1 term are very close in the series, particularly when differences in age distribution are considered.

377. When age-standardized percentage incidences were plotted in exposed and unexposed women of the three cohorts against time after irradiation, in no group was there evidence of an acceleration of breast cancer expression with dose. This result emphasizes two points: that expression of radiation-induced breast cancer may be influenced by the same physiological factors that affect the normal age-specific incidence rate of this tumour; and that an inverse relationship between dose and latency is highly unlikely for this neoplasm (see also [K39 and L32]).

C. TUMOURS OF THE THYROID

1. Direct studies

378. In their most recent published report, Shore et al. [S60] updated the follow-up to 1977 and reinvestigated several aspects of thyroid cancer induction by x rays in a series of subjects irradiated in childhood for alleged thymus enlargement [H18, H19, S38]. The subjects studied included 2856 irradiated and 5053 controls; 2652 and 4823, respectively, were followed for five or more years after the treatment (on the average, for 30 years).

379. Irradiation was performed with x-ray machines operating at various parameters of voltage and filtrations that were probably not very critical for assessment of the dose to the thyroid (in all cases, the skin dose was very close to the absorbed dose in the gland). The important factor was whether the gland was inside or outside the primary beam. Individual dose estimates were made on this basis, with other corrections. For 241 subjects, such estimate proved impossible, and they were excluded from studies involving analyses with dose.

380. Siblings of the irradiated subjects were the primary control, but comparisons were made also with cancer rates in upstate New York. The subjects were located by various means, and a questionnaire

was used to identify health problems, including tumours. Responses were obtained from 88% of the subjects. Only medically verified neoplasms were used in further considerations, and pathology reports were obtained for all cancers and about three-fourths of the nodules (which were benign). From the total person-years, five years were subtracted in each subject as the likely shortest latent period.

381. There were only small differences in some parameters characterizing the two groups. A large excess of thyroid cancer (P < 0.0001) was diagnosed in the irradiated groups (30 cases of various histological forms), and only 1 case in the controls (1.43 expected). The relative risk for the carcinomas, adjusted for sex, ethnicity and post-irradiation interval, was 49.1 (90% confidence limits 10.7-225) (p < 0.0001) when related to controls, or 44.6 (32.1-60.6) when related to the rate in the general population. There was also an excess of adenomas: 59 among irradiated against 8 among the controls (adjusted RR = 15 (90% confidence limits 8.1-27.7) (p < 0.0001). A separate comparison of cases with matched controls yielded similar odd ratios and p values for cancer as given above, but a somewhat lower estimate of relative risk for adenomas.

382. Doses in the thyroid ranged from 0.05 to 11 Gy, with a weighted average of 1.38 Gy and 62% of individual doses below 0.5 Gy. An absolute risk analysis of the dose-response relation (Figure XXVII)

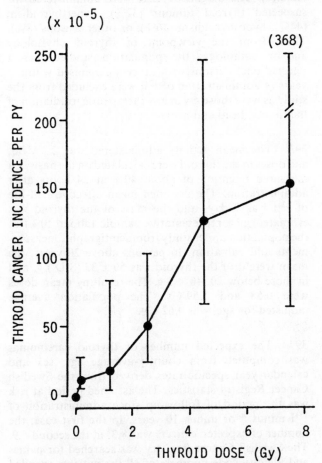

$(\times 10^{-5})$

Figure XXVII. Thyroid cancer incidence per person year (PY) as a function of the radiation dose in the thyroid. Rates adjusted for sex, ethnicity and interval after irradiation. Error bars represent 90% confidence limits.
[S60]

was undertaken with 6 and 12 dose categories, controlling for sex, ethnicity, and interval since irradiation. A linear regression (Mantel regression coefficient) yielded a coefficient of 3.46 ($\pm$ 0.82 S.E.) 10^{-4} Gy^{-1} a^{-1} (P < 0.0001) (5.25 and 2.05 for females and males, separately). Fitting the data to a linear-quadratic model, by iteratively weighted least square regression analysis, resulted in a highly significant linear term (P < 0.0001) and a non-significant dose-squared term (P > 0.4). When the so-called ridge regression analysis was applied, the linear term retained its predictive power, but the quadratic term was even farther removed from significance. The Cox regression analysis used for calculation of RR-model coefficients yielded for cancer a strong linear component (P < 0.00001) and an insignificant quadratic one (P = 0.08). The value of the relative increment coefficient was 0.0058% of the control frequency per Gy.

383. For adenomas, the risk expressed in absolute terms yielded a linear dose-response with a coefficient of 5.7 ($\pm$ 1.2 S.E.) 10^{-4} Gy^{-1} a^{-1} (7.7 for males and 3.6 for females) significant at P < 0.00001. In a linear-quadratic fit, the linear coefficient was 3.8 ($\pm$ 1.4) 10^{-4} Gy^{-1} a^{-1}; that for the quadratic term was negative, -0.04 ($\pm$ 0.004) 10^{-4} Gy^{-2} a^{-1}, and the relationship was downward concave. A strong linear component (P < 0.00001) and a significant quadratic component (P < 0.01) with a negative coefficient, were obtained for the risk expressed in relative terms. A simple linear regression yielded a relative increment coefficient of 0.0044% of the control frequency per Gy.

384. Of 2358 subjects with doses below 6 Gy, 51% were irradiated once, 39% twice and in 10% of cases the dose was split into 3 to 11 fractions. No influence of the dose per fraction, number of fractions and interval between fractions was found for carcinomas or adenomas. Tumour appearance as a function of time seemed to decrease slightly beyond 25 years post-irradiation, but still after 40 years there were excess tumours. The data were not a good fit to the relative risk projection model, but an adequate fit was obtained to the absolute risk model. The latent periods of thyroid carcinomas and adenomas did not show any relationship with the dose.

385. In conclusion, these data, derived from a cohort irradiated in infancy, show a dose-response relationship with a strong contribution of the linear terms, lack of demonstrable dose-squared terms, and lack of dose-fractionation effects. A paradox was also noted, in that irradiation seemed to multiply the sex-specific "spontaneous" risk, while, at the same time, the results fitted an absolute, but not a relative, risk projection model.

2. Indirect evidence

386. Among the studies on thyroid cancer reviewed in annex G of the 1977 UNSCEAR report [U6] none seems to qualify for the derivation of the dose-response relationship or for testing of various models. However, when the risk coefficients for irradiated

children are considered (see Table 10 in annex G of the same report) they seem to fall within a rather close range, although the average estimates of dose for each group vary from 0.065 to about 10 Gy. This would suggest a dose-response relationship close to linearity, a suggestion that must be taken with caution owing to the great uncertainties in retrospective dose estimates in all studies, and to the genetic, demographic and geographic differences between the series.

387. Modan [M25], and later Ron and Modan [R29, R45], followed up children irradiated for tinea capitis in their childhood. The last paper in the series [R45] summarizes the results for the follow-up period 1950-1978. All individuals were irradiated between 1948 and 1960 at an average age of 7. The majority (96%) were treated between 1 and 15 years, and over 50% between 3 and 8 years. Only 6% were irradiated more than once.

388. The final cohort study included 10,842 irradiated persons (IS) and 10,842 non-irradiated tinea-free subjects matched for age, sex, country of origin and year of immigration to Israel (PC). A second control group was composed of 5400 siblings (SC), non-irradiated and tinea-free. All groups were equally divided by sex. By the end of 1978, the three groups had accumulated 244,909, 245,435 and 121,854 person-years at risk, respectively. The average follow-up interval was 22.8 years. The dose to the thyroid was estimated to range from 0.043 to 0.16 Gy, with a mean of 0.096 Gy.

389. The following numbers of cancers were found in the three groups: IS, 29; PC, 6; SC, 2. They were ascertained from the Israel Cancer Registry with an efficiency of recovery of about 80%. The relative risk of thyroid cancer, estimated by using the Mantel-Haenszel method for cumulative data, amounted for the whole group to 5.4 (95% confidence interval 2.7-10.8). The absolute risk may be estimated betweeen 12 and 14 $10^{-4} Gy^{-1} a^{-1}$, depending upon the efficiency of detection assumed (100 or 80%, respectively). There was a clear influence of sex upon the incidence, the relative risk and absolute risk ratios females:males being 1.2 and 3.8, respectively. Subjects in the age bracket 0-5 years were twice as sensitive as those in the 9-15 years group. A significant ethnic difference was also seen because the children of Moroccan and Tunisian origin (contributing about one-half of the total) had an absolute risk twice as high, and a relative risk 6-9 times higher than the rest of the cohort.

390. The $\dot{F}_{TA}$ from this study is about 3-4 times higher than that derived by Shore et al. [S60] for a cohort with an average dose of 1.38 Gy. This however, does not indicate that the risk is truly higher at the lower dose of about 0.1 Gy, because the tinea capitis sample is composed entirely of people of Jewish origin. From the results of Shore et al. [S38], it follows that this factor alone could account for a two-fold difference, and the contribution of individuals of Moroccan and Tunisian origin may have added another factor of 2. Any systematic bias in dose estimates due to inadvertent movements of children during irradiation would have resulted in higher, and not lower, doses to the thyroid.

391. In summary, therefore, a similar value of $\dot{F}_{TA}$ for thyroid cancers in a cohort of children who received a thyroid dose of about 0.1 Gy, and in another cohort with doses ranging from 0.17 to 7.5 Gy, strongly supports the conclusion that the dose-response relationship for thyroid cancer may be essentially linear. Concurrent irradiation of the hypophysis with higher doses (of the order of 0.5 Gy) has been suggested as a possible explanation for this unique observation. However, only an increased secretion of thyroid stimulating hormone (TSH) would be expected to enhance the risk of thyroid carcinoma, while irradiation of the hypophysis would be expected to result in a decreased secretion. Data from an experiment aiming at answering this question are also in conflict with the explanation referred to above [L29]. A smaller group of 2213 children [S36] irradiated to induce epilation did not produce an excess of thyroid cancer. However, because of the low statistical power of the study, this result is consistent with reported values of $\dot{F}_{TA}$.

392. Holm [H17] published a retrospective study on patients given ^{131}I for diagnosis of thyroid diseases in the Stockholm area in 1952-1965. The population consisted of 10,133 persons, of average age 44 years, followed for an average period of 18 years after administration of the nuclide. Of these, 95% received ^{131}I when 20 years or older (2086 males and 8047 females). The diagnostic tests were administered for suspected thyroid tumour (32%); hyperthyroidism (44%); hypothyroidism (16%); or other reasons (8%). Thus, from the viewpoint of thyroid physiology and/or pathology, the population studied was a selected one. Persons with cancers diagnosed within 5 years of administration of ^{131}I were excluded from the study as were those given any therapeutic irradiation of the thorax, head and neck.

393. The mean activity administered was 2.2 MBq, and doses to the thyroid were calculated on the basis of a measured retention of about 40% at 24 hours after administration. The assumed mean effective half-life of ^{131}I was 7 days and the mass of the thyroid was estimated in a representative sample (about 10%) of the population under study from scintigraphic measurements and palpation. In persons above 20 years, the mean weight of the thyroid was 50 ± 33 (S.D.) g, and in those below 20, 10 ± 5 g. The resulting mean doses were 0.58 and 1.59 Gy. The population average (adjusted for age) was 0.62 Gy.

394. The expected number of thyroid carcinomas was computed from country-average age, sex and calendar-year specific rates derived from the Swedish Cancer Registry statistics. The assumed period at risk was the period of follow-up since administration of ^{131}I minus 5 or minus 10 years. In the first case, the number of expected cancers was 8.3, in the second 5.9. The Swedish Cancer Registry was searched for names and identity code numbers of all the patients enrolled in the study. Nine cancer diagnoses among them were identified and 8 confirmed. Thus, there was no excess cancer among the subjects given diagnostic amounts of ^{131}I.

395. Holm et al. [H17] compared the number of cancers diagnosed with estimated numbers calculated from UNSCEAR risk coefficients of 5000-15,000 cases 10^{-6} Gy^{-1} [U6] (derived predominantly from surveys on children) or from Hiroshima and Nagasaki surveys [U6] of 1400 10^{-6} Gy^{-1}. In the first case, the number of expected cancers would be 47-124, which is obviously very different from the observed 9 cases. For the second alternative, the authors quote a figure of 19 cases, which they claim to be not significantly different from the 9 cancers diagnosed.

396. However, when the lack of the excess incidence in that study was compared [N10] with the expectation in adults, taking the risk for adults to be one-half that in children [S60], to account for the age-related lower sensitivity, the difference appeared statistically significant on two tests applied. This would suggest that the effectiveness of ^{131}I for induction of thyroid carcinomas is lower, at least by a factor of 2. The question whether this is a true dose-rate effect, and to what extent other factors play a role, cannot be answered at present.

397. Several factors, separately or in combination, could be responsible for the difference between the predicted and the observed numbers of cancers. First, the linearity of the dose-response relationship in Figure XXVII may be more apparent than real, because the positive dose-squared term for initiation and the negative term for cell killing may compensate each other. Secondly, the subjects are a selected unhealthy population, with a high percentage of thyroid involvement, to whom specific rates of thyroid cancer induction, valid in the general population, may not apply. Thirdly, the treatment given after the diagnosis (surgery, thyroid hormones) could have suppressed the risk. This appears rather unlikely, as more than half the patients were not given any treatment and the nine with diagnosed cancers were treated with hormones (2 cases) and surgery (4 cases), which did not prevent the manifestation of tumours. Fourthly, a non-uniformity of dose distribution from ^{131}I in pathologically enlarged glands could be another confounding factor. Fifth, it cannot be excluded that risk coefficients are being compared for populations which may differ in their average iodine uptake and hence in activity of the thyroid and hypophysis (TSH stimulation). Finally, other dietary or environment-related factors could further confound the comparison.

398. In summary, two studies on humans [R45, S60] argue persuasively that the contribution of the linear term is very strong in the dose-response relationship for induction of carcinomas of the thyroid. This is also the conclusion to be drawn from the experiments on rats by Lee et al. [L29] discussed in chapter IV. If this conclusion were true, a dose-rate effect, should not be expected. However, the results of Holm's study [H17] are not consistent with this picture. Further investigations in this field are certainly called for.

D. CANCER OF THE RESPIRATORY TRACT

399. Induction of lung cancer has been discussed repeatedly in many UNSCEAR reports [U6, U7, U9-U12, U24] and risk estimates were given based on various groups' findings ([U6], annex G). Most of the data on lung cancer induced by external irradiation appeared unsuitable for analysis of the dose-response relation. The most numerous group, the atomic bomb survivors, is still affected by uncertainties in organ dosimetry. As a result, there are large statistical uncertainties in excess rates in various exposure categories ([U6], annex G).

400. The most interesting case for a discussion of the shape of dose-response relationships is the prolonged exposure of miners to radon and its daughter products. The difficulties in this case are:

(a) The long period of exposure, often at a variable rate. Exposures toward the end of the follow-up period are increasingly less effective, in view of the long latent period of these tumours;

(b) Possible changes in susceptibility with age, which is itself a variable correlated with the length of the exposure;

(c) Possible interaction of radon and its daughters with other factors, particularly smoking habits of miners [A8, A16, W17];

(d) The dosimetry, which is based either on measured concentration of potential alpha-energy in the air $(WL)^d$ or on estimates of radon concentrations, on the assumption of some degree of radon-daughter product equilibrium. Translation of these quantities into an absorbed dose in the cells at risk (basal layers of bronchial epithelium) is uncertain, but a recent ICRP review [I4] gives, for mining conditions, a range of about 3 to 8 mGy per WLM. The use of cumulative WLM as an indirect measure proportional to dose is probably adequate for discussions of the derived dose-response relationships.

1. The risk expressed in absolute terms

401. In Newfoundland, a group of 2120 fluorspar miners were exposed to an accumulated mean exposure to radon of about 550 WLM. They were followed for about 25 years and those who accumulated more than 1 WLM had a relative risk of cancer of the respiratory tract of 5.58 (95% C.L. 4.54-6.72). The absolute annual excess risk coefficient amounted to 6 (4.6-7.5) cases per 10^6 PY per WLM. The excess lung cancer incidence rose roughly in proportion to the exposure [M5].

402. Several studies were published on the epidemiology of cancer of the respiratory tract among uranium miners in the United States. The 1977 UNSCEAR report [U6] reviewed those by Archer et al. [A8] and by Lundin [L18]. To sum up the situation, the study by Archer [A8] referred to 3366 white and 780 non-white miners who had worked one or more months in underground uranium mining before 1 January 1964. Mortality analysis was terminated on 30 September 1968, and only 1% of people

---
^{d}See footnote c.

enrolled were lost from the survey. The death certificates of those deceased before the closing date were obtained. There was a substantial excess of deaths (437 observed versus 276.6 expected) among which there were 70 cancers of the respiratory system against 11.7 expected (p < 0.01). The diagnoses were ascertained using all sources of evidence (clinical findings, x rays, autopsy, histology, biopsy, cytology, sputum analysis). Numerous cancers occurred after 1968, or were evaluated as probable ones. These were not used in the assessment of risk or for characterization of the dose-response relationship [B20].

403.   The exposure was assessed by radon daughter measurements (nearly 43,000 from 1951 through 1968 in approximately 2500 mines). Measurements taken in a mine over yearly periods were averaged, but, in many instances, exposure over a number of years could only be estimated approximately, particularly in the early years of highest exposure. In addition, a fraction of miners had a history of hard-rock mining, before the work in uranium mines, which also required approximate assessment. Cumulative radon daughter exposure values were calculated with the above approximations for each miner and for each month of his employment.

404.   Person-months of risk of dying by single calendar year, for 5-year age groups, and for each time interval after the start of underground uranium mining, were calculated by a modified life table technique. These values were related to cumulative radon daughter exposure in WLM. Individuals who were lost to follow-up were considered to be alive throughout these analyses. A miner often contributed person-months to more than one exposure category if during the course of employment he passed from one category to the next. The expected number of deaths was calculated by applying the specific rates for age, race, calendar year and cause of death for white United States males to the appropriate number of person-years at risk.

405.   The number of expected and observed cancers of the respiratory tract as a function of cumulative exposure in WLM during the whole period of observation was converted to incidence rate by BEIR [B20], weighing the incidence in each group of white miners by its inverse variance. The fit was as shown in Figure XXVIII. Consistency with linearity is evident and the slope is about $3 \cdot 10^{-6}$ person-year WLM^{-1} for the whole range of exposure.

406.   There were confounding variables, like cigarette smoking, metropolitan versus non-metropolitan residence, possible mis-classification of miners into exposure categories, and dependence of WLM calculations on quality of the work histories, which could have distorted the data to some extent. It is difficult to see what their combined effect could have been. However, the authors suggest that the influence of these variables should not basically alter the trend of the dose-response relationship. Also, the excess of cancer cases even in the 120-359 WLM category is beyond doubt.

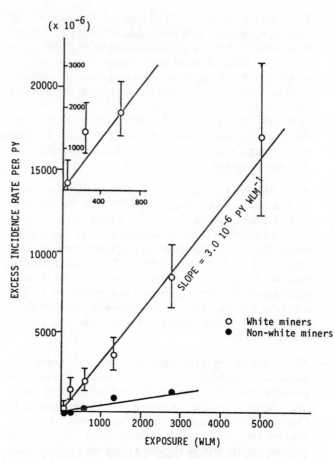

Figure XXVIII.   Dose-response relationships for lung cancer in uranium miners in the United States. Error bars include 90% range based on Poisson statistics. Modified from [B20].

407.   The mortality study of the uranium miners from the United States was extended to September 1974 [A16] with essentially the same methodology as in a previous study [A8]. Lung cancer rates were calculated for eight exposure categories and for the time after starting uranium mining. The total number of person-years at risk was 62,556; the average period of work in uranium mines was 9 years; the mean accumulated exposure was 820 WLM; and the average follow-up period was 19 years. The incidence rate increased approximately linearly up to 480 WLM, then the slope of the response decreased to give a lower risk per WLM, a feature possibly related to cell killing, which was also seen in the series from Czechoslovakia [S3]. Miners exposed to higher rates were usually followed for longer times, and most miners were middle-aged when they entered the occupation. Cigarette smoking, and constitutional factors such as stature and eye pigmentation were found to be correlated with the effect. Stature was thought to be correlated to lung volume in the sense that, for the same work at comparable oxygen consumption, a smaller lung volume means enhanced ventilation rate and higher lung doses. More recently, uranium miners from the United States have been followed through 1977 [W13], but the data, as reported, do not provide new information, as all uranium miners examined by the United States Public Health Service medical survey team were already considered in the study by Archer et al. [A16].

408. The data from the United States miners were tested by Myers and Stewart [M43] for their fit to various dose-response functions. The fit was made to an equation of the form $\dot{I}_{TA}(WLM) = a + bE^j$ where $\dot{I}_{TA}$ is the annual net incidence rate (10^{-6} a^{-1}) and E the cumulative exposure in WLM. The j exponent was fixed at 1.0, 0.5 and 0.25, and maximum likelihood estimates were obtained in each case for a and b. Allowing all parameters to produce a maximum likelihood estimate led to a preferred value of j not significantly different from unity and to a positive value of a, indicating that an excess cancer of the lung may obtain even in the absence of radon exposure. A linear fit to the data was found to be the best, with $b = 3.5 \; 10^{-6} \; WLM^{-1} \, a^{-1}$.

409. The latent period from the start of the exposure to diagnosis was examined as a function of the age at the start [A16]. It declined from about 45 years to about 10 years in those who started mining at 20 or 60 years, respectively. Smokers usually had a shorter induction time (see annex L of the 1982 UNSCEAR report [U24] for a discussion of the influence of tobacco smoke). There was also a shorter latent period associated with higher exposure rates, which appeared to contribute to shortening more than cumulative exposure.

410. Sevc, Kunz and Placek [S3] reported on lung cancer incidence among uranium miners in Czechoslovakia. The number of miners was not specified, but the group was similar in the number of people to that studied by Lundin et al. [L18, L19] in the United States, which consisted of 3366 workers. According to [I5], the study was based on about 60,000 person-years at risk, and a follow-up in the range of 21-26 years, 10 years of average working period in the mines and a mean cumulated exposure of 310 WLM. Fifty-six per cent of these miners started uranium mining between 1948 and 1952 inclusive (group A), the rest between 1953 and 1957 inclusive (group B). Miners were also subdivided into 3 age groups at the start of exposure: < 29 years (45%), 30-39 years (28%), and > 40 years (27%). The age structure in groups A and B was very similar. Each age group was subdivided into eight exposure sub-groups, the exposures being expressed as WLM. The numbers in each sub-group were approximately equal. Exposure estimates were based on about 120,000 radon concentration measurements made since 1948. Estimates of potential alpha energy concentration were made from radon measurements by choosing average values of equilibrium between radon and its decay products, typical for given ventilation conditions and practices (which were available from records) and radon daughter measurements which were introduced in 1960. Attempts were made to estimate the variability of dose measurements. The rates of exposure accumulation in the three age groups were comparable.

411. In each sub-group of miners (belonging to each exposure category and age group), the expected rate of lung cancer was calculated by year from the beginning of exposure up to 31 December 1973, on the basis of age- and calendar-specific lung cancer mortality rates for Czechoslovakia. A statistically significant excess

(at 5% level) started to appear in the 100-149 WLM category.[e] The presumption of linearity for the dose-response relationship in group A (start of the exposure 1948-1952, follow-up 21-26 years) could not be rejected at the 5% level of significance.

412. The same data [S3] were fitted by Myers and Stewart [M43] to quasi-threshold functions of probit and logistic response on the logarithm of cumulative WLM. When results were tested by means of χ^2 distribution for significance of deviations from these assumed functions, the χ^2 values were tenable at $P = 0.98-0.99$. However, the quasi-threshold was less than 3 WLM. Thus, the mathematical analysis, using maximum likelihood as the criterion, does not provide any reason to reject linearity, for which the χ^2 test gives a P value of 0.82.

413. Cumulative exposure E (WLM) and lung cancer incidence (I_{TA}) in group A were also fitted by Jacobi [J4] to a function of the form $I_{TA} = a \; E \; e^{-kE}$. A better fit was obtained than that resulting from assumption of linearity throughout the whole range of exposures. The most likely estimates of a and k were 320 excess cases $10^{-6} \; WLM^{-1}$ and $6 \; 10^{-4} \; WLM^{-1}$, respectively.

414. The excess cumulative cancer incidence in the various age groups shows that for the older age group the incidence was significantly elevated (5% level) at 100 WLM or more. For the two younger groups, this significance was reached at exposures above 150 WLM. The risk per unit exposure (WLM) increased with age, with some irregularity of response in miners who were older than 40 at the beginning of the exposure. In the younger age groups, linearity, with different slopes, could not be rejected at the 5% level of significance. The differences in incidence between the groups disappeared above 300 WLM.

415. Cigarette smoking did not appear to be a confounding variable because it was not dependent on exposure categories, although it was correlated with age. From random sampling, the frequency of smoking was similar to that in the country for which specific mortality rates were used for computation of the expected numbers of cancers. Also, hard-rock mining was not a complicating factor in assessment of the exposure.

416. In another paper, Kunz et al. [K22] studied the excess lung cancer incidence in miners in Czechoslovakia over the period 1948-1975 and related their findings to different time distributions of exposure. The previously mentioned group A composed of miners who started work between 1948 and 1952 was followed for 26 years on average. The cohort was divided into five exposure categories and also, according to duration of exposure, as short (4.0-7.9; mean 5.6 years), intermediate (8.0-11.9; mean 9.5) and long (> 12; mean 14). The same group was also divided alternatively, according to exposure rate, into group II with nearly constant accumulation rate; group I for which the earlier rates of exposure were higher than

---

[e]More recently, it has been reported [S51] that the excess is already significant at an average exposure of 72 ± 2 WLM.

231

later ones; and group III where the rate of accumulation increased with time and reached highest values in recent years.

417. The additional lung cancer incidence for the group as a whole, when related to duration of exposure and its cumulated values, is shown in Figure XXIX. For the group as a whole, a linear exposure-

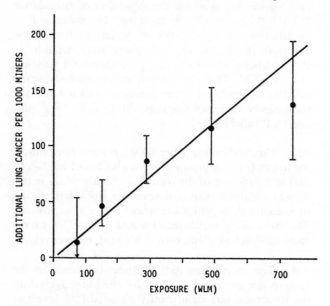

Figure XXIX. Relationship between additional lung cancer frequency and cumulated exposure in all uranium miners from Czechoslovakia. Error bars represent 95% confidence limits. [K22]

response relationship cannot be rejected, but there is some suggestion of saturation at the highest values of WLM. When divided into three groups in relation to the duration of exposure, the two groups with shorter exposure showed saturation very clearly. The early exposure rates in both groups with shorter duration of exposure at which a significant deviation from linearity occurs corresponds to about 50 WLM a^{-1}. The lower incidence resulted from a diminished excess of small-cell undifferentiated cancer. The groups with uniform and decreasing rate of accumulation showed linearity of the response, whereas that with the increasing rate showed a breakdown of the response in the highest exposure category (> 400 WLM). This decrease of the incidence was also due to diminished occurrence of small-cell undifferentiated cancer. A similar influence of exposure rate to radon daughters upon lung cancer incidence was observed in experiments on rats by Chmelevsky et al. [C34] (already discussed in chapter IV).

418. Since all Czechoslovak miners started exposure in 1948-1952, those accumulating their exposure over a shorter period did not have a shorter follow-up, and therefore the lower incidence in the two groups of 9.5 and 5.6 years of mean exposure duration cannot result from the shorter time available for manifestation of the effect (truncation due to long latency and short follow-up). A more likely explanation would be a killing effect on the transformed cells, which becomes manifest at an exposure rate of about 50 WLM per year. However, a shorter survival of miners at high exposures was also

suggested [J7]. Thus, lung cancer induction by alpha-particles of radon daughter products can be described by equation (3.1), with the proviso that the proportionality constant of the cell-killing term is dose-rate dependent. The slopes of the exposure-response relationships for different times of accumulation in the low-dose region were very similar. The effect of exposure rate cannot be easily separated from the effects of time course in groups that differ in respect of the rate of accumulation of WLM. Both the exposure rate and latency effects may play a role in the decreased incidence for the 400 WLM category of group III.

419. Horacek and Sevc [H25] studied the relationships between incidence (per 10^3, I_{TA}) of various histological forms of respiratory cancer in uranium miners from Czechoslovakia and the exposure (E, in WLM). For all miners, a function of the type $I_{TA} = 0.16 E$ gave a good fit to the data, and absence of a threshold could not be excluded. For epidermoid-type lung cancer, the relationship was different, and a regression line of the form $I_{TA} = aE + c = 0.15 E - 11.2$ could be fitted up to 700 WLM (c was significantly different from zero). Thus, the analysis suggests the presence of a threshold of about 75 WLM. There was also a small excess—unrelated to exposure—of other histological types of lung cancer the statistical significance of which cannot be assessed from the report [H25].

420. It is interesting to note that basically the same picture was obtained for the miners whose exposure began at ages less than 40 years. For those above 40 years, the relationship for epidermoid-type lung cancer was again linear with threshold ($I_{TA} = 0.13 E - 21.7$), suggesting a threshold of a similar magnitude, but a steeper linear rise of incidence with exposure up to 700 WLM. For small undifferentiated cancer, the excess at about 60 WLM was already close to $60 \; 10^{-3}$ cases and rose much less steeply to $80 \; 10^{-3}$ cases at about 300 WLM, with a decline to about $40 \; 10^{-3}$ cases at about 500 WLM. Other histological types also showed an increased incidence to about $40 \; 10^{-3}$ cases at 300 WLM, with a decline to very low levels at 500 WLM; however, the form of the ascending branch of the curve cannot be derived from the report.

421. The relationships of these findings to smoking could not be studied, due to lack of relevant information. The reasons why the two main histological types of pulmonary cancer should have different forms of the dose-response relationship (presence or lack of threshold) and different age dependence, are unknown. However, there is a causal link between development of epidermoid lung cancer and metaplastic changes in the bronchial epithelium [S58, S61]. The intensity with which noxious factors (e.g., tobacco smoke, radon exposure) act upon exposed individuals is probably related to the speed with which metaplasia develops. Therefore, at lower exposure rates, development of metaplasia and epidermoid cancer may simply be delayed. The percentage of the small undifferentiated and epidermoid cancers varied strongly with numerous factors, such as calendar time, age at diagnosis, and length of exposure. The epidermoid cancers usually appeared later, and at higher exposures, than the oat-cell undifferentiated carcinomas. All

these circumstances call for great caution in accepting a threshold-type relation for epidermoid lung cancer in uranium miners, particularly because the analysis of a similar type of cancers induced in rats exposed to radon decay products [C34] (see IV.B.6) did not suggest any threshold above a few WLM. A detailed study of the latent periods for the two types of cancer could give some insight into the problem.

422. By far the largest study on the mortality of miners, including that from lung cancer, was recently reported by Müller et al. [M70] from Ontario, Canada. Out of several groups of miners engaged in mining various minerals, excess of lung cancer mortality was found in three: uranium miners, gold miners, and those mining a mixed assortment of minerals. The dose-response study described below refers only to uranium miners, for whom radon daughters in the air could be envisaged as the sole causative factor. The group included all full- and part-time underground uranium miners with mining experience of one month or more. They were followed from 1 January 1955 through 31 December 1981. The cohort numbered 15,984 men, with an average follow-up of 15 years, average duration of exposure of 2 years, mean accumulated exposure of 60 WLM, and a total of 241,942 person-years at risk. The exposures to ^{222}Rn daughters were calculated in WLM from area monitoring and occupancy data from 1955 through 1967 and, starting in 1968, from personal exposure records. For each miner, upper and lower best estimates were derived, called "special" and "standard WLM", respectively. It was postulated that the most likely true exposure would fall within these boundaries.

423. Deaths among cohort members due to respiratory cancers were identified via the Canadian Mortality Data Base, utilizing death certificates. The expected number of deaths was calculated using age and calendar mortality rates for the male population of Ontario. Smoking habits were not taken into account, but, according to the authors, there were good reasons to suppose that the miners did not differ in this respect from the reference population. Among the uranium miners there was a highly significant excess of cancers of the respiratory tract (121 observed against 70.5 expected; $P < 10^{-9}$).

424. When the absolute attributable risk was calculated in 6 exposure groups according to a linear model, the intercept did not differ significantly from zero, irrespective of whether a zero, 5- or 10-year lag in exposure against effect was assumed. The slopes of I_{TA} as a function of WLM varied between 2.0-2.8 10^{-6} WLM^{-1} for "special" WLMs and 4.8-7.2 10^{-6} WLM^{-1} for the "standard" WLMs (at 3 different lag intervals). The slopes were significant at $P < 0.001$. An example of a dose-response relationship is presented in Figure XXX. In terms of the absolute attributable risk, the slope was significantly greater, by a factor of about 6, for those who lived to age 55 or more than for those who died at younger ages. Thus, all dose-response relationships were well described by a non-threshold linear function. A single relative risk model described the relationship for all attained ages (see paragraph 428).

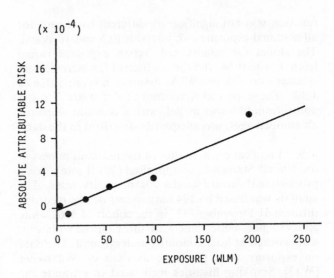

Figure XXX. Dose-exposure relationships for lung cancer incidence in uranium miners from Ontario, Canada, who had no prior exposure in gold mines. Exposure is expressed in WLM "standard" units.
[M70]

425. Preliminary data were reported from Sweden on lung cancer induction in iron-ore miners exposed to relatively low levels of radon daughters. A typical rate of exposure is 2 to 6 WLM per year of underground work, presumably rather constant over the last 60 years [R35, R36]. The group consists of 1435 miners born between 1880 and 1919, known to be alive on 1 January 1920. The mortality analysis dealt with the cohort alive on 1 January 1951 (1294 men) and covered the period through 31 December 1976.

426. The analysis [R36] is almost a life-long follow-up. Details and accuracy of exposure evaluation are not known. The estimates of exposure ranged from 2 to 300 WLM, the average being about 90 WLM. Detailed histories of smoking were available for each miner, and the expected numbers of lung cancers were calculated from the calendar- and age-specific cancer rates for smokers and non-smokers in Sweden. The interesting feature of this study is the very long latent period, with a minimum of 20-29 years after the start of mining and a mean of about 40 years.

427. From this series, only limited data have been published [R41] concerning the dose-response relationship. The earlier report [R36] states that "... the preliminary data show a reasonable dose-response relationship over the range of cumulative exposure from 2 to 300 Working Level Months (WLM). The significant point is that in the lowest dose range we do get a significant excess of lung cancer at about 25 WLM. So we have some indication that at these low doses and dose rates there is a significant lung cancer risk as the linear dose-response would have predicted."

2. The risk expressed in relative terms

428. The lung cancer risk of Canadian uranium miners was also expressed in terms of a relative increment versus exposure. The intercept of the

function was not significantly different from zero for all assumed exposure-risk intervals (0.5 and 10 years). The slopes for relative risk versus exposure varied from 0.51 to 0.54, and the coefficient for increment of spontaneous risk per WLM assumed a single value of 1.3%. The slope was significant at $P < 0.001$. Thus, a non-threshold linear model, with a constant slope for all attained ages, was adequately described in the data.

429. Lung cancer mortality of the uranium miners in the United States was re-appraised [W17] using Cox's proportional hazard model for mortality rates. The analysis was based on 194 lung cancer deaths recorded through 31 December 1977 in the cohort of 3362 white and 780 non-white miners in the Colorado plateau, who worked at least 2 months underground. The data on exposure were the same as used by Waxweiler [W13]. Smoking histories were used to estimate the total number of cigarettes smoked until the exposure cut-off (1968).

430. When considered in terms of the relative risk (RR), various specific models were tested which treated the exposure to ^{222}Rn decay product and smoking as additive or synergistic factors. The best fit to the data by the maximum likelihood method was obtained by a synergistic model of the form:

$$RR = (1 + a \ WLM)(1 + b \ packs) \qquad (5.1)$$

where WLM and packs are accumulated exposure to ^{222}Rn daughters and estimated total number of cigarette packages smoked up to 10 years before the miners' current age, respectively. The fit yielded $a = 0.31 \ 10^{-2} \ WLM^{-1}$ and $b = 0.51 \ 10^3 \ pack^{-1}$ and was significantly improved over that obtained when exposure to ^{222}Rn decay products was taken alone. Several additive models could be rejected. For exposure to ^{222}Rn decay products alone the dose-response model is a non-threshold linear one.

431. An ICRP Task Group [I5] re-calculated the lung cancer risk among United States, Czechoslovak and Canadian miners in terms of the relative risk. The ratios of the coefficient for the linear slope of the exposure-response relationships, i.e., the relative increment of spontaneous lung cancer risk per unit of exposure are as follows: United States, 0.5-1.0; Czechoslovakia, 1.0-2.0 and Canada 0.5-1.3 per cent per WLM. These values are much closer to each other than the respective values of the coefficient $\dot{F}_{TA}$ (in terms of the absolute attributable risk) of 3-8, 10-25 and 4-10 10^{-6} WLM per year. The relative risk per WLM also becomes slightly less at high accumulated exposures.

432. Data on induction of lung cancer are practically limited to prolonged exposure to alpha particles emitted by short-lived radionuclides attached to dust particles or as free ions in air passage ways (trachea, bronchi). Moreover, the available data refer to miners among whom a majority are tobacco smokers. The latter factor may act synergistically with radiation in inducing bronchial neoplasms ([U24], annex L). There were also other factors in the working environment of miners whose co-carcinogenic or promoting effects upon lung cancer induction could not be completely discarded. Attempts at dissociating these from radon decay products and tobacco effects have been so far unsuccessful. Whatever the limitations of the five studies discussed, they imply basic agreement with expectations of the linear non-threshold model, irrespective of whether the risk is expressed in absolute or relative terms.

E. BONE SARCOMA

433. The available information on induction of bone sarcoma by bone-seeking radionuclides has already been reviewed by UNSCEAR ([U6], annex G), which also discussed many experiments performed on animals ([U6], annex I). Relevant new information on animals is discussed in chapter IV of the present annex.

1. Direct studies

434. A group of dial painters who acquired various amounts of ^{226}Ra and ^{228}Ra has now been followed for more than five decades [E3, E4, R18-R20, R34] and has provided knowledge of average doses to bone and to endosteal tissue, in which the cells at risk are thought to be located. Average doses from radium isotopes in man can be calculated with reasonable accuracy for groups of subjects who acquired their body burdens 50 or 60 years ago [R18-R20]; however, the precision of individual estimates is difficult to appraise.

435. The ^{226}Ra and ^{228}Ra body burdens were measured in most of the individuals (in some of them on numerous occasions) and the initial skeletal uptake was estimated using Norris' [N7] empirical retention function for radium in man. The average skeletal doses of alpha radiation from both isotopes of radium and their daughter products were computed by integrating the retention function from the mid-point of exposure to the end of follow-up, and dividing the released energy by the average skeletal mass.

436. A large group of these subjects (dial painters) has been followed for more than 45 years and the estimated cumulative incidence should be very close to the complete life-long effect of the radionuclides. It is still uncertain whether the group might be selected for dose, i.e., whether or not the subjects with symptoms are grouped preferentially in higher dose categories where skeletal effects (including bone-sarcoma) occur more frequently [M29].

437. Rowland et al. [R34, R46] analysed the dose-response relationships for bone sarcoma in this population. Female dial painters were selected from the total group and were followed until 31 December 1979. Among 1468 individuals with a measured body content of radium, 42 bone sarcomas were found, whereas 0.4 were expected on age- and time-specific rates for white females in the United States. However, among all recognized sarcoma cases, the body burdens were not measured in about one-third of cases [R46]. Excess of sinus and mastoid carcinomas was also reported and they were thought to arise from irradiation of the lining epithelium by ^{222}Rn and decay products accumulating in the cavities. Their number

was too small and dosimetry too uncertain for any reasonable discussion of dose-response relationships.

438. The numbers of cases per person-year at risk were calculated as a function of the systemic intake of radium (activity of ^{226}Ra + 2.5 activity of ^{228}Ra; it had been shown [R18] that for induction of osteosarcomas in man ^{228}Ra is 2.5 times more effective per unit activity than ^{226}Ra). All cases with systemic intakes greater than about 10 kBq were used for the fit. The breakdown of cases into 14 intake groups was made in such a way that 3 strata covered each order of magnitude (Figure XXXI) from about 10 kBq up to about 1 GBq. Mean intakes were calculated either as simple weighted means or as roots of mean weighted squares. The former was used when linear, and the latter when quadratic, functions were fitted to the independent variable. Values of $0.7 \cdot 10^{-5}$ and $1.75 \cdot 10^{-5}$ were taken as expected (control) incidence rates for the two modes of treatment mentioned above.

439. Various forms of general initial activity (A)-incidence-rate expression $\dot{I}_{TA} = (a_0 + a_1A + a_2A^2)e^{-\beta_1 A}$ were fitted to the data and tested by χ^2 statistics for goodness of fit. Fitting of 13 data points was carried out by a general weighted least-squares procedure. A quadratic initiation + killing expression gives the best fit (P = 0.73). Arbitrary selection of a positive a_1 still gave an acceptable fit (P = 0.05) of $a_1 = 1.3 \cdot 10^{-5}$. The parameters of the equation $\dot{I}_{TA} = (a_0 + a_2A^2) e^{-\beta_1 A}$ are: $a_2 = (7.0 \pm 0.6) \cdot 10^{-8}$ and $\beta_1 = (1.1 \pm 0.1) \cdot 10^{-3}$, where A is the initial systemic intake of activity.

440. The pure quadratic and linear-quadratic functions give a similar response at higher intakes, but differ markedly in the region of about 4 MBq intake. To change the response from quadratic to linear while retaining a good fit, three additional sarcomas would have to appear in the years to come in the low-dose region where no sarcoma has yet been seen. This, the authors judge as quite improbable (although the activity distribution among unmeasured sarcoma cases is not known). Arbitrary changes of intake ranges did not alter the fact that dose-squared plus killing functions always gave the best fit to the data; only in isolated categorizations of the intake could a linear fit not be discarded.

441. When the dependence between radium intake and time of sarcoma appearance was examined, an inverse relationship was found between intake and maximum or mean (but not minimum) induction period. The numbers of observed and predicted bone sarcomas as a function of time after intake were in good agreement, suggesting that the risk is rather constant over 65 years after intake. No bone sarcoma has been observed among the 1680 measured cases (all categories) with intakes of less than about 2 MBq. The conclusion is, therefore, that the life-span probability of bone sarcoma induction below this level of intake must be very small. The authors calculated that after an intake of about 40 kBq ^{226}Ra over one year, the corresponding lifetime risk of bone sarcoma was $5 \cdot 10^{-14}$ and $1.3 \cdot 10^{-5}$ per year, for the quadratic and linear-quadratic dose-response functions, respectively.

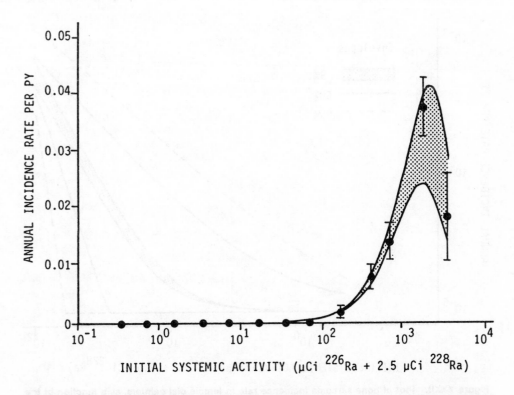

Figure XXXI. A semi-logarithmic plot of bone sarcoma incidence rate as a function of systemic intake for female dial painters employed before 1950, showing a dose-squared exponential fit. The shaded band indicates the range covered by the fitted function when the coefficients are allowed to vary by ± 1 S.D. Error bars represent the binomial standard errors of the observed incidences.
[R34]

442. Schlenker [S50], assumed a binomial distribution to calculate the probability of observing a number of bone sarcomas greater than predicted by the relationship $\dot{I}_{TA} = (a_0 + a_2 A^2) - \exp \beta_1 A$ in the zero range, i.e., for the activity A below about 4 MBq where no tumours were actually seen. For the dose-response curve itself, the probability was 50%. For pairs of curves delineating the 68% and 95% confidence limits (Figure XXXII) there is a corresponding chance that the true number of tumours lies between the two predictions. The curves enveloping the 95% confidence interval span a factor of 90 and their widest distance gives a feeling for the uncertainty in the estimated dose-response relationship at low activities of radium systemic uptake.

443. Because of the inverse relationship between activity and latent period, it might be expected that the upward concavity of the dose-response curve would result from the choice of the variable (rate per year) and would vanish when expressed as cumulative incidence. In annex H of the 1972 UNSCEAR report ([U7], Figure IX), the results of the follow-up through 1969, expressed in this way, showed a downwards concave dose-response relationship. In 1972, Mays and Lloyd [M11] investigated the dose-response relationship for all United States subjects containing radium in their bodies, thus continuing the combined MIT and the Argonne series updated to May 1971. In all, 762 individuals below 200 Gy average skeletal dose were included, 48 of whom developed bone sarcomas. The dose-incidence relationship had a linear trend with a slope of 0.46% per Gy. However, the probability of seeing the deficit of cases below 10 Gy as observed, on the basis of the regression analysis,

was less than 0.1. Mole [M29] plotted, as a function of dose, the cumulative incidence of bone sarcoma per 10^3 individuals for the group of dial painters who started work before 1930 [M27] and who were followed through 1972 [A10]. He assumed equal effectiveness of doses from both radium isotopes, as quoted in [A10]. Functions of incidence I_{TA} against dose (D) in Gy, of the form $I_{TA} = a_2 D^2 e^{-\beta_1 D}$ and $I_{TA} = a_1 D e^{-\beta_1 D}$ gave fits of comparable goodness (P = 0.26 and 0.45, respectively). The fit to a linear equation is

$$I_{TA}(D) = (111 \pm 22)10^{-4} \, D \, e^{-(8.5 \pm 2.2)10^{-3}D} \quad (5.2)$$

characteristic of the linear model for high-LET radiation, which could be used for interpretation of the data on incidence. The slope gives the risk of bone sarcoma from the absorbed dose from radium alpha-radiation. Very low values of β_1 cannot be interpreted in terms of a very high lethal dose to the transformed cells for a variety of reasons, including the long duration of exposure with possible repopulation of the irradiated cell pool.

444. Schlenker [S50] approached the same problem theoretically by calculating the life-time probability I_{TA} of bone sarcoma, corrected for the presence of competing risks, expressed as a function of time-average tumour rate from ^{226}Ra + ^{228}Ra derived from Rowland's equation referred to above [R18]. Thus,

$$I_{TA} = \int_A^{100} da \, \dot{I}_{TA} \, e^{-\int_A^a (I_{TA} + \dot{S}_a) \, da} \quad (5.3)$$

where A is the age at exposure; a is the age in years; $\dot{I}_{TA}$ is the time average tumour rate, equal to zero

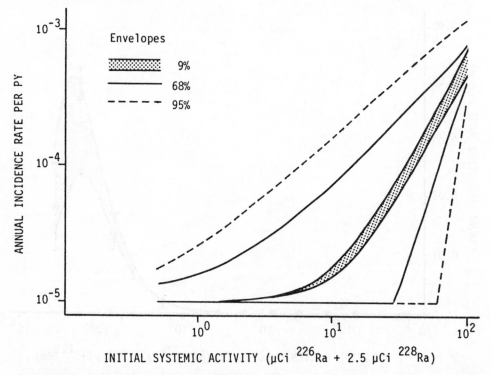

Figure XXXII. Plot of bone sarcoma incidence rate in female dial painters, as a function of the initial intake of radium. Three pairs of curves denote probabilities that the true number of bone sarcomas, in the region of intake where no tumours were observed, falls within the calculated envelopes [S50]. The shaded area covers two standard deviations on either side of the dose-response curve $\dot{I}_{TA} = (a_0 + a_2 A^2) e^{-\beta_1 A}$, as calculated from the standard errors of the parameters [R34].

until a five-year latent period has passed and constant thereafter; and $\dot{S}_a$ is the death rate from all other causes as a function of age.

445. For single ^{226}Ra intakes at ages 20, 45 and 70 years, the results are presented in Figure XXXIII,

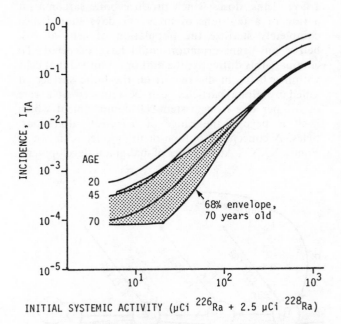

INITIAL SYSTEMIC ACTIVITY (μCi ^{226}Ra + 2.5 μCi ^{228}Ra)

Figure XXXIII. Predicted life-time incidence of bone sarcoma in the presence of competing risks, as a function of a single intake of ^{226,228}Ra.
[S50]

together with 68% confidence limit envelopes for a 70-year-old. For other ages, the envelopes are very similar. It is quite obvious that an approximately linear dose-response for cumulative incidence I_{TA} against intake of activity into the blood might be the prevailing trend over the range from about 200 kBq to about 8 MBq. This conclusion, of course, excludes neither the possibility of a "practical threshold" nor the absence of a life-shortening effect such as that referred to above, nor that a dose-squared relationship may be fitted into the envelopes.

446. The linear trend of bone sarcoma incidence (I_{TA}) against alpha-ray dose in the human skeleton is in accordance with the bulk of the evidence from animal experiments, as reviewed in chapter IV. However, more refined analyses of bone sarcoma integral tumour rates, induced in beagles by ^{239}Pu injections, support a dose-squared dependence of the rate [P17, W14]. For radionuclides emitting low-LET particles like ^{90}Sr, an upwards concave dose-response relationship was invariably observed [M12-M14].

447. Several thousand patients in the Federal Republic of Germany were given repeated intravenous injections of ^{224}Ra in the course of therapy for tuberculosis and ankylosing spondylitis. In contrast with ^{226}Ra, ^{224}Ra, with its short half-life of 3.64 days, decays on the surface of bone where it becomes deposited early after injection due to rapid ionic exchange. The fraction of the mean dose to the skeleton delivered by ^{224}Ra to the target cells is much

higher than that for ^{226}Ra. The effectiveness of the mean skeletal dose is therefore about 7 times higher for ^{224}Ra. The patients were of both sexes and included adults as well as juveniles. The most recent report on these patients through 1980 [M57] includes 218 juveniles and 680 adults. Bone sarcomas had appeared in 35 patients injected as juveniles and in 18 adults. The follow-up times ranged from 0 to 36 years; deaths accounted for most of the short follow-up times, whereas 582 patients were followed for more than 19 years and 78% were still alive in 1980. The mean skeletal doses from a-particles were estimated to be 10.98 and 2.05 Gy in juvenile and adult, respectively; the corresponding injection spans averaged 11 and 6 months. Virtually all bone sarcomas are ascribed to radiation, as only 0.2 cases would be expected, based on general population rates.

448. The shortest appearance times were 3.5 and 5 years in juvenile and adult patients, respectively; the corresponding average values were 10.4 ± 5.1 and 11.6 ± 5.2 years, and were not significantly different. The time distribution was similar to that for leukaemias in atomic bomb survivors, as described for those exposed within 1500 m of ground zero by Bizzozero et al. [B82] for which the average appearance time was 9 years. The peak of bone sarcoma appearance was 6-8 years. No additional cases were discovered since the previous report in 1974 [S21]. It may be concluded, therefore, that by 25-30 years after injection the vast majority of bone sarcomas have already become manifest.

449. There was some tendency towards a lower risk of bone sarcoma per unit dose with advancing age at injection, but this could be an artifact due to uncertainties in dosimetric assumptions, a possibly non-linear response, or a more pronounced fractionation of injected activity in juveniles. Fractionated administration appeared more effective; a protracted weekly administration over a few years carries a 5-times greater risk per unit dose than single injection [S18]. This observation is in agreement with studies on mice injected with ^{224}Ra in various fractionation schemes [L20, M67]. Original data from reference [S18] were examined [P8] for partial correlations between the increment of incidence per unit dose, average injection span and the average skeletal dose. Significant positive correlations were found between the span and dose, and also between the incidence increment and the span. The correlation between the increment of incidence and the fractionation span itself was non-significant (in fact it was negative) when the above partial correlations were accounted for. Thus, the suggestion of an increased effectiveness of fractionated versus single administration of ^{224}Ra, based upon human experience, appears unfounded. The dose-response relationship for bone sarcoma incidence in the treated patients was compatible with linearity. The slopes for juveniles and adults differ by a factor not greater than 2 (Figure XXXIV, [S21]). However, a dose-squared trend of the effect could not be rejected on statistical grounds. No carcinomas of the head sinuses were observed in patients injected with ^{224}Ra due to lack of sufficiently long-lived radon nuclides in the thorium decay series.

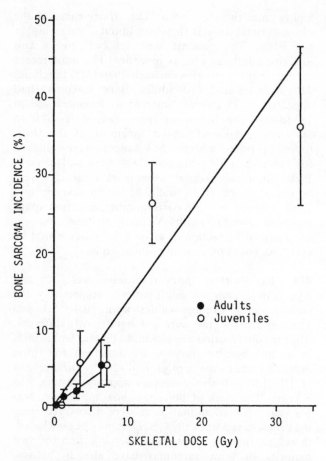

Figure XXXIV. Bone sarcoma incidence versus skeletal dose from ^{224}Ra. For the linear non-threshold lines shown the cumulative risk of bone sarcoma during 14-21 years post-exposure is 0.7% (adults) and 1.4% (juveniles) per unit average skeletal dose.
[S21]

450. Schlenker [S50] calculated the dose-response relationship for ^{224}Ra-induced osteosarcoma cases. For incidence I_{TA} (uncorrected for competing risks) in subjects older than 16 years at injection, the function had the form $I_{TA} = 1 - e^{-3.0 \ 10^{-5} A}$. At the widest separation, the 95% confidence limits span a range of 750, reflecting much less information at low doses for ^{224}Ra than for $^{226+228}$Ra. This can be explained by the smaller number of cases and shorter follow-up times.

2.   The model of Marshall and Groer

451.   Theories of bone sarcoma induction were developed in the past [B21, M26] but the most comprehensive one based on human epidemiological data has been presented by Marshall and Groer [M4]. They based their model on several observations. The first is that a linear dose-response relationship gave a poor fit to the incidence rate of bone sarcoma versus dose (bone averaged) from ^{226}Ra and ^{228}Ra, as discussed in detail by Rowland [R18-R20]. There were no cases of osteosarcoma below 9 Gy, and pure linearity of incidence rate versus dose was therefore highly unlikely on statistical grounds. They postulated, therefore, that two events produced by alpha radiation in a cell at risk are necessary to initiate the malignant transformation.

452.   Marshall and Groer assumed that there are about 10^{11} cells at risk in the endosteum of a "reference man". These cells are subject to sarcoma initiation in two steps, but also to cell killing, the killing being by a factor of 10^5 more probable than initiation (D_0 for the cells must be of the order of 1 Gy). Thus, doses which produce bone sarcoma (at a rate of a few tens of mGy per day) should also completely sterilize the population of cells at risk before any transformation could have occurred. To eliminate this difficulty, the authors assumed that cells within a 0-10 μm distance from the bone surface, if killed by alpha particles, can be replaced at a rate of 0.1 per day from a stem-cell compartment which itself is beyond the range of 5.7 MeV alpha particles. A conceptual outline of the model is shown in Figure XXXV. At all stages of malignant development,

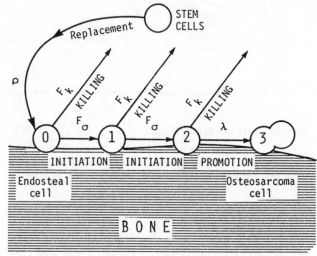

Figure XXXV.   Schematic representation of the Marshall and Groer [M4] model of bone sarcoma induction by alpha particles. An original endosteal cell is initiated twice and promoted to become an osteosarcoma cell; cells killed at any stage before promotion are replaced by stem cells. The rate of killing, F_k, is 10^5 times larger than the rate of initiation $F\sigma$ (F = endosteal dose rate). The rates of replacement ρ and of promotion λ are independent of radiation dose.

the cells are at risk of killing, which is proportional to their numbers (M_0, M_1, M_2) and to the dose rate F. The dose rate in turn is proportional to the content of radium per unit mass of the diffuse radium component in bone. The fully transformed cells (M_3) promoted to cellular division are not assumed to be at significant risk for cell killing due to a rapid multiplication of the clone and escape of the tumorous cells from the volume irradiated by alpha particles.

453.   To summarize, the model incorporates the following parameters:

(a)   initiation probability per cell per unit dose (σ);

(b)   killing probability per unit dose (k);

(c)   number of cells at risk (s);

(d)   promotion probability per unit time (λ);

(e)   replacement probability of killed cells (ρ);

(f)   growth time of a tumour to become recognizable (g);

(g) dose rate (F) proportional to activity per body weight (c).

These parameters were incorporated in a set of differential equations to give a probability of appearance, P(t), of an osteosarcoma per unit time per individual and unit activity of radium reaching the blood stream. The values of ρ, σ and s were held fixed, and initiation probability, promotion rate, tumour growth time and dose rate were adjusted through a solution of the model by best fit of the data obtained from observation of individuals with radium body burdens followed through December 1973 at the Argonne National Laboratory [A10].

454. From the solution of the model for man, it follows that the time of sarcoma appearance after radium uptake should increase with decreasing values of the intake q reaching a constant plateau at about 30-35 years at the level of 40 kBq per kg body weight. The theory predicts [G23, M4] an enhanced effect on bone sarcoma induction by fractionated administration of a short-lived bone-seeking alpha emitter. The existence of such a phenomenon was, in fact, suggested when bone sarcoma incidence was studied after injections of ^{224}Ra. When the isotope was administered over one month, the incidence was lower than that seen after prolonged (average 2 years) administration of the nuclide (P = 0.16) [S18]. The lower sarcoma incidence in this case should result, according to Marshall and Groer [G23, M4], from suppression of the population of viable endosteal cells M_0 by very high dose rates delivered over short intervals (the empirical basis to support this contention is open to critique, see paragraph 449).

455. The theory fits satisfactorily the preliminary data on the induction of bone sarcoma by ^{226}Ra in Utah beagles, in which the cumulative incidence reaches a plateau of about 92%, a factor of 3-4.5 higher than in man. The parameters of the theory, which give a good fit to the experimental situation, were rather similar to those for man, with the exception of higher promotion and initiation rates (both roughly by a factor of 10). Reasons for this interspecies difference in initiation probability are not clear.

456. Marshall and Groer [M4] correctly stated that fit of the model to the measured data does not prove correctness of the postulates. Some results of the theory were not envisaged a priori, e.g., the plateau of incidence rate at high doses (Figure XXXVI). This point of agreement enhances the credibility of the theory. However, in the light of the evidence that the cumulative incidence of ^{226}Ra-induced bone sarcoma, both in man and in beagles, can be reasonably approximated by a linear model, the basic assumption of two-hit initiation is open to question. A model similar to that of Marshall and Groer, but postulating a one-hit initiation has been proposed [P23]. The model explains the non-linear part of the activity-incidence rate curve by the promoting action of alpha radiation exerted via repopulation of the target cell pool (osteogenic cells).

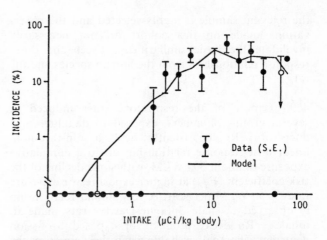

Figure XXXVI. The cumulative incidence of osteosarcomas in man versus the total intake (μCi per kg body weight) of radium-226 plus radium-228. Up to about 1 μCi per kilogram body weight systemic intake the slope of the line, according to the model of Marshall and Groer [M4], is close to 1.

F. INTERSPECIES COMPARISONS

457. In numerous instances in the course of the review of experimental (chapter IV) and human data (chapter V), qualitative similarities have been pointed out between animal and human data that may usefully be summarized here. From such comparisons, the pattern seems to emerge that the shape of dose-response relationships may be basically similar in various species.

458. Thus, the linear non-threshold type of dose-response relationship for female mammary carcinoma induced by x rays finds its counterpart in the results of studies on at least four strains of rats: (a) the Sprague-Dawley females irradiated externally by x rays and/or gamma rays, and internally by β particles from tritium; the linearity applies to adenomas but the results for adenocarcinomas are also consistent with the notion; (b) females of the WAG/Rij rat strain and the AC strain irradiated externally with x rays showing linearity for adenomas and carcinomas, respectively; and (c) non-inbred female rats irradiated from a β-particle source also showing a linear rise of incidence of mammary carcinomas. The dose-response curve for mammary carcinomas induced in BALB/C mice by gamma rays shows irregularities that defy any possible comparison.

459. A strong linear component is manifest in the non-threshold dose-response relationship for x-ray induced thyroid carcinoma in man; effects of dose-fractionation are virtually absent. Data on Long-Evans rats, even if the number of animals is limited and the observations were terminated 2 years after irradiation, are compatible with linearity. They also show a lack of a pronounced dose-rate effect, as shown by the comparison of x-ray and ^{131}I dose-response curves. The absence of an excess of thyroid cancers in humans exposed to diagnostic quantities of ^{131}I is not consistent with the above observation, but

239

the relevant sample is highly selected and the observations made on this cohort do not necessarily invalidate the basic similarities between the dose-response relationships from the human species and the rat.

460. Cancer of the respiratory tract induced in several groups of miners, exposed to daughter products of ^{222}Rn, consistently yields a non-threshold linear dose-response relationship up to a cumulative exposure of about 300 WLM, with some decline of the risk coefficient (F_{TA}) at higher exposures or exposure rates > 50 WLM per year. A very similar relationship is observed in male Sprague-Dawley rats made to inhale ^{222}Rn decay products or exposed to fission neutrons. The analogy holds when the data from the two species are analysed in terms of both the absolute and the relative risk model.

461. Dose-response relationships for bone sarcoma induced by long-lived isotopes of radium in man, beagles and mice are compatible with linearity between dose and cumulative incidence over the initial part of the curve. In all three species a decline of the tumour yield is seen at high and very high doses in the skeleton. In the three species there is also a pronounced inverse relationship between dose (or initial activity in the body) and the latent period.

462. In summary, it appears that the shape of the dose-response relationship for radiation-induced cancer of some organs in man generally follows the pattern seen in a number of experimental animal species. This qualitative finding will have to be verified in the light of future data. The similarity may not be surprising for those types of human malignancies that have a reasonable counterpart in other mammalian species, in view of the basic similarity of patho-physiological phenomena on which rests the rationale of using experimental animals to predict the response of man. However, the regularities pointed out do not imply that data from experimental animals may be used to derive risk coefficient applicable to man, because, so far, such similarities may not be shown to apply to the quantitative expression of the carcinogenic effect in various species.

G. SUMMARY AND CONCLUSIONS

463. Epidemiological data useful for an analysis of the shape of the dose-response relationships for radiation-induced cancer are limited. This applies to external and internal, to instantaneous and prolonged exposures. Caution should therefore be exercised in formulating broad generalizations. Several factors are known to affect the magnitude of the neoplastic response. Among those identified, age at irradiation, sex and genetic or ethnic characteristics are of importance, but the extent to which these factors may affect the form of the dose-response curves is almost totally unknown. For some tumours, e.g., cancer of the lung, the characteristics of the environment and the living habits may consistently affect the expression of malignancies.

464. With the Hiroshima and Nagasaki atomic bomb dosimetry still uncertain, the epidemiological information on leukaemia incidence in the survivors cannot yet be fully utilized. Information on induction of leukaemia derived from the follow-up of spondylitis patients is insufficient to allow firm conclusions as to the most likely form of the dose relationship, particularly because leukaemia incidence in this group may have been influenced to an unknown extent by dose-fractionation effects. Therefore, further discussion of dose-response relationships must be postponed until new information on the atomic bomb survivors becomes available.

465. Regarding breast cancer, there is no suggestion of a threshold for low-LET radiation; either a pure linear relationship with dose or one with a small dose-squared term might apply. This conclusion is supported by the small or absent effect of dose fractionation and by the lack of a detectable relationship of latency to dose. For this tumour, there is, however, a pronounced variation of the risk with the age at exposure, as women in the age range of 0-30 years are at the highest risk.

466. Dose-response relationships for carcinoma of the thyroid have a strong linear component and the data do not suggest a threshold. There appears to be no inverse relationship between latency and dose and this is consistent with the observed linearity. Infants and children are more susceptible to cancer of the thyroid than grown-up persons. Dose-rate effects cannot be excluded, and data on patients given ^{131}I for diagnostic purposes might be interpreted in this way; however, other interpretations are also possible, particularly since dose-rate effects have not been seen in recent animal experiments. The induction of benign thyroid adenomas is linearly related with x-ray doses at low doses, but with a decrease of the slope at doses above 1 Gy.

467. The available data on lung cancer induced by exposure to radon and its decay products in mines show, without exception, linear exposure-response relationships, with a decreasing slope at the highest exposure rates (above 50 WLM per year); there is no indication of a threshold. This type of relationship has also been consistently observed for airborne short-lived a-emitting radionuclides in animal experiments. For low-LET radiation the form of the dose-response curve is essentially unknown.

468. Alpha-emitting bone-seeking radionuclides, such as ^{226}Ra and ^{228}Ra, may induce bone sarcoma in man with a significantly elevated frequency at mean skeletal doses above 10 Gy. Plotting the incidence or incidence rate against cumulative dose results in relationships that may be interpreted as either linear or quadratic. In the latter case, below about 10 Gy there is a significant deficit of tumours when a linear interpolation to zero dose is attempted and I_{TA} fits very well a dose-squared model with a cell-killing term. In this case, linearity may be rejected. It appears impossible at present to decide whether linear or quadratic models, or a combination of both, provide better fits to incidence (I_{TA}) versus dose from radium

isotopes over the initial portion of the curve. Animal experiments suggest linearity. Bone sarcomas induced in man and animals by a-emitting bone seekers show a pronounced inverse relationship of latency to dose. The deficit of tumours in man, at the lowest end of the scale mentioned above, could therefore reflect an apparent "practical" threshold, and a decreasing tumour-related life shortening with lowering of the dose.

469. A dose-response relationship for bone sarcoma induced in man by short-lived a-emitters (^{224}Ra) is compatible with linearity, even though alternative models may not be excluded. The latent period for bone sarcoma appears to be rather short; the age at the beginning of exposure has no strong influence. There are no human studies of bone sarcoma caused by low-LET irradiation. However, irradiation of experimental animals by β-emitting bone seekers (^{45}Ca, ^{90}Sr, ^{89}Sr) invariably resulted in upwards concave relationships and a pronounced inverse relationship between dose and latent period. It would be expected that the same kind of relationship might also apply to man.

470. In summary, the model applying to the dose-response relationship for leukaemia is unknown and must remain so until new dose-incidence data for atomic bomb survivors become available. The reviewed evidence suggests that incidence of lung, mammary and thyroid cancers is probably related with dose by a generalized linear or linear-quadratic relationship. However, dose-incidence information is not available for lung cancers after low-LET and for breast and thyroid after high-LET irradiation.

471. In a comparison of data from experimental animals, reviewed in chapter IV, and from human epidemiological studies in the present chapter, UNSCEAR has identified a number of tumours for which the dose-response relationships appear to follow the same basic pattern in various species. Such a comparison will have to be verified as more data are accumulated. In any case, the qualitative similarity of the induction kinetics does not justify any simple quantitative extrapolation of incidence data from animals to man.

VI. SUMMARY

472. In order to estimate the absolute risk of radiation-induced cancer (number of induced tumours per million people exposed per unit dose, i.e., cases 10^{-6} Gy^{-1}), or the relative increase of tumour frequency per unit dose over the "natural" incidence at low doses and dose rates, two types of information are required: first, empirical data on the incidence of various forms of malignancy at relatively high doses where observations have actually been made; second, knowledge of the mathematical form of the relationships linking the incidence of cancers with the dose of radiation. Such data would allow predictions to be made of the cancer incidence at doses (and perhaps also at dose rates) very much lower than those at which direct observations in man have been gathered.

473. When the incidence of a given tumour in exposed animal or human populations is followed as a function of increasing dose, several observations may usually be made. At relatively low doses (at about 0.1 Gy of sparsely-ionizing radiation), only seldom (and then mostly in controlled animal experiments) can a statistically significant increase of cancer or leukaemia be shown. At higher doses (up to a few Gy, but with considerable differences between different tumours), the incidence of such malignancies may be shown statistically to exceed the level observed in non-exposed control populations, following some increasing function of the dose. At still higher doses (many Gy), the incidence gradually starts to fall off because of cell killing. Dose-response relationships of this type, going through a maximum at some intermediate dose, are often found in experimental animals. They are termed "biphasic".

474. A common interpretation attached to such a shape advocates the concurrent presence of two different phenomena: (a) a dose-related increase of the proportion of normal cells that are transformed into malignant ones; and (b) a dose-related decrease of the probability that such cells may survive the radiation treatment. Both these phenomena are normally operating in the region of doses where data are available, but to a different degree for various doses and different types of cancer. What may happen at the low doses, where direct information is lacking, may only be inferred from a combination of empirical data and theoretical assumptions, linked together into some models of radiation action.

475. The models referred to are simplified semi-quantitative representations of complex biological phenomena. Present knowledge of the mechanisms of carcinogenesis, including radiation carcinogenesis, is inadequate to design comprehensive models accounting for all physical and biological factors known to influence the induction of cancer. To avoid some of the complications involved, UNSCEAR suggests that the range of doses over which extrapolations may meaningfully be performed should be limited to low and intermediate doses. Under these conditions, it seems likely that no serious distortions would result from other radiation effects, called non-stochastic, that are observed when doses exceed fairly high thresholds, typical for each tissue and each effect.

476. The formulation and analysis of models of radiation carcinogenesis must rely on a few basic assumptions, as follows:

(a) The observed dose-response relationships for clinically visible tumours in vivo approximately reflect the relationships between dose and frequency of the initial triggering events in the cells where cancer will eventually arise, despite host reactions and the effect of latency, which may modify such relationships to some degree. This assumption is based on the overall similarity of the dose-response curves for cancer induction with those of various other cellular effects of radiation. UNSCEAR postulates this concept simply as a working hypothesis;

(b) Cancer initiation is basically a unicellular process occurring at random in single cells. This is also a working hypothesis that has not yet definitely been proved. However, evidence to the contrary, i.e., that cancer initiation takes place in several cells, is not entirely convincing. The uni-cellular theory of cancer induction is compatible with the notion that some, still ill-defined, influences resulting from irradiation of other neighbouring cells or other organs may modify the probability of an initiated cell to develop into an overt malignancy. Firm biological evidence in favour of this latter notion is very fragmentary;

(c) Absence of a dose threshold is characteristic of many, if not all, tumours. For some animal tumours (e.g., tumours of the ovary or thymic lymphoma of the mouse) threshold-type dose-response relationships are observed. In other cases (e.g., tumours of the skin) cancer is only induced with great difficulty, i.e., after high doses of radiation. In still others (i.e., epidermoid lung cancer in man) the data are unclear, owing perhaps to a short follow-up of the patients. However, in spite of these exceptions, absence of a threshold dose for the development of cancer is assumed by UNSCEAR as a working hypothesis for the time being;

(d) Susceptibility of an irradiated animal or human population to tumour induction is assumed to follow a unimodal distribution. Although genetic predispositions to the development of some forms of malignancy are well documented (see annex A), efforts to show that such phenomena apply also to radiation-induced human cancer have not been successful so far. Therefore, pending further studies, the same unimodal distribution of susceptibilities to the induction of cancer in irradiated and non-irradiated populations is also provisionally accepted as a working proposition.

477. On the above assumptions, it is possible to infer likely shapes for the dose-response relationships of radiation-induced cancer. Such inferences rely on the analysis of various other radiation effects observed at the cellular level. These effects involve the cells' genetic material, which is also thought to be the primary target for cancer initiation. The production of mutations and chromosomal aberrations in somatic and germinal cells, and the oncogenic transformation in vitro of mammalian cell lines, are examples of such effects. If cancer induction in vivo involves mechanisms similar to, or related with, those underlying the effects listed above, one would expect all these phenomena to respond similarly in respect of changes in dose, dose rate and fractionation. As such similarities have actually been observed, it may be possible to extrapolate the shape of dose-response relationships between such effects and the phenomenon of cancer induction.

478. Three basic non-threshold models of radiation action as a function of dose have been discussed with respect to such cellular effects and to cancer induction: the linear, the linear-quadratic and the pure quadratic. Notwithstanding some exceptions, these may provide a general envelope for a variety of radiation-induced end-points at the cellular level, as well as for tumour induction in experimental animals and human populations.

479. The vast majority of dose-response curves for induction of point mutations and chromosomal aberrations by sparsely-ionizing x and gamma rays may be described by a linear-quadratic model. For the same end-points, when cell killing is corrected for, a linear model usually applies to densely-ionizing neutrons or alpha particles. As a rule, for a number of chromosomal structural abnormalities, curvilinearity (upward concavity) is observed for low-LET radiation, while, for the same effects and a wide range of doses, linearity prevails for high-LET particles. Linearity of the dose-response for somatic mutations and terminal chromosomal deletions has been found in some cell lines, even for low-LET radiation, but these findings are relatively infrequent.

480. Approximate estimates of proportionality constants linking the chromosomal effects with the dose or its square may be obtained experimentally. They allow the frequency of such effects to be predicted at low doses and dose rates from observations at higher doses. For cancer induction, however, only fragmentary information supports the notion that similar quantitative relationships with the dose might apply. UNSCEAR has estimated that if the risk of tumour induction at 1 or 2 Gy of sparsely-ionizing radiation (at high dose rate) were extrapolated linearly down to zero dose, this procedure would over-estimate the risk by a factor of perhaps up to 5 in typical situations.

481. Over the last few years much information on radiation-induced oncogenic transformation of mammalian cells has become available. The cancerous nature of the transformed cells is shown by the fact that after transformation in vitro they are able to form malignant tumours upon transplantation into an animal of the same species. Transformation in vitro is therefore regarded as a model, albeit a simplified one, of radiation carcinogenesis at the cellular level. Cells exposed in vitro to sparsely-ionizing radiation 24 hours after seeding are transformed according to complex kinetics that cannot be fitted to models used for other cellular effects. Moreover, fractionation of the dose (below 1.5 Gy total) enhances transformation, which effect is contrary to what would be predicted by a linear-quadratic model. If similar phenomena would apply to the induction of cancer in vivo, extrapolation to low doses and dose rates might result in a significant under-estimate of the risk. Further research is needed to elucidate these phenomena, but several experiments indicate that the observations on in vitro systems referred to above may result from non-typical conditions of cellular growth during the early periods after establishment of the culture. Actually, irradiation of non-dividing cells or cells under exponential conditions of growth (which are thought to be more representative of an asynchronously dividing cell population) produces results that are compatible with those obtained for other cellular effects; thus, for example, high-dose-rate gamma irradiation results in a greater frequency of transformation than low-dose-rate exposure.

482. There are indications that when cells are irradiated with neutrons, low-dose-rate or dose fractionation may increase the rate of transformation, even at low doses; however, whereas some observations on tumour induction in experimental animals clearly support these findings, others do not. In other experiments, enhanced transformation by neutron fractionation or protraction were seen only at intermediate and high doses. In view of the scarcity of such data, and of the uncertainties regarding the mechanisms involved, further research is needed before enhancement of cancer induction by neutron fractionation and protraction (relative to single or high-dose-rate exposure) may be accepted for the purpose of risk assessment. Such a possibility should, however, be kept in mind even though the theoretical basis to explain such phenomena is uncertain at present.

483. Recent experimental findings on radiation-induced tumours in experimental animals have not substantially changed the main conclusions reached in annex I of the 1977 UNSCEAR report. Most data support the notion that dose-response relationships for x and gamma rays tend to be curvilinear and concave upward at low doses. Under these conditions, tumour induction is dose-rate dependent, in that a reduction of the dose rate, or fractionation, reduces the tumour yield. A linear extrapolation of the risk from doses delivered at high rates to zero dose would thus, as a rule, over-estimate the real risk at low doses and dose rates. However, in one experimental mammary tumour system (matched by epidemiological data on human breast cancer) x and gamma radiation produced a linear dose-response with little fractionation and dose-rate dependence. This was recognized as an exception in the 1977 UNSCEAR report. It appears likely that a similar dose-response relationship could also apply to the induction of thyroid cancers, but the data are too limited to permit any definite conclusion to be drawn in this respect.

484. For densely-ionizing neutron irradiation, tumour induction in animals follows, in general, a very nearly linear curve at the lower end of the dose scale and shows little dependence on dose rate. In some cases, however, enhancement upon fractionation (and possibly protraction) has been noted. Above about 0.1 Gy or so, the curve tends to become concave downward, markedly in some cases. Under these conditions, a linear extrapolation of the risk down to zero dose from intermediate or high doses and dose rates would involve a variable degree of under-estimation.

485. Having reviewed existing data on dose-response relationships for radiation-induced tumours in man, UNSCEAR considers that this whole matter must be treated with caution because at the present time observations are fragmentary. Those for neutrons are totally absent, and definitive data for atomic bomb survivors at Hiroshima and Nagasaki are still not available. For example, dose-response information for sparsely-ionizing radiation have not been reported for lung and bone tumours, and data for densely-ionizing radiation have not been reported for thyroid and mammary cancer. For sparsely-ionizing radiation, in some cases (lung, thyroid, breast), the data available are consistent with linear or linear-quadratic models. For breast cancer, however, predominant linearity may apply, as the incidence is little affected by dose fractionation. Linearity of the response for lung cancer after irradiation by alpha particles from radon decay products does not contradict the above statement, because with alpha particles the dose-squared component is practically absent. Some doubts still remain, however, as to osteosarcoma induced by bone-seeking alpha- or beta-emitting radionuclides. However, in spite of the fragmentary character of the human data, a general picture may be emerging from which several tentative conclusions can be derived.

486. For sparsely-ionizing radiation, linear extrapolation from about 2 Gy down would not over-estimate the risk of breast and possibly thyroid cancer. It would slightly over-estimate the risk of leukaemia, and it would definitely over-estimate the risk of bone sarcoma. For lung cancer, lack of direct evidence does not permit any assessment to be made of the magnitude of the over-estimate.

487. For densely-ionizing radiation, the risk of lung cancer from accumulated exposures to radon decay products at low dose rates from 300 WLM down (roughly corresponding to 20 to 50 Sv) would not be over- or under-estimated by linear extrapolation. However, extrapolation from observations made at higher cumulative exposures might result in a significant under-estimation due to observed flattening (saturation) of the dose-response curve in this region. It should be stressed that absolute risk coefficients derived for male miners, of whom a high proportion are smokers, should not be applied to the general public without due corrections for various factors (intensity of smoking, lung ventilation rate, presence of other contaminating pollutants, etc.) that are thought to increase the risk in the miners.

488. The incidence of bone sarcoma after internal irradiation by alpha particles from long-lived bone-seeking radionuclides is distorted by the existence of a pronounced inverse relationship between accumulated dose and latent period. This results in an apparent threshold at low doses, and in a reduced loss of life span per induced tumour, as a function of decreasing dose, down to zero loss at low doses. If this is a correct explanation for the upward concavity of the dose-response relationship, a linear extrapolation from a few tens of gray mean skeletal dose down to the gray or milligray region would grossly over-estimate the risk.

489. No human data for induction of breast cancer and leukaemia by densely-ionizing radiations are available at present and, therefore, no direct inferences can be made about risk extrapolation to the low-dose domain. On the basis of general knowledge, if the risk at intermediate doses could be derived from data on sparsely-ionizing radiation (suitably corrected for the higher effectiveness of the densely-ionizing particles), a linear extrapolation down to low doses might either under-estimate or correctly estimate the real risk in these cases.

490. For radiation-induced cancers of other organs, only experimental data are available. For sparsely-ionizing radiations upward concave curvilinear dose-response relationships with pronounced dose-rate and fractionation effects are usually found. If similar curves should apply to cancers in man, a linear extrapolation of risk coefficients (obtained at the intermediate dose region after acute irradiation) to the low dose and low dose rates, would very likely overestimate the real risk, possibly by a factor of up to 5. For densely-ionizing radiation, should relevant values become available, a linear extrapolation would probably under-estimate the risk.

491. Upon close inspection, some regularities seem to emerge that may indirectly help in assessing the character of dose-response relationships in man. A similarity of the shape of the relationships was noted between man and experimental animals for tumours of several organs for which reasonably good information exists. These are: mammary and thyroid cancers (low-LET radiations), and lung and bone cancers (high-LET radiations). Should this pattern be confirmed, knowledge of epidemiogical studies in man at intermediate or high doses, and of the shape of the dose-response relationships from several animal species, might make it possible to assess the bias introduced by linear extrapolation of the risk coefficients to low doses.

VII. RESEARCH NEEDS

492. At the conclusion of this analysis, it appears quite obvious that there exists a wide intellectual gap between the abstract and general nature of the models discussed and the very complex biological reality, particularly in respect of the molecular mechanisms of tumour induction that are gradually being uncovered. Assigning a biological meaning to the numerical constants of the models, searching for the compatibility between the mechanisms identified and the models' predictions, and formulating new models based on hard data rather than on a priori generalizations, are the formidable tasks facing this type of research today. Any advancement in the field of radiation carcinogenesis will presumably come in parallel with progress in tumour biology, of which the former is only a special aspect. Within these very general guidelines, specialized studies in the following subjects could be valuable and UNSCEAR would like to recommend them to the attention of the interested research worker:

(a) Studies on the nature of the cellular and sub-cellular changes involved in the transformation of normal into cancerous cells. These should aim at establishing and possibly identifying the stages in the induction process that have been postulated. Within these studies, the mechanisms of oncogenic transformation on a wide range of cell types in vitro, and the influence of the main radiobiological variables on the form of the relevant dose-effect relationship, should have a special place, because the biological end-point in question is probably very relevant to the initiation of cancer. Studies on the relationship between transformation of cells to a potentially malignant state in vitro, and the production of malignancies in vivo, should be particularly pursued. Mechanisms by which sub-transformation and potential transformation damage is repaired in cells after exposure to low- and high-LET radiation should also be explored.

(b) In experimental animals, a better understanding of the pathogenesis of radiation-induced tumours should allow the formulation of quantitative models more firmly founded than those available so far. More attention than in the past should be paid to the end-points tested and to the experimental design which will allow a correct statistical analysis of the experimental data. In particular, studies should aim at elucidating the mechanisms by which radiation interacts with oncogenes and the genetic material. Recommendations in respect of experimental work on animals were formulated in annex I of the 1977 UNSCEAR report and, in view of the rather slow rate of accumulation of the data for such long-term effects, many of these recommendations are still valid at present. Particular attention should be devoted to studies in the range of low doses. Comparative studies would be useful of dose-response relationships for those tumours that presumably represent adequate models for human malignancies, and especially those for which quantitative information on dose-response relationships is likely to become available in man in the not too distant future. Studies could usefully be devoted to the RBE of different types of low- and high-LET radiation, particularly in those instances where reliable epidemiological information does not exist, as is now the case for fast neutrons. A subject which remains to be explored in greater depth is that of effects of exogenous and endogenous factors on the shape of dose-response relationships for radiation-induced cancer, particularly the influence of the immunological state and the effects of promoting and inhibitory factors. Another important subject concerns the mechanisms by which downward-concave dose-response curves and enhanced fractionation (or protraction) effects are seen after various doses of neutrons.

(c) In human populations, the follow-up of groups already under study should be continued as a matter of high priority. New studies on groups that might potentially yield further information should also be considered and, if warranted, carefully undertaken. The topics on which further information would be required are, in general, the following:

(i) The shape of the dose-response relationships for a wide spectrum of tumours and an extended range of doses, with special attention to the correct assessment of doses, as well as its distribution in space and time;

(ii) The time distribution of the latent periods for tumours with long latencies;

(iii) The existence and the possible form of a relationship between the length of the latent period and the magnitude of dose;

(iv) The influence of age, sex, genetic factors and some habits (e.g., smoking) on the quantitative characteristics of dose-response relationships and the resulting variability in risk estimates;

(v) The adequacy with which relative and absolute risk models for different cancers permit projection of the risk for long periods after irradiation.

T a b l e   1

Observed (O) and expected (E) breast cancers with relative risk estimates as a function of radiation dose for the interval 10-34 years after radiation treatment for mastitis
[S16]

A.   Analysis of persons with average dose to both breasts

Dose range (Gy)	Mean dose (Gy)	Breast cancer			
		PY a/	O b/	E c/	RR d/
4.50-12.00	5.84	974	4	1.79	2.24
3.50-4.49	3.92	693	4	1.27	3.14
2.50-3.49	2.94	1084	9	3.09	2.91
1.50-2.49	1.93	2971	12	5.22	2.30
0.40-1.49	1.12	2620	7	4.78	1.47
Control		15767	28	28.0	1.0

B.   Analysis of single breasts with total dose per breast

Dose range (Gy)	Mean dose (Gy)	Breast cancer			
		PY a/	O b/	E c/	RR d/
6.00-14.00	8.00	1328	2	1.12	1.78
4.00-5.99	4.67	3183	7	2.58	2.71
3.00-3.99	3.49	2430	11	1.96	5.60
2.00-2.99	2.49	3271	11	2.73	4.03
0.60-1.99	1.50	1843	2	1.47	1.36
Control		37857 e/	31	31.0	1.0

a/ For benign tumours no latent period was assumed, so the person-years at risk include the full interval 1-34 years after irradiation for the single breast analyses.
b/ Observed cancers.
c/ Expected values were calculated by the combination x^2 method, with adjustment for age at irradiation and yearly intervals since irradiation, and were standardized so that O/E = RR = 1 in the control group.
d/ Relative risk.
e/ Observed cancers and person-years at risk for control group in this analysis include 392 non-irradiated breasts (with three cancers) of women with unilateral irradiation.

T a b l e   2

Curve-fitting analyses of breast cancer data
from Massachusetts fluoroscopy series
[L22]
(All parameters are scaled by a factor of 10^6)

Model	Parameter $\underline{a}/$	Massachusetts fluoroscopy series			
		Estimate ± S.D.	Goodness of fit		
			x^2	df	P
Linear	α_1	560±120	1.6	4	0.81
Linear-quadratic	α_1 α_2	450±300 29± 76	1.5	3	0.68
Linear + killing	α_1 β_2	450±230 0 $\underline{b}/$	1.6	3	0.66
Linear-quadratic + killing	α_1 α_2 β_2	450±860 29±570 0 $\underline{b}/$	1.5	2	0.47
Quadratic	α_2	130± 40	3.0	4	0.56
Quadratic + killing	α_2 β_2	220±140 (1.6±2.2)10^4	2.5	3	0.48

$\underline{a}/$ The dimensions of the parameters are as follows:
  α_1: 10^{-6} a-1 Gy-1
  α_2: 10^{-6} a-1 Gy-2
  β_2: 10^{-2} Gy-2.

$\underline{b}/$ The best-fitting parameter would be negative; the value of zero
results from the prior constraint that the parameter be non-negative.

246

Curve-fitting analyses of breast cancer data from Rochester mastitis series
[L22]
(All parameters are scaled by a factor of 10^6)

Model	Parameter $\underline{a}/$	Mean doses bo both breasts				Curves for dose to single breast			
		Estimate ± S.D.	Goodness of fit			Estimate ± S.D.	Goodness of fit		
			x^2	df	P		x^2	df	P
Linear	α_1	560±150	2.0	4	0.74	390±180	12.8	4	0.012
Linear-quadratic	α_1	560±430				390±540			
	α_2	0 $\underline{b}/$	2.0	3	0.57	0 $\underline{b}/$	12.8	3	0.005
Linear + killing	α_1	860±290				980±370			
	β_2	$(1.8±1.4)10^4$	1.2	3	0.75	$(3.4±1.6)10^4$	3.9	3	0.27
Linear-quadratic + killing	α_1	320±1140				780±1480			
	α_2	370±690				100±660			
	β_2	$(4.8±4.0)10^4$	1.1	2	0.58	$(4.2±4.9)10^4$	3.9	2	0.14
Quadratic	α_2	110±600	5.5	4	0.29	55± 49	27.0	4	0.00002
Quadratic + killing	α_2	550±170				470±210			
	β_2	$(5.6±1.5)10^4$	1.2	3	0.75	$(6.6±2.4)10^4$	4.1	3	0.25

$\underline{a}/$ See footnote $\underline{a}/$ in Table 2.
$\underline{b}/$ The best-fitting parameter would be negative; the value of zero results from the prior constraint that the parameter be non-negative.

REFERENCES

A1 Aalen, O. Nonparametric inference in connection with multiple decrement models. Scand. J. Stat. 3: 15-27 (1976).

A2 Abrahamson, S. and S. Wolff. The analysis of radiation-induced specific locus mutations in the mouse. Nature 264: 715-719 (1976).

A3 Abrahamson, S. Mutation process at low or high radiation doses. p. 1-8 in: Biological and Environmental Effects of Low-Level Radiation, Vol. I. IAEA, Vienna, 1976.

A4 Albert, R.E., F. Burns and R. Shore. Comparison of the incidence and time patterns of radiation-induced skin cancers in humans and rats. p. 499-506 in: Late Biological Effects of Ionizing Radiation. Vol. II. IAEA, Vienna, 1978.

A7 Anderson, T.W. Radiation exposures of Hanford workers: a critique of the Mancuso, Stewart and Kneale report. Health Phys. 35: 743-750 (1978).

A8 Archer, V.E., J.K. Wagoner and F.E. Lundin. Lung cancer among uranium miners in the United States. Health Phys. 25: 351-371 (1973).

A10 Argonne National Laboratory. Exposure data for radium patients, Appendix A (p. 177-229), ANL-75-3, part II (1975).

A13 Arlett, C.F. and J. Potter. Mutation to 8-azaguanine resistance induced by gamma-radiation in a Chinese hamster cell line. Mut. Res. 13: 59-65 (1971).

A14 Asquith, J.C. The effect of dose-fractionation on gamma-radiation induced mutations in mammalian cells. Mut. Res. 43: 91-100 (1977).

A16 Archer, V., E.P. Radford and O. Axelson. Factors in exposure-response relationships of radon daughter injury. Conference/Workshop on Lung Cancer Epidemiology and Industrial Applications of Sputum Cytology, November 1978. Colorado School of Mines Press, Golden, Colorado 1979.

A17 Adams, L.M. and R.L. Ullrich. Survival of mammary epithelial cells from virgin female BALB/c mice following in vivo gamma irradiation. Radiat. Res. 91: 409 only (1982).

A18 Albert, R.E., F.J. Burns and E.V. Sargent. Skin tumorigenesis by multiple doses of electron radiation in the rat. (Abstract) Radiat. Res. 87: 453 only (1981).

B1 Bajerska, A. and J. Liniecki. A variability of proliferation kinetics of rabbit lymphocytes in vitro. Mutat. Res. 60: 225-229 (1979).

B2 Bajerska, A. and J. Liniecki. The yield of chromosomal aberrations in rabbit lymphocytes after irradiation in vitro and in vivo. Mutat. Res. 27: 271-284 (1975).

B3 Bettega, D., P. Calzolari, P. Pollara et al. In vitro cell transformation induced by 31 MeV protons. Radiat. Res. 104: 178-181 (1985).

B4 Baral, E., L.E. Larsson and B. Mattsson. Breast cancer following irradiation of the breast. Cancer 40: 2905-2910 (1977).

B5 Barendsen, G.W. Mechanism of action of different ionizing radiations on the proliferative capacity of mammalian cells. p. 167 in: Advances in Theoretical and Experimental Biophysics, Vol. I. (A. Cole, ed.). M. Dekker, New York, 1967.

B6 Barendsen, G.W. Radiosensitivity of tumours and related cells in culture. Biomedicine 26: 259-260 (1977).

B7 Barendsen, G.W. Fundamental aspects of cancer induction in relation to the effectiveness of small doses of radiation. p. 263-276 in: Late Biological Effects of Ionizing Radiation. Vol. II. IAEA, Vienna, 1978.

B9 Barendsen, G.W. RBE-LET relations for induction and reproductive death and chromosome aberrations in mammalian cells. p. 55-68 in: Proceedings of the Sixth Symposium on Microdosimetry, Brussels, May 1978 (J. Booz and H.G. Ebert, eds.). Harwood Academic Publ., London, 1978.

B10 Barendsen, G.W. Characteristics of cell survival curves for different radiations in relation to iso-effect curves for fractionated treatments of a rat rhabdomyosarcoma. p. 270-279 in: Cell Survival after Low Doses of Radiation: Theoretical and Clinical Implications. The Institute of Physics and John Wiley and Sons, London, 1975.

B11 Barendsen, G.W. Influence of radiation quality on the effectiveness of small doses for induction of reproductive death and chromosome aberrations in mammalian cells. Int. J. Radiat. Biol. 36: 49-64 (1979).

B12 Barendsen, G.W. Quantitative biophysical aspects of response of tumours and normal tissues to ionizing radiations. Curr. Top. Radiat. Res. Quart. 9: 101-108 (1973).

B14 Barrett, J.C., T. Tsutsui and P.O.P. Ts'o. Neoplastic transformation induced by a direct perturbation of DNA. Nature 274: 229-232 (1978).

B15 Bauchinger, M. Strahleninduzierte Chromosomen-Aberrationen. p. 127-180 im: Handbuch der Medizinischen Radiologie (D. Olsson et al., eds.), Band 4/3. Springer Verlag, Berlin, 1972.

B16 Baum, J.W. Population heterogeneity hypothesis on radiation-induced cancer. Health Phys. 25: 97-104 (1973).

B17 Beebe, G.W., H. Kato and C.E. Land. Studies of the mortality of A-bomb survivors. 6. Mortality and radiation dose, 1950-1974. Radiat. Res. 75: 138-201 (1978).

B18 Beebe, G.W., C.E. Land and H. Kato. The hypothesis of radiation-accelerated aging and the mortality of Japanese A-bomb victims. p. 3-28 in: Late Biological Effects of Ionizing Radiation. Vol. I. IAEA, Vienna, 1978.

B19 Bedford, J.S. and H.G. Griggs. The estimation of survival at low doses and the limits of resolution of the single-cell-plating technique. p. 34-39 in: Cell Survival after Low Doses of Radiation: Theoretical and Clinical Implications. The Institute of Physics and John Wiley and Sons, London, 1975.

B20 BEIR Report. The Effects on Population of Exposure to Low-Level of Ionizing Radiation. Report of the Advisory Committee on the Biological Effects of

Ionizing Radiation. National Academy of Sciences, National Research Council, Washington, D.C., 1972.

B21 Burch, P.R.J. Radiation carcinogenesis: a new hypothesis. Nature 185: 135-142 (1960).

B23 Boer, P. de, P.P. van Buul et al. Chromosomal radiosensitivity and karyotype in mice using cultured peripheral blood lymphocytes and comparison with this system in man. Mutat. Res. 42: 379-394 (1977).

B24 Boice, J.D., M. Rosenstein and E.D. Trout. Estimation of breast doses and breast cancer risk associated with repeated fluoroscopic chest examinations of women with tuberculosis. Radiat. Res. 73: 373-390 (1978).

B25 Boice, J.D. jr., C.E. Land, R.E. Shore et al. Risk of breast cancer following low-dose radiation exposure. Radiology 131: 589-597 (1979).

B26 Boice, J.O. and R.R. Monson. Breast cancer in women after repeated fluoroscopic examinations of the chest. J. Natl. Cancer Inst. 59: 823-832 (1977).

B27 Boag, J.W. The statistical treatment of cell survival data. p. 40-53 in: Cell Survival after Low Doses of Radiation: Theoretical and Clinical Implications. The Institute of Physics and John Wiley and Sons, London, 1975.

B28 Bond, V.P., C.J. Shellabarger, E.P. Cronkite et al. Studies on radiation-induced mammary gland neoplasia in the rat. V. Induction by localized radiation. Radiat. Res. 13: 318-328 (1960).

B29 Borek, C., E.J. Hall and H.H. Rossi. Malignant transformation in cultured hamster embryo cells produced by x-rays, 430 keV mono-energetic neutrons and heavy ions. Cancer Res. 38: 2997-3005 (1978).

B33 Borek, C. and E. Hall. Transformation of mammalian cells in vitro by low doses of x rays. Nature 243: 450-453 (1973).

B34 Borek, C. In vitro cell transformation by low doses of x-irradiation and neutrons. p. 309-326 in: Biology of Radiation Carcinogenesis (J.M. Yuhas et al., eds.). Raven Press, New York, 1976.

B36 Boutwell, R.K. The function and mechanisms of promotion of carcinogenesis. Crit. Rev. Toxicol. 4: 419-443 (1974).

B41 Brewen, J.G., R.J. Preston, K.P. Jones et al. Genetic hazards of ionizing radiations: cytogenetic extrapolations from mouse to man. Mutat. Res. 17: 245-254 (1973).

B42 Bridges, B.A. and J. Huckle. Mutagenesis of cultured mammalian cells by x-irradiation and ultraviolet light. Mutat. Res. 10: 141-151 (1970).

B43 Broerse, J.J., S. Knaan, D.W. van Bekkum et al. Mammary carcinogenesis in rats after x- and neutron-irradiation and hormone administration. p. 13-28 in: Late Biological Effects of Ionizing Radiation, Vol. II. IAEA, Vienna, 1978.

B45 Broerse, J.J. and G.W. Barendsen. Relative biological effectiveness of fast neutrons for effects on normal tissues. Curr. Top. Radiat. Res. Quart. 8: 305-350 (1973).

B46 Brouty-Boye, D. and J.B. Little. Enhancement of x-ray-induced transformation in C3H-T10-1/2 cells by interferon. Cancer Res. 37: 2714-2716 (1977).

B47 Brown, J.M. The shape of the dose-response curve for radiation carcinogenesis. Extrapolation to low doses. Radiat. Res. 71: 34-50 (1977).

B48 Brues, A.H. Biological hazards and toxicity of radioactive isotopes. J. Clin. Invest. 28: 1286-1296 (1949).

B49 Brues, A.H. Critique of the linear theory of carcinogenesis. Science 128: 693-699 (1958).

B56 Burns, F.J., P. Strickland, M. Vanderlaan et al. Rat skin tumour incidence following single and fractionated exposures to proton radiation. Radiat. Res. 74: 152-158 (1978).

B57 Burns, F.J. and M. Vanderlaan. Split-dose recovery for radiation-induced tumours in rat skin. Int. J. Radiat. Biol. 32: 135-144 (1977).

B58 Burns, F.J., R.E. Albert, I.P. Sinclair et al. The effect of a 24 hour fractionation interval on the induction of rat skin tumours by electron radiation. Radiat. Res. 62: 478-487 (1975).

B59 Burns, F.J., R.E. Albert and R.D. Heimbach. RBE for skin tumours and hair follicle damage in the rat following irradiation with alpha particles and electrons. Radiat. Res. 36: 225-241 (1968).

B60 Busch, H. (ed.) The Molecular Biology of Cancer. Academic Press, New York, 1974.

B61 Buul, P.P. van. A comparative study of the frequency of radiation-induced chromosome aberrations in somatic and germ cells of the rhesus monkey (maccaca mulatta). Mutat. Res. 36: 223-236 (1976).

B62 Bragin, Yu. N. and I.V. Filyushkin. The basis of the theory of dual action of radiation (in Russian). Third All-Union Conference on Microdosimetry, June 1979. Abstracts, Moscow, 1979.

B63 Borek, C. X-ray induced in vitro neoplastic transformation of human diploid cells. Nature 283: 726-778 (1980).

B64 Borek, C. Neoplastic transformation following split doses of x rays. Br. J. Radiol. 50: 845-846 (1979).

B65 Borek, C., R. Miller, C. Pain et al. Conditions for inhibiting and enhancing effects of the protease inhibitor antipain on x-ray induced neoplastic transformation in hamster and mouse cells. Proc. Natl. Acad. Sci. U.S.A. 76: 1800-1803 (1979).

B71 Barrett, J.C., B.D. Crawford and P.O. Ts'o. The role of somatic mutation in a multistage model of carcinogenesis. in: Mammalian Cell Transformation by Chemical "Carcinogens". (N. Mishra et al., eds.). Senate Press, New Jersey, 1980.

B72 Barrett, J.C. Cell transformation, mutation and cancer. in: The Use of Mammalian Cells for Detection of Environmental Carcinogens, Mechanisms and Application. Gann. Monograph on Cancer Res. (C. Heidelbeyer et al., eds.). (in press).

B73 Borek, C. Hormone and nutritional factors as regulators of X ray-induced transformation. (Meeting abstract.) Long Term Normal Tissue Effects of Cancer Treatment, Bethesda, 1981.

B74 Borek, C., R.C. Muller, C. Geard et al. In vitro modulation of oncogenesis and differentiation by retinoids and tumor promoter. (Meeting abstract). p. 113 in: Cocarcinogenesis and Biological Effects of Tumor Promoters. German Cancer Research Center, Heidelberg, 1980.

B76 Borek, C. Radiation oncogenesis in cell culture. p. 159-232 in: Advances in Cancer Research. (G. Klein and S. Weinhouse, eds.), Vol. 37, Academic Press, New York, 1982.

B77 Bartlett, D.T. A review of Japanese bomb dosimetry. Radiat. Prot. Dosim. 2: 127-139 (1982).

B79 Borek, C. and E.J. Hall. Induction and modulation of radiogenic transformation in mammalian cells. p. 291-302 in: Radiation Carcinogenesis: Epidemiology and Biological Significance. (J.D. Boice and J.F. Fraumeni, eds.). Raven Press, New York, 1984.

B82 Bizzozero, O.J., K.G. Johnson and A. Ciocco. Radiation related leukemia in Hiroshima and Nagasaki 1946-1964. New Engl. J. Med. 274: 1095-1101 (1966).

B83 van Bekkum, D.W. and P. Benovelzen. The concept of gene transfer misrepair mechanism of radiation carcinogenesis may challenge the linear extrapolation model of risk estimation for low radiation doses. Health Phys. 43: 231-237 (1982).

B84 Barlow, R.E., D.J. Bartholomew, J.M. Bremner et al. Statistical inference under order restrictions; the theory and application of isotonic regression. John Wiley and Sons, New York, 1972.

B85 Brooks, A.L., S.A. Benjamin, R.K. Jones et al. Interaction of ^{144}Ce and partial hepatectomy in the production of liver neoplasms in the Chinese Hamster. Radiat. Res. 91: 573-588 (1982).

B86 Broerse, J.J., L.A. Hennen, M.J. van Zwieten et al. Mammary carcinogenesis in different rat strains after single and fractionated irradiations. p. 155-168 in: Neutron Carcinogenesis (J.J. Broerse and G.B. Gerber, eds.) EUR-8084 (1982).

B87 Brooks, A.L., S.A. Benjamin, F.F. Hahn et al. The induction of liver tumours by ^{239}PuO$_2$ particles in the Chinese hamsters. Radiat. Res. 96: 135-161 (1983).

B88 Bird, R.P. Biophysical studies with spatially correlated ions. 3. Cell survival studies using diatomic deuterium. Radiat. Res. 78: 210-223 (1979).

B89 Balcer-Kubiczek, E.K. and G.H. Harrison. Oncogenic transformation of C3H/10T1/2 cells by x rays, fast-fission neutrons and cyclotron-produced neutrons. Int. J. Radiat. Biol. 44: 327-386 (1983).

B90 Borek, C. and E.J. Hall. Effect of split doses of X rays on neoplastic transformation of single cells. Nature 252: 499-501 (1974).

B91 Backer, J.M., M. Boerzig and I.B. Weinstein. When do carcinogen-treated 10T1/2 cells acquire the commitment to form transformed foci? Nature 299: 458-460 (1982).

B92 Broerse, J.J., L.A. Hennen, M.J. van Zwieten et al. Dose-effect relations for mammary carcinogenesis in different rat strains after irradiation with X rays and mono-energetic neutrons. p. 507-520 in: Proceedings of an IAEA/WHO Symposium on the Biological Effects of Low-Level Radiation with Special Regard to Stochastic and Non-Stochastic Effects. IAEA, Vienna, 1983.

B93 Boice, J.D., N.E. Day, D. Andersen et al. Cancer risk following radiotherapy of cervical cancer: a preliminary report. p. 161-179 in: Radiation Carcinogenesis: Epidemiology and Biological Significance (J.D. Boice and J.F. Fraumeni, eds.). Raven Press, New York, 1984.

B95 Burch, P.R.J. Problems with the linear-quadratic dose-response relationship. Health Phys. 44: 411-413 (1983).

B96 Borek, C., W.F. Morgan, A. Ong et al. Inhibition of malignant transformation in vitro by inhibitors of poly(ADP-ribose) synthesis. Proc. Natl. Acad. Sci. U.S.A. 81: 243-247 (1984).

B97 Borsa, J., M.D. Sargent, M. Einspenner et al. Effects of oxygen and misonidazde on cell transformation and cell killing in C3H10T1/2 cell by x rays in vitro. Radiat. Res. 100: 96-103 (1984).

B98 Brenner D.J. and M. Zaider. Modification of the theory of dual radiation action for attenuated fields. II. Application to the analysis of soft x-ray results. Radiat. Res. 99: 492-501 (1984).

B99 Bond, V.P. The conceptual basis for evaluating risk from low-level radiation exposure. p. 25-62 in: Critical Issues in Setting Radiation Dose Limits. NCRP Proceedings No. 3 (1982).

C1 Chadwick, K.H. and H.P. Leenhouts. The effect of an asynchronous population of cells on the initial slope of dose-effect curves. p. 57-63 in: Cell Survival after Low Doses of Radiation: Theoretical and Clinical Implications. The Institute of Physics and John Wiley and Sons, London, 1975.

C2 Chadwick, K.H. and H.P. Leenhouts. A molecular theory of cell survival. Phys. Med. Biol. 18: 78-87 (1973).

C7 Chadwick, K.H. and H.P. Leenhouts. Dose-effect relationship for malignancy in cells with different genetic characteristics. p. 327-340 in: Late Biological Effects of Ionizing Radiation. Vienna, IAEA, 1978.

C9 Chen, P.C., M.F. Lavin, C. Kidson et al. Identification of ataxiateleangiectasia heterozygotes, a cancer prone population. Nature 274: 484-486 (1978).

C10 Chu, E.W.Y. Mammalian cell genetics. III. Characterization of x-ray-induced forward mutations in Chinese hamster cell cultures. Mutat. Res. 11: 23-24 (1971).

C15 Clifton, K.H. and J.J. Crowley. Effects of radiation type and dose and the role of glucocorticorids gonadectomy and thyroidectomy in mammary tumour induction in mammotropin-secreting pituitary tumour-grafted rats. Cancer Res. 38: 1507-1513 (1978).

C16 Coggle, J.E. and D.M. Peel. The relative effects of uniform and non-uniform external radiation on the induction of lung tumours in mice. p. 83-94 in: Late Biological Effects of Ionizing Radiation. IAEA, Vienna, 1978.

C18 Covelli, V., P. Metalli and B. Bassani. Decreased incidence of reticulum cell carcoma in whole body irradiated and bone marrow shielded mice. Br. J. Cancer 31: 369-371 (1975).

C19 Covelli, V., P. Metalli, G. Briganti et al. Late somatic effects in syngeneic radiation chimaeras: II. Mortality and rate of specific diseases. Int. J. Radiat. Biol. 26: 1-15 (1974).

C20 Cox, R., J. Thacker, D.T. Goodhead et al. Mutation and inactivation of mammalian cells by various ionising radiation. Nature 267: 425-427 (1977).

C21 Cox, R. and W.K. Masson. Changes in radiosensitivity during the in vitro growth of diploid human fibroblasts. Int. J. Radiat. Biol. 26: 193-196 (1976).

C22 Cox, R. and W.K. Masson. X-ray survival curves of cultured human diploid fibroblasts. p. 217-222 in: Cell Survival after Low Doses of Radiation: Theoretical and Clinical Implications. The Institute of Physics and John Wiley and Sons, London, 1975.

C23 Cox, R., J. Thacker and D.T. Goodhead. Inactivation and mutation of cultured mammalian cells by aluminium characteristic ultrasoft x rays. II. Dose response of Chinese hamster and human diploid cells to aluminium x rays and radiations of different LET. Int. J. Radiat. Biol. 31: 561-576 (1977).

C24 Cox, R. and W.K. Masson. Do radiation-induced thioguanine-resistant mutants of cultured mammalian cells arise by HGPRT gene mutations or X-chromosome rearrangement? Nature 276: 629-630 (1978).

C29 Committee on the Biological Effects of Ionizing Radiation. The Effects on Populations of Exposure to Low Levels of Ionizing Radiation. National Academy of Sciences. Washington, D.C. 1980.

C32 Cairns, J. The origin of human cancers. Nature 289: 353-357 (1981).

C33 Clark, E.P., G.M. Hahn and J.B. Little. Hyperthermic modulation of X-ray-induced oncogenic transformation in C3H10T1/2 cells. Radiat. Res. 88: 619-622 (1981).

C34 Chmelevsky, D., A.M. Kellerer, J. Lafuma et al. Pulmonary neoplasms in the Sprague-Dawley rat after radon inhalation—a maximum likelihood analysis. Radiat. Res. 91: 589-614 (1982).

C36 Chmelevsky, D., A.M. Kellerer, J. Lafuma et al. Maximum likelihood estimation of the prevalence of nonlethal neoplasms. An application to radon daughter inhalation studies. Radiat. Res. 91: 589-614 (1982).

C37 Cathers, L.E. and M.N. Gould. Human mammary cell survival following ionizing radiation. Int. J. Radiat. Biol. 44: 1-16 (1983).

C38 Chmelevsky, D., A.M. Kellerer, J. Lafuma et al. Comparison of the induction of pulmonary neoplasms in Sprague-Dawley rats by fission neutron and radon daughters. Radiat. Res. 98: 519-535 (1984).

D3 Di Majo, V., M. Coppola, S. Rebessi et al. Dose-response relationship of radiation-induced Harderian gland tumours and myeloid leukaemia of the CBA/Cne mouse. J. Natl. Cancer Inst. 76: 955-963 (1986).

D4 Dolphin, G.W. A review of in vitro dose-effect relationships. p. 1-8 in: Mutagen-Induced Chromosome Damage in Man (H.J. Evans and D.C. Lloyd, eds.). Edinburgh University Press, Edinburgh, 1978.

D7 Durand, R.E. and R.M. Sutherland. Effects of intercellular contact on repair of radiation damage. Exp. Cell. Res. 71: 74-80 (1972).

D8 Durand, R.E. and R.M. Sutherland. Intercellular contact: its influence on the D_q of mammalian survival curves. p. 237-247 in: Cell Survival after Low Doses of Radiation: Theoretical and Clinical Implications. The Institute of Physics and John Wiley and Sons, London, 1975.

D9 Dilman, V.M. A mutation-metabolic model of cancer development and of the progression of the malignant process (in Russian). p. 3-16 in: Voprosy Onkologii, Vol. 22, No. 8.

D13 Di Paolo, J.A., A.J. De Marinis, C.H. Evans et al. Expression of initiated and promoted stages of irradiated carcinogenesis in vitro. Cancer Lett. 14: 243-249 (1981).

D14 Darby, S.C. and J.A. Reissland. Low levels of ionizing radiation and cancer—are we underestimating the risk? J.R. Statist. Soc. A: Part 3, 144: 298-331 (1981).

D15 DeMott, R.K., R.T. Mulcahy and K.H. Clifton. The survival of thyroid cells following irradiation: a directly generated single-dose survival curve. Radiat. Res. 77: 395-403 (1979).

D16 Doniach, I. Effects including carcinogenesis of ^{131}I and x-rays on the thyroid of experimental animals: a review. Health Phys. 9: 1357-1362 (1963).

D17 Doll, R. and R. Peto. Epidemiology of cancer. p. 4.51-4.79 in: Oxford Textbook of Medicine (D.J. Wheatherall et al., eds.). Oxford University Press, Oxford, 1984.

D18 Day, N.E. Radiation and multistage carcinogenesis. p. 437-443 in: Radiation Carcinogenesis: Epidemiology and Biological Significance. (J.D. Boice and J.F. Fraumeni, eds.). Raven Press, New York, 1984.

D19 Di Paolo, J.A., C.H. Evans, A.J. De Marinis et al. Inhibition of radiation-initiated and -promoted transformation of Syrian hamster embryo cells by lymphotoxin. Cancer Res. 44: 1465-1471 (1984).

E2 Elkind, M.M. The initial part of the survival curve. Implications for low dose, low dose-rate radiation responses. Radiat. Res. 71: 9-23 (1977).

E3 Evans, R.D. The effects of skeletally deposited a-ray emitters in man. Br. J. Radiol. 39: 881-895 (1966).

E4 Evans, R.D., A.T. Keane and M.M. Shanahan. Radiogenic effects in man of long term skeletal a-irradiation. p. 431-486 in: Radiobiology of Plutonium (B.J. Stover and W.S.G. Jee, eds.). J.W. Press, Salt Lake City, 1972.

E6 Evans, C.H. Lymphotoxin, an immunological hormone with anticarcinogenic and anti-tumor activity. Cancer Immunol. Immunother. 12: 181-190 (1982).

E8 Evans, J.H. and Vijayalaxmi. Induction of 8-azaguanine resistance and sister chromatid exchange in human lymphocytes exposed to mitomycin C and X rays in vitro. Nature 292: 601-605 (1981).

E9 Elkind, M.M., A. Han and C.K. Hill. Error-free and error-prone repair in radiation-induced neoplastic cell transformation. p. 303-318 in: Radiation Carcinogenesis: Epidemiology and Biological Significance (J.D. Boice and J.F. Fraumeni, eds.). Raven Press, New York, 1984.

E10 Elkind, M.M. Repair processes in radiation biology. Radiat. Res. 100: 425-449 (1984).

F1 Faber, M. Radiation carcinogenesis and the significance of some physical factors. p. 149-159 in: Radiation-Induced Cancer. IAEA, Vienna, 1969.

F2 Fertil, B., P. Deschavanne, B. Lachet et al. Survival curves of neoplastic and non-transformed human cell lines: statistical analysis using different models. p. 145-156 in: Proceedings of the Sixth Symposium on Microdosimetry, Brussels, May 1978 (J. Booz and H.G. Ebert, eds.). Harwood Academic Publishers, London, 1978.

F3 Fialkow, P.J. Clonal origin of human tumours. Cancer Reviews 458: 283-321 (1976).

F4 Fialkow, P.J. Clonal origin and stem cell evolution of human tumours. p. 439-453 in: Genetics of Human Cancer (J.J. Mulvihill et al., eds.). Raven Press, New York, 1977.

F5 Fialkow, P.J., R.W. Sagebiel, S.M. Gastler et al. Multiple cell origin of heriditary neurofibromas. N. Engl. J. Med. 284: 298-300 (1971).

F6 Fialkow, P.J. The origin and development of human tumours studied with cell markers. N. Engl. J. Med. 291: 26-35 (1974).

F7 Filyushkin, J.V. Microdosimetric determination of radiation quality factors. Sov. At. Energy 40: 227-233 (1976).

F8 Finkel, M.P., B.O. Biskis and P.B. Jinkins. Toxicity of radium-226 in mice. p. 369-391 in: Radiation-Induced Cancer. IAEA, Vienna, 1969.

F10 Friedman, J.M. and P.J. Fialkow. Viral tumourgenesis in man: cell markers in condylomata acuminata. Int. J. Cancer 17: 57-61 (1976).

F12 Filyushkin, I.V., I.M. Petoyan. Mathematical model of carcinogenic action of radiation. Radiobiologiya 24: 481-488 (1984). (in Russian).

F13 Farber, E. and R. Cameron. The sequential analysis of cancer development. Adv. Cancer Res. 31: 125-226 (1980).

F14 Farber, E. Chemical carcinogenesis. New Eng. J. Med. 305: 1379-1389 (1981).

F15 Fisher, P.B., R.A. Mufson, I.B. Weinstein et al. Epidermal growth factor, like tumor promoters, enhances viral and radiation-induced cell transformation. Carcinogenesis 2: 183-187 (1981).

F16 Fry, R.J.M., R.D. Ley, D. Grube et al. Studies on the multistage nature of radiation carcinogenesis. p. 155-165 in: Carcinogenesis, Vol. 7 (Hecker et al., eds.). Raven Press, New York, 1982.

F18 Frankenberg-Schwager M., D. Frankenberg, D. Blöcher et al. The linear relationship between DNA double-strand breaks and radiation dose (30 MeV electrons) is converted into a quadratic function by cellular repair. Int. J. Radiat. Biol. 37: 207-212 (1980).

F19 Freeman, M.L., E. Sierra and E.J. Hall. The repair of sublethal damage in diploid human fibroblasts: a comparison between human and rodent cell lines. Radiat. Res. 95: 382-391 (1983).

F20 Farber, E. The multistep nature of cancer development. Cancer Res. 44: 4217-4223 (1984).

F21 Filyushkin I.V. and I.M. Petoyan. An assessment of carcinogenic action of radiation at the cellular level. Radiobiologiya 22: 781-786 (1982). (in Russian).

F22 Fry, R.J.M. Relevance of animal studies to the human experience. p. 337-396 in: Radiation Carcinogenesis: Epidemiology and Biological Significance. (J.D. Boice and J.F. Fraumeni, eds.). Raven Press, New York, 1984.

G5 Gilbert, E.S. and S. Marks. An analysis of the mortality of workers in a nuclear facility. Rad. Res. 79: 122-148 (1979).

G9 Goodhead, D.T. Inactivation and mutation of cultured mammalian cells by aluminium characteristic ultrasoft x rays. III. Implications for theory of dual radiation action. Int. J. Radiat. Biol. 32: 43-70 (1977).

G10 Goodhead, D.T. and J. Thacker. Inactivation and mutation of cultured mammalian cells by aluminium characteristic ultrasoft x rays. I. Properties of aluminium x rays and preliminary experiments with Chinese hamster cells. Int. J. Radiat. Biol. 31: 541-559 (1977).

G11 Goodhead, D.T., J. Thacker and R. Cox. The conflict between the biological effects of ultrasoft x rays and microdosimetric measurements and application. p. 829-843 in: Proceedings of the Sixth Symposium on Microdosimetry, Brussels, May 1978 (J. Booz and H.G. Ebert, eds.). Harwood Academic Publishers, London, 1978.

G12 Gorlin, R.J. Monogenic disorders associated with neoplasia. p. 169-178 in: Genetics of Human Cancer (J.J. Mulvihill et al., eds.). Raven Press, New York, 1977.

G14 Gould, M.N. and K.H. Clifton. Evidence for a unique in situ component of the repair of radiation damage. Rad. Res. 77: 149-155 (1979).

G15 Gould, M.N., R. Jirtle, J. Crowley et al. Reevaluation of the number of cells involved in the neutron induction of mammary neoplasms. Cancer Res. 38: 189-192 (1978).

G16 Gray, L.H. Cellular radiation biology. p. 725 in: Proceedings of the 18th Annual Symposium on Fundamental Cancer Research. University of Texas and M.D. Anderson Hospital. Williams and Williams, Baltimore, 1965.

G17 Groer, P.G. Dose-response curves from incomplete data. p. 351-358 in: Late Biological Effects of Ionizing Radiation, Vol. II. IAEA, Vienna, 1978.

G18 Groer, P.G. Dose-response curves and competing risks. Proc. Natl. Acad. Sci. U.S.A. 75: 4087-4091 (1978).

G19 Groer, P.G. Correction to dose-response curves and competing risks. Proc. Natl. Acad. Sci. U.S.A. 76: 1524 (1979).

G23 Groer, P.G. and J.H. Marshall. A model for the induction of bone cancer by radium-224. p. 201-209 in: Biological Effects of radium-224 (W.A. Muller and H.G. Ebert, eds.). Martinus Nijhoff Medical Division, The Hague/Boston, 1978.

G24 Glass, H.B. and R.K. Ritterluff. Mutagenic effect of a 5-r dose of x rays in Drosphila melanogaster. Science 133: 1366 (1961).

G25 Gofman, J.W. The question of radiation causation of cancer in Hanford workers. Health Phys. 32: 612-639 (1979).

G26 Guernsey, D.L., C. Borek and I.S. Edelman. Crucial role to thyroid hormone in X-ray-induced neoplastic transformation in cell culture. Proc. Natl. Acad. Sci. U.S.A. 78: 5708-5711 (1981).

G27 Guernsey, D.L., A. Ong and C. Borek. Thyroid hormone modulation of X-ray-induced in vitro neoplastic transformation. Nature 288: 591-592 (1980).

G28 Geard, C.R., M. Rutledge-Freeman, R.C. Miller et al. Antipain and radiation effects on oncogenic transformation and sister chromatic exchanges in Syrian hamster embryo and mouse C3H10T1/2 cells. Carcinogenesis 2: 1229-1233 (1981).

G29 Goodhead, D.T., R.J. Munson, J. Thacker et al. Mutation and inactivation of cultured mammalian cells exposed to beams of accelerated heavy ions. IV. Biophysical interpretation. Int. J. Radiat. Biol. 37: 135-167 (1980).

G30 Gould, M.N. Radiation initiation of carcinogenesis in vivo: a rare or common cellular event. p. 347-358 in: Radiation Carcinogenesis Epidemiology and Biological Implications. Proceedings of a Symposium. (J.D. Boice and J.F. Fraumeni, eds.). Raven Press, New York, 1984.

G31 Geard, C.R., R.D. Colvett and N. Rohrig. On the mechanics of chromosome aberrations: a study with single and multiple spatially associated protons. Mutat. Res. 91: 81-89 (1980).

G32 Goodhead, D.T. An assessment of the role of microdosimetry in radiobiology. Radiat. Res. 91: 45-76 (1982).

G33 Guerrero, I., A. Villasante, V. Corces et al. Activation of a c-K-ras oncogene by somatic mutation in mouse lymphomas induced by gamma radiation. Science 225: 1159-1162 (1984).

G34 Goodhead, D.T. Deduction from cellular studies of inactivation, mutagenesis and transformation. p. 369-386 in: Radiation Carcinogenesis: Epidemiology and Biological Significance. (J.D. Boice and J.F. Fraumeni, eds.). Raven Press, New York, 1984.

G35 Gragtmans, N.J., D.K. Myers, J.R. Johnson, et al. Occurrence of mammary tumours in rats after exposure to tritium β rays and 200 kVp x rays. Radiat. Res. 99: 636-650 (1984).

G36 Gart, J.J. Statistical analyses of the relative risk. Environ. Health Perspect. 32: 157-167 (1979).

H1 Han, A. and M.M. Elkind. Transformation of mouse C3H10T1/2 cells by single and fractionated doses of x-rays and fission-spectrum neutrons. Cancer Res. 39: 123-130 (1979).

H2 Hall, E.J. Biological problems in the measurement of survival at low doses. p. 13-24 in: Cell Survival after Low Doses of Radiation: Theoretical and Clinical Implications. The Institute of Physics and John Wiley and Sons, London, 1975.

H6 Haynes, R.H. The influence of repair processes on radiobiological survival curves. p. 197-208 in: Cell Survival after Low Doses of Radiation: Theoretical and Clinical Implications. The Institute of Physics and John Wiley and Sons, London, 1975.

H8 Hill, R.P., B.F. Warren and R.S. Bush. The effect of intercellular contact on the radiation sensitivity of KHT sarcoma cells. Radiat. Res. 77: 182-192 (1972).

H9 Hirai, M. and S. Nakai. Dicentric yields induced by x-radiation and chromosome arm number in primates. Mutat. Res. 43: 147-158 (1977).

H10 Hornsey, S. The radiation response of human malignant melanoma cells in vitro and in vivo. Cancer Res. 32: 650-651 (1972).

H11 Hulse, E.V., R.H. Mole and D.G. Papworth. Radiosensitivity of cells from which radiation-induced skin tumours are derived. Int. J. Radiat. Biol. 14: 437-444 (1968).

H12 Hulse, E.V. and R.H. Mole. Skin tumour incidence in CBA mice given fractionated exposure to low-energy β particles. Br. J. Cancer 23: 452-463 (1969).

H13 Hulse, E.V. Incidence and pathogenesis of skin tumours in mice irradiated with single external doses of low energy β particles. Br. J. Cancer 21: 531-547 (1967).

H14 Han, A. and M.M. Elkind. The effect of radiation quality and repair processes on the incidence of neoplastic transformation in vitro. p. 621-626 in: Radiation Research (S. Okada et al., eds.). J.A.A.R., Tokyo, 1979.

H15 Hoel, D.G. and H.E. Walburg. Statistical analysis of survival experiments. J. Natl. Cancer Inst. 49: 361-372 (1972).

H17 Holm, L.E. Incidence of malignant thyroid tumors in man after diagnostic and therapeutic doses of iodine-131. Epidemiologic and Histopatiologic study. Radiumhemmet, Karolinska Hospital, Stockholm 1980.

H18 Hempelmann, L.H., J. Pifer, G. Burke et al. Neoplasms in persons treated with x rays in infancy for thymic enlargement. A report of the third followup survey. J. Natl. Cancer Inst. 38: 317-341 (1967).

H19 Hempelmann, L.H., W. Hall, M. Phillips et al. Neoplasms in persons treated with x rays in infancy: fourth survey in 20 years. J. Natl. Cancer Inst. 55: 519-530 (1975).

H20 Hutchinson, G.B., B. MacMahon, S. Jablon et al. Review of report by Mancuso, Stewart and Kneale of radiation exposure of Hanford workers. Health Phys. 37: 207-220 (1979).

H21 Hall, E.J. and R.C. Miller. The how and why of in vitro oncogenic transformation. Radiat. Res. 87: 208-223 (1981).

H22 Han, A. and M.M. Elkind. Enhanced transformation of mouse C3H10T1/2 cells by 12-O-Tetradecanoyl-phorbol-13-acetate following exposure to x-rays or to fission-spectrum neutrons. Cancer Res. 42: 477-483 (1982).

H23 Holtzman, S., J.P. Stone and C.J. Shellabarger. Radiation-induced mammary carcinogenesis in virgin, pregnant, lactating and postlactating rats. Cancer Res. 42: 50-53 (1982).

H25 Horacek, J. and J. Sevc. Histological types of pulmonary carcinoma after long-term exposure to radiation. Studia Pneumol. Phtiseol. Cechoslov. 40: 324-328 (1980).

H26 Hill, C.K., F.M. Buonaguro, C.P. Myers et al. Fission-spectrum neutrons at reduced dose-rates enhance neoplastic transformation. Nature 298: 67-69 (1982).

H27 Haynes, R.H. The interpretation of microbial inactivation and recovery phenomena. Radiat. Res. Supp. 6: 1-29 (1966).

H28 Hall, E.J., H.H. Rossi, M. Zaider et al. The role of neutrons in cell transformation research. II. Experimental. p. 381-395 in: Neutron Carcinogenesis. Proceedings of a Symposium. (J.J. Broerse and G.B. Gerber, eds.). EUR-8084 (1982).

H29 Hoel, D.G. and H.E. Walburg, Jr. Statistical analysis of survival experiments. J. Natl. Cancer Inst. 49: 361-372 (1972).

H30 Hill, C.K., A. Han, F. Buonaguro et al. Multifractionation of cobalt-60 gamma rays reduces neoplastic transformation in vitro. Carcinogenesis 5: 193-197 (1984).

H31 Hirakawa, T., T. Kakunaga, H. Fujiki et al. A new tumor-promoting agent, dihydroteleocidin-B, markedly enhances chemically-induced malignant cell transformation. Science 216: 527-529 (1982).

H32 Hendry, J.H. and B.I. Lord. The analysis of the early and late response to cytotoxic insults in the haemopoietic cell hierarchy. in: Cytotoxic Insult to Tissue (Plotten and Hendry, eds.). Churchill and Livingstone, Edinburgh, 1983.

H33 Hulse, E.V., S.Y. Lewkowicz, A.L. Batchelor et al. Incidence of radiation induced skin tumours in mice and variations with dose rate. Int. J. Radiat. Biol. 44: 197-206 (1983).

H34 Hill, C.K., A. Han and M.M. Elkind. Protracted exposures to fission-spectrum neutrons increase neoplastic transformation. in: Proceedings of the Seventh International Congress of Radiation Research. (J.J. Broerse, G.W. Barendsen et al., eds.) Martinus Nijhoff Publishers, Amsterdam, 1983. Also: Int. J. Rad. Biol. 46: 11-15 (1984).

H35 Hall, T.D. The interpretation of exponential dose-effect curves. Bull. Math. Biophys. 15: 43-47 (1953).

H36 Hill, C.K., B.A. Carnes, A. Han et al. Neoplastic transformation is enhanced by multiple low doses of fission-spectrum neutrons. Radiat. Res. 102: 404-410 (1985).

H37 Han, A., C.K. Hill and M.M. Elkind. Repair processes and radiation quality in neoplastic transformation of mammalian cells. Radiat. Res. 99: 249-261 (1984).

I1 International Commission on Radiological Protection. Recommendations of the International Commission on Radiological Protection. ICRP Publication 9. Pergamon Press, Oxford, 1966.

I2 International Commission on Radiological Protection. Recommendations of the International Commission on Radiological Protection. ICRP Publication 26. Pergamon Press, Oxford, 1977.

I3 International Commission on Radiological Protection. Biological effects of inhaled radionuclides. ICRP Publication 31. Annals of the ICRP. Pergamon Press, Oxford, 1980.

I4 International Commission on Radiological Protection. Limits for Inhalation of Radon Daughters by Workers. ICRP Publication 32. Pergamon Press, Oxford, 1981.

I5 International Commission on Radiological Protection. Exposure and lung cancer risk from indoor exposure to radon daughters. A Task Group Report, to appear in Annals of the ICRP, 1986.

I6 International Commission on Radiological Protection. Bases for developing a unified index of harm. ICRP Publication 45. Annals of the ICRP, 1985.

J1 Jablon, S. and H. Kato. Studies of the mortality of A-bomb survivors. 5. Mortality and radiation dose, 1950-1970. Radiat. Res. 50: 649-698 (1972).

J4 Jacobi, W. Carcinogenic effects of radiation on the human respiratory tract. In: Radiation Carcinogenesis. (A.C. Upton, ed.). Elsevier North-Holland, New York, 1983.

J6 Jirtle, R.L., P.M. DeLuca and M.N. Gould. The survival of parenchymal hepatocytes exposed to 14 MeV neutrons. Radiat. Res. 91: 409-410 (1982).

J7 Jacobi, W. Expected lung cancer risk from radon daughter exposure in dwellings. p. 31-42 in: Proc. Int. Conf. on Indoor Air Quality. Stockholm, August 1984. Swedish Council for Building Research. Stockholm, 1984.

J8 Jacobi, W., H.G. Paretzke and F. Schindel. Lung cancer risk assessment of radon-exposed miners on the basis of a proportional hazard model. p. 17-22 in: Occupational Radiation Safety in Mining. Proceedings of the International Conference. Vol. I. (H. Stocker, ed.). Canadian Nuclear Association, Toronto, 1985.

K1 Kaplan, E.L. and P. Meier. Non-parametric estimation from incomplete observations. J. Am. Stat. Assoc. 53: 457-481 (1958).

K2 Kellerer, A.M. Statistical and biophysical aspects of the gamma-ray survival curve. in: Cell Survival after Low Doses of Radiation: Theoretical and Clinical Implications (J. Alper, ed.). The Institute of Physics and John Wiley and Sons, London, 1975.

K3 Kellerer, A.M., E.J. Hall, H.H. Rossi et al. RBE as a function of neutron energy. II. Statistical analysis. Radiat. Res. 65: 172-186 (1976).

K4 Kellerer, A.M. and H.H. Rossi. The theory of dual radiation action. Curr. Top. Radiat. Res. Quart. 8: 85-158 (1972).

K5 Kellerer, A.M. and H.H. Rossi. A generalized formulation of dual radiation action. Radiat. Res. 75: 471-488 (1978).

K6 Kellerer, A.M. and H.H. Rossi. Biological implications of microdosimetry II: spatial aspects. p. 331-351 in: Proceedings of the Fourth Symposium on Microdosimetry, Verbania-Pallanza, September 1973. EUR-5122 (1974).

K7 Kellerer, A.M. and H.H. Rossi. RBE and the primary mechanism of radiation action. Radiat. Res. 47: 15-34 (1971).

K8 Kellerer, A.M. Radiation carcinogenesis at low doses. p. 405-422 in: Proceedings of the Sixth Symposium on Microdosimetry, Vol. I, Brussels, May 1978 (J. Booz

and H.G. Ebert, eds.). Harwood Academic Publishers Ltd., London, 1978.

K10 Kennedy, A.R., S. Modal, C. Heidelberger et al. Enhancement of x-ray transformation by 12-O-tetra-decanoylphorbol-13-acetate in a cloned line of C3H mouse embryo cells. Cancer Res. 38: 439-443 (1978).

K12 Klein, J.C. The use of in vitro methods for the study of x-ray-induced transformation. p. 301-308 in: Biology of Radiation Carcinogenesis (M.J. Yuhas et al., eds.). Raven Press, New York, 1976.

K16 Knaap, A.G.A. and J.W.I. Simons. A mutational assay system for L5178 Y mouse lymphoma cells using hypoxanthineguanine phosphoribosul transferase (HG-PRT) deficiency as marker. The occurrence of a long expression time for mutations induced by x rays and EMS. Mutat. Res. 30: 97-109 (1975).

K17 Kneale, G.W., A.M. Stewart and T.F. Mancuso. Reanalysis of data relating to the Hanford study of the cancer risks of radiation workers. p. 387-412 in: Late Biological Effects of Ionizing Radiation, Vol. II. IAEA, Vienna, 1978.

K20 Knudson, A.G., Jr. Germinal and somatic mutations in cancer. p. 367-371 in: Human Genetics (S. Amendares and R. Lisker, eds.). Excerpta Medica, Amsterdam, 1977.

K21 Korner, I., M. Walicka, W. Malz et al. DNA repair in two L5178 Y cell lines with different x-ray sensitivities. Stud. Biophys. (GDR) 61: 141-149 (1977).

K22 Kunz, E., J. Sevc, V. Placek et al. Lung cancer in man in relation to different time distribution of radiation exposure. Health Phys. 36: 699-706 (1979).

K24 Kal, H.B. Effects of protracted gamma irradiation on cells from a rat rhabdomyosarcoma treated in vitro and in vivo. p. 259-269 in: Cell Survival after Low Doses of Radiation: Theoretical and Clinical Implications. The Institute of Physics and John Wiley and Sons, London, 1975.

K25 Kasuga, T., T. Sado, Y. Noda et al. Radiation-induced tumours in C57BLf/6JNrs [SPF] and C3Hf/HeMsNrs [SPF] strain male mice. p. 29-41 in: Late Biological Effects of Ionizing Radiation, Vol. II. IAEA, Vienna, 1978.

K26 Kennedy, A.R., M. Fox, G. Murphy et al. Relationship between x-ray exposure and malignant transformation in C3H10T1/2 cells. Proc. Natl. Acad. Sci. U.S.A. 77: 7262-7266 (1980).

K27 Kennedy, A.R., G. Murphy and J.B. Little. Effect of time and duration of exposure to 12-O-Tetradecanoyl-phorbol-13-acetate on X ray transformation of C3H10T1/2 cells. Cancer Res. 40: 1915-1920 (1980).

K28 Kinsella, A.R. Do chromosomal rearrangements represent a rate-limiting step in carcinogenesis? (Meeting abstract). J. Supramol. Struct. Suppl. 15: 214 (1981).

K29 Kinsella, A.R. and M. Radman. Tumor promoter induces sister chromatid exchanges: Relevance to mechanisms of carcinogenesis. Proc. Natl. Acad. Sci. U.S.A. 75: 6149-6153 (1978).

K30 Kennedy, A.R. and R.R. Weichselbaum. Effects of dexamethasone and cortisone with X-ray irradiation on transformation of C3H10T1/2 cells. Nature 294: 97-98 (1981).

K31 Kennedy, A.R. and J.B. Little. Actinomycin D suppresses radiation transformation in vitro. Int. J. Radiat. Biol. 38: 465-468 (1980).

K32 Kneale, G.W., T.F. Mancuso and A.M. Stewart. Hanford radiation study III: a cohort study of the cancer risks from radiation to workers at Hanford (1944-77 deaths) by the method of regression models in lifetables. Brit. J. Int. Med. 38: 156-166 (1981).

K33 Kaplan, H.S. and M.B. Brown. A quantitative dose-response study of lymphoid tumor development in irradiated C57 Blade mice. J. Natl. Cancer Inst. 13: 185-208 (1952).

K34 Kerr, G.D. Findings of a recent ORNL review of dosimetry for the Japanese atomic-bomb survivors. ORNL/TM-8078 (1982).

K35 Kennedy, A.R. and J.B. Little. Effects of protease inhibitors on radiation transformation in vitro. Cancer Res. 41: 2103-2108 (1981).

K36 Kucerova, M., A.J.B. Anderson, K.E. Buckton et al. X-ray-induced chromosome aberrations in human peripheral blood leucocytes: the response to low levels of exposure in vitro. Int. J. Radiat. Biol. 21: 389-396 (1972).

K37 Kalbfleisch, J.D. and R.L. Prentice. The statistical analysis of failure time data. John Wiley and Sons, New York, 1980.

K38 Kellerer, A.M. and D. Chmelevsky. Analysis of tumor rates and incidences. A Survey of Concepts and Methods. p. 209-231 in: Proceedings of the European Seminar on Neutron Carcinogenesis. (J.J. Broerse and G.B. Gerber, eds.) EUR-8084 (1982).

K39 Kato, H. and W.J. Schull. Studies of the mortality of A-bomb survivors. 7. Mortality, 1950-1978: Part I. Cancer Mortality. Radiat. Res. 90: 395-432 (1982).

K40 Kato, H., C.C. Brown, D.G. Hoel et al. Studies of the mortality of A-bomb survivors. 7. Mortality, 1950-1978: Part II. Mortality from causes other than cancer and mortality in early entrants. Radiat. Res. 91: 243-264 (1982).

K41 Kellerer, A.M., Y.M.P. Lam and H.H. Rossi. Biophysical studies with spatially correlated ions. 4. Analysis of cell survival data for diatomic deuterium. Radiat. Res. 83: 511-528 (1980).

K42 Kato, H., K. Kopecky and D. Preston. Radiation mortality among A-bomb survivors. 1950-1982. Technical Report. (Personal communication)

L1 Land, C.E. and D.H. McGregor. Breast cancer incidence among atomic bomb survivors: implications for radiobiologic risk at low doses. J. Natl. Cancer Inst. 62: 17-21 (1979).

L3 Leenhouts, H.P. and K.H. Chadwick. An analysis of radiation-induced malignancy based on somatic mutation. Int. J. Radiat. Biol. 33: 357-370 (1978).

L4 Lea, D.E. Action of radiations on living cells. University Press, Cambridge, 1962.

L6 Lehnert, S. Relation of intracellular cyclic AMP to the shape of mammalian cell survival curves. p. 226-236 in: Cell Survival after Low Doses of Radiation: Theoretical and Clinical Implications. The Institute of Physics and John Wiley and Sons, London, 1975.

L7 Leonard, H. and G.B. Gerber. The radiosensitivities of lymphocytes from pigs, sheep, goat and cow. Mutat. Res. 36: 319-332 (1976).

L8 Lever, W.F. Histopathology of the skin. Pitman Medical Publ. Co. London/A. Lippincott Co. Philadelphia, 1967.

L9 Liniecki, J., A. Bajerska, K. Wyszynska et al. Gamma radiation-induced chromosomal aberrations in human lymphocytes; dose-rate effects in stimulated and non-stimulated cells. Mutat. Res. 43: 291-304 (1977).

L10 Little, J.B. Quantitative studies on radiation transformation with the A31-11 mouse BALB/3T3 cell line. Cancer Res. 39: 1474-1480 (1979).

L12 Lloyd, D.C., R.R. Purrott, G.W. Dolphin et al. Chromosome aberrations induced in human lymphocytes by neutron irradiation. Int. J. Radiat. Biol. 29: 169-182 (1976).

L13 Lloyd, D.C., R.J. Purrott, G.W. Dolphin et al. The relationship between chromosome aberrations and low-LET radiation dose to human lymphocytes. Int. J. Radiat. Biol. 28: 75-90 (1975).

L15 Lloyd, E.L., H.A. Gemmell, C.B. Henning et al. Transformation of mammalian cells by alpha particles. Int. J. Radiat. Biol. 36: 467-478 (1979).

L16 Lloyd, E.L., H.A. Gemmell and C.B. Henning. Supression of transformed foci induced by alpha radiation of C3HT101/2 cells by untransformed cells. ANL-78-65, Part II (1979).

L18 Lundin, F.E., J.K. Wagoner and V.E. Archer. Radon daughter exposure and respiratory cancer, quantitative and temporal aspects. U.S. Department of Health, Education and Welfare, Public Health Service, National Institute of Occupational Safety and Health, National Institute of Environmental Health Sciences joint monograph no. 1. Springfield, 1971.

L19 Lundin, F.E., V.E. Archer and J.K. Wagoner. An exposure-time-response model for lung cancer mortality in uranium miners: effects of radiation exposure, age and cigarette smoking. p. 243-264 in: Proceedings of the Conference on Energy and Health, Alta, Utah, June 1978. (N.E. Breslow et al. eds.). SIAM Publishers, Philadelphia, 1979.

L20 Luz, A., W.A. Müller, W. Gossner et al. Estimation of tumour risk at low dose from experimental results after incorporation of short-lived bone-seeking alpha emitters radium-224 and thorium-227 in mice. p. 171-181 in: Biological and Environmental Effects of Low-Level Radiation. IAEA, Vienna, 1976.

L22 Land, C.E., J.D. Boice, R.E. Shore et al. Breast cancer risk from low-dose exposures to ionizing radiation: results of parallel analysis of three exposed populations of women. J. Natl. Cancer Inst. 65: 353-376 (1980).

L23 Little J.B., H. Nagasanra and A.R. Kennedy. DNA repair and malignant transformation: effect of x-irradiation, 12-O-tetradecanoylphorbol-13-acetate, and protease inhibitors on transformation and sister-chromatid exchanges in mouse 10T1/2 cells. Radiat. Res. 79: 241-255 (1979).

L24 Land, C.E. and J.E. Norman. Latent periods of radiogenic cancers occurring among Japanese A-bomb survivors. p. 29-47 in: Late Biological Effects of Ionizing Radiation, Vol. II. IAEA, Vienna 1978.

L26 Little, J.B. Influence of noncarcinogenic secondary factors on radiation carcinogenesis. Radiat. Res. 87: 240-250 (1981).

L27 Loewe, W.E. and E. Mendelsohn. Revised dose estimates at Hiroshima and Nagasaki. Health Phys. 41: 663-666 (1981).

L29 Lee, W., R.P. Chiaccierini, B. Shleien et al. Thyroid tumours following iodine-131 or localized x-irradiation to the thyroid and the pituitary glands in rats. Radiat. Res. 92: 307-319 (1982).

L30 Loewe, W.E. A-bomb survivor dosimetry update. Paper presented at the Third International Symposium on Radiation Protection, Inverness, Scotland, 1982.

L32 Land, C.E. and M. Tokunaga. Induction period. p. 421-436 in: Radiation Carcinogenesis: Epidemiology and Biological Significance. (J.D. Boice and J.F. Fraumeni, eds.) Raven Press, New York, 1984.

L33 Lin, S.L., M. Takii and P.O.P. Ts'o. Somatic mutation and neoplastic transformation induced by (methyl³H) thymidine. Radiat. Res. 90: 142-154 (1982).

L34 Lemotte, P.K., S.J. Adelstein and J.B. Little. Malignant transformation induced by incorporated radionuclides in BALB/3T3 mouse embryo fibroblasts. Proc. Natl. Acad. Sci. U.S.A. 79: 7763-7767 (1982).

L35 Little, J.B., B.N. Grossman and W.F. O'Toole. Induction of bronchial cancer in hamsters by polonium-210 alpha radiation. Radiat. Res. 43: 261-262 (1970).

L36 Lloyd, D.C. and A.A. Edwards. Chromosome aberrations in human lymphocytes: effect of radiation quality, dose and dose rate. p. 23-49 in: Radiation-Induced Chromosome Damage in Man. Alan R. Liss Inc., New York, 1983.

M1 MacKenzie, I. Breast cancer following multiple fluoroscopies. Br. J. Cancer 19: 1-8 (1965).

M2 Major, I.R. and R.H. Mole. Myeloid leukaemia in x-ray irradiated CBA mice. Nature 272: 455-456 (1978).

M3 Mancuso, T.F., A. Stewart and G. Kneale. Radiation exposures of Hanford workers dying from cancer and other causes. Health Phys. 33: 369-385 (1977).

M4 Marshall, J.M. and P.G. Groer. A theory of the induction of bone cancer by alpha radiation. Radiat. Res. 71: 149-192 (1977).

M5 Morrison, H.I., R.M. Semenciw, Y. Mao et al. Lung cancer mortality and radiation exposure among the Newfoundland fluorspar miners. p. 365-368 in: International Conference on Occupational Radiation Safety in Mining (H. Stocker, ed.). Canadian Nuclear Association, Toronto, 1985.

M6 Marx, J.L. Tumour promotion: carcinogenesis gets more complicated. Science 201: 515-518 (1978).

M7 Matanoski, G.N., R. Seltser, P.E. Sartwell et al. The current mortality rates of radiobiologists and other physician specialists: specific causes of death. Am. J. Epidemiol. 101: 199-210 (1975).

M8 Mayneord, W.V. The time factor in carcinogenesis. The 1977 Sievert Lecture. Health Phys. 34: 297-309 (1978).

M9 Mayneord, W.V. and R.H. Clarke. Carcinogenesis and radiation risk: a biomathematical reconnaissance. Br. J. Radiol. Supplement 12: 11-12 (1975).

M10 Mayneord, W.V. and R.H. Clarke. Time and dose in carcinogenesis. RD/B/N-3940 (1978).

M11 Mays, C.W., G.N. Taylor, W. Stevens et al. Bone sarcomas at low doses of α-radiation in beagles. p. 9-14 in: COO-119-254 (1979).

M12 Mays, W.C. and R.D. Lloyd. Predicted toxocity of ^{90}Sr in humans. p. 181-205 in: Proceedings of the Second International Conference on Strontium Metabolism. CONF-720818 (1972).

M13 Mays, C.W. and R.D. Lloyd. Bone sarcoma risk from ^{90}Sr. p. 352-375 in: Biomedical Implications of Radiostrontium Exposure (M. Goldmann and L.K. Bustad, eds.). Symposium Series 25, CONF-710201 (1972).

M14 Mays, C.W. and R.D. Lloyd. Bone sarcoma incidence versus alpha particle dose. p.409-430 in: Radiobiology

of Plutonium (B. Stover and W.S.S. Jee, eds.). J.W. Press, Salt Lake City, 1972.

M16 McCulloch, E.A. and J.E. Till. The sensitivity of cells from normal mouse bone marrow to gamma-radiation in vitro and in vivo. Radiat. Res. 16: 822-832 (1962).

M17 McGregor, D.H., C.E. Land and K. Choi. Breast cancer incidence among atomic bomb survivors, Hiroshima and Nagasaki 1950-1969. J. Natl. Cancer Inst. 59: 799-811 (1977).

M18 McNulty, P.J., C.H. Nauman, A.H. Sparrow et al. Influence of x-ray dose fractionation on the frequency of somatic mutations induced in Tradescantia stamen hair. Mutat. Res. 44: 235-246 (1977).

M19 Metalli, P., V. Covelli and G. Silini. Dose-incidence relationships of reticulum cell sarcoma in mice. Observations and hypotheses at the cellular level. p. 341-349 in: Late Biological Effects of Ionizing Radiation. Vol. II. IAEA, Vienna, 1978.

M20 Metalli, P., G. Silini, V. Covelli et al. Late somatic effects in syngeneic radiation chimaeras: III. Observations on animals repopulated with irradiated marrow. Int. J. Radiat. Biol. 29: 413-432 (1976).

M21 Millar, B.C., E.M. Fielden and J.L. Millar. Interpretation of survival-curve data for chinese hamster cells, line V-29, using the multitarget, multitarget with initial slope and α, β equations. Int. J. Radiat. Biol. 599-603 (1978).

M22 Miller, D.R. A note on independence of multivariate lifetimes in competing risks models. Am. Stat. 5: 576-579 (1977).

M23 Miller, R. and E.J. Hall. X-ray dose fractionation and oncogenic transformations in cultured mouse embryo cells. Nature 272: 58-60 (1978).

M25 Modan, B., D. Baidatz, H. Mast et al. Radiation-induced head and neck-tumours. Lancet 1: 277-279 (1974).

M26 Mole, R.H. Bone tumour production in mice by strontium-90: further experimental support for two-event hypothesis. Br. J. Cancer 17: 524-531 (1963).

M27 Mole, R.H. Personal communication.

M28 Mole, R.H. The sensitivity of the human breast to cancer induction by ionizing radiation. Br. J. Radiol. 51: 401-405 (1978).

M29 Mole, R.H. Carcinogenesis by thorotrast and other sources of irradiation, especially other α-emitters. Environ. Res. 18: 192-215 (1979).

M30 Mole, R.H. Letter to the editor. Lancet 1: 1155-1156 (1978).

M31 Mole, R.H. Ionizing radiation as a carcinogen: practical questions and academic pursuits. Br. J. Radiol. 48: 157-169 (1975).

M32 Mole, R.H. Pathological findings in mice exposed to fission neutrons in the reactor CLEEP. p. 117-128 in: Biological Effects of Neutron and Proton Irradiations. IAEA, Vienna, 1964.

M33 Momeni, M.H. Competitive radiation-induced carcinogenesis: an analysis of data from beagle dogs exposed to radium-226 and strontium-90. Health Phys. 36: 295-310 (1979).

M35 Mulvihill, J.J. Genetic repertory of human neoplasia. p. 137-144 in: Genetics of Human Cancer (J.J. Mulvihill, R.W. Miller and J.F. Fraumeni, eds.). Raven Press, New York, 1977.

M36 Munson, R.J. and D.T. Goodhead. The relation between induced mutation frequency and an examination of experimental data for eukaryotes. Mutat. Res. 42: 145-160 (1977).

M37 Muramatsu, S. and O. Matsuoka. Comparative studies of radiation-induced chromosome aberrations in several mammalian species. p. 229-236 in: Biological and Environmental Effects of Low-Level Radiation, Vol. I. IAEA, Vienna, 1976.

M39 Myrden, J.A. and J.E. Hiltz. Breast cancer following multiple fluoroscopies during artificial pneumothorax treatment for pulmonary tuberculosis. Can. Med. Assoc. J. 100: 1032-1034 (1969).

M40 Myrden, J.A. and J.J. Quinlan. Breast carcinoma following multiple fluoroscopies with pneumothorax treatment of pulmonary tuberculosis. Ann. Royal Coll. Phys. Surg. Can. 7: 45 (1974).

M41 Miller, R., E.J. Hall and H.H. Rossi. Oncogenic transformation of mammalian cells in vitro with split doses of x rays. Proc. Natl. Acad. Sci. U.S.A. 76: 5755-5758 (1979).

M43 Myers, D.K. and C.G. Stewart. Some health aspects of Canadian uranium mining. AECL-5970 (1979).

M45 Mole, R.H. Bone tumour production in mice by strontium-90: further experimental support for a two-event hypothesis. Br. J. Cancer 17: 524-531 (1963).

M46 Muller, H.J. Advances in radiation mutagenesis through studies on Drosophila. p. 313-321 in: Proc. 2nd Int. Conf. Peaceful Uses of Atomic Energy. Vol. 22, Geneva 1958.

M47 Mole, R.H. Carcinogenesis as a result of two independent rare events. p. 161-165 in: Cellular Basis and Aetiology of Late Somatic Effects of Ionizing Radiation (H.J. Harris ed.). Academic Press, London, 1963.

M49 Muller, R.C., R. Osman, M. Zimmerman et al. Sensitizers, protectors and oncogenic transformation in vitro. Int. J. Radiat. Oncol. Biol. Phys. 8: 771-775 (1982).

M50 Moolgavkar, S.H. and A.G. Knudson. Mutation and cancer: A model for human carcinogenesis. J. Natl. Cancer Inst. 66: 1037-1052 (1981).

M51 Mulcahy, R.T., M.N. Gould and K.H. Clifton. The survival of thyroid cells: in vivo irradiation and in situ repair. Radiat. Res. 84: 523-528 (1980).

M52 Mole, R.H. Dose-response relationships. p. 403-420 in: Radiation Carcinogenesis: Epidemiology and Biological Implications. (J.D. Boice and J.F. Fraumeni, eds.), Raven Press, New York, 1984.

M57 Mays, C.W. and H. Spiess. Bone sarcomas in ^{224}Ra patients. p. 241-252 in: Radiation Carcinogenesis: Epidemiology and Biological Significance. (J.D. Boice and J.F. Fraumeni, eds.), Raven Press, New York, 1984.

M58 Mahler, P.A., M.N. Gould, P.M. De Luca et al. Rat mammary cell survival following irradiation with 14.3 MeV neutrons. Radiat. Res. 91: 235-242 (1982).

M60 Mahler, P.A., M.N. Gould and K.H. Clifton. Kinetics of in situ repair in rat mammary gland cells. Radiat. Res. 91: 409 only (1982).

M61 Moskalev, Yu.i., L.A. Buldakov, V.N. Iljin et al. Study of the dose-effect relationship from the standpoint of radiation hygiene. Med. Radiologia 4: 74-82 (1982) (in Russian).

M62 Maisin, J.R., A. Wambersie, G.B. Gerber et al. The effects of a fractionated gamma irradiation on life shortening and disease incidence in BALB/c mice. Radiat. Res. 94: 359-373 (1983).

M63 Maisin, J.R., A. Wambersie, G.B. Gerber et al. Life shortening and disease incidence in BALB/c mice following a single d(50)-Be neutron or gamma exposure. Radiat. Res. 94: 374-389 (1983).

M64 Mole, R.H., D.G. Papworth and M.J. Corp. The dose-response for x-ray induction of myeloid leukaemia in male CBA/H mice. Br. J. Cancer 47: 285-291 (1983).

M65 Mole, R.H. and I.R. Major. Myeloid leukaemia frequency after protracted exposure to ionizing radiation: experimental confirmation of the flat dose-response found in ankylosing spondylitis after a single treatment course with x rays. Leukaemia Res. 7: 295-300 (1983).

M66 Mole, R.H. and J.A.G. Davids. Induction of myeloid leukaemia and other tumours in mice by irradiation with fission neutrons. p. 31-42 in: Neutron carcinogenesis (J.J. Broerse and G.B. Gerber, eds.). EUR-8084 (1982).

M67 Müller, W.A., A. Luz, E.H. Schäffer et al. The role of time-factor and RBE for the induction of osteosarcomas by incorporated short-lived bone-seekers. Health Phys. 44 Suppl. 1: 203-212 (1983).

M68 Moskalev, Yu.I. and V.N. Strelcova. Radiation carcinogenesis from the standpoint of radiological protection. Energoizdat, Moscow, 1982 (in Russian).

M69 Mays, C.W. Discussion of paper by O.G. Raabe [R40] in: Health Phys. 44: Suppl. 1: 46-47 (1983).

M70 Müller, J., W.C. Wheeler, J.F. Gentleman et al. Study of mortality of Ontario miners. p. 335-343 in: Proc. Int. Conf. on Occupational Radiation Safety in Mining. Vol. I. (H. Stocker, ed.). Canadian Nuclear Association, Toronto, 1985.

M71 Moskalev, Yu.I. and I.A. Milovidova. Induction of mammary tumours in rats by single and fractionated β irradiation from strontium-90 and yttrium-90. Radiobiologija 23: 54-58 (1983).

N1 National Council on Radiation Protection and Measurements. Influence of dose and its distribution in time on dose-effect relationships for low-LET radiations. NCRP-R-64 (1980).

N2 Nauman, C.H., A.G. Underbrink and A.H. Sparrow. Influence of radiation dose rate on somatic mutation induction in Tradescantia stamen hairs. Radiat. Res. 62: 79-96 (1975).

N3 Nelson, W. Theory and applications of hazard plotting for censored failure data. Technometrics 14: 945-966 (1972).

N4 Neyman, J. Public health hazards from electricity-producing plants. Science 195: 754-758 (1977).

N5 Nowell, P.C. The clonal evolution of tumour cell populations. Science 194: 23-28 (1976).

N6 Nowell, P.C. and L.J. Cole. Hepatomas in mice: incidence increased after gamma irradiations at low dose rates. Science 148: 96-97 (1965).

N7 Norris, W.P., T.W. Speckman and P.F. Gustafson. Studies on metabolism of radium in man. Am. J. Roentgenol. Radium Ther. Nucl. Med. 73: 785-802 (1955).

N8 Norris, G. and S.L. Hood. Some problems in the culturing and radiation sensitivity of normal human cells. Exp. Cell Res. 27: 48 (1962).

N9 Nolibé, D., R. Masse and J. Lafuma. The effect of neonatal thymectomy on lung cancers induced in rats by Plutonium Dioxide. Radiat. Res. 87: 90-99 (1981).

N10 National Council on Radiation Protection and Measurements. Induction of thyroid cancer by ionizing radiation. NCRP Report No. 80 (1985).

O1 Okada, S., H.B. Hamilton, N. Egami et al. A review of thirty years study of Hiroshima and Nagasaki atomic bomb survivors. J. Radiat. Res. (Tokyo): 16 (Suppl.): 1-164 (1975).

P2 Parfenov Yu, D. Mathematical dose-effect models in studies of cancerogenesis. Vopros. Onkol. 32(1): 9-22 (1986) (in Russian).

P7 Paterson, M.C., A.K. Anderson, B.P. Smith et al. Enhanced radiosensitivity of cultured fibroblasts from ataxia teleangiectasia heterozygotes manifested by defective colony forming ability and reduced DNA repair replication after hypoxic gamma-irradiation. Cancer Res. 39: 3725-3734 (1979).

P8 Pochin, E.E. Personal communication (1986).

P11 Polednak, A.P. Bone cancer among female radium dial workers. Latency periods and incidence by time after exposure: brief communication. J. Natl. Cancer Inst. 60: 77-82 (1978).

P15 Puck, T.T., D. Morokovin, P. Marcus et al. Action of x rays on mammalian cells. II. Survival curves of cells from normal human tissues. J. Exp. Med. 106: 485-500 (1957).

P17 Peterson, A.V., R.L. Prentice and P. Marek. Relationship between dose of injected ^{239}Pu and bone sarcoma mortality in young adult beagles. Radiat. Res. 90: 77-89 (1982).

P18 Peto, R., M.C. Pike, N.E. Day et al. Guidelines for simple, sensitive significance tests for carcinogenic effects in long-term animal experiments. p. 311-423 Annex to IARC Monographs on the Evaluation of the Carcinogenic Risk of Chemicals to Humans, Suppl. 2. Long-term and short-term Screening Assays for Carcinogena: A Critical Appraisal. IARC. Lyon, 1980.

P19 Peto, R. Guidelines on the analysis of tumour rates and death rates in experimental animals. Br. J. Cancer 29: 101-105 (1974).

P20 Prosser, J.S., D.C. Lloyd, A.A. Edwards et al. The induction of chromosome aberrations in human lymphocytes by exposure to tritiated water in vitro. Rad. Prot. Dosim. 4: 21-26 (1983).

P21 Papworth, D.G. and E.V. Hulse. Dose-response models for the radiation-induction of skin tumours in mice. Int. J. Radiat. Biol. 44: 423-431 (1983).

P22 Petoyan, I.M. and I.V. Filyushkin. Theoretical model of radiation-induced cancer. Radiobiologiya 24: 481-488 (1984) (in Russian).

P23 Petoyan, I.M. and I.V. Filyushkin. A mathematical model of the carcinogenic effect of osteotropic alpha emitters. Radiobiologiya 25: 356-361 (1985). (in Russian).

R1 Ramzaev, P.V., M.N. Troitzaia, A.P. Ermolaieva et al. Supra-linear effects of small doses of ionizing radiation. p. 140-144 in: Proc. 8th All-Union Conference on Radiation Hygiene. Leningrad, 1978. (in Russian).

R2 Reif, A.E. Radiation carcinogenesis at high dose-response levels: a hypothesis. Nature 190: 415-417 (1961).

R3 Reissland, J.A. An assessment of the Mancuso study. NRPB-R79 (1978).

R4 Reassessment of Atomic Bomb Radiation Dosimetry in Hiroshima and Nagasaki. Proceeding of a Workshop held at Nagasaki on 16-17 February 1983. Radiation Effects Research Foundation. Hiroshima, 1983.

R5 Richold, M. and P.D. Holt. The effect of differing neutron energies on mutagenesis in cultured Chinese hamster cells. p. 237-244 in: Biological Effects of Neutron Irradiation. IAEA, Vienna, 1974.

R6 Reassessment of Atomic Bomb Radiation Dosimetry in Hiroshima and Nagasaki. Proceeding of a Workshop held at Nagasaki on 8-9 November 1983. Radiation Effects Research Foundation. Hiroshima, 1984.

R7 Robinson, V.C. and A.C. Upton. Competing-risk analysis of leukaemia and non-leukaemia mortality in x-irradiated, male RF mice. J. Natl. Cancer Inst. 60: 995-1007 (1978).

R8 Rose, D.M. An investigation of dependent competing risks. Unpublished dissertation, University of Washington, 1973.

R9 Rosenblatt, L.S., N.H. Hetherington, M. Goldman et al. Evaluation of tumour incidence following exposure to internal emitters by application of the logistic dose-response surface. Health Phys. 21: 869-875 (1975).

R12 Rossi, H.H. and A.M. Kellerer. Biological implications of microdosimetry. I: temporal aspects. p. 315-330 in: Proceedings of the Fourth Symposium on Microdosimetry, Verbania-Pallanza, September 1973. EUR-5122 (1974).

R15 Rossi, H.H. Biophysical implications of radiation quality. p. 994-997 in: Radiation Research, Biomedical, Chemical and Physical Perspective (O. Nygaard et al., eds.). Academic Press, New York, 1975.

R16 Rossi, H.H. Interrelation between physical and biological effects of small radiation doses. p. 245-251 in: Biological and Environmental Effects of Low-Level Irradiation. IAEA, Vienna, 1976.

R17 Rossi, H.H. and A.M. Kellerer. Radiation carcinogenesis at low doses. Science 175: 200-204 (1972).

R18 Rowland, R.E., A.F. Stehney and H.F. Lucas, Jr. Dose-response relationships for female radium dial workers. Radiat. Res. 76: 368-383 (1978).

R19 Rowland, R.E., P.M. Failla, A.T. Keane et al. Some dose-response relationships for tumour incidence in radium patients. p. 1-17 in: ANL-7760 (1970).

R20 Rowland, R.E., P.M. Failla, A.T. Keane et al. Tumour incidence in radium patients. p. 1-8 in: ANL-7860 (1971).

R21 Rowland, R.E. The risk of malignancy from internally deposited radioisotopes. p. 146-155 in: Radiation Research, Biomedical, Chemical and Physical Perspectives (O.F. Nygaard et al., eds.). Academic Press, New York, 1975.

R24 Russell, W.L. Mutation frequencies in female mice and the estimation of genetic hazards of radiation in women. Proc. Natl. Acad. Sci. U.S.A. 74: 3523-3527 (1977).

R25 Russell, W.L. Discussion of the paper by S. Abhamanson. p. 17 in: Biological and Environmental Effects of Low-Level Radiation, Vol. I. IAEA, Vienna, 1976.

R26 Russell, W.L. Criticism of a current model for estimating genetic risks of radiation. p. 121-123 in: Biology Division Annual Progress Report, 1 July 1974 to 30 June 1975. ORNL-5072 (1975).

R28 Raabe, O.G., S.A. Book and N.J. Parks. Bone cancer from radium: canine dose response explains data for mice and humans. Science 208: 61-64 (1980).

R29 Ron, E. and B. Modan. Benign and malignant thyroid neoplasms after childhood irradiation for tinea capitis. J. Natl. Cancer Inst. 65: 7-11 (1980).

R30 Raaphorst, G.P., E.L. Azzam and J. Borsa. Enhancement by BUdR of x-ray-induced cell killing and oncogenic transformation in cultured C3H10T1/2 cells. (abstract) Radiat. Res. 87: 498 (1981).

R31 Rubin, H. Is somatic mutation the major mechanism of malignant transformation? J. Natl. Cancer Inst. 64: 995-1000 (1980).

R32 Raabe, O.G., N.J. Parks and S.A. Book. Dose-response relationships for bone tumors in beagles exposed to ^{226}Ra and ^{90}Sr. Health Phys. 40: 863-880 (1981).

R33 Radford, E.P., R. Doll and P.G. Smith. Mortality among patients with ankylosing spondylitis not given X-ray therapy. New Engl. J. Med. 297: 572-576 (1977).

R34 Rowland, R., A.F. Stehney and H.F. Lucas. Dose-response relationships for radium-induced bone sarcomas. Health Phys. 44: 15-31 (1983).

R35 Radford, E.P. Radon daughters in the induction of lung cancer in underground miners. p. 151-163 in: Banbury Report 9: Quantification of Occupational Cancer. Cold Spring Harbor Laboratory, New York, 1981.

R36 Radford, E.P. Radiogenic cancer in underground miners. p. 225-230 in: Radiation Carcinogenesis: Epidemiology and Biological Significance. (J.D. Boice and J.F. Fraumeni, eds.), Raven Press, New York, 1984.

R37 Rossi, H.H. Consideration on the time factor in radiobiology. Radiat. Environ. Biophys. 20: 1-9 (1981).

R38 Rossi, H.H. Biophysical studies with spatially correlated ions. I. Background and theoretical considerations. Radiat. Res. 78: 185-191 (1979).

R39 Robertson, J.B., A. Koehler, J. George et al. Oncogenic transformation of mouse BALB/3T3 cells by plutonium-238 alpha particles. Radiat. Res. 96: 261-274 (1983).

R40 Raabe, O.G., S.A. Book and N.J. Parks. Lifetime bone cancer dose-response relationships in beagles and people from skeletal burdens of ^{226}Ra and ^{90}Sr. Health Phys. 44: Suppl. 1: 33-48 (1983).

R41 Radford, E.P. and K.G. St.Clair Renard. Lung cancer in Swedish iron miners exposed to low doses of radon daughters. New Engl. J. Med. 310: 1485-1494 (1984).

R42 Robertson, M. Oncogenes and multistep carcinogenesis. Brit. Med. J. (Clin. Res.) 287: 1084-1086 (1983).

R43 Rossi, H.H. and E.J. Hall. The multicellular nature of radiation carcinogenesis. p. 359-368 in: Radiation Carcinogenesis: Epidemiology and Biological Significance. (J.D. Boice and J.F. Fraumeni, eds.). Raven Press, New York, 1984.

R44 Ransom, J.H., C.H. Evans, A.E. Jones et al. Control of the carconogenic potential of ^{99m}Technetium by the immunologic hormone lymphotoxin. Cancer Immunol. Immunother. 15: 126-130 (1983).

R45 Ron, E. and B. Modan. Thyroid and other neoplasms following childhood scalp irradiation. p. 139-152 in: Radiation Carcinogenesis: Epidemiology and Biological Significance. (J.D. Boice and J.F. Fraumeni, eds.). Raven Press, New York, 1984.

R46 Rowland, R.E. and H.F. Lucas, Jr. Radium-dial workers. p. 231-240 in: Radiation Carcinogenesis: Epidemiology and Biological Significance. (J.D. Boice and J.F. Fraumeni, eds.). Raven Press, New York, 1984.

S2 Sanders, B.S. Low-level radiation and cancer deaths. Health Phys. 34: 521-538 (1978).

S3 Sevc, J., E. Kunz and V. Placek. Lung cancer in uranium miners and long-term exposure to radon daughter products. Health Phys. 30: 433-437 (1976).

S4 Scott, D., H. Sharpe, A.L. Batchelor et al. Radiation-induced chromosome damage in human peripheral blood lymphocytes in vitro. I. RBE and dose rate studies with fast neutrons. Mutat. Res. 17: 377-383 (1969).

S5 Scott, D. and T.R.L. Bigger. The relative radiosensitivities of human, rabbit and rat-Kangaroo chromosomes. Chromosoma 49: 185-203 (1974).

S7 Segaloff, A. and H.M. Pettigrew. Effect of radiation dosage on the synergism between radiation and estrogen in the production of mammary cancer in the rat. Cancer Res. 38: 3445-3452 (1978).

S8 Seltser, R. and P.E. Sartwell. The influence of occupational exposure to radiation on the mortality of American radiologists and other specialists. Am. J. Epidemiol. 81: 2-22 (1965).

S10 Shellabarger, C.J. and R.W. Schmidt. Mammary neoplasia in the rat as related to dose of partial-body irradiation. Radiat. Res. 30: 497-506 (1967).

S11 Shellabarger, C.J., J.P. Stone and S. Holtzman. Rat differences in mammary tumour induction with estrogen and neutron irradiation. J. Natl. Cancer Inst. 61: 1505-1508 (1978).

S12 Shellabarger, C.J. Modifying factors in rat mammary gland carcinogenesis. p. 31-44 in: Biology of Radiation Carcinogenesis (J.M. Yuhas et al., eds.). Raven Press, New York, 1976.

S13 Shellabarger, C.J., V.P. Bond, E.P. Cronkite et al. Relationship of dose of total body cobalt-60 radiation to incidence of mammary neoplasia in female rats. p. 161-172 in: Radiation-Induced Cancer. IAEA, Vienna, 1969.

S14 Shellabarger, C.J., E.P. Cronkite, V.P. Bond et al. The occurrence of mammary tumours in the rat after sublethal whole-body irradiation. Radiat. Res. 6: 501-512 (1957).

S15 Shellabarger, C.J., R.D. Brown, A.R. Rao et al. Rat mammary carcinogenesis following neutron- or x-irradiation. p. 391-401 in: Biological Effects of Neutron Irradiation. IAEA, Vienna, 1974.

S16 Shore, R.E., L.H. Hempelmann, E. Kowaluk et al. Breast neoplasms in women treated with x rays for acute post-partum mastitis. J. Natl. Cancer Inst. 59: 813-822 (1977).

S17 Sinclair, W.K. The shape of radiation survival curves of mammalian cells cultured in vitro. p. 21-43 in: Biophysical Aspects of Radiation Quality. IAEA, Technical Report Series No. 58. Vienna, 1966.

S18 Spiess, H. and C.W. Mays. Protraction effect on bone sarcoma induction of radium-224 in children and adults. p. 437-450 in: Radionuclide Carcinogenesis (C.L. Sanders et al., eds.). U.S. Atomic Energy Commission, 1973.

S19 Sparrow, A.H., A.G. Underbrink and H.H. Rossi. Mutations induced in tradescantia by small doses of x-rays and neutrons analysis of dose-response curves. Science 176: 916-918 (1972).

S20 Sparrow, H.H., L.A. Schairer and R. Villalobos-Pietrini. Comparison of somatic mutation rates induced in tradescantia by chemical and physical mutagens. Mutat. Res. 26: 265-276 (1974).

S21 Spiess, H. and C.W. Mays. Bone cancers induced by ^{224}Ra (Th X) in children and adults. Health Phys. 19: 713-729 (1970).

S25 Suzuki, F. H. Hoshi and M. Horikawa. Repair of radiation-induced lethal and mutational damage in Chinese hamster cells in vitro. Jap. J. Genetics 54: 109-119 (1979).

S26 Sutherland, R.M. and R.E. Durand. Cell contact as a possible contribution to radiation resistance of some tumours. Br. J. Radiol. 45: 788-789 (1972).

S27 Sutherland, R.M. and R.E. Durand. Radiation response of multicell spheroids: an in vitro tumor model. Curr. Top. Radiat. Res. Quart. 11: 87-139 (1976).

S33 Szumiel, J. Requirements for potentiation of radiation effect by a platinum complex. Int. J. Radiat. Biol. 33: 605-608 (1978).

S36 Shore, R.E., R.E. Albert and B.S. Pasternack. Follow-up study of patients treated by x-ray epilation for tinea capitis. Arch. Environ. Health 31: 21-28 (1976).

S37 Shellabarger, C.J., D. Chmelevsky and A.M. Kellerer. Induction of mammary neoplasms in the Sprague-Dawley rat by 430 keV neutrons and x rays. J. Natl. Cancer Inst. 64: 821-833 (1980).

S38 Shore, R.E., E.D. Woodard, B.S. Pasternack et al. Radiation and host factors in human thyroid tumours following thymus irradiation. Health Phys. 38: 451-465 (1980).

S39 Sax, K. The time factor in x ray production of chromosome aberrations. Proc. Natl. Acad. Sci. U.S.A. 25: 225-233 (1939).

S40 Sax, K. An analysis of x-ray induced chromosomal aberrations in Tradescantia. Genetics 25: 41-68 (1940).

S43 Straus, D.S. Somatic mutation, cellular differentiation and cancer causation. J. Natl. Cancer Inst. 67: 233-241 (1981).

S44 Suzuki, N., M. Watanabe and M. Horikowa. Studies of radiation-induced carcinogenesis. p. 568 (Meeting abstract). Proc. of the Jap. Cancer Assoc. Tokyo, 1980.

S45 Siminovitch, L. On the nature of hereditable variation in cultured somatic cells. Cell 7: 1-11 (1976).

S46 Straume, T. and R.L. Dobson. Implications of new Hiroshima and Nagasaki dose estimates: cancer risks and neutron RBE. Health Phys. 41: 666-671 (1981).

S48 Sasaki, S. and T. Kasuga. Life-shortening and carcinogenesis in mice irradiated neonatally with x rays. Radiat. Res. 88: 313-325 (1981).

S49 Smith, P.G. and R. Doll. Mortality among patients with ankylosing spondylitis after a single treatment course with X rays. Brit. Med. J. 284: 449-460 (1982).

S50 Schlenker, R.A. Risk estimates for bone. p. 153-163 in: Critical Issues in Setting Radiation Dose Limits. Proceedings of the Seventh Annual Meeting of the NCRP. NCRP Proceedings 3 (1982).

S51 Sevc, J., V. Placek and P. Vernerova. Malignant tumour in lungs and inhalation radiation exposure. Prac. Lek. 34: 266-269 (1982). (in Czech).

S52 Shellabarger, C.J., D. Chmelevsky, A.M. Kellerer et al. Induction of mammary neoplasms in the ACI rat by 430-keV neutrons, X-rays and diethylstilbestiol. J. Natl. Cancer Inst. 69: 1135-1146 (1982).

S53 Storer, J.B. Associations between tumour types in irradiated BALB/c female mice. Radiat. Res. 92: 396-404 (1982).

S54 Sanders, C.L., G.E. Dagle, W.C. Cannon et al. Inhalation carcinogenesis of high-fired ^{238}PuO$_2$ in rats. Radiat. Res. 71: 528-546 (1977).

S55 Scarpelli, D.G. Recent developments toward a unifying concept of carcinogenesis. Ann. Clin. Lab. Sci. 13: 249-259 (1983).

S56 Sandberg, A.A. A chromosomal hypothesis of oncogenesis. Cancer Cytogenet. 8: 277-285 (1983).

S57 Storer, J.B. and R.L. Ullrich. Life shortening in BALB/c mice following brief, protracted or fractionated exposures to neutrons. Radiat. Res. 96: 335-347 (1983).

S58 Saccomano, G., V.E. Archer, O. Auerbach et al. Age factor in histological type of lung cancer among uranium miners. A preliminary report. p. 675-679 in: International Conference on Radiation Hazards in Mining: Control, Measurements and Medical Aspects. (M. Gomez, ed.). Soc. of Mining Engineers of American Institute of Mining, Metallurgical and Petroleum Engineers, New York, 1981.

S59 Schull, W.J. Atomic bomb survivors: patterns of cancer risk. p. 21-36 in: Radiation Carcinogenesis: Epidemiology and Biological Significance. (J.D. Boice and J.F. Fraumeni, eds.). Raven Press, New York, 1984.

S60 Shore, R.E., E. Woodard, N. Hildreth et al. Thyroid tumours following thymus irradiation. J. Natl. Cancer Inst. 74: 1177-1184 (1985).

S61 Saccomano, G. Cancer of the lung in uranium miners. p. 203-204 in: International Conference on Radiation Hazards in Mining (M. Gomez, ed.). Society of Mining Engineers of American Institute of Mining, Metallurgical and Petroleum Engineers, New York, 1981.

S62 Storer, J.B. and T.J. Mitchell. Limiting values for the RBE of fission neutrons at low doses for life shortening in mice. Radiat. Res. 97: 396-406 (1984).

T3 Thorn, M. Personal communication (1986).

T4 Terzaghi, M. and J.B. Little. Oncogenic transformation in vitro after split-dose x-irradiation. Int. J. Radiat. Biol. 29: 583-587 (1976).

T5 Terzaghi, M. and J.B. Little. Repair of potentially lethal radiation damage in mammalian cells is associated with enhancement of malignant transformation. Nature 253: 548-549 (1975).

T6 Terzaghi, M. and J.B. Little. Oncogenic transformation in vitro by x rays: influence of repair processes. p. 327-334 in: Biology of Radiation Carcinogenesis (J.M. Yuhas et al., eds.). Raven Press, New York, 1976.

T7 Terzaghi, M. and J.B. Little. X-irradiation-induced transformation in a C3H mouse embryo-derived cell line. Cancer Res. 36: 1367-1374 (1976).

T8 Thacker, J. The involvement of repair processes in radiation-induced mutation of cultured mammalian cells. p. 612-620 in: Proceedings of the 6th International Congress of Radiation Research, Tokyo, May 1979. (S. Okada et al., eds.). Jap. Assoc. for Radiation Research, Tokyo, 1979.

T9 Thacker, J., A. Stretch and M.A. Stephens. The induction of thoguanine resistant mutations of chinese hamster cells by gamma rays. Mutat. Res. 42: 313-326 (1977).

T10 Thacker, J. and R. Cox. Mutation induction and inactivation in mammalian cells exposed to ionizing radiation. Nature 258: 429-431 (1975).

T11 Terasima, T., M. Yazukawa and M. Kimura. Radiation-induced transformation of 10T1/2 mouse cells in the plateau phase: post-irradiation changes and serum dependence. Gann. 72: 762-768 (1981).

T12 Tokunaga, M., J.E. Norman, Jr., M. Asano et al. Malignant breast tumours among atomic bomb survivors, Hiroshima and Nagasaki, 1950-1974. J. Natl. Cancer Inst. 62: 1347-1359 (1979).

T15 Trosko, J.E. and C.C. Chang. Environmental carcinogenesis: an integrative model. Quart. Review of Biol. 53: 115-141 (1978).

T17 Tanooka, H. and K. Tanaka. Evidence for single-cell origin of 3-methyl-cholantrene-induced fibrosarcomas in mice with cellular mosaicism. Cancer Res. 42: 1856-1858 (1982).

T18 Thacker, J., A. Stretch and D.T. Goodhead. The mutagenecity of a-particles from plutonium-238. Radiat. Res. 92: 343-352 (1982).

T19 Thacker, J. and A. Stretch. Recovery from lethal and mutagenic damage during post-irradiation holding and low dose-rate irradiations of cultured hamster cells. Radiat. Res. 96: 380-392 (1983).

T20 Thomson, J.F., F.S. Williamson, D. Grahn et al. Life shortening in mice exposed to fission neutrons and gamma rays. I. Single and short-term fractionated exposure. Radiat. Res. 86: 559-572 (1981).

T21 Thomson, J.F., F.S. Williamson, D. Grahn et al. Life shortening of mice exposed to fission neutrons and gamma rays. II. Duration-of-life and long-term fractionated exposures. Radiat. Res. 86: 573-579 (1981).

T22 Taylor, G.N., C.W. Mays, R.D. Lloyd et al. Comparative toxicity of Ra-226, Pu-239, Am-241, Cf-249 and Cf-252 in C57Bl/Do black and albino mice. Radiat. Res. 95: 584-601 (1983).

T23 Tokunaga, M., C.E. Land, T. Yamamoto et al. Breast cancer among atomic bomb survivors. p. 45-56 in: Radiation Carcinogenesis: Epidemiology and Biological Significance. (J.D. Boice and J.F. Fraumeni, eds.). Raven Press, New York, 1984.

T24 Terasima, T., M. Yasukawa and M. Kimura. Neoplastic transformation of plateau-phase mouse 10T1/2 cells following single and fractionated doses of x rays. Radiat. Res. 102: 367-377 (1985).

T25 Thomson, J.F., F.S. Williamson and D. Grahn. Life shortening in mice exposed to fission neutrons and gamma rays III. Neutron exposures of 5 and 10 rads. Radiat. Res. 93: 205-209 (1983).

T26 Thomson, J.F., F.S. Williamson and D. Grahn. Life shortening in mice exposed to fission neutrons and γ rays. V. Further studies with single low doses. Radiat. Res. 104: 420-428 (1985).

U2 Ullrich, R.L. and J.B. Storer. Influence of gamma-ray irradiation on the development of neoplastic disease. II. Solid tumours. Radiat. Res. 80: 317-324 (1979).

U3 Ullrich, R.L. and J.B. Storer. Influence of gamma-ray irradiation on the development of neoplastic disease. III. Dose rate effects. Radiat. Res. 80: 325-342 (1979).

U4 Ullrich, R.L., M.C. Jernigan and J.B. Storer. Neutron carcinogenesis. Dose and dose-rate effects in BALB/c mice. Radiat. Res. 72: 487-498 (1977).

U5 Ullrich, R.L., M.C. Jernigan, G.E. Cosgrove et al. The influence of dose and dose-rate on the incidence of neoplastic disease in RFM mice after neutron irradiation. Radiat. Res. 68: 115-131 (1976).

U6 United Nations. Sources and Effects of Ionizing Radiation. United Nations Scientific Committee on the Effects of Atomic Radiation 1977 report to the General Assembly, with annexes. United Nations sales publication No. E.77.IX.1. New York, 1977.

U7 United Nations. Report of the United Nations Scientific Committee on the Effects of Atomic Radiation to the General Assembly, with annexes. Volume I: Levels, Volume II: Effects. United Nations sales publication No. E.72.IX.17 and 18. New York, 1972.

U9 United Nations. Report of the United Nations Scientific Committee on the Effects of Atomic Radiation. Official Records of the General Assembly, Twenty-fourth Session, Supplement No. 13 (A/7613). New York, 1969.

U10 United Nations. Report of the United Nations Scientific Committee on the Effects of Atomic Radiation. Official Records of the General Assembly, Twenty-first Session. Supplement No. 14 (A/6314). New York, 1966.

U11 United Nations. Report of the United Nations Scientific Committee on the Effects of Atomic Radiation. Official Records of the General Assembly, Nineteenth Session, Supplement No. 14 (A/5814). New York, 1964.

U12 United Nations. Report of the United Nations Scientific Committee on the Effects of Atomic Radiation. Official Records of the General Assembly, Seventeenth Session, Supplement No. 16 (A/5216). New York, 1962.

U13 Underbrink, A.G. and A.H. Sparrow. The influence of experimental endpoints, dose, dose rate, neutron energy, nitrogen ions, hypoxia chromosome volume and ploidy level on RBE. p. 185-214 in: Biological Effects of Neutron Irradiation. IAEA, Vienna, 1974.

U14 Upton, A.C., V.K. Jenkins, H.E. Walburg Jr. et al. Observations on viral, chemical and radiation-induced myeloid and lymphoid leukaemia in RF mice. Natl. Cancer Inst. Monogr. 22: 329-347 (1966).

U15 Upton, A.C., F.F. Wolff, J. Furth et al. A comparison of the induction of myeloid leukaemias in x-irradiated RF mice. Cancer Res. 18: 842-848 (1958).

U16 Upton, A.C., M.L. Randolph and J.W. Conklin. Late effects of fast neutrons and gamma rays in mice as influenced by the dose rate of irradiation: induction of neoplasia. Radiat. Res. 41: 467-491 (1970).

U17 Upton, A.C. Radiobiological effects of low doses. Implications for radiological protection. Radiat. Res. 71: 51-74 (1977).

U18 Upton, A.C. The interplay of viruses and radiation in carcinogenesis. p. 895-908 in: Radiation Research, Biomedical, Chemical and Physical Perspectives (O. Nygaard et al., eds.). Academic Press, New York, 1975.

U19 Underbrink, A.G., A.M. Kellerer, R.E. Mills et al. Comparison of x-ray and gamma-ray dose response curves for pink somatic mutations in tradescantia clone 02. Radiat. and Environ. Biophysics 13: 295 ff (1976).

U20 Ullrich, R.L. and J.B. Storer. Influence of gamma-irradiation on the development of neoplastic disease in mice. I. Reticular tissue tumors. Radiat. Res. 80: 303-316 (1979).

U21 Ullrich, R.L., M.C. Jernigan and L.M. Adams. Induction of lung tumors in RFM mice after localized exposures to x rays or neutrons. Radiat. Res. 80: 464-473 (1979).

U22 Ullrich, R.L. Effects of split doses of x rays on neutrons on lung tumor formation in RFM mice. Radiat. Res. 83: 138-145 (1980).

U23 Ullrich, R.L. Tumor induction in BALB/c mice after fractionated or protracted exposures to fission-spectrum neutrons. Radiat. Res. 97: 587-597 (1984).

U24 United Nations. United Nations Scientific Committee on the Effects of Atomic Radiation 1982 Report to the General Assembly, with annexes. Ionizing Radiation: Sources and Biological Effects. United Nations sales publication No. E.82.IX.8. New York, 1982.

U25 Ullrich, R.L. Tumour induction in BALB/c female mice after fission neutron or gamma irradiation. Radiat. Res. 93: 506-515 (1983).

U26 Ullrich, R.L. Tumour induction in BALB/c mice after fractionated or protracted exposures to fission-spectrum neutrons. Radiat. Res. 97: 587-597 (1984).

U27 Underbrink, A.G., F.M. Edwards, W.R. Lower et al. Absence of detectable fractionation effects in trades-cantia somatic mutations for an x ray dose of 5 rad. Radiat. Res. 101: 170-176 (1985).

U28 Ullrich, R.L. The rate of progression of radiation-transformed mammary epithelial cells is enhanced after low dose rate neutron irradiation. Radiat. Res. 105: 68-75 (1986).

U29 Umeda. M, K. Tanaka and T. Ono. Effect of insulin on the transformation of BALB/3T3 cells by x-irradiation. Gann 74: 864-869 (1983).

V1 Vanderlaan, M., F.J. Burns and R.E. Albert. A model describing the effects of dose and dose-rate on tumour induction by radiation in rat skin. p. 253-263 in: Biological and Environmental Effects of Low-Level Radiation, Vol. II. IAEA, Vienna, 1976.

V2 Vilenchik, M.M., T.M. Tretyak, V.M. Lobachev et al. The similarity of circular dichorism spectrum of DNA of aged animals or irradiated by γ rays. Dokl. Akademii Natl. SSSR 259: 1488-1490 (1981). (in Russian)

V3 Vilenchik, M.M. Spontaneous instability and plasticity of DNA in vivo: recombination between the nuclear and mitochondrial DNA and its biological importance. Usp. Sovr. Biologii 99(2): 194-211 (1985).

V4 Vogel, H.H. and R. Zaldivar. Neutron-induced mammary neoplasms in the rat. Cancer Res. 32: 933-938 (1972).

V5 Vogel, H.H. Jr. High-LET irradiation of Sprague-Dawley female rats and mammary neoplasm induction. p. 147-162 in: Late Biological Effects of Ionizing Radiation, Vol. II. IAEA, Vienna, 1978.

V6 Vilenchik, M.M. Modification of carcinogenic and antitumour radiation effects (biomedical aspects). Medicina, Moscow, 1985. (in Russian)

V9 Vogel, H.H. Jr. and H.W. Dickson. Mammary neoplasia following acute and protracted irradiation with fission neutrons and ^{60}Co gamma-rays. (Abstract). Radiat. Res. 87: 453-454 (1981).

V10 Vogel, H.H. Jr. and J.E. Turner. Genetic component in rat mammary carcinogenesis. Radiat. Res. 89: 264-273 (1982).

V11 Vulpis, N., G. Panetta and L. Tognacci. Radiation-induced chromosome aberrations in radiological protection. Dose-response curves at low dose-levels. Int. J. Radiat. Biol. 29: 595-600 (1976).

W6 Weichselbaum, R.R., J. Epstein, J.B. Little et al. In vitro cellular radiosensitivity of human malignant tumours. Eur. J. Cancer 12: 47-51 (1976).

W7 Weichselbaum, R., J. Epstein and J.B. Little. In vitro radiosensitivity of human diploid fibroblasts derived from patients with unusual clinical responses to radiation. Radiology 121: 479-482 (1976).

W8 Whittemore, A.S. Quantitative theories of oncogenesis. Adv. Cancer Res. 17: 55-88 (1978).

W9 World Health Organization. Cancer incidence in five continents. IARC, Lyon, 1982.

W12 Walinder, G., C.Y. Jonsson and A.M. Sjöden. Dose-rate dependence of the goitrogen stimulated mouse thyroid. A comparative investigation of the effects of roentgen, ^{131}I and ^{132}I irradiation. Acta Radiol., Ther. 11: 24-36 (1972).

W13 Waxweiler, R.J., R.J. Roscoe, V.E. Archer et al. Mortality follow-up through 1977 of the white underground uranium miners cohort examined by the United States Public Health Service. p. 823-830 in: Proc. Int. Conf. on Radiation Hazards in Mining. (M. Gomez, ed.), Society of Mining Engineers, New York, 1981.

W14 Whittemore, A.S. and A. McMillan. Osteosarcomas among beagles exposed to Pu-239. Radiat. Res. 90: 41-56 (1982).

W15 Wesch, A., G. van Kaick, W. Riedel et al. Recent results of the German Thorotrast Study—statistical evaluation of animal experiments with regard to the non-radiation effects in human thorotrastosis. Health Phys. 44, Suppl. 1: 317-321 (1983).

W16 Woch, B., A.G. Underbrink, J. Huczkowski et al. Effects of dose fractionation in Tradescantia stamen hairs after high and intermediate doses of x-irradiation. Radiat. Res. 90: 547-557 (1983).

W17 Whittemore, A.S. and A. McMillan. Lung cancer mortality among U.S. uranium miners: a reappraisal. J. Natl. Cancer Inst. 71: 489-499 (1983).

W18 Watanabe, M., M. Horikawa and O. Nikaido. Induction of oncogenic transformation by low doses of x rays and dose-rate effect. Radiat. Res. 98: 274-283 (1984).

W19 Wrenn, M.E., G.N. Taylor, W. Stevens et al. Summary of dosimetry, pathology and dose-response for bone sarcomas in beagles injected with ^{226}Ra. p. 43-45 in: Research in Radiobiology. University of Utah, School of Medicine, Radiobiology Division. Annual Report C00-119-258. Salt Lake City, Utah, 1983.

Y1 Yuhas, J.M. Dose-response curves and their modification by specific mechanisms. p. 51-65 in: Biology of Radiation Carcinogenesis (J.M. Yuhas et al., eds.), Raven Press, New York, 1976.

Y2 Yuhas, J.M. Recovery from radiation—carcinogenic injury to the mouse ovary. Radiat. Res. 60: 321-332 (1974).

Y3 Yang, T.C.H. and C.A. Tobias. Radiation and cell transformation in vitro. p. 417-461 in: Advances in Biological and Medical Physics, Vol. 17, 1980.

Y5 Yang, T.C., J. Howard, L. Craise et al. Effects of energetic silicon ions, UV radiation and X rays on neoplastic cell tranformation and mutation. Radiat. Res. 91: 412-413 (1982).

Z1 Ziemba-Zoltowska, B., E. Bocian, O. Rosiek et al. Chromosome aberrations induced by low doses of X-rays in human lymphocytes in vitro. Int. J. Radiat. Biol. 37: 231-236 (1980).

ANNEX C

Biological effects of pre-natal irradiation

CONTENTS

Introduction

1. A study entitled "Developmental effects of irradiation in utero" was presented in annex J of the 1977 UNSCEAR report [U2]. It reviewed most of what was known at the time concerning such effects, both in experimental animals and in man, but since the amount of information on the former exceeded by far that on the latter, the study dwelt largely on the experimental animal data.

2. Since then, new information has become available, relating particularly to man, which has highlighted the need to focus discussion on the human experience and to draw on any data that might set more precisely in perspective the effects and risks of irradiation in utero. Moreover, effects such as tumour induction, which have been discussed elsewhere, need to be re-examined in light of the new data if overall risk estimates for man are to be attempted. These considerations have prompted UNSCEAR to undertake the present study entitled "Biological effects of pre-natal irradiation".

3. As reflected by its title, the study is meant to be more comprehensive than the earlier one, including effects such as tumour induction and other long-term sequelae of irradiation which were specifically excluded from the 1977 study [U2]. It is also aimed at drawing conclusions concerning the potential for practical applications, insofar as the data will allow. As the previous study adequately covered the fundamental aspects of the subject, the present one will simply point out how the new data would alter previously drawn conclusions. (Data pertaining to genetic damage induced by irradiation in utero, damage induced before fertilization, and some special effects such as the induction of XO females, are to be found in annex A to the present report.)

4. In the 1977 report [U2] the subject was divided, mainly as a matter of convenience, into general chapters covering the methodological aspects and the mechanisms of action of radiation effects in utero. The substantive data were mostly reviewed in separate sections covering the pre-implantation period, the period of major organogenesis, and the fetal period. Within each section, lethal, teratological, developmental and other effects were considered, information on animals and man being grouped for the purpose of showing qualitative similarities. Such a treatment may not always adequately reflect the complications of the biological models and the variability of the data, but any alternative sub-division of the subject matter would also have its limitations. The format used did, however, offer the advantages of setting the observations in some reasonable sequence with respect to embryonic and fetal development, thereby allowing individual discussions of each major class of effect, by drawing together all observations pertaining to the same stage of development.

5. In the present study, the matter is reviewed again by pre-natal stages in animals and man, in order to facilitate projections across species. This way of ordering the subject does not imply that all such projections may be legitimate and justified. On the contrary, as emphasized repeatedly in the 1977 study, such projections (and particularly the more quantitative ones) should not be undertaken without due regard for the specific characteristics of the biological systems under comparison.

6. As in the 1977 study, the present one will consider separately subjects such as modifying factors, internal irradiation and tumour induction because the relevant information does not apply specifically to any developmental stage but often refers to the whole pre-natal period.

7. Although the main aim of the study is to review the published data with a view to assessing radiation effects in man, this is made difficult by the nature of most of the work available, which is usually directed towards studying the mechanisms of development rather than the radiobiologically important variables, such as dose and time. It should be noted that quantitative information on dose-effect relationships and on the influence of dose rate and radiation quality (which is the most valuable for the Committee's own purposes) is still scanty, particularly at the low doses. Moreover, it is often buried under observations on the pathogenesis of malformations or the morphology of malformed tissues. This, together with the lack of systematic information on species, tissues and effects, may in some instances cause this new study to fall short of its aim. However, in view of the interest that the field continues to command, of the new data available, and of the relatively high risk that exposure of the conceptus in utero might entail under certain conditions, the re-consideration of old data and the discussion of new data is amply justified.

I. BASIC INFORMATION ON THE HUMAN EMBRYO AND FETUS

8. In order to set the following text in perspective with respect to its main aim, it is important to review some basic information on the normal development of the human embryo and fetus. (As a general reference on this subject see [H27].) After a short introduction on the main phases of pre-natal development in various mammalian species, therefore, the present chapter will focus particularly on the human central nervous system (CNS), which is known in man to be most susceptible to radiation-induced pre-natal damage. New data on the gross development and the biochemical events taking place in human ontogenesis will be outlined, together with modern acquisitions on the histogenesis of the brain structures. For the same purpose, a short section will also be devoted to the etiology and epidemiology of malformations in man, as a background to the risk evaluations discussed later (see chapter VIII).

A. THE MAIN PHASES OF PRE-NATAL DEVELOPMENT

9. The development of the conceptus in mammals is usually (and very schematically) divided into three major phases: the pre-implantation phase, the period of major organogenesis and the phase of fetal development. Implantation of the early embryo into the uterine mucosa marks the separation between the first two periods. Although implantation is given in the reports at a certain day post conception (p.c.), it should be remembered that the complete process, from the initial contact of the blastocyst with the uterine wall to its firm attachment through the erosion of the uterine epithelium by the trophoblast and the establishment of a placental blood flow, may last from one to one and a half days in the mouse and a few days in man. A clear-cut separation between the embryonic and the fetal periods is even more difficult since the transition is marked by the end of differentiation and the growth of the newly formed organs in an animal which has attained the characteristic morphological features of the species. It is estimated that by the end of the embryonic period, that is by the 8th post-ovulatory week, the human embryo (measuring about 30 mm in crown-rump length and weighing 2-2.7 g) already possesses more than 90% of the more than 4500 structures described in the adult body [O8].

10. Thus, the conventional limits of the three developmental periods, which are given for various animal species in Table 1, should only be regarded as rough approximations. A tabulation of times for the development of morphological characters in some mammals is also to be found in [S84] and [M57].

11. The division into the three phases mentioned above corresponds approximately with significant differences of developmental events in the embryo. It is also suitable for a description of radiation effects, which are very different in nature and degree within the three phases. For example, death in utero is generally characteristic of irradiation in the pre-implantation phase, while neo-natal death and malformations are associated particularly with irradiation during organogenesis. Irradiation during the fetal stage does not normally lead to gross malformations in the teratological sense, but rather to maldevelopment of tissues and defects of growth, particularly in the CNS and gonads. At high doses, it may lead to death. A systematic description of pre-natal effects of radiation supporting these conclusions is to be found in the 1977 UNSCEAR report [U2]. That report emphasized, by means of examples referring to different animal species and various types of effects, that the outcome of a given radiation exposure in respect to both dose and time is highly dependent on the developmental characteristics of each species. This condition makes it difficult to extrapolate the type and degree of radiation-induced effects across species and to formulate generalized and particularly quantitative conclusions. However, as the developmental physiology is similar, some useful comparisons may be made.

B. NORMAL DEVELOPMENT OF THE HUMAN EMBRYO, PARTICULARLY OF THE CNS

12. In order to assess whether or not there are periods of high susceptibility in human development in regard to any toxic agent, it is important to time the effects induced in relation to the menstrual cycle or to fertilization. A precise mapping of developmental events is still, however, a major unresolved issue in human embryology, because experimental studies are not possible and because one must rely on approximate estimates of the date of conception. Gross measurements, histological investigations and biochemical analyses on autopsy material have usually been employed to this end, although, more recently, direct measurements in vivo have become possible. Up-to-date observations on the early development of the human brain and information on the staging system of human embryology are to be found in several references [M49, O7, O8]. The last of these also provides an annotated list of the chief sources of recent information on the development of various structures of the human body.

1. Gross measurements

13. It should be realized that neither the weight nor the length of an embryo are an adequate guide to developmental status and therefore should not be taken as a "stage", which is a term based on the overall morphology of the embryo and not on any single measurement. Kobyletzki and Gellen [K27] investigated the phase of development of 555 human embryos (morphologic development, fresh weight, crown-rump length) obtained from legal terminations of early pregnancies and correlated it with the duration of pregnancy, age and weight of the mother, parity and number of abortions. They found it impossible to correlate the phase of development in any single case to a reasonable degree of precision and, as a consequence, to predict periods of gestation where the product of conception might be at a higher risk of exogenous embryotoxic agents.

14. The normal and abnormal development of early human embryos was also studied by Nishimura and collaborators. In a first publication [N5] containing data on 1213 intact embryos, standards of normal development (with respect to crown-rump length, body weight and external form) were established which were thought to be more reliable than the standards usually cited. Remarkable variation was noted between clinical age and these growth indicators. It was concluded, therefore, that the general developmental stage was more reliably established by such objective parameters than by the clinically established age. Dead embryos were more frequent in women with genital bleeding during pregnancy. The prevalences of externally malformed embryos were 2.35% (44/1870) at Carnegie stages [O8] 16-18, and 2.12% (46/2169) at stages 19-23 [N14]. Malformations observed included exencephaly, cyclopia, myeloschisis, cleft lip and various limb abnormalities. It was noted that the incidence of most of these defects was far higher than that observed in newborn infants. In a second paper [N6] reporting on 90 normal specimens from healthy pregnancies at Carnegie stages 7-13, they correlated clinically assessed age and growth and found remarkable individual variability in embryos at stages 11-13, but an overall accordance with observations published by other investigators.

15. Jakobovits et al. [J9] also addressed the problem of establishing reliable standards of the rate of growth of human embryos and fetuses. The material examined comprised 354 embryos and fetuses ranging from 20 to 200 mm crown-rump length, obtained by therapeutic abortion in three different countries. Comparison of the measurements taken with the widely used standards of Streeter [S55] (see Table 2) indicated that the discrepancy observable at the embryonic stages diminishes gradually into the fetal period and eventually becomes quite insignificant. The discrepancies may be explained on the ground that Streeter's material [S55] contained data on a significant number of spontaneous abortions in the early embryonic period when the fetal age may be misjudged by the possible occurrence of menstruation after fertilization. The embryos would then be judged to be younger than their real age. When the number of embryos below the standard morphological age for their ovulation age is compared with the number of those above standard, it is found that the morphological development of a large proportion of malformed embryos is below standard [N14]. The paper by Jakobovits et al. [J9] discusses the sources of variability between and within series and concludes that the standards of intra-uterine growth must be considered of limited value in correlating age and measurements in single cases.

16. Skidmore [S43] also examined the crown-rump length of 483 fixed human embryos (Carnegie stages 6-23) and calculated the median and predicted mean length. The results were compared with those of others and found to be in good agreement. Weight standards for the whole body and organs in human fetuses below 500 g (or 200 mm of crown-rump length) were described by Tanimura [T15].

17. In a study of a few hundred staged human embryos examined for a variety of gross and microscopic morphological features, Moore et al. [M30] investigated the significance of a relationship between estimated post-ovulatory age and size or maturity of the embryos, as well as the timing of the development of major landmarks. They concluded that the embryo develops to 1 mm at the 28th post-menstrual day, after which its crown-rump length increases at the rate of approximately 0.7 mm per day up to 80 mm. Coital and post-ovulatory ages estimated from menstrual data correlated significantly ($P < 0.001$) with crown-rump length and the Carnegie stage system. However, the post-ovulatory age, even after adjustment for lack of synchrony between menstrual period and time after ovulation, showed high variability (standard deviation, 10.5 days) indicating poor predictability for single specimens. On the other hand, morphological features appeared within a narrow interval. The data showed that during the portion of embryogenesis studied (up to about 100 days of post-ovulatory age), there is a close synchrony of events, each of which occurs very rapidly in an apparently stereotyped sequence with little statistical variation. The time of normal development may be determined accurately if the date of a single or most likely fertile coitus is known. To assess embryonic age in individual cases on the basis of menstrual data, however, is a very unreliable system of dating.

18. With the development of new ultrasonic techniques, it is now possible to measure in vivo embryonic development as a function of pre-natal age in order to compare such findings with length/age tables in current embryological usage and to score for the presence of congenital malformations [C21, C22]. Drumm and O'Rahilly [D16] made one such comparison on a sample of 44 normal women studied between 33 and 86 days from ovulation. They concluded that, in the embryonic period proper (i.e., up to 8 post-ovulatory weeks), the measurements in vivo give a slightly greater length for a given age than those normally assigned in embryology, possibly due to differences between in vivo and post-mortem length or to imprecision in estimating the data from anamnestic findings. At later stages in the period investigated (early fetal) a good correspondence was found between in vivo ultrasonic and morphological measurements on fixed specimens.

19. Dobbing and Sands [D17] analysed, as a function of pre- and post-natal age, the changes of biparietal diameter, head circumference and brain weight in man. The shape of the curves was shown to be different for each parameter and the differences were compared and justified. The significance of these findings in relation to limiting influences, such as nutritional deficiencies, and to the capacity for recovery, was discussed. Jordaan [J7] also investigated the relationships between body and brain weight as a function of intra-uterine age in man and showed that the ratio of brain/body weight is a useful index for appraising the quality of growth in cases at risk of intra-uterine growth retardation.

20. Burdi et al. [B14] examined organ weight patterns in the course of human fetal development. They studied 80 singleton abortuses assessed as being morphologically normal and typical for age, covering a period between 13 and 31 weeks of fertilization. They obtained regression formulae characterizing the growth of 10 selected fetal organs relative to total body weight (Table 3). According to these authors, fetal body weight (rather than the more commonly used crown-rump length or age since last menstruation) appears to be the best reference parameter for assessing the growth of the various organs and for working out quantitative formulae for such growth. Data analysis showed that, of the 10 organs monitored, the brain was the organ the weight of which is most highly correlated with the changes of either crown-rump length or total body weight.

21. In a series of 72 autopsies, Friede [F8] timed some readily identifiable histological landmarks useful for dating cerebellar development between 24 weeks of gestation and 13 months of life and compared histological events in the cortex with overall weight data for the cerebellum. This work shows that by the 9th post-natal month the human cerebellum has attained only 50% of its adult weight, and up to about this time active growth of the molecular cell layer takes place to its adult dimension. The doubling of the cerebellar weight after the 9th post-natal month is probably due more to a continuing process of myelin formation in the white matter than to continued cell proliferation in the cortex.

22. Table 4, taken from O'Rahilly [O8], summarizes information of a quantitative and morphological nature on the sequence of developmental stages in the human embryo. The author, among other points, emphasizes that the most useful single measurement for assessing the age of an embryo or fetus is the crown-rump length, which is found to agree closely with that determined ultrasonically [D16]. Alternatively, the greatest length of the embryo may be used, which is a practicable measurement from 2 post-ovulatory weeks (stage 6) through the remainder of the embryonic and also in the fetal period [O11]. The 23 stages mentioned in Table 4 refer to the embryonic period only, because no staging system has yet been devised for the fetus. Finally, embryonic ages are now expressed in post-ovulatory weeks or days; little or no attention is paid in modern embryological work to menstrual data.

23. The ectodermal tissue that will eventually form the various brain structures may be identified in the human embryo at about 6 days after conception [O7]. It appears as a neural plate which develops into a neural groove at about 18 days. By day 20 [M49] the three major portions of the brain (the prosencephalon, the mesencephalon and the rhombencephalon) can be identified. The neural groove becomes a neural tube at about 22 days p.c. The open ends of this structure soon close. As the tube grows in length and thickness, it flexes, particularly at the rostral end, while other structures (otic vesicle, optic vesicle) begin to appear. By stage 15 (about 5 weeks p.c.), the neural tube is well differentiated and the embryonic cortical zones, which will finally give rise to the cerebral hemispheres, begin to form [S21].

2. Cellular phenomena

24. The cellular events leading to the formation of the brain cortex in mammals have now been described in considerable detail [S21]. In order to understand these events it is necessary to have in mind the morphology of the embryonic cortical zones mentioned in the previous paragraph and shown in Figure I. The following zones may be recognized: (a) a ventricular zone, made by the ventricular cells which replace the spongioblasts and the germinal cells; (b) a marginal zone, the outermost cell-sparse zone from which cell nuclei are excluded during their movements; (c) an intermediate zone, developing between the previous two, as postmitotic neurons move outwards and afferent axons grow between regions; and (d) a subventricular zone, situated at the junction between the ventricular and the intermediate zones, containing cells giving rise to the macroglia and special classes of neurons.

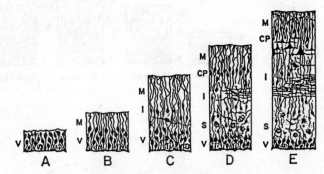

Figure I. Semi-diagrammatic drawing of the development of the basic embryonic zones and the cortical plate. Abbreviations: CP, cortical plate; I, intermediate zone; M, marginal zone; S, subventricular zone; V, ventricular zone.
[S21]

25. According to the descriptions of Sidman and Rakic [R23, S21], which integrate previous observations, the whole process of cell migration and cortical development in man may be summarized in a number of stages, as in Figure II (approximate gestational ages in weeks given in parentheses):

Stage I (7-10). This is characterized by the initial formation of the cortical plate, starting with the migration outward of post-mitotic ventricular cells to form a new accumulation of cells (neocortical plate) which is several layers of cells deep by the end of the stage.

Stage II (10-11). There is a primary condensation of the cortical plate which becomes thicker and more compact. Neurons in the plate are immature and their elongated axis is oriented perpendicularly to the surface of the cortex. Migration of cells to the cortical plate from the ventricular zone through the fibre-rich intermediate zone slows down by the 11th week.

Stage III (11-13). The cortical plate becomes subdivided between an external zone of cells with densely packed nuclei and an inner zone with widely spaced large nuclei. The maturation of early migrated cells and the addition of new immature neurons from a new wave of migration accounts for this bilaminate structure of the cortical plate.

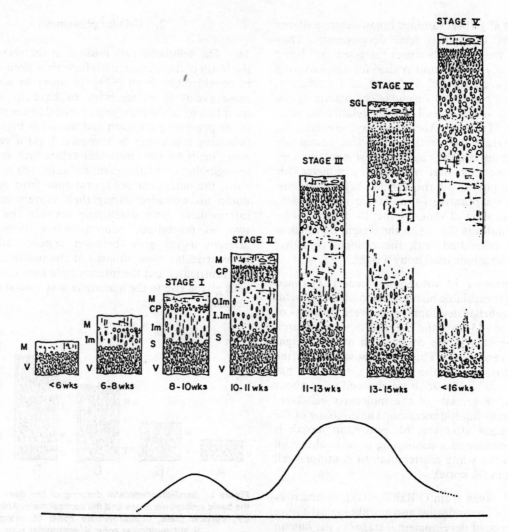

Figure II. Semi-diagrammatic drawing of the human cerebral wall at various gestational ages listed in fetal weeks below each column. The stages refer specifically to an area arbitrarily chosen midway along the lateral surface of the hemisphere. Because there is a gradient of maturation, as many as 3 of 5 stages of cortical development may be observed in different regions of neocortex in the same fetal brain. The extreme right column shows a large interruption in the intermediate zone to signify that the full thickness of the cerebral wall has increased compared to earlier stages. The curve in the lower part of the figure represents roughly the time and relative magnitude of the waves of proliferation and migration of neuronal cells. Abbreviations: CP, cortical plate; Im, intermediate zone; I.Im and O.Im, inner and outer intermediate zones, respectively; M, marginal zone; SGL, subplate granular layer; S, subventricular zone; V, ventricular zone; wks, age in fetal weeks.

[S21]

Stage IV (13-15). There is a progressive thinning of the ventricular zone as many of its cells move outwards and less of the remaining continue to divide. The cortical plate becomes at the same time more homogeneous in appearance, due possibly to an enlargement of the neurons. As relatively few cells enter the cortical plate, its separation from the intermediate zone appears sharper. The intermediate zone has in the meantime become over 5 mm thick.

Stage V (16-after birth). This stage, lasting well into post-natal life is not precisely defined and includes a large range of interrelated developmental events. There is controversy as to the amount and length of neuronal migration during this stage. Although proliferation of the ventricular zone is decreased by the fifth month, many neurons which had been generated earlier are still in the process of migrating to the cortical plate. There is evidence that the subventricular

zone persists as a germinal area and continues to produce medium-sized and small neurons as well as an increasing number and variety of glial cells, and that these processes of cell production may continue up to the middle of gestation. Cell migration, on the other hand, may continue throughout the first year of extra-uterine life, but the extent and the timing of these processes of cell production and migration are still uncertain.

26. The curve in the lower part of Figure II is meant to represent, roughly, the two waves of proliferation and migration of neuronal cells, the first one being of shorter duration and involving less cells than the second. These waves are taking place in the human cerebral cortex around stage I and stages II-IV, respectively.

27. In the developing cortex of the cerebellum, cell relationships are very similar, but the migration of granular cell neurons proceeds from the external surface inwards past the dendrites and somas of the Purkinje cells, guided by the radial arrangements of the Bergmann glial fibres. There are also other special migration patterns applying to some zones of the CNS.

28. It is not yet clear whether cell migration might involve the same mechanisms during the initial stages of cortex development, or during later stages when cells move along distances of several millimetres. However, it is now well established that migrating neurons find their way to the cortex by following the radially oriented fibres of the glial cells as guides. The later generated cells take positions external to those of their predecessors and the final position of cell elements along the radial sectors may be influenced by afferent axons. Cell surface properties may be involved in controlling migration, but their nature still remains undefined [R24].

29. Another paper by Rakic [R9] added important details to the basic phenomena described, which are of significance in respect to the specificity of origin and interconnections of neurons. A systematic analysis of the neuron division and migration carried out by ³H-thymidine labelling in the Rhesus monkey has made it possible to establish that successive generations of neurons originating in a given location at the ventricular surface migrate along the same glial fibres and settle themselves eventually in the same radial cortical column. Thus, the glial fibres, in addition to directing neuronal migration, may be of importance in preserving the topographical, and therefore functional, relationship of clonally related neurons. They are also important in reproducing the mosaicism of the ventricular zone in which neurons originate at the level of the expanded surface of the cerebral cortex. It is not known whether the killing of glial cells may impair the orderly migration of the neurons. In summary, although migration of cells from one part of the body to another is a common phenomenon in ontogenesis, there are unique features associated with cell migration taking place in the developing brain. First, as it only occurs after the last cell division, it involves neurons that will not reproduce any longer. Secondly, it involves active cell movement following selected pathways along the glial fibres. Finally, it exhibits precise space and time dependencies [R24].

30. In addition to neuroblast division, migration and differentiation, neuronal death has been shown to play a role in shaping the final morphology and function of the adult brain. Various types of programmed neuronal death have been described in various animal species [C17]. One is related to the target area to be connected by certain types of neurons and is to some extent adjustable to the size of this area; another is related to the elimination of errors that may occur in connecting various areas of the brain; a third relates to the selective response of neurons to circulating hormones; and a fourth is under tight genetic control. Although there is doubt whether, and to what extent, all these types may be present in the developing

mammalian brain, it appears that programmed death of neurons is directed to the adjustment of each neuronal population to the size or functional needs of its projection field and to the elimination of neurons whose axons have grown to the wrong target or to the wrong region within the target area. Other regressive events leading to the elimination of some neuronal connections initially formed, without death of the parent cell, are also known, and they appear to be directed to the fine tuning of neuronal wiring. All these phenomena are now recognized to play a major role in the final maturation of the CNS, but nothing is known yet about their possible relationship or importance to radiation-induced cell killing.

3. Biochemical development

31. Brain maturation may also be followed by mapping of biochemical events as a function of time. Howard et al. [H14] studied the content of desoxyribonucleic acid (DNA) in 28 human fetal brains at between 10 and 31 weeks of gestation from surgical specimens obtained in Sweden and in the United States. The cerebrum and cerebellum were analysed separately and, in addition to DNA and ribonucleic acid (RNA), cholesterol was also estimated as an index of the biochemical maturation of the organs. The total content of DNA in the cerebrum increased exponentially between 10 and 14 weeks of gestation, after which the rate gradually declined to a linear function; there was no sign that growth would stop up to 31 weeks of gestation (Figure III). By contrast, the DNA content of the cerebellum kept increasing exponentially throughout the same period (Figure IV).

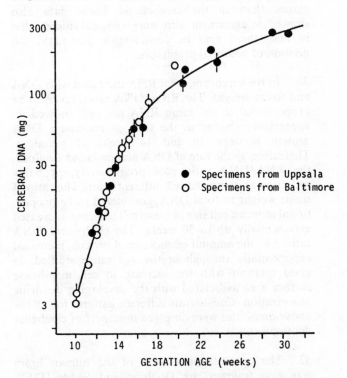

Figure III. The increase of total cerebral DNA during development of the human fetus. Ordinates: DNA in mg on a logarithmic scale; abscissae: age in weeks from the onset of the last menstrual period, estimated from body weights according to Streeter. Each circle represents one brain. Data from [H14].

269

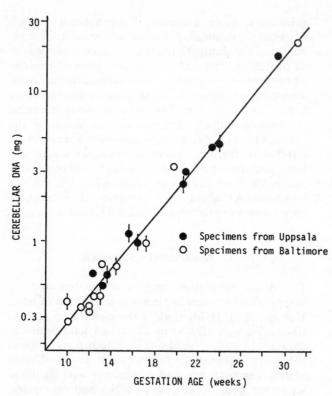

Figure IV. The increase in total cerebellar DNA during development of the human fetus. Each circle represents one brain. Data from [H14].

- ● Specimens from Uppsala
- ○ Specimens from Baltimore

On the assumption that the increase in DNA may roughly correspond to an increase in the number of nuclei, the different patterns of growth of the cerebrum and cerebellum were interpreted to show that in some areas of the cerebrum cell division may be terminated earlier than in the cerebellum. These data also showed, in agreement with morphological studies, that in man there may be considerable post-natal cell division of neuronal precursors.

32. In the cerebrum, total RNA increased with DNA and tissue weight. The RNA/DNA ratio, taken to be proportional to the mean RNA per cell, showed no appreciable change at the time of maximum DNA growth between 10 and 14 weeks of gestation. Thereafter, as the rate of DNA accumulation declined, the RNA/DNA ratio rose progressively, probably reflecting an increased cell differentiation. The ratio of tissue weight to total DNA, considered to be proportional to mean cell size or mean cell territory, increased exponentially up to 30 weeks. The cholesterol/DNA ratio, i.e., the amount of cholesterol per cell, increased exponentially throughout the age range studied, in good relation with the increase in cell membrane surface area associated with the developing dendritic arborization. Consistently different patterns for all the above quantities were observed in respect of cerebellar development.

33. The quantitative growth of the human brain was also followed by Dobbing and Sands [D12]; 139 human samples, ranging in age from 10 weeks gestation to 7 years post-natal, were studied, together with 9 adult brains. The whole brain and the three major regions (forebrain, stem, cerebellum) were examined separately for weight, DNA, cholesterol and water content, in order to describe quantitatively the spurt in brain growth. The weight of the whole brain and its parts followed a sigmoid trend with time, with a cut-off point between 18 and 24 months of post-natal life for whole brain and forebrain. The cut-off point for the cerebellum was a little earlier than that of the whole brain. The cerebellum appeared to start growing later and to come to a plateau earlier than the rest of the brain. Cellularity (as expressed by the amount of DNA per g of tissue) in the forebrain and in the stem decreased as a function of age up to birth, due to disproportionately rapid growth of cell size, cell branching and myelination. In the cerebellum, however, cellularity increased until after birth, owing mainly to a rapid rate of cell multiplication.

34. Total cell number increased in an approximately sigmoid fashion as a function of time in the whole brain and all its regions. In the whole brain the cut-off point marking the levelling-off of the sigmoid curve occurred at around 18 post-natal months. Cerebellar cell growth started later and finished earlier, while the forebrain curve bent over at about 2 years of age. Figure V shows a semi-logarithmic plot of total DNA (proportional to total cell number) in the human forebrain between about 10 weeks of gestation and 4 months post-natal. The first of the two growth phases was thought to reflect rapid neuronal proliferation, the later, shallower, part was attributed to glial proliferation. The sharp bend of the curve at about 18 weeks of gestation does not imply that neuronal proliferation is stopped completely at this time, nor that glial cell division does not occur before, but rather that the rate at which the two processes proceed is sufficiently different to be reflected in the overall curve. The similarity of these data with the earlier ones reported by Howard et al. [H14] and shown in Figure III is remarkable. Figure VI summarizes, for the three different brain regions, the values of total DNA content as a function of fetal and post-natal ages, expressed as percentage of adult DNA values.

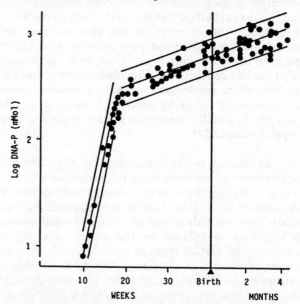

Figure V. Total DNA-P (proportional to total number of cells) in the human forebrain from ten gestational weeks to four post-natal months, showing the two-phase characteristics of pre-natal cell multiplication.

[D12]

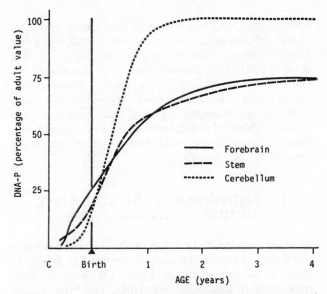

Figure VI. Relative values for DNA-P (proportional to total number of cells) in three human brain regions.
[D12]

35. The cholesterol content is taken as an index of myelination. For cholesterol, the growth spurt was less sharply defined and extended for whole brain, forebrain and stem well into 3 or 4 years after birth, possibly up to 5 years. The cerebellum seemed to accumulate this substance faster compared with other regions of the brain.

36. The paper by Dobbing and Sands [D12] adds considerably to the previous one by Howard et al. [H14]. It establishes a growth spurt for human brain development centred around the time of birth, but extending from mid-pregnancy well into the second post-natal year and beyond. This is at variance with what happens in other species: for example, the growth spurt is essentially post-natal in the rat, pre-natal in the guinea pig and perinatal in the pig. Data referring to the timing of the brain growth spurt in various mammalian species taken from another paper of Dobbing [D13] are shown in Figure VII. Dobbing and Sands [D12] commented on the length of human fetal brain development in comparison with that of other species and on the timing of the various processes in relation to noxious influences such as malnutrition. They specifically drew attention to the striking correlation between the high rate of multiplication of neurons between 10 and 18 weeks of gestation and the period of maximum sensitivity for radiation-induced small head size and mental retardation shown by Miller and Blot [M20] in children exposed in utero during the bombing of Hiroshima and Nagasaki. Mole [M10] also emphasized this correlation. Although it has long been known that the time of major organogenesis of a structure coincides with its maximum sensitivity to irradiation [U2], the observation of Dobbing and Sands [D12] is important in human radiobiology because it provides a cellular basis for the occurrence of mental retardation.

37. Dobbing and Sands [D18] investigated the mechanisms for the vulnerability of developing rat brain. Starting from the notions that the brain is especially vulnerable to growth retardation during the growth spurt, and that any deficit imposed at this time cannot be recovered at later stages, even if the

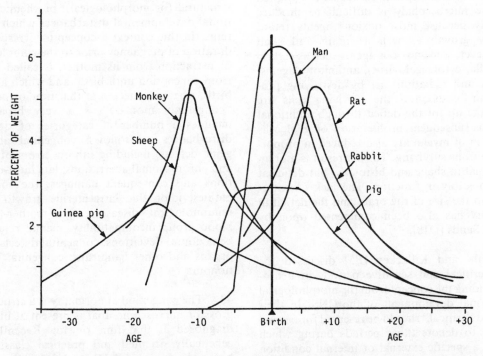

Figure VII. The total brain growth spurts of 7 mammalian species expressed as first-order derivative curves of the increase in weight with age. It should be noted (Figure VI) that different regions of the brain develop at different times. Weights are expressed as weight gain as a percentage of adult weight for each unit of time. The units of time for each species are as follows: guinea pig, days; rhesus monkey, 4 days; sheep, 5 days; pig, weeks; man, months; rabbit, 2 days; rat, days.
[D13]

271

restrictive action is over, they attempted to study whether growth retardation might be due to a chronological delay of the growth spurt complex or, instead, to a lesser extent of the growth spurt occurring at a fixed chronological time. They examined, as a function of time before and after birth, the changes in weight, DNA and cholesterol concentration in the brains of either normal or undernourished growth-retarded animals and showed that these components of the brain growth spurt were determined by the chronological and not by the developmental age. Thus, the brain has a once-only opportunity to grow correctly and when such opportunity is restricted the damage directly or indirectly induced may not be recovered at later stages.

38. In a review of the effects of early nutrition on CNS growth, Winick et al. [W13] pointed out that the series of critical periods occurring during brain development make this organ particularly sensitive to lack of nutrients. During the post-natal proliferative growth of some mammalian species, including man, malnutrition may interfere with cell division. In the pre-natal life of the rat, maternal under-nutrition blocks cell division in the fetal brain, whereas uterine vascular insufficiency does not. This suggests that there may be different types of intra-uterine growth failure. In man, severe malnutrition retards placental cell division and may affect fetal brain development. However, the study of these effects is difficult because of the lack of appropriate biochemical markers to assess fetal growth in utero. A later chapter by Dobbing [D13] also reviewed the problem of brain vulnerability to the lack of nutrients in relation to structural development.

39. In a short communication, Edwards [E7] pointed out that true microcephaly is difficult to produce experimentally because most noxious agents retard general body growth as well as brain and skull growth. However, some noxious agents such as certain viruses (rubella, cytomegalovirus), antimitotic agents, hyperthermia and radiation, act by destroying proliferating neuroblasts, and the surviving cells are unable to make up for the deficit through additional divisions. The subsequent proliferation of glial cells and production of myelin are also reduced in proportion to the neurons surviving. The net result is a brain which is normal in shape and histology, but deficient in size and possibly in function. The lack of correlation between the size of the brain and the deficit in mental activity has also been commented upon by Dobbing and Sands [D18].

40. Erzurumlu and Killackey [E5] discussed the presence of critical and sensitive periods in neurobiology, extending the concept from the morphological to the functional development of the CNS. In their view, the word "critical" should be reserved for normal development, to denote those periods during which the action of a specific external or internal condition or stimulus is required for the normal progress of development; "sensitive" periods, however, are times in development during which a given system is highly susceptible to the effects of harmful agents. This term refers, therefore, to the realm of teratology. In connection with such critical and sensitive periods, the authors discussed the effects of nutritional and hormonal deficiencies, of the exposure to toxins or other harmful agents, and of stimuli deprivation during development. They showed that it is at the time of the fastest rate of growth of a given structure that vulnerability is at its maximum. They also illustrated, with practical examples, a general theoretical approach to the problem of critical periods and an analysis of a system's organization and rate of development in relation to such periods.

C. EPIDEMIOLOGY AND AETIOLOGY OF HUMAN ABNORMALITIES

41. To keep the findings in a proper perspective when discussing radiation-induced developmental defects in man, it is important to know the natural birth prevalence of congenital anomalies. The brief outline of the epidemiology and aetiology of congenital anomalies given below is based on general references [C11, C14, C18, I5, K32, L4, M45, N9, N10, S38, U5, V5, V8] which contain compilations of numerous original literature reports, in addition to original material. No effort is made to review individual reports independently, since the object of the exercise is simply to provide some indications of the nature and order of magnitude of the baseline occurrence of human anomalies.

1. Terms and concepts

42. The term "congenital anomaly" is used by the World Health Organization (WHO) [W26] in the International Classification of Diseases (ICD) to designate structural (or morphological), biochemical and functional developmental disturbances which occur in the fetus (in this context a conceptus, irrespective of the duration of pregnancy prior to the complete expulsion or extraction from its mother, is called fetus [W26]) from conception until birth, and which are present at birth, whether detected at that time or not. The term "congenital anomaly" is a very broad one and includes a number of categories of developmental disturbances, as follows: congenital abnormalities; genic defects, including inborn errors of metabolism and chromosomal aberrations; late intra-uterine infections and consequent damages, the so-called fetopathies; idiopathic intra-uterine growth retardation; immunological diseases, e.g., mother-fetus rhesus blood group incompatibility; mental retardation and behavioural deviations; congenital defects of the sense organs and other handicaps; congenital hernias; and tumours.

43. The congenital abnormality is a structural defect, gross or microscopic, that is present at birth, whether diagnosed at that time or not. Recently, a pathogenetically oriented and practical classification has been recommended [S77] for defects of morphogenesis (i.e., congenital abnormalities) as follows:

(a) Malformation: a morphological defect of an organ, part of an organ, or larger region of the body resulting from an intrinsically abnormal developmental process;

(b) Disruption: a morphological defect of an organ, part of an organ, or a larger region of the body resulting from the extrinsic breakdown of, or an interference with, an originally normal developmental process;

(c) Deformation: an abnormal form, shape, or position of a part of the body, caused by mechanical forces;

(d) Dysplasia: an abnormal organization of cells into tissue(s) and its morphological result(s), that is, the process (and the consequence) of dys-histogenesis.

44. Pathogenetically, it is necessary to separate isolated and multiple patterns of morphological defects within congenital abnormalities [C18]. For example: isolated cleft lip, with or without cleft palate, may represent a homogeneous group of congenital abnormalities of similar origin. However, cleft lips with other, different, congenital abnormalities may occur as part of multiple congenital abnormalities in a number of diseases of different origin. Thus, the combination and joint evaluation of isolated and multiple congenital abnormalities is the cause of serious confusion both in research and in clinical practice.

45. Isolated congenital abnormalities are the consequences of developmental disturbances of single localized errors in morphogenesis. This category involves single, complex (more abnormalities in one organ or organ system), sequential (one defect with its subsequently derived secondary defects in later morphogenesis) and polytopic field defects (a pattern of defects derived from the disturbance of a developmental field). A multiple congenital abnormality is a concurrence of two or more morphogenetic errors of different sites in the same person. Within this category, syndromes (patterns of multiple anomalies thought to be causally related), associations (non-random patterns of two or more anomalies presumed to be pathogenetically related) and random combinations are usually distinguished.

2. Birth prevalence of congenital abnormalities

46. The baseline birth prevalence of all congenital abnormalities in man is difficult to assess for a variety of reasons. First, as is well known, the affected newborns seen at birth are only the survivors of pre-natal selection, i.e., of a much greater number of abnormal fetuses which occurred at one or another stage of pre-natal development. Therefore, only their point prevalence at birth (and not time incidence) can be determined for a majority of congenital abnormalities; recently, the former has been designated as birth prevalence. Second, some classes of abnormalities (e.g., coarctation of aorta, teeth abnormalities) cannot be scored at birth or are fewer at birth than after a few years, i.e., their point prevalences would be higher by 50 to 100% if cases could be followed up for a few years. However, the rate of these late-diagnosed cases may permit estimates of prevalence at birth. Third, the prevalence of other abnormality types (e.g., ventricular septal defect or undescended testicle) may be higher at birth than later, owing to spontaneous recovery. Fourth, a large group of congenital abnormalities such as congenital dislocation of the hip or phenylketonuria has only a "theoretical" birth prevalence because, due to neo-natal screening, at least in some countries, the development of these conditions may be prevented by special treatment or diet. The method of scoring (birth or death certificates, hospital records, special anomaly registries, surveillance or monitoring systems), the variable sizes of the samples, the variability of the definition and classification of congenital anomalies and the diagnostic criteria between different observers, differences in reference unit (affected individual or congenital anomaly) are important factors influencing the estimates. To these should be added other confounding demographic factors (age, parity), ethnic group, the family genetic background, and the socioeconomic characteristics of the parents (e.g., social class). Finally, there is the additional variability related to the geographical location, the season of the year, and the time span covered by the investigators. All these factors explain the difficulty in comparing the figures reported in the literature.

47. It is not surprising, therefore, that the figures found or cited in the references given [C11, C14, C18, I5, K32, L4, M45, N9, N10, S38, U5, V5, V8] are very variable from a low of 1.0% of all liveborns to a high of 8.5% in total births (i.e., still- and live-births) in the United States [M45]. Recent Hungarian estimates suggest that, for the group of conditions designated by ICD codes 740 to 759 (in chapter XIV of the ICD entitled "Congenital anomalies"), the prevalences are 6.1% and 6.0% in total births and live-births, respectively. If the entities covered by the ICD codes 550 (inguinal hernia), 553 (umbilical hernia) and 227-228 (congenital tumours)—which many teratologists consider as congenital anomalies—are included, then the figures become 7.2% and 7.3%, in live- and total births, respectively. In the prospective United States study [M45] which aimed at as complete an ascertainment of all congenital anomalies as possible (and in which the liveborn children were followed up to one year of age), the prevalence (including ICD entries 740-759, 550, 552, 227-228) was 8.5% of total births.

48. It is worth stressing the fact that in both the Hungarian and the United States data, musculoskeletal and skeletal anomalies are the predominant contributors to the total. Foremost among them, especially in Hungary, is congenital dislocation of the hip. Anomalies of the integument constitute about 10% of the total in the United States and about 1% in Hungary. (For detailed comparisons between the Hungarian and the United States data, see chapter I of the annex A to the present report.) Since a truly representative figure, applicable in a global context, for the prevalence of all congenital anomalies is difficult to arrive at, and in view of the differences existing between different studies (some, genuine differences between populations and some due to different degrees of ascertainment), a round figure of 6% of total births for the prevalence of congenital anomalies with medical consequences, is adopted in the present study, to provide a general frame of reference for discussions. It is realized that this

estimate might become higher if anomalies ascertained later in post-natal life, minor structural blemishes or conditions of little medical significance, low birth weight, mental retardation and other congenital handicaps (not always accurately ascertained) are also included.

49. As a result of progress in epidemiological expertise, birth prevalences of specific types of congenital abnormalities are less variable. In fact, a number of well-defined and easily diagnosed congenital conditions (e.g., cleft lip, spina bifida, anal atresia) have approximately similar birth prevalences in several countries. Furthermore, birth prevalences of different types of congenital abnormalities show a surprisingly narrow range of random fluctuation within the same country or region [I9]. Congenital anomalies are usually listed according to the anatomical structures affected and they are grouped together, although they may have quite different pathogenetic mechanisms. Therefore, a pathogenetically oriented classification system is very much needed.

50. The approximate birth prevalences of all isolated common major congenital abnormalities are shown in Tables 5, 6 and 7. Table 5 is based on a study of a series of consecutive births in 24 centres organized by WHO in 1961-1964 [S38]. In this study, a similar approach was used in all the participating centres and the outcome of a total of 421,781 pregnancies was investigated. The study indicated geographical variations of birth prevalences of congenital abnormalities depending on ethnic-genetic, territorial-environmental, demographic and social (health service, etc.) circumstances. Some congenital abnormalities were not investigated in the WHO study. In these cases, the data of other important epidemiological studies were taken into consideration. These figures are indicated by asterisks in Table 5 and the references are in [C18]. Table 6 shows the data from Hungary where birth prevalences were obtained by the same method (ad hoc epidemiological studies) and by the same staff in a population of 10.7 million between 1963 and 1974. Over this period, the prevalence of congenital abnormalities was studied continuously. The variability of the estimates as a function of time was surprisingly small. Table 8 (modified from a review of Villumsen [V8]) expresses the proportion of congenital abnormalities in various anatomical structures as a percentage of all abnormalities scored, and shows a range of values which is comparable to that seen in Tables 5 to 7.

3. The aetiology of human congenital abnormalities

51. As mentioned earlier, there are a number of ways of classifying congenital abnormalities, e.g., according to their severity (lethal, major, mild, minor), occurrence (common, moderately frequent, rare), teratological manifestation (zygopathy, embryopathy, fetopathy) and aetiology. Their classification according to aetiology, which is considered below, distinguishes between those of simple genic origin; those due to the interaction between hereditary, mainly polygenic, liability and environmental triggering factors; those due to

chromosomal aberrations; those brought about by the action of environmental, including teratogenic and maternal, factors; and finally, a heterogeneous class of abnormalities of unknown origin [K32].

52. Mutant genes, autosomal or gonosomal, recessive and dominant, may be the cause of congenital abnormalities, mainly congenital malformation syndromes. The occurrence of each single mutant gene in the population at large may be small, but since these mutant genes are numerous (a few thousand have been described in the McKusick catalogue [M47]), their overall effect in the population may be important. Their variability in penetrance, their rarity, and the differences in clinical severity of their manifestations (expression) account for the difficulties in estimating the frequency of the relevant malformations. Figures between 0.5 and 10 per 1000 births have been provided, but the extreme values may reflect overassignment or incomplete ascertainment of cases to this class. Taking intermediate values of 2.25 per 1000 [C11] or 5 per 1000 children born with a serious disorder [W27], it may be calculated that of the order of 3.8 and 8.3 (i.e., as an average round figure 6%) of all congenital abnormalities may be of genic (or monolocal, monogenic or Mendelian) origin in North America and Europe (2.25/60 = 3.8%; 5.0/60 = 8.3%; average between 3.8 and 8.3% = ~6%). Inclusion of still-births in these estimates would make little change as the major part of congenital abnormalities in the still-born is not of genic origin.

53. To the second class of abnormalities belong all those for which twin and familial studies indicate a complex aetiology explained by the multifactorial-threshold model [C18]. These congenital abnormalities depend on a polygenic disposition interacting with a variety of mostly unknown environmental factors. For congenital abnormalities belonging to this class, the findings pointing to genetic disposition in the various major types and the genetic mechanism underlying their appearance have been discussed by Carter [C11]. According to a WHO study [S38], there are 11 most common congenital abnormalities, that is, those exceeding the rate of 1 per 1000 births. Their detailed break-down is given in Table 5. Comparable data for Hungary, where the situation has been followed carefully, are given in Table 6 [C18]. In this country, for example, the total prevalences of congenital anomalies are 73.6 and 71.8 per 1000 total or live-births, respectively [C19]. Table 6 shows that, for 9 out of the 11 conditions, the most likely explanation is the multifactorial aetiology. The overall point prevalence of these 9 in Hungary is 54.0 per 1000 births, that is 73% of all congenital abnormalities in that country, as shown in Table 6 (54.0/73.6 = 73%). (The figure of 54.0 is obtained by adding the prevalences for: neural tube defects (2.9), ventricular septum defects (2.1), cleft lip ± cleft palate (1.0), congenital hypertrophic pyloric stenosis (1.5), undescended testicles (3.6), hypospadias (2.2), congenital dislocation of the hip (28.0), structural talipes equinovarus (1.3) and congenital inguinal hernia (11.4)). It should be borne in mind, however, that the number of cases with treated congenital dislocation of the hip is extremely high in central and eastern Europe. Recently figures of

the order of about 5 per 1000 for congenital dislocation of the hip have been published in western and northern Europe. Taking this into consideration, the proportion of the 9 isolated common congenital abnormalities becomes 42% of all congenital abnormalities, as a minimal figure (54.0—28.0 + 5.0 = 31.0 out of 73.6 is 42%). Furthermore, only structural talipes equinovarus was evaluated within groups of varus, valgus and other deformities of feet with a figure of 28.8 per 1000 births. Also, about 3.5% of male new-borns have undescended testicle(s) at birth, but nearly 80% of these descend spontaneously within the third month. Finally, some moderately frequent isolated congenital abnormalities (e.g., cardiovascular malformations with a birth prevalence of 5 per 1000 (i.e., one-half of 10.6 minus 2.1)) may belong to this class. Taking all these considerations into account, a total prevalence of 30 per 1000 births, i.e., about 50% of all congenital anomalies, appear to be a reasonable estimate for this class (i.e., 50% of 60/1000).

54. In the third class belong those due to chromosomal abnormalities. The most recent UNSCEAR review of the total frequency of chromosomal abnormalities in newborns (which includes a total of 67,014 karyotyped cases) [U5] points to a birth prevalence of 0.63%. Not all of these would carry visible malformations, but assuming that roughly 50% do, it may be estimated [W27] that the contribution of this class to the total abnormalities in man may be of the order of 5% $(3.1/10^3 \div 60/10^3 = 5\%)$. This figure would negligibly increase when still-births are included. It hardly needs to be stressed that chromosomal abnormalities are more frequent early in pregnancy. The review [U5] indicates that about 15% of recognized conceptions will lead to spontaneous abortion (early and intermediate fetal deaths) and about one-third of the aborted fetuses will carry some kind of chromosomal aberrations [H18, H21]. Germinal chromosomal mutations occur in about 5% of recognized conceptions [H22, W26]. The rate of embryonic loss between conception and recognized pregnancy is unknown, but is generally agreed to be very high [K39]: of the order of 40% between conception and 20 weeks of pregnancy [M7] and of the order of 10% between 10 and 18 weeks [G16]. These figures indicate that most conceptual losses must occur before pregnancy has been diagnosed, and often before the first missed period. The occurrence of abnormalities in the spontaneously aborted fetuses is also much higher than that seen in new-borns, which points to the role of fetal death in selecting morphologically and chromosomally abnormal fetuses.

55. The fourth class of abnormalities is that induced by environmental factors, many of which have been suspected (but less often proved) to induce teratogenic effects in utero. The list that follows is taken from Kalter and Warkany [K32], who gave a detailed discussion with references. Among environmentally induced congenital abnormalities, it is worth separating maternal conditions from teratogens, because the importance of the former is probably underestimated, while that of the latter may be exaggerated. Maternal diseases (e.g., diabetes mellitus, phenylketonuria, some hormonally functioning tumours and perhaps hypo-

gonadism) belong to the group of maternal conditions. Maternal infection (e.g., rubella and varicella which can cause embryopathy and fetopathy, and cytomegalovirus and toxoplasmosis, which may damage the fetus) is a condition which is intermediate between the maternal and the teratogenic factors, because the infectious agents may sometimes cause congenital abnormalities without affecting the mother. Considering all maternal factors together, probably 3.5% of congenital abnormalities could be attributed to this group of causes.

56. Among chemicals, pharmaceutical drugs seem to have the greatest practical significance as teratogens. At present, the list of teratogenic drugs involves thalidomide, androgens, anticancer and immunosuppressive cytotoxic and antifolic-acid derivates, synthetic female sex hormones, anticonvulsants (including hydantoin, trimethadion, valproic acid and other derivatives), anticoagulants, large doses of vitamin A and its derivatives, lithium and penicillamine. The mild effect of tetracyclin (teeth discoloration), and the reversible goitre after excess maternal ingestion of iodide or propylthiouracil, have also been discussed. However, the suspicion of teratogenicity for many of these drugs has not been confirmed. Among nutritional factors, the ingestion of alcoholic drinks during pregnancy has the greatest importance owing to the fetal alcohol syndrome. Of a long list of environmental substances, at present only mercury is considered to be a demonstrated human teratogen [K32].

57. Specificity is an important attribute of teratogenesis because nearly all known teratogens cause characteristic multiple congenital abnormalities, i.e., syndromes. Many other conditions or agents may, of course, have non-teratogenic effects on the fetus; for example, hyperthyroidism and lupus erythematoides as well as occupational exposure to anaesthetics may increase the rate of fetal death, while active and passive smoking during pregnancy may cause a significant reduction of weight in newborns. To give an approximate figure for the birth prevalence of environmentally induced anomalies is very difficult because any agent administered in high amounts could be toxic and could retard the development of human fetuses or cause fetal loss. On the other hand, several environmental factors could have a triggering effect on a number of common or moderately frequent congenital abnormalities of polygenic origin. Estimates of the causal role of teratogens vary between 1 and 5% of all congenital abnormalities. Thus, it is estimated that roughly 6% of congenital abnormalities might be caused by environmental (including maternal) factors.

58. In summary, it is clear that, on the basis of their aetiology, the congenital abnormalities can be subdivided into those due to (a) major genes, 6% of the total prevalence of 60/1000; (b) multifactorial causation, 50% of the total; (c) chromosomal anomalies, 5% of the total; and, (d) environmental, including maternal factors, 6% of the total. It can be inferred that about 30% of the abnormalities scored at birth have no known cause at present.

D. CONCLUSIONS

59. The development of the mammalian conceptus may be divided approximately into three major phases: the pre-implantation phase, lasting from fertilization to the settling of the embryo into the uterine mucosa; the phase of major organogenesis, which extends in man to approximately the 8th week post-ovulatory; and the phase of fetal development, lasting from about 9 weeks until birth. The timing and developmental details of each phase, however, differ greatly in various species and may considerably influence the outcome of a given radiation exposure. Quantitative extrapolations across species are therefore unwarranted.

60. The developing human brain appears to be vulnerable to irradiation. In order to assess the existence and extent of special sensitivity periods, it is important to map the development of the nervous system in relation to time. To this end, time after ovulation is a more reliable parameter than time after menstruation. There is, however, no single quantitative parameter to describe the developmental age of an embryo or fetus. Although the length of the embryo is statistically well correlated with its age and developmental status, it is, in any single case, of limited value for predictive purposes. It has, however, the advantage of being directly measurable in vivo using non-destructive ultrasonic techniques. These give information that is in close agreement with measurements taken on embryological samples. There are standardized systems of staging embryonic development, based on the overall morphology of the embryo, by which the major landmarks of organogenesis may be characterized with sufficient precision.

61. The formation of the human brain has recently been described in considerable detail according to the major stages of organogenesis, the cellular kinetics of the developing structures and the overall biochemical maturation of the various structures as a function of time. The major features are: the division of undifferentiated neural cells in the ventricular zone; the migration of post-mitotic cells to the cortical zones according to precise sequences of time and programmed spatial arrangements; the establishment of functional connections between neurons and glial cells and between neurons in various areas of the brain; and the presence of selective mechanisms to adjust the size and functions of the nerve cells in relation to their areas of projection and to neuronal wiring. All these phenomena and their temporal sequence determine, to a large extent, the final outcome of a radiation exposure of the developing brain.

62. It has been confirmed that the period of maximum sensitivity of the brain structures corresponds to the period of maximum activity in neural cell production between about 8 and 16 weeks post-fertilization in man. It is also apparent that brain histogenesis and maturation take place in various animal species at different times and that in man the maturation of the CNS extends from the embryonal well into the fetal and even the post-natal ages. This accounts for the different sensitivity of the brain structures in various species to the damaging action of radiation. Also, different parts of the brain develop and mature at different times, so that one should expect different periods of sensitivity for the functions associated with each of these structures. In contradistinction with what happens in rodents, the development and maturation of the human brain cortex lasts relatively longer than the major organogenesis of the brain: this may explain why, in man, disturbances of higher nervous functions are relatively more common after irradiation than is gross teratological damage.

63. The following concepts, derived from what is currently known about human brain development, structure and function, should be emphasized for their importance in respect of radiation effects. First, the neurons are perennial cells: they are generated once and for all in the course of cortex histogenesis and their inactivation by the action of radiation (or any other embryotoxic agent) is likely to result in permanent loss of mental functions. Secondly, brain structures are arranged in anatomical centres related to specific functional activities; inactivation of these centres is likely to result in a deficiency of the specific functions. These functions are not recovered by repopulation of glial cells. Thirdly, the brain functions are critically dependent on the establishment of special connections between neuronal cells in various parts of the CNS. A programmed sequence of events allows the cellular architecture to be established according to precise spatial and temporal arrangements. Interference by radiation, or other agents, in such a highly structured developmental plan is likely to result in a disruption of the neuronal connections, with the related functional loss.

64. The incidence of congenital abnormalities in the human species is highly dependent on the method and the time of scoring. They are found in about 6% of new-born individuals. Very roughly, they may be classified according to their etiology into those of simple genic origin (about 6% of all malformations at birth); those having a complex multifactorial origin (about 50%); those due to chromosomal defects (about 5%); and those known to be associated with various environmental factors (around 6%). Finally, there is a large class comprising about one-third of all abnormalities visible at birth which includes all those without an apparent cause. Radiation-induced malformations must be viewed against this background of naturally occurring conditions.

65. Children seen to be malformed at birth are only the survivors of a much greater number of malformed embryos or fetuses that have died at some stage in the intra-uterine development. If scoring is done on grown-up children the incidence of malformed ones is higher than at birth. Incidence figures are highly dependent on the method of scoring, on the size of the sample and on diagnostic criteria. The ethnic group, the familial genetic background, the age, parity and social class of the parents, the geographic location, the season of the year are also important sources of variability for malformation incidence. For the purpose of this study it is assumed that approximately 6% of all new-born children are affected by structural

abnormalities that are sufficiently severe to disturb their physical well-being and in some cases to decrease their viability.

II. THE PRE-IMPLANTATION PERIOD

66. It is very difficult to study, in man, events taking place in the conceptus before implantation. This is because there is no way of knowing whether fertilization has taken place, until the most sensitive radioimmunoassay tests show an increased concentration of human chorionic gonadotropin (HCG) in urine, thus indicating trophoblastic activity. It is widely believed, however, that many pregnancies end in embryonic losses before pregnancy has been clinically diagnosed and often before the first missed menstruation [G16, K39, M7]. These considerations explain why direct human observations of the pre-implantation stages are very rare for both normal development or after embryotoxic treatments. Of necessity, therefore, one must rely on observations in experimental animal systems. The short duration of the pre-implantation phase relative to the total duration of pregnancy in man, and the high rate of embryonic loss during this phase, must be kept in mind in order to assess appropriately any radiation effects that may be induced during this period of development. The scope and the limitations of model systems in teratology have been discussed in a paper by Beck [B29].

67. From its previous analysis, based exclusively on animal data, UNSCEAR concluded [U2] that death of the embryo was the most conspicuous effect to be seen after irradiation in the pre-implantation phase. Reduction of body growth and induction of malformations were not reported after irradiation at this stage of development. Chromosomal damage in the irradiated blastomeres, leading to degeneration of the primitive cells, is the major mechanism responsible for the killing of the embryo. Substantial differences in sensitivity were noted depending on the various species and as a function of time from fertilization in the early segmentation stages. In the mouse, the rodent species to which most data referred, data in good agreement pointed to a risk coefficient for killing of zygotes soon after fertilization, of the order of 1 Gy^{-1}. The following text updates these conclusions by review of the new findings on in vitro and in vivo systems.

A. EXPERIMENTS IN VITRO

68. Since the 1977 UNSCEAR report [U2], the culture in vitro of fertilized mammalian oocytes up to defined stages in their development has been widely used in many laboratories, both as a means to investigate mechanisms of damage in the pre-implantation stage and as a useful test of effects induced by radiation when administered alone or in combination with other embryotoxic agents. The main advantages of this technique are: incubation under well-defined conditions; careful timing of the treatments; good plating efficiency and capacity for further differentiation; and possibility to reimplant the blastocysts

into foster mothers to follow their further development [J15, S19]. The reports dealing with mechanisms will be examined here, while the work in which in vitro culture of embryos has been used simply as a test for embryotoxicity will be reviewed in VI.B.

69. Alexandre [A3] irradiated 2-cell or morulae mouse embryos (x rays, doses from 0.5 to 10 Gy) and cultured them in order to follow the percentage of embryos that would reach the blastocyst stage at various times post-irradiation. The most significant effect for irradiation of 2-cell embryos was the inhibition of primary differentiation shown by the failure of the embryo to proceed to the blastocyst stage. No embryo reached such a stage after a dose of 4 Gy. X rays administered to advanced morulae did not inhibit primary differentiation, although they did affect, eventually, the hatchability of the blastocysts. In a subsequent paper [A4], the same author showed that the reduced capacity to reach the stage of blastula after irradiation at the 2-cell stage was the result of early killing of cells. In fact, blastocysts from irradiated embryos contained a smaller number of cells. A lack of inner cell mass and its derivatives in further development was the end-effect of irradiation for both the 2-cell and morula-stage embryos.

70. Two papers by Pedersen et al. [P1, P2] showed that early mammalian embryos possess the enzymes required to perform excision repair of DNA damaged by ultraviolet (UV) light. Embryo cells maintained a relatively constant level of excision repair capacity until the late fetal stages, when such capacity was lost. However, there seemed to be no simple relationship between these changes in repair capacity and the known changes in the radiation sensitivity of embryos and fetuses.

71. In a small series of experiments, Jacquet et al. [J1] followed, as a function of time after fertilization, the development in vitro of cultured mouse embryos that had been irradiated with a series of x-ray doses (from 0.25 to 1 Gy) 2.3 or 6.7 hours after induced ovulation. The authors concluded that the sensitivity of the mouse egg was high at the pronuclear stage before DNA synthesis began, when doses of 0.2 Gy were sufficient to increase pre-implantation loss. These results in vitro parallel earlier in vivo findings by Russell and Montgomery [R20] who reported that the sensitivity to radiation-induced killing and to chromosome loss was very high shortly after sperm entry, and again at the early pronuclear stage, but became low in a late pronuclear stage. Jacquet's findings [J1] are at variance, however, with those of Schlesinger [S4] who found no difference in the radiosensitivity at any time during the first day after fertilization.

72. Jacquet et al. [J10] also reported on a preliminary study of the synthesis of DNA in mouse zygotes. They irradiated, with a range of x-ray doses (0.25 to 1.0 Gy), superovulated mice at the time of fertilization, at the beginning and at the maximum of DNA synthesis, and at the beginning of the first cleavage metaphase. On the day following irradiation the embryos were collected and classified as either uncleft

or 2-cell embryos; the latter were followed for a further 7 days. The pronuclear stage was found to be the most sensitive: irradiation at this time resulted in high mortality prior to first cleavage and at the 8-cell (1 Gy) or morula (0.5, 0.25 Gy) stages. Hatching of the blastocysts and attachment to the bottom of the culture flasks with the formation of a normal inner cell mass (which phenomena are referred to by the authors as "implantation") were also impaired. Cytogenetic studies on metaphase chromosomes also confirmed the well-established notion [U2] that embryonic death is attributable to chromosomal damage.

73. Domon [D10] analysed the cell-cycle-dependent radiosensitivity of BDF_1 mouse 2-cell embryos. The cell cycle of these embryos lasts 18 hours and is characterized by a long $G_2 + M$ of 14 hours and an S phase of 4 hours, a figure that is shorter than in other cases [M47, S70]. The author followed, as a function of time, the changes of the dose needed to prevent 50% of the cells from reaching the blastocyst stage (LD_{50}) and found that the LD_{50} varied within a factor of about 6. The LD_{50} of the embryos was about 2 Gy during the S phase and increased sharply in early G_2 ($\sim$ 6 Gy); resistance gradually dropped (to $\sim$ 1 Gy) as they progressed to M. Domon concluded that the position in the cell division cycle at the time of irradiation is a major determinant for the in vitro response of the early embryo to irradiation. The range of variation of the radiosensitivity values observed within the cell cycle appears, indeed, much larger than the range of radiosensitivities of pre-implantation embryos in different developmental stages (see Table 4, annex J, in [U2]). One-cell-stage mouse embryos were also found to be more sensitive than two-cell stages in experiments by Ku and Voytek [K18].

74. Domon [D11] also measured the dose required to prevent development of 50% of the embryos to blastocysts during 5 days of culture in vitro of pronuclear mouse embryos irradiated at various times during the cell cycle. This dose was found to vary from 1 to 2 Gy during the time from G_1 to the first cleavage. Pronuclear embryos were found to be more sensitive to radiation than embryos in the 2-cell stage [D10]. However, when radiosensitivity was related to the number of blastomeres, the pronuclear embryos appeared to be as sensitive as the 2-cell ones. It was concluded that the proportion of cells of various cell-cycle ages in the conceptus governed radiosensitivity during the early cleavage stages.

75. Yamada et al. [Y3] addressed the problem of the rapid changes in radiosensitivity, observed in the fertilized ovum during the time from fertilization to first cleavage, by the use of a mouse in vitro fertilization system. They found that the LD_{50}, as defined by Domon [D15], varied rapidly and extensively over a range of about 40 to 400 R. Sensitivity was relatively low soon after sperm entry and became progressively high (40 R) 4 to 6 hours after insemination, just before pronuclear formation. In the later pronuclear stage (12 hours after fertilization) sensitivity became low (400 R), only to rise again just before first cleavage.

76. In another paper by the same group [M48], mature sperm, eggs just before insemination and zygotes in the early pronuclear stage were exposed to x rays (40 R) and then cultured in vitro. The control non-irradiated zygotes, and those derived from irradiated sperm and eggs, progressed to the metaphase stage in over 90% of the cases by 15-17 hours from insemination. By this time, however, about 40% of the 1-cell eggs were still at the pronuclear stage, following irradiation in the early pronuclear phase. There was often a delay of chromatin condensation in one of the two pronuclei. In agreement with these observations, the incidence of chromosomal aberrations in first-cleavage metaphases of zygotes was much higher (20%) when irradiation took place on the zygotes than when it was carried out in sperm (2.9%) or unfertilized eggs (11.0%).

77. A series of papers by a group in the Federal Republic of Germany dealt with mechanisms of radiation damage during the initial phases of mammalian embryonic development. One of these papers [M11] showed that pre-implantation mouse eggs irradiated with x rays or neutrons in the G_2 phase of the 2-cell stage contained micronuclei and chromosomal aberrations when they reached the 4- and 8-cell stages. Micronuclei were more numerous in the 8-cell embryos, while chromosomal aberrations (particularly of the chromatid type) appeared more numerous in the 4-cell stage. As micronuclei derive from acentric fragments following chromosomal aberrations, the sequence of events would thus be logically explained.

78. Other papers [M32, M34] described the cell kinetic events following irradiation of the G_2 phase of the 2-cell mouse embryo. Doses of x rays between 0.12 and 1.88 Gy were delivered to such embryos, and their development up to blastocysts was followed as a function of time. A dose-related impaired hatching of blastocysts, and a reduced number of cells per blastocyst, were observed. Recovery and survival of irradiated embryos was also found. Moreover, normal, healthy mice could be produced by blastocyst transfer into foster mothers even after 0.94 and 1.88 Gy. A radiation-induced G_2 block of the cells, leading to a disturbance of cell progression along the cycle, was described. Hypodiploid cells were seen in later cell cycles, presumably related to the loss of genetic material induced by chromosomal aberrations. A finer analysis of the radiation-induced G_2 block after irradiation of embryos in various stages of development and of the resulting effects was also published by the same group [M12].

79. The DNA amounts and cell cycle phases were studied in mouse embryos after administering a dose of 1.88 Gy to 1- or 2-cell mouse embryos [M13]. Blastocyst formation was more impaired (28% of control) following irradiation of the 1-cell than of the 2-cell embryos (73% of controls) and cell death was mostly responsible for the impairment of the embryonic development. Cell death was well correlated with the presence of micronuclei after irradiation, and both phenomena were most evident after irradiation of the 1-cell zygote than of the 2-cell embryos.

80. The cell proliferation in vivo and in vitro of pre-implanted mouse embryos was investigated from 2 to 144 hours after conception [S70] by measuring the number of cell nuclei, the DNA content of the cells and the mitotic and labelling indices. After the first cell cycle the length of the S phase remained constant at about 7 hours, while G_1 and G_2 varied considerably. The increase in the number of cells was exponential from 31 to 72 hours after fertilization, but the rate of growth during this time was slower in vitro than in vivo. Also, the proliferation rate slowed down as the development proceeded to blastocyst. Although, in general, development was judged to be slightly faster in vivo, the phenomena were found to be very comparable under both conditions: this is evidence that the technique of in vitro culture is suitable for studying early kinetic events in the developing embryo.

81. Molls et al. [M47] compared, by using cytofluoro-metric techniques, the progression through the first few cell cycles of pre-implantation mouse embryos of the Heiligenberger and NMR1 strains. Ova fertilized in vivo during a short mating period were followed up to about 4 days from conception and the duration of the cell cycle phases was estimated at various times directly from the DNA histograms. Differences between the two strains were mainly in the length of the $G_2 + M$ phases. In both strains, the length of S increased from the first to the second cell cycle and the G_1 periods of the second and third cycle were very short. The increase in total cell number was exponential by the third cycle, with some differences in the rate of proliferation between the two strains. By the end of the pre-implantation development, when embryos reached the stage of hatched blastocysts, growth started to decline. The differences found were considered to be strain-specific and not due to the methods used for DNA measurements or to the different degree of synchrony of the embryos in the two strains.

82. In experiments on the preservation of mouse stocks by low-temperature storage of early embryos, Whittingham et al. [W11] kept 8-cell embryos in liquid nitrogen at $-196°$ C. They were exposed to various levels of background radiation ranging from 1.8 to 84 times the "normal" background, for periods ranging from 6 to 29 months. The capacity of these embryos to reach the blastocyst stage in vitro or to reach fetal or live-born stages when transferred to recipient females were the end-points used to assess the effects. Comparisons with non-frozen or short-term frozen controls were also made. The low-temperature treatment itself was responsible for a marked loss of viability, so that when all data were pooled, only about 20-30% of the embryos originally frozen were recovered as fetuses or live-borns. By comparison with this high rate of loss, the effect of background was absent or non-significant. Only the embryos kept for 29 months at 84 times the control background showed a slight reduction of implanted and live fetuses. However, even this effect was of doubtful significance in view of the lack of any relationship with the time of storage.

83. When assessing the usefulness of techniques of assay in vitro for exposure of embryos in vivo, direct comparisons by the evaluation of similar end-points are of importance. In this respect, it is appropriate to cite a paper [F2] which escaped the previous UNSCEAR review [U2]. In these experiments, 2-day-old mouse embryos of the 129/SvSl strain were obtained by hormonally-induced superovulation. They were treated with increasing exposures from 220-kVp x rays (from 6 to 1455 R) either in vitro or directly in the superovulated females. Embryos were then removed from these females within 2 hours and cultured in vitro up to blastulation under conditions similar to those used for the embryos irradiated in vitro. Blastulation occurred in about 80% of cultured sham-irradiated control embryos. It was found, in essence, that under all conditions the inhibition of blastocyst development by irradiation was dose-related. However, the exposure required to inhibit blastulation of 50% of the embryos was about 300 R for irradiation in vitro and about 600 R for irradiation in vivo.

84. After 48 hours of culture, embryos that had blastulated were again transplanted into pseudo-pregnant females which were killed 15 days later for scoring of implantation scars, resorptions and fetuses (weight, gross abnormalities, skeletal abnormalities). Approximately 70% of implanting control blastocysts developed into fetuses. After in vitro exposures in excess of 73 R, significantly fewer fetuses developed. Exposures of the order of 170 R resulted in no fetal development at all, and those of about 270 R resulted in no implantation. Following in vivo irradiation, fetal development occurred up to 388 R. No more or no different gross and skeletal abnormalities were observed significantly above the control level after either in vitro or in vivo exposure. As to weight changes, an impairment occurred in fetuses developing from trans-planted embryos irradiated in vitro with 73 R or more. It was concluded that the lower susceptibility to radiation damage found for embryos irradiated in vivo was due either to direct embryo shielding or to a protective physical or metabolic mechanism provided by the maternal tissues and operating within the 2-hour interval between irradiation and transfer to culture. However, the details given in the paper [F2] about radiation dosimetry and the use of exposures, rather than absorbed doses, render any quantitative assessment of these data rather problematic.

B. EXPERIMENTS IN VIVO

85. By comparison with reports on irradiation in vitro, the reports on in vivo treatment of pre-implantation stages are few. In a series of papers on the effects of gamma rays and helium ions on embryonic rats (0.5-6.0 Gy), Ward et al. [W1] exposed pregnant animals on one of days 4 to 9 of gestation (the pre-implantation stage ends in the rat at about day 7) and scored the embryo survival at 20 days p.c., as a function of the embryo position in the uterus. They found that embryos located in the ovarian or in the cervical ends of the uterus had higher rates of mortality than their litter-mates implanted in the middle part of the uterine horns. This conclusion was true for both radiations and for all irradiation times. The influence on survival of the uterine position

increased with the dose of radiation and with the number of implants, so that with high doses and a crowded uterus the probability of survival of embryos in the least advantageous positions could be as low as one-half of that of the litter as a whole. Irradiation under hypoxic conditions also led to a high rate of killing of embryos implanted in the cervical end of the uterine horns: this suggested that the selective distribution of intra-uterine deaths could not be attributed to a state of relative hypoxia. The non-random distribution of the killing effect was in contrast with the random occurrence of the gross morphological abnormalities to be seen in the irradiated litters.

86. In another experiment [S4], pregnant mice were exposed to 100 R of x rays at various hours in the first day of gestation and the fetuses were scored at term for death during the pre-implantation or early post-implantation stages. An increased rate of both types of death was induced by the treatment, accompanied by an increase in the mean fetal weight and a decreased incidence of malformations. Changing the irradiation time did not affect survival of the animals at term. At various times after irradiation, the embryos were tested by the eosin Y supravital staining method to assess cell viability. The relative frequency of viable and dead cells in normal or irradiated embryos was found to be comparable at 1, 2 and 3 days. At 4 days of gestation, an increased proportion of dead cells was noted in both the control and irradiated embryos: this was taken as evidence of the occurrence of cell death as a normal mechanism in the course of mammalian development. At this time, irradiation caused a decrease in the percentage of embryos reaching the blastocyst stage and a decrease in the number of cells per embryo. The authors noted that the lack of a significant increase in the percentage of dead cells in irradiated mice could be due to the high variability of the findings masking the killing effect of radiation or to the fact that cell death may become manifest only after the fourth day of gestation. This research is broadly in agreement with many other experiments [U2] confirming that embryonic death is the main effect found after pre-implantation irradiation. However, the single exposure used, the short time tested, the lack of a precise timing for mating, and the non-specificity of the techniques used, render these conclusions of rather limited significance.

87. Roux et al. [R21] investigated the effect of 0.05, 0.1, and 0.25 Gy of gamma radiation administered in single doses to Wistar rats 9 or 16 hours after mating. At 9 hours, DNA synthesis had not yet begun, and at 16 hours was still taking place in the ovum. The pregnant females were killed on the 21st day of gestation for counting of the total number of implantation sites, the number of live fetuses, resorption sites (embryonic death between 7 and 12 days) and dead fetuses (death after day 12). Live fetuses were also weighed and examined for malformations of the head and skeleton. The pre-implantation embryonic mortality, the mean weight of the fetuses and the sex ratio were not significantly changed by the radiation treatment. There were also no differences in the type and incidence of malformations in the various experimental groups. However, mortality (both embryonic

and fetal) was increased by the radiation exposure, without any significant difference between the two irradiation times. At 0.05 Gy the increased mortality only occurred at the fetal stage; at 0.1 Gy both the embryonic and fetal mortality were enhanced, but the latter more than the first; at 0.25 Gy the stage of conceptus at death depended on irradiation time, because embryonic mortality was always increased, although much more in the 16-hour group, while fetal mortality was only increased in the 9-hour group. These results are in agreement with previous ones in showing that mortality, rather than malformation induction, is the prevalent effect of irradiation during the pre-implantation stage. They are, however, at variance with the previously discussed notion [U2] that pre- and early post-implantation death is generally seen under such conditions of exposure. As to the dependence of mortality on irradiation time, the present series [R21] shows a complex relationship between dose and time at irradiation.

88. Aldeen and Konermann [A2] treated pregnant mice by a single exposure of 300 R x rays 1, 2 and 3 days p.c. and dissected the uteri 6 days p.c. The mean number of implantation sites was found to be 9.67 per female in the controls and 8.00, 6.63 and 7.00 per female in animals irradiated 1, 2 and 3 days p.c., respectively. Among 22 implants that were examined histologically after irradiation on day 1 p.c., no living embryo could be detected; the same was true of 19 implants on day 2 and 11 implants on day 3 after irradiation. The percentage of resorptions was lowest on day 1 after irradiation (31.8%) and highest (94.7%) on day 2. Cytological and histochemical criteria were used to assess the state of the decidua, which was either normal or only marginally affected on day 2 after irradiation, concomitantly with the peak of embryonic deaths. From this the authors concluded that direct embryonic killing, and not maternal effects, were involved in the damage described.

89. Zhou and Wang [Z3] submitted mouse embryos in the pre-implantation period to single or fractionated exposures of radiation (gamma rays, 100 R). Among early effects, they reported an increased mortality (as evidenced by an increased number of dead fetuses and resorption sites) and a decreased mean fetal weight of irradiated litters.

C. CONCLUSIONS

90. The latest information on the effects of embryo irradiation during the pre-implantation stages does not include data for man. In the last few years, techniques of embryo culturing in vitro have been widely employed in experimental animals to study a variety of problems, mostly dealing with the mechanisms of radiation damage during this stage. For such problems, in vitro culture offers significant technical advantages and results that are qualitatively comparable with those obtainable in vivo. The similarity of the findings between in vitro and in vivo analyses does not extend, however, to the quantitative aspects of

radiation damage; conclusions drawn in vitro may not easily be extrapolated to in vivo irradiation. Another condition that impedes generalizations across species is that the latest data refer only to mice and rats.

91. Experiments in vitro have made it possible to ascertain that the sensitivity of the embryos is highest for irradiation of the pronuclear stage. They show quite conclusively that there are oscillations in the response of the embryos related to the cell division cycle. Doses as low as 0.2 Gy have been reported to cause statistically significant embryo killing at the time of maximum sensitivity before DNA synthesis begins. However, the variability of doses required to kill one-half of the cultured embryos (LD_{50}) spans a factor of about 10 among different phases in the mitotic cycle and different mitotic cycles. The formation of blastocysts is more damaged when irradiation takes place at the 1-cell than at the 2-cell stage, and there is a good correlation between the death of the embryo after irradiation and the occurrence in it of chromosomal abnormalities. Irradiation also disturbs the kinetics of cell progression, mostly through a variation of the duration of G_1 and G_2 phases.

92. Irradiation of the 2-cell embryo results in a dose-related block to proceed to the blastocyst stage. Doses of a few Gy are needed to stop completely 50% blastocyst formation. As the embryo maintains a reasonable degree of synchrony during the first few segmentation divisions, its sensitivity may be analysed as a function of cell cycle phases. Under these conditions, the changes of embryo sensitivity result in LD_{50} values ranging from 1 to 2 Gy (irradiation in M and S) and 6 Gy (irradiation in G_2). A G_2 block of the cell cycle has also been described for irradiation at this stage. Hatching of blastocysts is, in general, a more sensitive end-point. Cell killing by induction of chromosomal aberrations appears to be the cause of a decreased rate of growth of the irradiated embryo and, ultimately, of the embryonic mortality. As the number of cells in the embryo increases, the dose needed to stop embryonic development to a given stage appears also to increase. However, for irradiation at a given stage, the apparent radiosensitivity of the embryo to killing increases with the time intervening between irradiation and the scoring of the effect.

93. Experiments in vitro have documented the existence of some strain-related variability in the rate of progression of the embryo through the initial developmental stages in the mouse. There may also be differences in the intrinsic radiosensitivity of early mouse embryos of the same strain irradiated in vitro or in vivo, the latter condition being apparently less damaging. Transplantation into foster-mothers of embryos irradiated and cultured in vitro allows the surviving embryos to complete their development to normal animals. Such experiments have confirmed that loss of viability is the only effect to be seen for treatment during the pre-implantation stages at the two-cell stage or later. Weight changes in the survivors could be secondary to the killing of some of the conceptuses in polytocous animals. Radiation-induced teratological effects in excess of the natural level have not been documented.

94. Experiments on rodent embryos irradiated in vivo have confirmed the above in vitro conclusions, at least qualitatively. Embryonic killing emerges in vivo as the major effect of irradiation. It appears to be due to an action on the embryos that is direct and not mediated through disturbances of the formation of the placenta. In vivo, relatively small doses (0.05 Gy) have been reported to result only in fetal mortality, but after higher doses (0.1 Gy) embryonic mortality is also affected. Oscillations of embryonic radiosensitivity would appear, on the whole, to be less prominent for irradiation in vivo: this could, however, be due to the lesser degree of synchrony that obtains under these conditions.

III. THE PERIOD OF MAJOR ORGANOGENESIS

95. In its 1977 review [U2] UNSCEAR concluded that the most characteristic (but by no means the only) type of damage to be seen in mammalian embryos irradiated during the period of major organogenesis was the induction of malformations. The review discussed the conditions under which teratological damage became apparent and stated that, at least qualitatively, similar classes of malformations occurred in various animal species upon irradiation of comparable developmental stages. Inter- and intra-species variability was also reviewed on the basis of the data then available. The review discussed the presence and timing of the periods of maximum sensitivity for certain classes of malformations and observed that these maxima usually coincided with the major phase of morphogenesis of the relevant anatomical structures. It observed that, although the dose-response relationships for a given type of malformation were of the sigmoid type, grouping of embryologically or topographically related malformations or expressing the teratological damage as the ratio of malformed to normal animals, irrespective of the type and degree of malformations carried, tended to generate quasi-linear dose-effect relationships. Data then available concerning rodents (the projection of which to man would, however, be unwarranted) tended to yield estimates of the absolute increase of incidence of malformed fetuses per unit absorbed dose of the order of $5 \cdot 10^{-1}$ Gy^{-1} of low-LET radiation delivered at high dose rate. In man, an estimate of incidence of severe mental retardation per unit absorbed dose was tentatively set at 10^{-1} Gy^{-1}, based on the data from Hiroshima and Nagasaki. Other epidemiological surveys in man, after doses in the region of 0.01-2.0 Gy, were only of indirect value in excluding the possibility that at such doses the human embryo could be 10 times more sensitive than implied by the incidence of malformations at higher doses [U2].

96. The information that has since become available has added considerably to our knowledge of phenomena induced by irradiation in experimental animals, particularly in the CNS. New data have also been produced on the occurrence of mental deficiencies in children irradiated during the explosions at Hiroshima and Nagasaki. All the relevant material on malforma-

tions of the CNS in experimental animals is being reviewed here, partly because it would be difficult and repetitive to separate out from the various series data referring to either embryonic or fetal stages; and partly because mental retardation in man (which occurs especially at times which are at the borderline between the two developmental stages) is also treated here. It is recognized, of course, that cases of mental deficiency may also appear in children irradiated at times which are considered well within the fetal stage of development. However, by discussing all data together it is hoped to convey a more coherent picture of the malformations observed and of their incidence as a function of dose and time. The reader is referred to chapter I for a brief description of normal CNS development in animals and man.

A. DATA FROM ANIMALS

1. Skeletal malformations

97. Single exposures from ^{60}Co radiation, in the range from 50 to 500 R, were given to about 600 pregnant Swiss mice at 9, 10, 11 and 12 days of pregnancy [P3]. Starting from day 13, and up to day 18 p.c., the embryos and their placentas were weighed and examined. For irradiation on day 9, exposures below 150 R produced no significant deviations from controls, whereas higher exposures were lethal to the conceptus. For irradiation on day 10, an exposure of 100 R was the threshold for effects on the weight of the placenta. Malformations became apparent at 125 R. At 150-175 R, fetal mortality was over 60% and surviving fetuses were malformed. At 200 R, fetal loss approached 100%. On day 11 the feto-placental complex was reduced in weight at 75 R. At 200 R, pre-natal death was over 60%, and at 300 R it was close to 100%. On day 12 the weight of the conceptus and placenta declined between 125 and 450 R. Malformations were seen at 150 R, and 500 R produced total loss of the fetuses. The data were compounded into an overall model of action accounting for dose, time and type of effects.

98. Tribukait and Cekan [T3] carried out experiments on C3H mice, primarily to study the form of dose-effect relationships for malformations brought about by irradiation with single, fractionated or protracted doses during the period of major organogenesis. Pregnant females irradiated at 9 days p.c. with 180- or 250-kV x rays were killed at 18 days p.c. for examination of implantations, resorptions, living and dead fetuses and fetuses with gross external abnormalities. Skeletal and visceral malformations were also specifically studied, but the incidence of this latter class was too low and its scoring was later omitted. Single doses in the range of 0.125 to 2.5 Gy were delivered. In total, 50 malformed out of 1929 non-irradiated fetuses were found; 1320 malformations were seen in 3558 irradiated animals.

99. The frequency of malformations belonging to various classes was very different when all irradiated and non-irradiated animals were compared. In the vertebral column and ribs the frequencies were 32 and

44% in non-irradiated and irradiated, respectively; umbilical hernia was, respectively, 14 and 6%; digital malformations 8 and 6%; anophthalmia, and micro-ophthalmia and other malformations of the eye 8 and 18% (although coloboma was mostly seen in the irradiated mice). Tail malformations were, in both cases, 18%. Dose-response curves for resorptions and malformations were of the sigmoid type, with a very low incidence of the effects up to 0.75 Gy and a steep rise thereafter. Resorptions, in particular, with a control incidence of 10% did not show any clear trend with dose, up to about 1 Gy. Taking the various classes of malformations separately, absolute increases of incidence per unit absorbed dose of between 9 and 54% Gy^{-1} were observed in the steep region of the curves. Pooling all malformations, a 57% increase per Gy resulted, with practically 100% malformed animals at 2 Gy. For doses below 0.75 Gy, the absolute increase in the percentage of malformed mice would be 0.1% per 0.01 Gy (Figure VIII). Expressing the effect as number of malformations per fetus produced a similar pattern, with an initial increase to 1.4 malformations per animal up to 0.75 Gy and a further, steeper rise to 3 malformations per fetus up to the highest doses used.

100. Dose-fractionation experiments were also carried out [T3] in which the embryos received a total of 1.75 Gy, split into 2 fractions delivered at intervals between 15 minutes and 8 hours. Even taking into account that a decrease in the sensitivity of the system occurred over this time (resorptions dropped from 45 to 34% and malformations from 45 to 21% following single doses of 0.875 Gy) an interval of 15 minutes brought about a 30% reduction in the incidence of both effects, followed by an increase at 4-6 hours and a further decrease to near control values at 8 hours. This pattern is reminiscent of the two-dose recovery curves commonly described for many mammalian cells and tissues. Different responses as a function of fractionation time were noted for the various classes of malformation, those of the eye being apparently more spared by dose splitting than the skeletal ones.

101. Further experiments were conducted [T3] in which the same dose of 1.75 Gy was delivered at dose rates of 0.72, 0.055 and 0.015 Gy min^{-1}. The total incidence of malformations increased from 55 to 80% between the highest and the lowest dose rates tested, but different malformation types were differently affected, the external and the ocular malformations being practically unchanged and the skeletal ones essentially doubled. This finding is at variance with the majority of data discussed in the 1977 report [U2], but it is consistent with the notion that dose-rate changes and fractionation may affect various malformations differently. Cell kinetic data obtained by whole embryo preparations were also given in [T3], but the significance of such findings in relation to the problems at hand is not clear.

102. A thesis by Knauss [K8] contains accurate data on the dose-response relationships for mouse skeletal malformations induced by pre-natal exposure to radiation. Mice of the Heiligenberger strain were exposed at 7, 10 and 13 days p.c. to 150-kV x rays in the range of

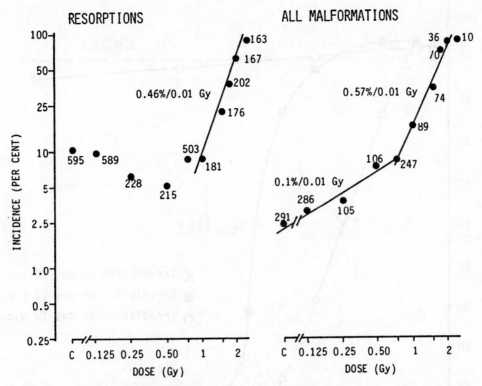

Figure VIII. Dose-response relationships on a log-log scale for resorption (left) and all malformations (right) incidence in mice irradiated at 9 days p.c. The number of observations is given for each experimental group.
[T3]

5-250 R and examined on day 19 p.c. for the presence of minor variants, abnormalities or major malformations of the skeleton, after staining with Alizarin S. The various types of effect were examined separately or jointly as a function of dose. The 7th day p.c. was the time at which the sensitivity appeared to be at its maximum; the minimum was at 13 days p.c. By considering each class of malformation (they were divided according to the various sections of the skeleton), quite pronounced threshold-type exposure-incidence curves were obtained. The data were also treated in such a way as to obtain estimates of fetuses without abnormalities or malformations (excluding the variants). They were plotted, as a function of dose, as in Figure IX. That figure shows that exposures of the order of about 80 or 140 R would be needed to induce malformations in 50% of the irradiated fetuses at 7 or 10 days, respectively. The difference is due mainly to the wider threshold observed at 10 days p.c. These experiments are to be regarded as a further confirmation of the non-linearity of the dose-response relationship for the induction of malformations at the most sensitive stages in development.

103. These and other experiments were later included in a review by Konermann [K12] from which Figure X is taken. The experimental points in this figure are based on 500 to 800 mice each. By plotting the incidence of gross skeletal malformations as a function of x-ray exposure on a semi-logarithmic graph, it is shown that the spontaneous incidence of 0.6% malformations is increased by a factor of 3 after an exposure of 5 R on day 7 p.c. The increase is due essentially to the contribution of malformations in the skull and the cervical column. The decrease in incidence from 5 to

25 R is attributed to the confounding influence of embryonic selection. An exposure of 25 R on day 10 p.c. doubles the incidence of malformations seen in the control mice, which is, however, unaffected by an exposure of only 12.5 R.

104. In the course of work on sensitivity analysis for an in vivo screening test for teratogens, Russell [R19] explored the possibility of using homeotic shifts in the quantitative configuration of the axial skeleton. Having ascertained that about 9 days p.c. was the optimum time for induction of changes in certain quantitative features of the axial skeleton of BALB/c mice, she irradiated pregnant mice at this particular stage (12.5, 25, 50 and 100 R). Fetuses were removed just before delivery and their axial skeleton was analysed. This inbred mouse strain shows a high degree of variability for several quantitative characters such as the numbers of ribs, costo-sternal junctions, pre-sacral vertebrae and sternebrae. Even the lowest exposure tested caused clearly discernible shifts in 3 of the 4 quantitative characters mentioned. By contrast, the morphological abnormalities of the axial skeleton showed much higher thresholds: of 10 abnormalities scored, none was induced at 12.5 R, and 1, 5 and 10 were induced at 15, 50 and 100 R, respectively.

2. Malformations of the eye

105. Cellular changes in the developing eye of embryonic mice irradiated on day 8 p.c. with 0.9 Gy of x rays were described by Balla and Michel [B1, B3]. The end-points scored on days 9 and 10 p.c. included eye size, mitotic activity, cell death and chromosomal

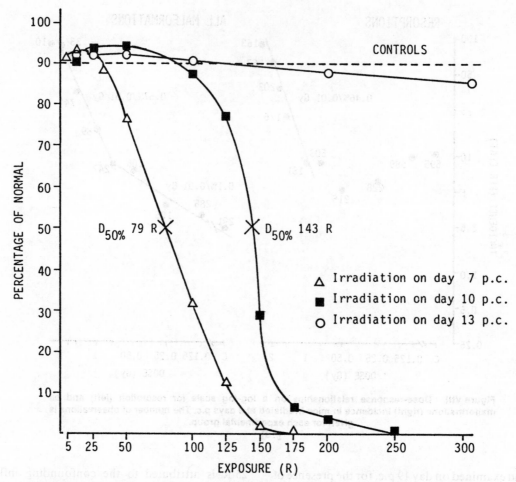

Figure IX. Percentage frequency of fetuses with normal skeletal structure, including variants, after x irradiation on days 7, 10 or 13 p.c., expressed in per cent of the total number of living fetuses on day 19 p.c.
[K12]

aberrations. The size of the eye vesicle was significantly reduced in the irradiated embryos, but was restored 24 hours later, except for a significant reduction of the lens size. In agreement with these findings, the total number of cells and the mitotic activity of the vesicle were decreased at the time of observation. The incidence of chromosomal aberrations in anaphase cells was increased in the irradiated eyes, as was the incidence of morphologically assessed cell death. Similar experiments were conducted on embryos at the 9th day of gestation. Cell death was scored at various times post-irradiation, up to 24 hours, and in different regions of the developing eye. The pattern of necrosis differed from that seen, for irradiation on day 8, and the rapid recovery occurring by 12 hours pointed to a high capacity for repair of this tissue [B2].

3. Malformations of the CNS

106. Although normal events in the development of the human nervous system have been mapped to a reasonable degree of precision (see chapter I), data on the effects of radiation directly on human material are virtually impossible to obtain. Thus, our knowledge of the pathogenesis of radiation-induced changes relies entirely on observations in experimental animals, mostly rodents. It may reasonably be assumed that, in

their main aspects and for their qualitative features, the effects observed on such animals are similar to those produced in man. Hicks and D'Amato [H15], in a review of the lethal and non-lethal cell changes of the nervous system, have attempted to show the good correspondence existing in respect of the underlying mechanisms between the laboratory animal and the human data. Brizzee et al. [B9] also published a brief review of data on the structural nervous system effects caused by irradiation in utero in both animals and man. In the following paragraphs, new data on this subject will be reviewed, with special reference to those appearing since about 1977. Further data on brain damage by chronically ingested radionuclides, particularly by tritium [V2, Z1, Z2], are discussed in chapter V.

(a) The mouse

107. Kameyama et al. [K3] studied the effect of 25 or 100 R x radiation on CF-1 mouse embryos exposed at 10, 13 or 15 days of gestation, in an attempt to obtain quantitative evidence of early effects on the undifferentiated matrix cells of the developing telencephalon. Of all gestational ages, the 13-day-old embryos were found to be the most sensitive in terms of lengthening of the cell-cycle time in thymidine-labelling experiments. An exposure-effect relationship between 10 and

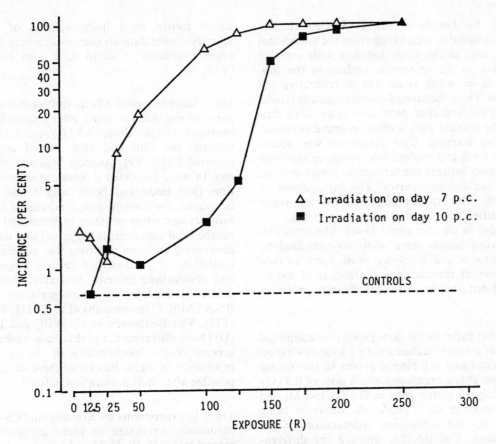

Figure X. The incidence of gross malformations in the mouse skeleton after various exposures
on days 7 or 10 p.c.
[K12]

150 R was also established at this age for mitotic delay
($G_2 + 1/2M$) of the matrix cells. The delay was found
to be directly related to the logarithm of exposure.
Extrapolation of this function to the lowest exposure
suggested that the apparent threshold for the effect
would be slightly lower than 10 R, thus confirming the
detectability of cell kinetic disturbances (the overall
significance of which is, however, difficult to assess) at
this exposure level. Other data on the cell cycle and
radiosensitivity of matrix cells in the brain of the
mouse fetuses at 13 days p.c. were also reported in an
abstract by Hoshino and Kameyama [H28].

108. Hayashi et al. [H2, H4, but particularly H9]
described pathological changes observable by light
and electron microscopy in the telencephalon of CF-1
fetal mice exposed to 25 R or 100 R on days 10, 13
and 15 p.c. The detectability and incidence of cells
with cytoplasmic inclusions by light microscopy was
increased when earlier developmental stages were
exposed. By electron microscopy, such inclusions could
be divided into cytoplasmic degeneration and phago-
cytosed neuronal cells; they preceded the appearance
of nuclear changes in the irradiated cells. Precise times
for the occurrence of all these changes, as a function
of dose and irradiation time, could be established.

109. Kameyama [K30] noted that the changes in the
radiation response of the matrix cells were not
apparently related with the decrease of the cells'
mitotic activity as a function of time. He pointed out
that the most sensitive period for these cells is when

the cortical plate begins to appear. According to the
author, this developmental stage in the mouse corresponds, approximately, to the 8th to 10th week of
gestation in man, based on the histogenic state of the
cerebral cortex.

110. Working on two different mouse strains (CF-1
and ICR), and with different gestation times (13 and
15 or 17 days), Hoshino et al. ([H12, H13], summarized
in [H18]), studied the changes in the architecture of
the cerebral cortex induced by 25 or 100 R. To do so,
they mapped the position of thymidine-labelled neurons
reaching various layers of the cortex by 4 weeks of
extra-uterine age. They recognized the presence of
specific changes in the various layers. The nature of
the changes was found to depend on irradiation time,
their severity on dose. In parallel experiments by
Hayashi et al. [H10], where cortical thickness, cell
density and dendritic arborization of pyramidal cells
were observed, it was found that 25 R did not cause a
decrease in the number of cortical cells, but resulted in
a developmental effect on the pyramidal cells whose
dendritic arborization was retarded. Ten roentgens,
given at 13 days p.c. to ICR mice, reduced the
branching indices marginally [H11].

111. Schmahl and his collaborators published a
valuable series of papers in which the mechanisms and
consequences of radiation-induced damage to the
CNS were analysed. In a first contribution [S7], they
reported on experiments in which NMRI mice received
2.0 Gy of x rays on day 12 p.c. and were examined on

285

day 18 p.c. for lesions of the CNS. Cell clusters (rosettes), presumably originating from the ependymal layer, were seen at this time, together with areas of necrosis close to the ventricular surface in the sub-ependymal layer, which is the site of reparative cell proliferation. These lesions had morphologically typical aspects and evolved after birth into cysts, with flattening of the cortical wall, without reactive processes such as glial scarring. Cyst formation was accentuated after birth and evolved into porencephaly with communication between the ventricular lumen and the surface of the cerebral cortex. The histogenesis of these events, with special emphasis on the topographical differences in the developing brain, was described also in another paper [S40]. Abnormalities of the nervous tissues were often accompanied by malformations of the overlying skull, such as dysdifferentiation of the cartilage, formation of hyperostosis, and disturbances of the calcification processes [S58].

112. Another paper by the same group [S5] attempted an analysis of cellular mechanisms by a joint evaluation of pathological and cell-kinetic events in the mouse telencephalon at late organogenesis. A dose of 0.95 Gy killed virtually all matrix cells in G_1, G_2 and M, and 50-75% of those in the S phase, the survivors being responsible for the subsequent regeneration of the damaged tissue. Cell labelling allowed the differentiation of two different pools of cells surviving in S, which contributed in different ways to the regeneration processes of the telencephalic roof after radiation injury. A later study on similarly treated mice [S49] described the generation times, potential doubling times, growth fraction and cell cycle stages of the neuroblasts and their alterations following irradiation.

113. Heinzmann [H3] studied, in the mouse, the dysplasia of the third cerebral ventricle induced by 1.9 Gy of x rays on the 12th day of gestation. Perinatal observations and observations at 20 months of age were conducted by gross, microscopic and ultrastructural techniques. Brain reduction and ventriculocele were carefully described and the genesis of the lesions discussed in its possible patho-physiological mechanisms. This author also described [H19] gross changes and alterations in the fine structure of the choroid plexus of mice, induced by doses of 0.95 and 1.9 Gy of x rays given to the 12-day fetus. These changes were found to persist throughout post-natal life up to the age of 20 months.

114. In related studies [H25], the same author described the normal functional activity of the mouse brain, from the 13th day of gestation up to post-natal ages, by injection of tritium-labelled deoxy-D-glucose and radioactivity measurements. He showed that tritium uptake differed considerably between tissue samples taken from various regions of the brain at various developmental times. He also compared the normal pattern of glucose incorporation into the brain structures with changes induced by x irradiation (0.9 and 1.9 Gy) given on the 12th day of gestation. It is difficult, however, to correlate such biochemical findings with the morphological effects of irradiation

which consist in a hydrocephalus of dose-related severity. Other data on the biochemistry of the mouse brain irradiated in utero have also been reported [V10].

115. Morphological effects (cell necrosis) in various parts of the brain 6 hours after irradiation with fast neutrons (single dose, 0.5 Gy) on C57BL/6 mice between the 13th and 18th day of gestation were reported [A15, V9]. Animals similarly irradiated on day 18 were examined 3 weeks after birth, at which time their body and brain weight was significantly decreased, for content and synthesis of DNA, RNA, histones and other proteins in brain and liver. These biochemical experiments suggested that damage to the developing brain by neutrons was associated with the inhibition of synthesis of certain histone fractions and non-histone proteins, probably resulting from a decreased capacity of amino-acylation by transfer RNA [A16]. (Timmermans et al. [T11], Tanaka et al. [T12], Van Beuningen et al. [V10] and Deroo et al. [D1] have also reported preliminary studies of various aspects of the biochemistry of the rat brain after irradiation in utero. Review of these data will only be possible after their publication in full.)

116. In experiments by Konermann [K34], mice were chronically irradiated in utero at various developmental stages (5-10, 11-15, 6-13 days p.c.) with a range of exposure rates from 40 to 80 R/day. These treatments induced compensatory proliferation reactions during the formation of the brain glia, and such reactions were more marked the more brain development was retarded [K11]. The lipid synthesis during the period of pre-myelination gliosis was also studied by spectrophotometric and histoautoradiographic analysis of the uptake of ^{3}H-mevalonic acid, ^{3}H-glucose and ^{32}P-sodium-phosphate in the brain. During the pre-myelination period, it was found that there was a very strict correlation between the lipid synthesis and the formation of glial cells. Such correlation was independent of the irradiation period and of the exposure rate and, since over-proliferation occurs at high doses, a rise of incorporation with increasing brain retardation (and therefore with dose) was documented. In various brain sections, in parallel with an increase of myelin density, a tighter packing of the oligodendrocytes responsible for brain myelination was also shown. From an overall evaluation of the findings, it was concluded that lipogenesis during pre-myelination occurs indirectly as a result of cell proliferation which leads, in the most developmentally retarded brains, to non-coordinated, over-compensatory reactions [K34].

117. Konermann and Schwald [K13] irradiated albino inbred mice at 13, 16, 18.5 and 22 days p.c. with 4 doses of x rays of between 0.5 and 3.0 Gy, and studied, by means of a microphotometric technique, the formation of the tigroid substance up to 80 days post-natally. The formation of this substance is thought to be related to, and reflected in, the maturation of the neurons. An irregular decrease with respect to controls of the tigroid density, which was dose- and stage-related, was observed in the irradiated animals. There were fluctuating responses also in

relation to the various brain regions examined (cortex, thalamus, cerebellum, hippocampus, gyrus dentatus, nucleus motorius trigemini) which were most pronounced during the critical periods of post-natal brain maturation of the various structures. The decrease of tigroid density was compensated at long term in the animals irradiated with the smallest dose, but with increasing doses the changes became either not compensated or progressive. Since the magnitude of the late responses decreased when the embryonic age at irradiation increased from 13 to 22 days p.c., the responses must either be extended through several cell generations or be induced to a lesser degree in the late pre-natal stages. In parallel with the responses of the tigroid substance during the second and third week after birth, there were also changes in the total content of RNA in the brain, which were again most pronounced for the earliest ages at irradiation. The overall meaning of these changes appears to be a retardation and stabilization of the brain maturation, but their significance remains to be fully evaluated and interpreted.

118. Treatment of mice in utero with fractionated doses between 3×1.05 and 3×1.33 Gy on gestational days 11-13 gave rise to rosette-like clusters of primitive cells resembling ependymal cells, dispersed within the brain cortex wall. These lesions appeared to be particularly abundant in the females, suggesting that the radiation treatment acted on differentiation steps that were specific for one of the sexes and fully developed already by the beginning of the fetal period prior to gonadal differentiation. It was speculated that lesions in the X chromosome would be involved in the development of such a specific dimorphic action, and that this pattern might only become apparent in the forebrain because of the relationship existing in this organ between cell necrosis and rosette development [S60].

119. Dimorphic lesions were described not only in the forebrain, but also in the epithalamus, as gross malformations appearing in the mouse at 18 days p.c., following a three-day fractionation treatment at doses between 0.95 and 1.35 Gy/day on days 11-13 p.c. [S61]. Two specific types of lesions regarding, respectively, the dorsal diencephalic sulcus and a narrowing of the epithalamus were recognized: it was shown that the second (and more severe) type of malformation is rather more common in female fetuses. Dose dependencies for the two lesion types were also described. The sexually dimorphic reaction pattern of these thalamic malformations cannot be explained by the fact that the relevant structures are in a different developmental stage in the two sexes at the time of irradiation; nor with a disturbance of perinatal hormone imprinting mechanisms in the CNS occurring in females more than in males. The authors believe that these malformations should be viewed together with other changes described in the neo-cortex [S60] and are the result of retrograde (cortico-thalamic) trans-synaptic degeneration, secondary to the cortical lesions. Epithalamic dysfunction in the immediate neo-natal period would then be responsible for the death of animals carrying preferentially the second type of lesions, which are the female animals.

120. In order to find some justification for such a preferential effect on female animals, Weber and Schmahl [W19] studied also the developmental profiles in mouse brain of the activities of a number of enzymes (alpha-galactosidase, hypoxanthine-guanine phosphoribosyltransferase and glucose-6-phosphate dehydrogenase) which are linked with the X-chromosome. The inactivation of this chromosome, which takes place at an early stage of development, leads to identical enzyme activities in male and female animals between 15 days p.c. and 64 days of post-natal age. These enzyme activities were studied in the brains of animals that had received 1.05 Gy three times, at 11, 12 and 13 days p.c. Treatment of the animals with this dosage (but not after 3×0.95 Gy or 3×1.15 Gy at the same ages) resulted in death of predominantly female offspring within 48 hours of birth [S59]. When the hypothesis was tested that such preferential mortality might be attributable to a reactivation of the inactive female X-chromosome in brain cells, it was found that, although the radiation-induced differences in enzyme patterns were quite remarkable, none of them was specific to either of the two sexes. It appeared unlikely, therefore, that the two phenomena might be at all correlated.

121. Schmahl et al. irradiated pregnant NMRI mice on gestational days 11-13 with 3×1.05 Gy and found that only the female offspring had an increased post-natal mortality within 2 days of birth [S59]. It should be noted that this effect was not observed with 3×1.18 Gy. However, within this narrow dose range, the only neuropathological difference between the treated groups was the occurrence of rosette-like lesions after 3×1.05 Gy, which were more abundant in females than in males. This was the reason to associate the post-natal mortality effect with rosette-like lesions in the brain [S60]. Weber and Schmahl [W20] investigated the weight of the brain, its protein content and the activities of two enzymes, acetylcholinesterase and Na,K-ATPase, at various post-natal ages up to 64 days. The treatment resulted in a 50% reduction of brain weight, as compared with controls, with accompanying alterations of the protein content. The activity of acetylcholinesterase was increased in treated offspring at all times, but the differences from control levels were not very high. The activity of Na,K-ATPase was changed slightly, but not significantly. Brain weight, protein content and enzyme levels were not different between male and female animals, either control or irradiated. Thus, these findings do not help in explaining the sex-specific difference.

122. Konermann [K11] exposed mice during organogenesis (6-13 days p.c.) or fetogenesis (14-18 days p.c.) to gamma rays (10-80 R/day) and studied the growth-retarding effect of the treatment on the brain. He found that under these conditions the capacity for compensating the brain growth deficit became smaller the later in development that irradiation took place. Even in the absence of appreciable embryo or fetus killing, the growth-retarding effect of the exposure continued at long term. Daily fractionated treatments at 6-10 days or 5-9 days p.c. resulted in death as well as in some deficit of brain weight. The uptake of

tritiated thymidine into brain DNA at birth was decreased in irradiated as compared with non-irradiated animals, but at the end of the first and at the end of the second weeks in neo-natal life it appeared to be increased. At this latter time the amount of uptake followed an increasing function of dose and, therefore, of the brain growth retardation. This abnormal response was interpreted as an overshoot in the recovery processes, due to the fact that microneuron and glial cell proliferation, which occurs during early post-natal development, is stimulated in inverse proportion to the radiation-induced killing of neurons.

123.   Other papers by Konermann et al. [K12, K36] summarized a variety of post-natal effects induced by pre-natal and perinatal x irradiation of the albino mouse brain with doses of 0.25-0.5 Gy. Biphasic patterns of increased brain cell proliferation occurred during the time of myelination gliosis after acute or daily fractionated exposure to radiation. Such overproliferation was, however, insufficient to make up for the loss of brain weight and was only confined to glial cells, so that the organ could not recover its specific functions. Other damages in the lipid uptake, myelination and formation of the tigroid substance were also reported. Biochemical and histochemical responses fluctuated with time, while structural and cytoarchitectural damage persisted in post-natal brain. The changes described were induced by irradiation throughout the advanced stages of intra-uterine and the post-natal development in the mouse, as might be expected from the normal pattern of development of the CNS in this species. Disruption of cerebellar architecture in mice given various doses of gamma rays from ^{137}Cs at birth (0.5 to 7 Gy) or on day 17 p.c. (2-4 Gy) was also described by Sasaki [S79]. The sensitivity of fetal mice appeared to be lower than that of mice irradiated post-partum. The changes described were of different severity and persisted at 900 days of age.

124.   As to functional effects, Minamisawa and Sasaki [M42] studied the electrocorticogram (ECG) of hybrid mice irradiated at 17 days p.c. or at birth with x rays (300 R). The ECGs were recorded on the freely moving animals by permanently implanted electrodes fixed over the surface of the visual cortex when the animals were 6-8 or 24-26 months of age. From the pattern of changes observed, the authors concluded that the adult and aged mice, irradiated when in utero or at birth, showed ECG responses that were characteristic of later ages in control groups. This was interpreted as evidence of an accelerated "aging" of the ECG pattern brought about by the radiation treatment. In its 1982 report [U5], UNSCEAR commented at length on the impossibility of defining "aging" at the tissue or organ level by means of any morphological or functional test.

(b)   The rat and the guinea-pig

125.   In an attempt to reconcile differences between morphological and teratological findings after x irradiation, Berry and Rogers [B15] provided a description of the development of the rat cerebral cortex, studied by labelling with tritiated thymidine between the 16th day

in utero and birth. They were able to establish that the neuroblasts present on days 16-17 migrated to infragranular layers V and VI; those found on day 18 to layer IV; and those found on days 19-21 to layers II and III. The ependymal cells retained a physical connection with the superficial and deep strata of the cortex by means of their long processes, which provided a channel through the cortex along which the neuroblasts migrated. Not until completion of migration did these cells separate from the ependymal processes to start differentiation. Therefore, in this species also the formation of brain cortex occurs from the inside out, as was later shown in primates and man (see I.B.2).

126.   In contrast with the paucity of data on the development of the cerebrum in the rat [B15, B30, B38], there is relatively more data available on cerebellar development [A12-A14, L10]. It may be deduced from the whole of the information cited that the growth spurts of the cerebrum and cerebellum are very similar in the rat and the mouse; and that while the cerebrum shows a sharp peak of mitotic activity around 14-15 days p.c., the cerebellum shows its most active wave of cell production 6-10 days after birth. Any study that does not take into account the peculiarities of each structure is therefore bound to be inaccurate, considering the developmental complexity of the phenomena described.

127.   Berry and Eayrs [B30] described the effect of x irradiation of the fetus (200 R) on the histogenesis of the cerebral cortex and the morphology of neurons. Exposure at 19 days of gestation resulted in widespread destruction of cortical cells 12 hours after irradiation, with signs of recovery and differentiation of the surviving neurons at 24 hours. Evidence was also found that under these conditions the ependymal layer had lost its capacity to contribute further, as in the normal situation, to the histogenesis of the cortex. A variety of morphological cell abnormalities were described in the irradiated neurons. The germinal layer, the mantle layer and the actively migrating cells appeared to be selectively destroyed, while cells which had completed migration remained relatively unharmed. The distribution pattern of dendrites appeared to be little affected by irradiation, although the number of primary dendrites and the amount of branching was less than normal, suggesting that the capacity of these cells to establish interconnections with incoming axons was greatly reduced.

128.   According to Semagin [S9], exposure of pregnant Wistar rats from day 16 of pregnancy to delivery into a ^{60}Co irradiation field between 0.0008 and 10 R/day (8 hours/day) reduced the whole-body weight of the new-born animals and increased significantly the absolute weight of the brain. The effect could not be attributable to oedema. Thickening of the cerebral cortex (in the absence of any microscopically detected destructive changes) was also described. The author attributed this finding to a stimulating effect of low-dose-rate irradiation on the cerebral cortex and was obviously aware of the peculiarity of this conclusion in the face of other experimental and clinical data. The same author [S75] irradiated 26 non-inbred rats

in utero on the 18th day of pregnancy (1 R) and tested them (together with 25 controls) for conditioned reflexes, starting at 45 days of age. In the irradiated animals, there was a slowing down in the consolidation of conditioned reflexes and a weakening of such reflexes. Conditioned natural reflexes were found to be more pronounced than in the controls, a phenomenon explained by an impairment in the co-ordination of movements. Irradiated animals also showed an increase in the magnitude of intersignal reflexes during conditioning of differentiated responses. In the author's opinion all these findings are evidence for the harmful effect of the radiation treatment.

129.   Inouye [I1] studied, in the cerebral cortex of rat embryos exposed to 200 R at 17 days p.c., the development of histopathological changes from 1 hour p.c. to late in post-natal life. Cell killing of the brain cortex was described as an early change which later resulted in profound disturbances of the fibre formation of the corpus callosum, with reduction of its size. These defects were also recognizable in irradiated animals which reached adulthood. As to the cortex, disturbances in cell migration were seen, resulting later in a hypoplasia of layers II-IV, abnormal branching and irregularity of the dentritic processes of pyramidal cells in layer V. Tridimensional reconstructions of various sections of the brain showed marked hypoplasia of the cortex, the basal ganglion and the thalamus.

130.   Following a suggestion that there may be species differences in the relative contribution of the different layers of the neocortex to the development of the corpus callosum, Jensen and Altman [J5] made use of the sterilizing effect of x irradiation given at various pre-natal ages to kill the late-generated neurons in the rat. They found that the late-generated neurons residing primarily in the supra-granular layers are essential for the formation of the corpus callosum. Reyners et al. [R29] irradiated with x rays on the 15th day p.c. rat embryos with doses of 0.1-0.5 Gy, and examined them at various times between 1 month and 2 years after irradiation. They found that the depth of the cingulum bundle, a myelinated substructure of the corpus callosum, was a sensitive indicator of radiation damage at doses of 0.2 Gy. The authors traced the origin of the anatomical damage to a disorder in the sequence of morphogenetic events, rather than to a process of radiation-induced cell killing.

131.   In experiments involving the use of ^{137}Cs gamma rays (1.75 ± 0.08 Gy) administered to pregnant Sprague-Dawley rats on gestation days 16-19 (day 1 was considered to be the morning after mating), Jensen and Killackey [J13] investigated the subcortical projection of cortical neurons that had been caused to take up an ectopic position by the radiation treatment. The study was carried out by a labelling technique with horse radish peroxidase applied when the rats had reached 30-80 days of age. It showed that the radiation treatment given before, during, or after the production of neurons destined for layer V in the neocortex and projecting to the spinal cord resulted in their abnormal location. One ectopic location, typical

of rats irradiated on or before day 17, was in clusters beneath the cortical white matter bordering the dorsomedial aspect of the lateral ventricle. The other location was between layer V and the pial brain surface, which was seen in rats exposed at any time between day 16 and 19. In spite of their abnormal position, all these neurons projected to a sub-cortical target appropriate for level V, indicating that neither the migratory path nor the final position of the neurons was essential for specifying their target. Furthermore, the fact that peri-ventricular ectopias occurred after irradiation on day 17 and earlier suggested that the projections of the cortico-spinal neurons are determined early in their individual ontogeny, prior to migration. In view of the high dose used, the importance of this paper lies more with the implications for mechanisms, rather than with any consideration of risk.

132.   Adult rats exposed in utero to x rays (0.09 to 0.49 Gy) on day 15 p.c. were killed at various ages for electron microscopic analysis of different brain parameters selected to provide quantitative information. The x-ray treatment reduced the body size of both nerve and glial cells in the central cortex and produced an increased packing density of these cells. The reduction in cell size appeared to be the primary factor in these changes because, when the data were appropriately corrected, the number of cells per unit volume of cortex was not significantly modified by the radiation treatment. It appeared as though the brain had suffered a sort of miniaturization process, rather than a loss of cells as a result of cell killing. Defects of synaptic arborization were also described. A dose-related decrease of blood capillaries in the cortex was reported from these studies, which, when appropriately corrected for the reduction in cortex thickness, became statistically significant at the dose of 0.49 Gy [R25].

133.   A comparison of the neuronal damage induced by irradiation in chick and rat embryos was attempted by Schneider and Norton [S8]. They carried out an analysis of cells at the telencephalic-diencephalic border on neurons which show morphologic similarities in the two species. Analysis involved nuclear size, the content of cytoplasmic acetylcholinesterase and the presence of several branched, spiny dendritic processes. These authors were able to establish that 1 Gy in the 7-day chick embryo had about the same effect as 1.25 Gy in the 15-day rat fetus. They interpreted the similarity of the response of an avian and a mammalian species to mean that maternal factors in mammals may be of little significance for the radiation response of these structures.

134.   A fair amount of information has also been reported in regard to cerebellar damage. Das [D3] exposed 18 days p.c. rat embryos to x rays (170 R) and collected specimens of the cerebellum at various times thereafter, from 1 hour to 30 days post-natally. Six hours after irradiation, the author described pyknosis of cells in the external granular layer along the posterior part of the cerebellum. The neuroblasts, that would later develop into Purkinje cells, were found arrested in their migratory pathway. Some recovery of the external granular layer was seen at later stages, but

an abnormal clustering of neuroblasts resulted as a permanent architectural abnormality during post-natal development. Malformation of the folia in the cerebellum, and the smaller size of this organ, were described as the long-term sequelae of the treatment.

135. Given that development of some brain structures continues in the rat well after birth [D19] it is not surprising that similar changes could also be induced by post-natal irradiation of the rat 5 days after birth. According to Korogodin and Korogodina [K14], animals exposed to various doses of ^{60}Co gamma rays, and killed at 30 days of age, showed disorganization in the location of the Purkinje cells which was dose-related with a maximum at the low lethal doses. Here again, the increase of disorganization was accompanied by a decrease of the cerebellar weight and an impairment of some electrophysiological parameters.

136. In experiments by Inouye [I6], a quantitative analysis was attempted of the cerebellar malformation induced by exposure to x rays (100 or 200 R) administered to pre-natal rats on one gestation day from 16 to 21 p.c. The changes described were those to be seen at 60 days of post-natal age in surviving animals. After the highest exposure, there was a slight reduction of the weight, but not of the width, of the organ. The dorso-ventral length of the cerebellum was reduced, the more so the earlier x irradiation had taken place. A description of the diameters and arrangements of hemispheres and lobules, as altered by the radiation treatment, was provided. Histo-logically, an ectopic appearance of Purkinje cells in either the granular cell layer or the white matter was seen in rats treated on days 20 or 21 p.c., but not for irradiation at earlier stages. The size and the archi-tectural disposition of the cerebellum after 100 R were only mildly altered.

137. Inouye and Kameyama [I7] studied the effects on the matrix cells in the cerebellum of rats exposed to several single doses of x rays ranging from 0.03 to 1 Gy. Exposure took place at 0, 3, 6, 10, 13 and 17 days of post-natal age. Animals were killed 6 hours after exposure and the organ was processed for scoring of the frequency of pyknotic cells in the external granular layer along the primary fissure. Pyknosis was significantly increased by the lowest dose level of 0.03 Gy. At all irradiation times, the incidence of pyknotic cells increased linearly with dose in the range of 0.03 to 0.25 Gy and then increased more rapidly at higher doses, suggesting a linear-quadratic trend. The highest response was seen in animals irradiated at 6 and 10 days of age.

138. A quantitative analysis of cerebellar develop-ment was performed by Inouye and Kameyama [I10] on F334/DuCrj male rats exposed between 0 and 17 days post-partum to single whole-body doses of 0.25, 0.5 and 1 Gy of x rays. When these animals reached the age of 8 weeks, they were killed and measured for body, brain and cerebellum weight. None of these parameters, nor their ratios, appeared to have been altered by the treatment. Microscopically, the only effect reported was a reduction of cell counts

in the molecular layer of the cerebellar decline. This was statistically significant only in animals given 1 Gy at 6 days of development and amounted to about 17%. There was no gross cortical abnormality to be observed in the cerebellum.

139. Concerning behavioural functional effects, ex-periments were reported in which rats were exposed at 17 days of gestation to x irradiation (150 R, 200-kVp) and males were reared after birth under enriched (EC), standard (SC) or impoverished environmental conditions (IC) for 30 days after weaning [S57]. Standard conditions implied large cages with three or four rats; impoverished conditions implied isolated cages with animals housed singly; and enriched conditions implied cages where many animals lived together and had various objects to play with, such as ladders, tubes, balls and boxes. The irradiated animals, together with an appropriate number of controls, were then tested in a maze for their performance, using a standardized behavioural technique. The effects of radiation and of the different environmental condi-tions were both significant in initial, repetitive and total error scores and running time. At later times, it was found that the differences between the EC-SC and EC-IC were significant in irradiated rats, whereas only the EC-IC difference was significant in controls. A 20% decrease in brain weight was present in irradiated animals, as compared with controls. X-irradiated animals, compared with controls, revealed a decrease in total protein, protein per gram of cortex, total benzodiazepine and muscarine receptor bindings and muscarine cholinergic receptor binding per milligram of protein in the cortex. However, all these indices were not significantly different in animals reared under different environmental conditions. Other experi-ments by the same group had shown that at 200 R the radiation effects were very evident and those of the environment virtually absent [K35], while at 100 R irradiation was essentially insignificant and environ-ment very important in respect of the performance of irradiated microcephalic animals [S73]. The conclusion from the experiments on the intermediate 150 R exposure was that environmental enrichment is a useful tool to alleviate the learning impairments induced by irradiation in pre-natal animals.

140. In other experiments by Tamaki and Inouye [T8], a facilitation of the avoidance behaviour was found in rats that had been exposed to x rays (200 R) on their 17th day of gestation. The primordial hippocampus of these animals showed extensive cellular damage. The facilitation described was thought to be a consequence of a strong tendency to running induced by the shock and was related to the hippocampal damage.

141. Bornhausen et al. [B17] studied the learning ability of rats and reported data on animals irradiated in utero on days 6-9 of pregnancy with 4 daily doses of 0.01 Gy. When tested at 4 months of age, using behavioural tests in which the performance require-ments were gradually increased, the animals showed a significantly impaired function, particularly when they were required to perform the most difficult tests.

Preliminary data were also reported by the same author [B40] on rats irradiated in utero on day 13 of pregnancy with doses of gamma rays from ^{137}Cs in the region of 0.15-0.9 Gy. In addition to showing a large variability of performance from one animal to another, the data indicated that performance deficits depended more on the time of exposure than on dose.

142. In another paper [M17], the locomotor damage present in adult rats after irradiation in utero (days 14-17 p.c.) was studied. Alterations in gait were found after 125 R given on days 14-16. Exposures of 50 R on day 14 and 125 R on day 17 induced no effect on locomotion. Hopping or alternating, waddling gait, accompanied by abnormal positions of the hind feet, resulted from such treatments. By histological examination of the brain, these effects could be traced back to lesions of the corpus callosum and the telencephalic commissures.

143. Hudson et al. [H5] reported that neo-natal x irradiation induces, at 7 days of age, changes in the metabolism of monoamines in the brain of rats. The concentrations of norepinephrine and serotonin increased in all the regions of the CNS showing rapid growth and proliferation of the axons, but not in the regions of the cell bodies from which these transmitters originate. The increase of the concentration was attributed to the increase in the rate of synthesis. These changes were to be seen up to about 3 weeks of age, but the monoaminergic system returned to normal when brain maturity was attained. Such changes were interpreted as reflecting a disturbance in the density of nerve endings in the regions where these terminate due to the radiation-induced disturbance in cell proliferation. Cerda et al. [C10] irradiated young rats at 5, 10 or 25 days of post-natal life with doses of 1-8 Gy of ^{60}Co gamma radiation and followed the fate of the DNA strand breaks in the brain cells between 1 and 180 minutes of irradiation. The number of breaks induced per gray was found to agree with earlier data on small intestine and spleen mouse cells. It was also found that by 30 minutes after treatment the radiation-induced double-strand breaks in the brain were repaired in all age groups tested.

144. Wanner and Edwards [W12] reported on a comparison of the effects of ^{60}C gamma radiation and hyperthermia in inducing retardation of brain growth in the guinea-pig. To this end, they exposed pregnant animals on the 21st day of pregnancy to gamma-ray doses of 0.32-3.75 Gy delivered at dose rates of 0.043, 0.069 or 0.125 Gy/minute; or to 42.5-43.5° C for one hour. The offspring were killed within 24 hours of birth for examination of the viscera and weighting of the body and brain. Doses of 0.04-0.99 Gy produced a dose-related, irreversible reduction of the brain weight, but had little effect on the weight of the body. Hyperthermia also resulted in microcephaly of the offspring. The relative effectiveness of the two agents was such that a dose increment of 0.525 Gy produced a brain weight loss equivalent to an elevation of the maternal temperature of 1° C. The dose threshold detected by this assay system was between 0.05 and 0.10 Gy of gamma radiation.

(c) Primates

145. In view of the difficulties in obtaining samples from irradiated human fetuses, observations on primates are of particular interest. Brizzee et al. [B8] reported on the gross and microscopic effects in some brain structures (visual cortex, hippocampus and others) of squirrel monkeys irradiated at each trimester of their pre-natal life with ^{60}Co gamma radiation (2 Gy). The total duration of pregnancy in these animals is 165 ± 5 days. In the visual cortex, animals irradiated during the last two trimesters and examined 2 days after birth showed a thinning and a decrease in the number of neurons per cubic millimetre of tissue, although neither of these effects was statistically significant. The spines in the dendrites of the giant Meynert neurons also showed some alterations. In the hippocampus, the thinning of the cortex and the loss of neurons in the irradiated monkeys was statistically significant, as were the alterations in the morphology of dendrites. In the three animals irradiated in the first trimester, gross abnormalities of the brain, urinary system and limbs were seen, but no microscopic observations of the brain were yet available. It is to be hoped that, with an improvement of the morphometric techniques, the careful quantitative evaluation of similar data on primates will facilitate the projection to man of findings from the widely studied rodent species.

146. In another paper by Brizzee and collaborators on the effects of pre-natal irradiation of the squirrel monkey [B10], various morphological and functional end-points were evaluated. Data were reported on 78 pregnant females, either controls or irradiated with ^{60}Co gamma rays (0.1, 1.0 and 2.0 Gy). Irradiation took place at 95 ± 5 days of gestation. Among all females, 55 live births and 23 infant deaths were recorded. Up to the time of reporting, the sex ratio and the percentage of infant mortality were not significantly different between controls and irradiated. On day 2, and during 30 days after birth, body weight, crown-rump length and head circumference were decreased in the offspring receiving 1 and 2 Gy. Various nervous reflexes were also disturbed, as were other tests of behavioural exploration and general motor activity. Temperature was significantly lower, and the respiration rate significantly higher, in these animals. Brain, cerebellum, pituitary and kidney weights were significantly lower after 2 Gy on day 2 after birth. Dendritic spine counts of cortical motor neurons were also significantly reduced after the same dose. The percentage of B lymphocytes with surface IgM and the total blood lymphocytes were decreased after 1.0 Gy at 1 year of age.

147. The same group [O2] reported on the effects of pre-natal ^{60}Co irradiation on the visual acuity, maturation of the retinal fovea and the striate cortex of squirrel monkey offspring receiving between 0.1 and 1.0 Gy at 80-90 days of gestation. The visual acuity of animals receiving 0.5 and 1.0 Gy was significantly lower than that of control animals or of those given 0.1 Gy; these changes were scored in the periods from birth to 30 days and from 30 to 90 days. Morphometric evaluations of the retina at 90 days of

age showed that pre-natal exposure, with a dose of 1.0 Gy, resulted in a significant difference in foveal cone density. In the brain there was a corresponding thinning of the foveal striate cortex at 90 days after 1.0 Gy. The cytoarchitecture of the cortex was also altered.

148. Finally, in another paper [O1], the effects of 0.5 and 1.0 Gy of gamma rays from ^{60}Co given to squirrel monkeys pre-natally between 80 and 90 days p.c. were reported. The animals were studied between birth and 3 months of age for a number of morphological and functional parameters. The circumference of the head, the crown-rump length and (to a lesser extent) the whole-body weight grew at a significantly slower rate after irradiation. The nervous activity of the monkey irradiated at both doses appeared to be less accurate and complete by comparison with that of the controls; the time required for the performance of reflexes and neuromuscular co-ordination was also lengthened. In visual orientation, discrimination and reversal learning, irradiated animals had a significantly decreased percentage of correct responses. Spontaneous light-dark activity was significantly increased in the dark session over that of control. Plasma cortisol was also significantly increased in the animals receiving 1 Gy.

4. Other types of malformations

149. A previously undescribed class of malformations of the skull was reported by Schmahl et al. [S58] on NMRI mice exposed in utero in the late organogenesis stages (11-13 days p.c.) to either a single (200 R) or fractionated (3 × 160 R) x-ray exposure. The developmental stage at irradiation appears to be a critical factor for observation of these effects, because irradiation during the early fetal period (14-16 days p.c.) did not influence the development of the neurocranium, irrespective of the dose applied. The malformations consisted of: (a) small nodules of cranial hyperostosis in up to 90% of the offspring; or (b) an excessive formation of bony tissues, a heterotopic chondrification of the neurocranial capsule in the parietal and occipital bones. Both classes of abnormalities occurred in the presence of a completely normal development of other cranial and facial bones. Malformations of type (b) extended deep into the forebrain and could be seen histologically only in about 10% of the offspring. A growth disturbance of both the mesenchymal skull primordium and the brain was thought to be at the origin of these overgrowth phenomena, in the sense that brain malformations producing a lower intracranial pressure may lead in turn to an abnormal growth activity of the skull sutures, stimulated by irradiation in a hyperplastic direction. For these effects, see also a paper by Meyer [M44].

150. Fractionated irradiation of pre-natal mice in late organogenesis at 11-13 days p.c. induced a marked incidence of hypotrichosis and alopecia in the offspring and led to severe ulcerative dermatitis, starting at 2 months of age. This effect had a marked prevalence for animals irradiated at least on the above days (other fractionation patterns were also tested extending over 11-16 and 14-16 days p.c.). There was

no apparent dose dependence for such an effect within the range of 2.4 to 7.2 Gy total dose, as incidences of ulcers of between about 39 and 48% were observed among the irradiated animals. No sex dependence was apparent, nor was any dependence on the conditions of the animals' housing. Internal organs showed no special sign of alterations, except for a higher incidence of amyloidosis. Keeping animals under germ-free conditions also did not alter the disease pattern or incidence [S62]. The intra-cutaneous administration of skin extracts from affected animals into non-irradiated ones resulted in a marked infiltration of leukocytes, suggesting that the pathogenesis of the lesions may involve a radiation-induced skin dysplasia which is followed by an endogenous leukotactic activity resembling human psoriasis [S63].

151. An observation by Michel and Fritz-Niggli [M8] should be mentioned for its general methodological relevance. These authors studied the effect that confinement and restraining of pregnant mothers (which is often necessary in the course of experimental work) may have on the incidence of malformations in the developing fetus. NMRI pregnant females on day 8 were restrained for 2 to 36 minutes; the fetuses they carried on day 13 had a significantly higher incidence of malformations of all types (but not of any single class). The effect was attributed by the authors to a hormonal discharge of the hypophysis-adrenocortical axis induced by the stress of confinement.

B. DATA FROM MAN

152. Müller and O'Rahilly [M57] published a histological study of a twin at stage 13 showing an opening of the neural tube, believed to be the earliest example of purely cerebral dysraphia recorded so far. The paper is valuable for its careful description of timing of morphological events and mechanisms resulting in anencephaly in man and for a comparison, by means of synoptic tables, of events and stages leading to similar types of malformations in the rat and mouse.

153. The information accumulated since 1977 on the occurrence in man of severe mental retardation following exposure at Hiroshima and Nagasaki is of great interest and must be reviewed in depth. In 1978, Ishikawa [I2] published what is essentially a case report on the long-term follow-up of four patients exposed pre-natally to the atomic explosions and followed for their psychological symptoms over a long time. These individuals had been exposed between 2 and 8 weeks of gestation at distances between 780 and 1180 m from the hypocentre and their mothers had all shown signs of acute radiation sickness. The subjects were between 1.3 and 2.0 kg of weight at birth and were later found to be microcephalic, and physiologically and mentally retarded. Degenerative signs and diseases, as described in the "Epidemiological study on microcephaly" [T5] were also found in these children. This small survey showed essentially that the state of these children was clinically serious and their prognosis over a long observation period of about 20 years should be considered as very severe.

292

154. Ishimaru et al. [I12] published a re-analysis of the anthropological measurements obtained at age 18 in children exposed in utero (and their controls) in Hiroshima and Nagasaki. The paper reported, as a function of dose, the height, body weight and head and chest circumference of these children. There was a statistically significant linear decrease of head and body size with T65 dose for both sexes and both cities (except for height in Nagasaki females), but the interrelationships between the various effects shown was not analysed. There was no apparent correlation between pre-natal age at exposure and head circumference. It should be noted, however, that head circumference was not adjusted for body size, and pre-natal age was treated as a continuous variable, without regard to discrete embryological events.

155. A discussion of the terms "microcephaly" and "mental retardation" is to be found in a paper by Dobbing [D21] who pointed out that such terms are used for conditions of different clinical severity in various reports. Radiation is very effective in producing small head size and mental handicap, but it is only one among many other agents that may cause similar effects. Actually, the precise developmental time at which an agent responsible for such effects is applied is often more important than the nature itself of the agent. Contrary to other teratological malformations, which are induced by a precise, momentary exposure to such agents, microcephaly and mental handicaps are characterized by relatively longer periods of developmental vulnerability lasting hours or days in rodents and other fast-growing species, and weeks or months in man and slowly growing animals. Unlike teratological defects which result in permanent lesions, brain growth disturbances may to some extent be remedied, and much more so the later the affected stage is and the earlier any remedial action is undertaken.

156. A study by Otake and Schull [O3] describes epidemiological findings in atomic bomb survivors in relation to dose and time, thus allowing some rough estimate of the rate of incidence of mental retardation. After exclusion of a few children from the in utero sample at the Radiation Effects Research Foundation (RERF), on account of wrong or incomplete information on date of birth and exposure of the mothers, the sample on which the study was based comprised 1599 children (1251 at Hiroshima and 348 at Nagasaki). For the purpose of the study, mental retardation was defined as incapability "to perform simple calculations, to make simple conversation, to take care of himself or herself, or if he or she was completely unmanageable or had been institutionalized". Most of the retarded children were never enrolled in public schools, but among the few who were, the highest IQ was 68.

157. The stages of pregnancy at the time of the bombing were re-assessed and expressed as the number of weeks elapsed from the presumed time of conception. The dose to the fetuses was expressed in terms of maternal kerma T65 rad, modified by the related attenuation factors for position of the fetus within the body of the mother (both at present under revision), because this was likely to remain, for some time, the only system of individual dose assessment. The alter-native provisional "free-in-air" doses available in 1983 did not appear to change greatly the form of the dose relationships or the estimates of incidence. A detailed account of the findings is given in Table 9.

158. Table 9 and Figure XI show a dose-related increased risk of mental retardation for gestational ages 8-15 weeks and also, to a lesser degree, for ages 16-25 weeks. Table 10 shows the statistical parameters for the evaluation of the relationships between mental retardation and fetal absorbed dose from reference [I11]. It shows that the absolute excess risk per unit absorbed dose for exposure at 8-15 weeks in both cities combined, when zero-dose cases are excluded, is $0.38 \pm 0.09 \text{ Gy}^{-1}$; this value is about 4 times greater than for exposures at 16 weeks and over. Statistical analysis showed that there was little or no suggestion of a non-linear component in the dose-response function at 8-15 weeks. The calculated regression suggests no threshold. Actually, a threshold of > 40 mSv may be excluded only with a probability of 0.20 [P17]. This is not true, in general, for the later exposure times, particularly after 25 weeks of conception, but here the dose-response relationship is weak and not significantly different from zero. Exclusion of 4 mentally retarded cases non-radiation-related (3 with Down's syndrome and 1 with infantile encephalitis) did not alter the above findings appreciably. Although children exposed in utero in the range between 2000 and 3000 m from the hypocentre were not included in this revision, ancillary evidence showed that there was no reason to suggest that the frequency of mental retardation in this group (approximately 5/601 or 0.8%) would be different from that found in the control group (9/1085 or 0.8%). As to the difference between observations in the two cities, the baseline values of 0.6% incidence of mental retardation at Hiroshima and 1.6% at Nagasaki are not significantly different but, if so, could not be explained on any known ground. Differences in other irradiation groups also remain unexplained. Moreover, if the absolute risk of mental retardation per unit dose seen in the more numerous Hiroshima series were used to predict the incidence among those exposed at Nagasaki, given the average dose received by that group, 4 to 9 cases (all ages included) would be expected to appear in that series; 4 cases were actually found.

159. Concerning any possible correlation between mental retardation and small head size, it has been reported [W22, W23] that about 10% of individuals having a head size two or more standard deviations below the mean of all those in the study sample were also mentally retarded. Data on the relationship between mental retardation and small head size are given in [O4]. This subject has been discussed separately by Mole [M9, M10, M21]. It appears that among the mentally retarded children, about 60% had a small head size. Thus, the association between the two conditions is not very close, owing presumably to the fact that loss of neuronal cells is compensated to some extent by over-proliferation of the glia, which may restore the size, but not the function, of the irradiated brain. There is no unequivocal evidence that other types of malformations may be increased in this population of children exposed in utero [M51, P16].

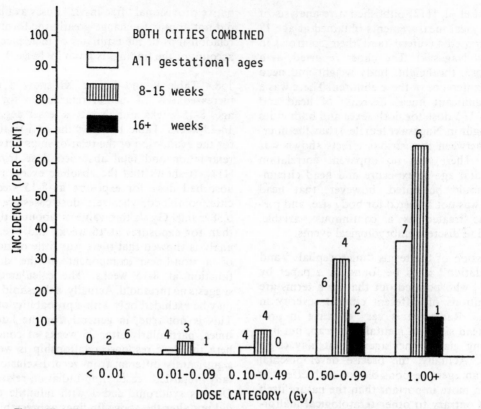

BOTH CITIES COMBINED

All gestational ages

8-15 weeks

16+ weeks

0   2   6   4   3   1   4   4   0   6   4   2   7   6   1

< 0.01   0.01-0.09   0.10-0.49   0.50-0.99   1.00+

DOSE CATEGORY (Gy)

Figure XI. The frequency of mental retardation among children exposed in utero during the atomic explosions in Japan, as a function of dose category and gestational age. (Both cities combined.)
[I11]

160. The existence in this series of a well-defined period of maximum susceptibility of the brain, taken in conjunction with the changing form of the dose-effect relationship as a function of the time at exposure, were discussed in the study by Otake and Schull [O3] in light of the findings reviewed in chapter I, section A. The evidence presented there shows that both proliferation and migration of neurons in the human forebrain are largely completed by the 16th week of gestation, although glial cell production may still continue in the brain cortex up to much later stages in development, with some uncertainty as to the timing and the actual extent of such processes. Also, any distinction between effects on cell proliferation, differentiation and migration is hard to make since these are not taking place at the same time but different cells in different stages are found in the cortex at the same time of development.

161. The apparent linearity of the response at 8-15 weeks warrants some discussion. In view of the non-stochasticity of the phenomena, which is reflected almost invariably in the animal experiments by the curvilinearity (upper concavity) of the dose-response relationships for malformations induced at well-defined developmental stages (see III.A), the finding of a linear trend with dose appears surprising. There are, however, possible explanations for it. Among them: the fact that many cellular events (division, differentiation, migration) may be variously contributing to the observed effect; the fact that the period between 8 and 15 weeks of gestation is very long and that the sensitivity of the neuroblasts and their functions may

change considerably during this time; the fact that the clinical conditions grouped under the definition of "mental retardation" may be of different severity, and that severity may change with dose; the fact that, in clinical judgement, severe mental retardation is an arbitrary cut-off point in the lower portion of a normal distribution curve; and the possible effect of the environmental conditions under which retarded individuals were kept from birth to diagnosis, which might themselves have affected the outcome of any given case. If any of the processes or conditions envisaged were characterized by a curvilinear relationship with dose, but if each of these relationships had different linear or quadratic components, it would still be possible for them to combine in a way that the overall effect might be seen as apparently linear. However, in the present state of knowledge, the linearity of dose-effect relationships from 8 to 15 weeks of gestation must be taken as observational evidence, since our capacity to interpret it in precise radiobiological terms may be inadequate given the complexity of the underlying phenomena.

162. The data reported by Otake and Schull [O3] show quite conclusively that the apparent absolute excess incidence of severe mental retardation per unit dose, under the exposure and observational conditions described, is of the order of $4 \, 10^{-1} \, Gy^{-1}$ at the peak sensitivity period, a figure greater than that given by UNSCEAR in its 1977 report [U2] which was averaged over the whole pregnancy and based on an earlier and much less refined analysis of the epidemiological evidence. They also show that the develop-

mental stages at 16 weeks or later, which coincide in man with the period of synaptogenesis, are distinctly less sensitive to the radiation insult (risk factor about 10^{-1} Gy^{-1}) and that the form of the dose-effect relationship for mental retardation induced at these stages does not exclude curvilinearity. This latter observation would be expected with a non-stochastic type of damage; the decreasing susceptibility with time is to be seen in the framework of the repeatedly discussed concept of maximum sensitivity periods and the time for the changing form of the response agrees closely with the nature and timing of developmental events in the brain cortex (see Figure V).

163. The results of an autopsy performed on a microcephalic child exposed in utero to the atomic bomb deserve some attention, even though they are so far only available in an abstract [N12]. As previously discussed, disturbance of neuronal migration may be an important cause of radiation-induced mental retardation. The morphological consequence of disturbed migration is, of course, the presence of heterotopic gray matter in the brain white matter. The importance of this case (the dose was estimated at 1.75 Gy) is due to the finding of massive inclusions of heterotopic gray matter in the brain hemispheres. This observation confirms in man observations in animals discussed in the 1977 UNSCEAR report [U5], showing the similarity of the basic mechanisms leading to brain abnormalities and the consequent functional defects in all mammals.

164. Another aspect of these findings which deserves mentioning is the relatively high frequency of mental retardation in the control children (of the order of 1%) over lower values reported from other sources. There is, of course a well-known geographic and ethnic variability in the natural incidence of malformations (see I.C.2), to which the high rate of first-cousin marriages in Japan at the time of the bombing may have contributed to some extent. Aside from this, however, the possible effect of malnutrition has been discussed, which was known to be prevailing in Japan towards the end of the Second World War [O4]. There are data on animals indicating that malnutrition may itself produce abnormal development of the brain and brain functions [D18, W13, W32], but no clear effect of synergism with radiation has so far been documented. The extent of malnutrition in the pregnant mothers, and its effect separate from that of radiation in producing mental disorders, would be difficult to quantify and resolve.

165. Another possible confounding factor could be anaemia induced in the pregnant mothers that were exposed to a relatively high radiation dose. While indirect effects on the fetus through the mother's state of health may not be definitely ruled out, particularly at high doses [U2], there are at least some grounds for believing that they may not have played a very major role. Actually, it is known that, to a large extent, lack of haemoglobin concentration or red blood cells in the mother's circulating blood may be compensated by physiological adaptation of the haemodynamic conditions. In addition, mothers carrying congenital anaemic diseases are not known to produce an abnormally high prevalence of mentally retarded off-spring. It seems likely, therefore, as a first approximation, that the high incidence of mentally handicapped children after irradiation in utero may be attributed to a direct action of radiation on the developing nervous structures of the conceptus.

166. A preliminary analysis of intelligence test scores on individuals exposed in utero at Hiroshima and Nagasaki has also been reported [S38]. In the words of the authors, the following is a summary of the major findings: "First, neither tests of skew nor graphical representation of the data suggest a commingling of distributions such as might arise through the inadvertent inclusion of a qualitative different group of individuals, that is unrecognized cases of mental retardation. Indeed, the cumulative distribution suggests a general phenomenon, a shift in the distribution of scores with exposure. Second, there is no evidence of a radiation-related effect on mental retardation or intellection generally for those individuals exposed in the first eight weeks of life. Third, the mean test scores but not the variances are consistently significantly heterogeneous among exposure categories for those individuals exposed at 8-15 weeks after conception, and less heterogeneous for those groups exposed at 16-25, or 26 or more weeks of age. Fourth, regression analyses indicate that among those in utero individuals exposed either at 8-15 or 16-25 weeks of gestational age a significant decrease in intelligence test score occurs with increasing exposure. This obtains whether the eight clinically diagnosed cases of mental retardation to which allusion has been made are or are not included. However, the shape of the dose-response curves appears different; it is linear-quadratic for the 8-15 week group and linear for the 16-25 week group. This is the opposite of the findings with respect to clinically diagnosed mental retardation in the Revised PE-86 sample. Finally, fifth, within the most sensitive group, that is, individuals exposed 8 to 15 weeks after conception, and with the better fitting model, the linear-quadratic, the diminution in intelligence score is 21-26 points per gray . . ." (at 1 Gy). Further analysis and evaluation of these data will have to be deferred until a definitive publication appears.

167. In the present state of knowledge, the action of radiation on the cortical brain function could be visualized as a dose-related shift towards lower values of the normal distribution of "intelligence" as assessed by conventional test scores. Such a shift would take an increasing percentage of individuals at the lower end of the distribution into a region where they would be clinically defined as mentally retarded. As might be expected of a true non-stochastic effect, both the probability of entering such a region and the severity of the retardation would thus be dose-dependent. However, as the clinical definition of mental retardation includes conditions of different severity, it would be difficult to predict the shape of the dose-response relationship for mental retardation. If such an interpretation is accepted, then "severe mental retardation" may be viewed as the extreme consequence of a dose-related loss of mental fuction. Accordingly, irradiation at low doses (say, 0.1 Gy of low-LET radiation) would not result in an increased probability of perfectly normal individuals becoming severely mentally retarded, but

rather in an increased probability that individuals who would otherwise develop to be at the lower tail of the distribution of intelligence test scores may suffer damage that would turn them into mentally retarded, according to the clinical definition of this term.

168. In view of the non-stochastic nature of the damage caused by irradiation in utero, one would expect conditions of lesser clinical importance than severe mental retardation to be present in the cohorts of Hiroshima and Nagasaki exposed pre-natally. In addition to the intelligence test scores mentioned above, it is known that clinical evidence collected from these children over the years is available in respect of a number of other topics, as follows: anamnestic observations, such as the occurrence of convulsions, diplopia, blurring of vision; observations on major landmarks of physical development, such as the ages when the children were able to stand up, to walk, to speak; information on school performance during elementary training (including periods of absence from school on account of disease or other causes), number and types of subjects taken at school with relevant scores over the years, performance as a function of age as the children moved to higher classes, behaviour of the children while attending school; and information on grip dynamometer studies and on repetitive action tests. All these data should give a fairly good representation of the development, neuro-muscular coordination and higher nervous function in the children [S78]. It is to be hoped that this material will be appropriately collated and analysed, because it may give information on man that is of the highest interest and obtainable directly.

169. Granroth [G8] reported a study based on the Finnish Register of Congenital Malformations, which has been in operation since 1963. Defects of the CNS (710 cases from 1965 to 1973 comprising: anencephaly, 199; spina bifida, 239; hydrocephaly, 216; microcephaly, 41; hydroanencephaly, 15) and polydactyly (259 cases, to provide an internal control by a malformation with a strong genetic background) were included. The study was based on a total number of 621,026 deliveries. The effect of radiation exposure (diagnostic x rays administered for medical reasons) on the occurrence of malformations was evaluated in terms of relative risk in a matched-pair case control study aimed at evaluating the association of defects with different types of x-ray examinations received by the mother before or during pregnancy. There was no statistically significant increased risk of malformations to the fetus from pelvis examination of the mother prior to pregnancy. As to examinations received during pregnancy, the risk of malformations after chest x rays was not significant, while for fetal x rays the risk of developing CNS malformations was 2.2 times higher than for those not receiving any examination. For polydactyly, the odds ratio was 1. For abdominal examination of the mother, the relative risk was found to be between 2 and 3 during the various trimesters of pregnancy, but the number of examinations was very small and did not allow any meaningful calculation to be made. In a careful discussion of these findings, the author concluded that the few associations found between congenital CNS defects and diagnostic x-ray

examinations could be explained either by chance (no statistical significance) or by the fact that the defect itself was the probable reason for the x-ray examination. It turned out, in fact, that, although the specific reasons for the examinations were not recorded in every case, the great majority of examinations were performed because of clinical suspicion of either maternal or fetal anomaly.

170. Preliminary data have also been reported of a prospective clinical study started in 1967 to provide advice to parents whose children were exposed in early pregnancy to diagnostic x-ray examinations [N2, N7]. In the course of the study, embryological observations after abortion are carried out and the children irradiated in utero are followed up clinically and genetically. Up to 1982, more than 200 cases had been collected and studies performed on 73 children up to 10 years. One publication dealing with this series [N8] provides useful information as to the time at which irradiation occurred, the doses received, chromosomal analyses of 28 irradiated children, and the instances in which spontaneous or induced abortion occurred. But it gives no information as to the number and type of malformations found in the irradiated children.

171. Further data [N11] on the 73 children followed to 10 years showed that, of those exposed in the dose range below 100 mGy, there were two malformations (3.4%) that could not be associated with radiation because exposure occurred before organogenesis. Another malformation (hypospadia and spina bifida occulta) was found on an aborted fetus: here the exposure time might correspond with the time of differentiation of the organs involved. However, the malformations found are not rare among those occurring naturally. In the dose range above 100 mGy, two embryological abnormalities were found at termination of pregnancy. Cytogenetic investigations on 30 exposed children were negative as were other investigations of 21 biochemical genetic markers carried out on a selected group of 19 children. The results of a wide range of pediatric and laboratory investigations appeared, on the whole, to be similarly negative.

172. The search for a possible increased incidence of disturbances in human development among children born in areas of high background has continued. In a paper from China, Lu [L1] reported on a survey of hereditary ophthalmopathies and congenital ophthalmic malformations in the Guangdong province, comparing two areas where the annual cumulative dose equivalents to the whole body were about 2.5 and 1 mSv, respectively. In the area of low background, 66 out of 13,987 children were found to carry eye malformations, to be compared with 99 out of 13,425 children living in the high-background area. The difference was not statistically significant. Two contributions from Ujeno examined the relationships between gonad dose in areas of Japan and the incidence of various conditions. The first paper [U6] dealt with the presence of Down syndrome and visible malformations among subjects born over a three-year period (1979-1981) in 46 prefectures, where the dose rates of natural background radiation varied between

about 0.4 and 0.9 mSv per year. Over 457,397 subjects included in the survey, there were no statistically significant correlations between dose and the incidence of the conditions examined. The second paper [U7] covered 11 prefectures having about the same spread of gonadal dose rates and 1,899,477 births between 1974 and 1976. The following chorionic diseases were examined: hidatidiform mole, malignant hidatidiform mole and chorionepithelioma. Of these, only the first two showed a statistically significant correlation with gonadal dose rate. However, when all diseases were pooled together the regression on dose was found to be non-significant.

173. Evidence of a decreased weight of female offspring born of mothers irradiated (mostly by thorax fluoroscopy) in the course of pregnancy was reported by Ilina [I8], but her findings are not sufficiently documented. Findings of doubtful significance on the incidence of human malformations were also reported in an abstract in 1972 [E1]. Since brain maturation continues beyond birth in man, data on exposure of juveniles are also of interest in a general sense, such as those reported by Glazunov and Tereshchenko [G14] and by Meadows et al. [M3]. Doses of many grays are, however, involved in this experience, and these are far beyond those of interest in the present context. In addition, the relatively low number of cases involved makes them unsuitable for the purpose of risk assessment.

C. CONCLUSIONS

1. Experimental animals

174. The current data on the irradiation of experimental animals during organogenesis have added significant details to the overall picture drawn by UNSCEAR in its 1977 report, but have not strikingly changed its main conclusions. They have confirmed that the effects resulting from irradiation of the mammalian conceptus during the phase of major organogenesis are characteristically teratological. They have also confirmed that such effects, most common in experimental animals, are essentially not seen in man. Teratogenic effects develop during the intra-uterine life as the growth of the organs proceeds, and they persist, if compatible with extra-uterine survival, during post-natal development. Malformations may also be accompanied by growth disturbances of the various structures or of the whole body. The period of main organogenesis of each structure (for example, the skeleton, the brain, the eye) coincides with the period of maximum sensitivity of that particular structure to the induction of malformations, in the sense that the dose needed to produce a given level of incidence of each malformation is lowest when the spurt of cell multiplication occurs in the relevant structure. Increasing the dose either before or after the peak sensitivity period may, however, result in the same type and degree of effect.

175. As organogenesis proceeds at different rates in different animal species, it is to be expected, and it is

actually found, that malformations of given structures occur in each species at a characteristic time from fertilization. There is, therefore, a very pronounced dependence of each kind and degree of malformation (for a given acute dose to the embryo) on the animal species and its developmental state at the time of irradiation. Spreading of the same dose over a longer period of time by fractionation or protraction tends to reduce the frequency of occurrence for each class of abnormalities below that expected from an equal exposure at the most sensitive stage.

176. The most recent data have added to the evidence that the form of the dose-effect relationship for each specific type of malformation is generally sigmoid, with the malformation rate per unit dose increasing as a function of dose. This evidence is in agreement with the expectation for effects of the non-stochastic type. It applies to the majority of cases when effects were accurately quantified over a sufficiently large range of doses, which happens particularly in the mouse. It also applies to effects as different as skeletal abnormalities or major malformations, disturbances of brain cell kinetics or pyknosis of cerebellar matrix cells. When irradiations at different developmental ages were compared, as for mouse skeletal malformations, the curvilinear form of the relationship was found to become more pronounced as development proceeds. This is also in agreement with the postulated non-stochasticity of the induction mechanisms.

177. Abnormalities of the mouse skeleton have been particularly well analysed, as they may be scored rather effectively and are fairly easily quantified. Although, in general, sigmoid dose-incidence curves adequately describe their induction pattern, the precise shape of the relationship is different for malformations found in different parts of the skeleton. Accordingly, dose-fractionation and dose-protraction regimes affect the various classes to different degrees, with results that may be difficult to predict in terms of the overall responses for the whole skeleton. To give some estimates of incidence, at the time of maximum sensitivity: in one strain of mouse acute exposures of the order of 5 R were found to triple the spontaneous incidence, although there was no further proportional increase, but rather a decrease, from 5 to 25 R. When the effect was examined in terms of the frequency of animals having a normal skeletal structure, no significant deviation from normal could actually be detected up to at least 25 R. In another strain the quantitative configuration of the axial skeleton appeared to be shifted by an exposure of 12.5 R.

178. Malformations of the CNS have been thoroughly investigated, although in this case the quantitative analysis of dose-response relationships has taken second place to the study of pathogenetic mechanisms. From the overall evidence available in experimental animals, it appears, however, that no effects having clearly pathological connotations have been reported for doses in the brain structures lower than about 0.1 Gy of low-LET radiation. The fairly extensive sets of observations on mice, rats and primates shows that,

depending on the time of pregnancy at irradiation, different structures may be affected, although the pattern appears to be fairly uniform in all species when irradiation takes place at similar stages.

179. In very schematic terms (but with many intermediate forms due to the fact that cells in the developing brain may be at different stages of development at any one time), damage to the developing brain cortex may be induced by a variety of mechanisms. Irradiation at the time of active division of the neuroblasts results in the production of fewer neurons and therefore in a loss of function. Damage to the neuroblasts may to some degree be compensated by a hyperplastic reaction of the glial cell which might restore the size, albeit not the function, of the irradiated structures. During the formation of the cerebral cortex, radiation may interfere with the migration of the neurons (by this time, cells are in a post-mitotic stage). Failure of the cells to reach the appropriate cortex layers causes them to be left behind in the white matter as displaced islands of gray matter, thus disrupting the final brain architecture. Radiation may also disturb the establishment of neuronal connections in neurons that are in the course of migration and are taking up their final position in the cerebral cortex. An impairment of the number of dendritic processes of the neurons, and of their secondary branching, results from irradiation interfering with synaptogenesis.

180. There are indications that each process may be differently affected by irradiation at the various developmental stages, the sensitivity of the neurons decreasing as their maturation proceeds; however, no systematic investigation of this point has been undertaken. In parallel, other processes of maturation, such as the myelination of the fibres or the formation of the tigroid substance in the neurons, may be altered. Glial cells may also be affected in both number and function. Qualitative data on these latter mechanisms are still insufficient and quantitative observations only refer to overall structures and not to specific cell types. In other sections of the CNS, such as the cerebellum, essentially similar effects have been described: however, they take place at times and with mechanisms that are characteristic of these structures.

181. Functional deficits resulting from structural damage in experimental animals have not been studied systematically and so far there has been little attempt to correlate precisely the lesions in given brain structures with the resulting loss of the functions under their control. In rodents, disturbances of conditional reflexes, impairment of learning ability and locomotor damage have been reported after various, but mostly fairly high, doses causing, or expected to cause, gross structural damage. Relatively minor functional deficits induced by irradiation in utero have been shown to be alleviated by stimulation of nervous and behavioural activity post-natally, although the more severe damage induced by the higher doses appears to be largely, if not wholly, irreparable. In primates, impairment of nervous reflexes, behavioural and motor activities, visual acuity and orientation and

neuro-muscular co-ordination have been described, but the documentation in this respect is only indicative and therefore insufficient.

2. Human observations

182. In man, teratological effects of the type described in experimental animals are uncommon. As to other abnormalities, a significant step forward has recently been made with a re-evaluation of clinical findings and doses in children exposed in utero during the atomic bombing of Hiroshima and Nagasaki. The latest data show that mental retardation is the most likely type of developmental abnormality to appear in the human species. Severe cases of mental retardation have been included in the study sample. The association between mental deficit and small head size is not very close. In essence, analysis as a function of time shows that the probability of radiation-related mental retardation is essentially zero with exposure before 8 weeks from conception, is maximum with irradiation between 8 and 15 weeks (at the time of rapid neuronal production and migration), and decreases between 16 and 25 weeks when glial cell proliferation and synaptogenesis occur. After 25 weeks and for doses below 1 Gy no case of severe mental retardation has been reported. Analysis as a function of dose shows that the incidence of severe mental retardation is apparently linear for irradiation between 8 and 15 weeks and curvilinear (concave upward) between 16 and 25 weeks. On the assumption that the induction of the effect is linear with dose, the probability of induction per unit absorbed dose at the time of the peak sensitivity is of the order of $4 \cdot 10^{-1} \, Gy^{-1}$ (fetal dose) and of the order of $10^{-1} \, Gy^{-1}$ between 16 and 25 weeks from conception.

183. These findings are important for a number of reasons. First, they emphasize that the most common types of malformation to occur in man are those of the brain cortex, resulting in severe mental deficit. Secondly, they extend to man the notion of a close correlation between the time of most active division of precursor cells of the cortical neurons and the time of maximum sensitivity of the brain cortex to radiation-induced malformations. Thirdly, they show that similar mechanisms of action as those experimentally seen in animals may be operating in the developing human brain, with due allowance for the time scale over which the relevant events occur in different species. Finally, they allow reasonable quantitative estimates of risk to be made for the induction of radiation-induced severe mental deficit in man. While not all aspects of the reported findings may be explained at the present state of knowledge, it is expected that they may have a significant impact in radiation protection in the exposure of pregnant women for occupational or medical reasons. Further developments in respect of functional disturbances of lesser severity than mental retardation may also come from studies currently under way on this cohort of people. Other newly reported observations on radiation-induced malformations in man are much less informative and essentially negative in showing any effect.

IV. THE FETAL PERIOD

184. The 1977 UNSCEAR report [U2] reviewed much information concerning irradiation during the fetal stage of development, pointing out the heterogeneity of the observations. It appeared that lethal effects and growth disturbances had been commonly described for irradiation at high doses, while teratogenic effects became increasingly difficult to document macroscopically as fetal development proceeded. Effects on the eye, the CNS and the gonads were the most commonly described consequences of irradiation during the fetal stage, in addition to a large variety of other effects, e.g., the haematological. The most recent literature has added considerably in some areas, such as the effects on the CNS and on the gonads, but little elsewhere. The effects on the CNS have been considered in III.A, although they actually start to occur at the borderline between the embryonic and the fetal period in man, and extend well into the latter. The present chapter groups the effects on the gonads and on the reproductive system (including external and internal exposure) and all other miscellaneous effects. It should be pointed out that in some experimental series, embryonal as well as fetal exposures are included.

A. EFFECTS ON THE GONADS AND REPRODUCTION

1. The mouse

185. In 1978, following other experiments previously discussed by UNSCEAR [U2], Nash and Sprackling [N1] reported on the reproductive capacity of animals belonging to 13 inbred mouse strains that had been exposed continuously, for a varying number of generations, to ^{60}Co gamma rays. Over the period the experiments lasted, the exposure rate changed between about 7.8 and 0.33 R per 22-hour day. Ancestral and direct exposure values were determined when the animals were removed at weaning from the irradiation chamber and tested for their reproductive performance, using standard tests, to measure percentage fertility, mean litter size and ratio of living to total embryos. Each female (irradiated or control) was classified as sterile or fertile. The latter were killed at the 10th day of pregnancy for scoring of the pregnancy outcome. This included counting, for each litter, the number of resorptions, the number of dead or live embryos, and the percentage of live to dead embryos.

186. The data showed [N1] that for ancestral exposures of 1100 R or greater nearly all females were sterile, but the incidence of sterility at exposures from zero to 200 R was little affected. Response to direct irradiation was found to be more pronounced, with extensive sterility (> 70%) at 200 R or above and no fertile females above 900 R. In the range of exposures below those that induced complete sterility, the overall fertility curves were found to be sigmoid, an observation indicating that this damage is of a cumulative type. Eleven out of the 13 strains studied showed a significant decrease in fertility with increasing ancestral

or direct irradiation. Analyses of variance were carried out to detect the presence of linear, quadratic and cubic components in dose-effect relationships, or possible strain differences which might be reflected on total litter size or on the ratio of living to total embryos. In each instance, strain effects were found to be significant. Litter size was more likely to be affected by radiation than the ratio of live to total embryos. Interpretation of these results is made difficult by the fact that the results of similar experiments reviewed previously by UNSCEAR [U2] do not compare in design with this series, so that it is not clear to what extent the differences might be attributable to the different designs or to the methods of scoring and analysis.

187. Adult female mice of the strain A/J received tritiated water by injection on the day of fertilization, so that the tritium content in the body water was brought promptly to levels of about 310, 31 and 3.1 kBq/ml. They were also started at the same time on drinking water containing about 480, 48 and 4.8 kBq per ml of tritium to maintain the initial levels during the entire periods of pregnancy and lactation. Female F_1 offspring thus exposed from conception to 14 days of age were killed at this time for counting the total number of oocytes in serial sections of their ovaries. It was calculated that the whole-body doses accumulated in the 33 days from conception to killing were from 0.79 Gy to 0.0079 Gy at the highest and lowest levels of contamination, respectively. The numbers of primary oocytes were lowered by the following percentages with respect to control: at 0.79 Gy, more than 90%; at 0.079 Gy, 30%; at 0.0079 Gy, 13%. It must be noted that the lowest level of tritium contamination is substantially below those previously reported to cause measurable biological effects in mammals. The dose-effect relationship was said to be exponential and without threshold within the dose interval referred to above, indicating that, in a female mouse exposed continuously from conception to 14 days of post-natal age, the level of tritium that may be expected to result in a 50% loss of the number of germ cells is about 74 kBq per ml body water, corresponding to 0.12 Gy [D8].

188. After reporting that a single injection of 5 MBq tritiated water/g body weight, given to pregnant mice on gestation day 9, reduced the reproductive performance of the offspring [T7], Török and Kistner examined this effect systematically as a function of the activity administered and of the day of administration [T1]. The injection time (a single intraperitoneal administration of 5 MBq/g to the mother, corresponding to a pre-natal dose of about 1.3 Gy) was varied between 5 and 13 days p.c. In addition, three activity levels were tested at this latter time (5, 2.5 and 0.625 MBq/g, corresponding to pre-natal doses of 1.3, 0.6 and 0.2 Gy, approximately). At 2 and 3 months of age the offspring were mated, in single pairs, with control mice of the other sex for 10 days consecutively and then separated. Mice were also set up for histological analysis of the gonads. Fertility was not influenced by treatment on gestation days 5 or 7, but starting from day 9 p.c. in females, and from day 11 p.c. in males, a 50-100% decline by comparison with

controls was found. Administration of tritium on gestation day 13 had the greatest effect. Male fertility was less affected. At 2 months of age, all males and 40% of the females were infertile, while at 3 months female fertility declined and male fertility tended to improve. These observations were broadly in accordance with histological findings. Analysis as a function of dose showed that the fertility of both sexes was affected by doses in excess of 0.5 Gy, while, at a constant dose rate, 3.3 Gy from HTO would be needed to decrease reproductive performance. The late organogenesis stages were found to be the most sensitive under these conditions.

189. Török et al. [T7] reported a significant decrease in the weight of brain and genital organs at 4.5 months in the offspring of NMRI mice given a single intra-peritoneal injection of tritiated water (2.6 MBq/g) at 9 days of pregnancy. The number of oocytes in the ovaries was reduced and the seminiferous epithelium of the male mice was considerably damaged. These mice had been found to be fertile at 2 months of age, while at the same age doses twice as large affected the fertility of females but not that of males, and doses four times as large resulted in sterility of both sexes. At 18 months of age, the ovarian tumour incidence of the controls (14%) was increased almost 5-fold (67%) by the administration of about 10 MBq/g of tritiated water. As to effects before or at birth, about 20 MBq/g at 7, 9 or 11 days p.c. resulted in 100% peri-natal mortality, increased resorption and stunting, but negligible incidence of gross external or skeletal malformations. Administration of tritium in excess of 37 MBq/g caused maternal death. In the offspring, damage to the prosencephalon and the gonads stood out generally as the most prominent histological finding.

2. The rat

190. Coffigny and his group [C5] reported on experiments in which pregnant (14 to 21 days p.c.) and new-born rats of up to 2 days of age received a single dose of 1.5 Gy of ^{60}Co gamma radiation. Neo-natal mortality, body weight and adult brain weight were investigated. Among the effects found, germ cell killing was particularly notable. This became the subject of another publication [C7] in which the observations were extended to animals irradiated between 10 days p.c. and 6 days after birth, with the same dose being delivered. When the male animals irradiated in utero reached adulthood, they were studied for testis weight and histological appearance, for the weight of the epididymis and seminal vesicles, and for testosterone plasma concentrations. Testis weight was found to be slightly reduced by irradiation at day 15, but progressively more so at later times, with a maximum between 18 days p.c. and 3 days after birth. A reduced number of spermatogenic cells in the seminiferous tubules accounted for the reduction in mass of the organs. The weight curve of the epididymis followed, in the main, that of the testis but the weight loss of the seminal vesicles was rather moderate. Testosterone secretion was not adversely affected, suggesting that the endocrine function of the testis is, on the whole, rather resistant, as might be expected.

191. The same conclusions were drawn from another study [C6] in which the adrenal activity of male and female rats was tested after 1.5 Gy administered on day 15 of gestation, the time when the hypothalamic nuclei and the pituitary and adrenal glands begin to differentiate. When the irradiated animals reached adulthood, their brain mass was severely decreased, both absolutely and in relation to the whole body mass. The weight of the pituitary and adrenal glands was also reduced absolutely, but not in relation to the whole-body weight. The functional activity of the hypothalamo-pituitary-adrenal axis, as measured by adrenal and plasma corticosterone levels, their diurnal variations, their response to stress or pharmacological challenge were found to be normal, in spite of the gross lesions of the brain and gonads.

192. Reported changes in the fertility of females irradiated during the stage of major organogenesis are scanty. Shapiro [S53] noted the occurrence of sterility in 36% of female animals that had exposures of 50 R at 9 days p.c. Tests conducted by Kakushine and Plodovskaya [K29] showed that 70% of rats exposed to 250 R on day 20 p.c. were sterile.

193. Pietrzak-Flis [P5] investigated the effects of low doses of tritiated water or organically bound tritium ingested chronically, on the number of oocytes in the ovaries of contaminated rats. After adjusting the ^{3}H concentration in water and food to levels that would give similar total ingestion, female rats were exposed starting 5 weeks before mating with a non-exposed male and up to the 21st day of life of their offspring. Female offspring of the F_1 and F_2 generation were sampled at 3 weeks of life for tritium analysis and oocyte counts. There was a close similarity of the doses calculated in different tissues between animals receiving tritiated water or organically bound tritium, although the contribution of the non-exchangeable tritium to the total dose was on average 3 to 7 times higher in animals fed tritiated food than in those drinking tritiated water. A lower (although not statistically significant) number of oocytes was found in contaminated females than in controls. On the basis of some simplifying assumptions, it was calculated that the mean dose to the ovaries was 73 mGy. This led to a 10% loss of oocytes, both in F_1 and in F_2 animals. It appeared, therefore, that the total absorbed dose, rather than the form under which tritium was administered, was the variable that mattered most for oocyte survival.

194. In a subsequent series of experiments [P15], the same author exposed rats continuously to a constant activity of tritium in the drinking water or to organically bound tritium from the time of conception of the F_1 generation through maturity. She calculated that the two groups of animals exposed to tritiated water had a mean absorbed dose rate in the ovaries of 7.25 ± 0.37 and 14.73 ± 0.79 mGy/day, respectively. The group receiving tritium-contaminated food received on average 4.84 ± 0.25 mGy/day. Female offspring were killed when 21 or 71 days old for oocyte counting. The reduction of the number of oocytes in the animals exposed to organically bound tritium was larger (for the same dose rate) than in the animals

exposed to tritiated water, and the dose-rate dependence of the reduction of small oocytes was of an exponential type. The damaging effect of tritium appeared to be higher between birth and 3 weeks of age than between 21 and 71 days of age. The highest sensitivity to tritium irradiation was seen in small oocytes and in oocytes with one complete layer of follicle cells; disappearance of these highly sensitive cells resulted, in turn, in an increased relative frequency of growing and large oocytes.

3. Other animals

195. Fractionated x-ray exposures (0.115 Gy per fraction given twice weekly up to 2 Gy) were administered to 12 female bonnet monkeys either between 48 and 104 days or between 77 and 133 days p.c. Follicle counting in the animals' ovaries was performed between 3 months and 1.6 years of their post-natal life. Animals exposed in the first group had a number of follicles approaching that of non-irradiated controls (about 2000), while the others revealed severe ovarian damage, abortive oogenesis, and reduction of the follicle counts to less than one-third of the normal. No other damage in any organ was found except in the ovary [A5, A6].

196. Data concerning gonadal damage by pre-natal irradiation are also available in the cow [E3]. Cows bearing conceptuses of varying ages from 40 ± 5 days p.c. (when gonadal sex differentiation occurs) to 270 ± 10 days (about 2 weeks before birth) were irradiated once with ^{60}Co gamma rays (300 R), an exposure known to be just below that likely to cause maternal death and gross abnormalities in the product of conception. This resulted in an absorbed dose in the fetal gonads estimated to be about 1 Gy. When female offspring reached about 10 months of age, their ovaries were histologically analysed to count the follicles in different stages of maturation. Primordial follicles were significantly lowered (to 64% of control) for exposure between 70 and 90 days of gestation. Since at this stage the germ cell population is characterized by a high proportion of mitotically active oogonia, it was deduced that this class of cells is the most vulnerable to radiation. Follicular development, however (as shown by counts of growing and vesicular follicles), was apparently unaffected by irradiation at all ages tested. Cows irradiated pre-natally under the same conditions at 80 ± 10 or 130 ± 20 days p.c. had a fertility rate and a reproductive performance that were not different from controls over at least five years of post-natal life and three pregnancies.

4. Interspecies comparisons

197. When Dobson et al. [D25] examined the effect of tritium on fertility by measuring the life-long reproductive capacity of treated mice, they found that reproduction was less affected than germ cell number. For doses causing early oocyte losses of 80-90%, the number of offspring only decreased by 20%. However, initial oocyte deficiencies of about 50% resulted in a premature end of reproductive life. Despite well-known differences between the radiosensitivity of human and mouse oocytes (see annex A), the authors attempted an extrapolation between the two species, using tritium data from monkeys. They concluded that pre-natal irradiation was likely to result in premature menopause in women and could possibly follow "relatively low exposures".

198. Two papers [D9 and E2] attempted some interspecies comparison of gonadal cell sensitivity in utero under internal and external conditions of exposure, respectively. Dobson et al. [D9] exposed mice from conception to 14 days of age to tritium in drinking water and established that the concentration required to cause 50% loss of oocytes under these conditions was about 74 kBq/ml of body water, delivering about 0.0056 Gy/day. Female germ cells of squirrel monkeys required an even lower level (about 19 kBq/ml) for the same end-point. Over the full 153 days of gestation of the species, this level would correspond to a total dose of 0.168 Gy, which might further drop to 0.056 Gy if the sensitivity of the oocytes were confined to the last third of gestation. These data are in sharp contrast with the well-known radioresistance of primary oocytes in monkeys and man to acute x-irradiation exposures. It must be assumed, therefore, that the germ cells in the fetal primate are going through a highly sensitive period of short duration, occurring probably around the middle of the last trimester of gestation in the monkey, at which time doses of less than 0.05 Gy are sufficient to cause 50% killing. It appears that in mice this stage of high sensitivity is maximum between 5 and 19 days post-partum, a time at which susceptibility is also high in respect of the toxicity of the polycyclic aromatic hydrocarbon 3-methylcholanthrene. Similarities between rodent and primates, and between radiation and chemically related sensitivity, suggest that there may also be a highly vulnerable period for the oocytes of the human fetus located approximately at the middle of the third trimester of pregnancy, which might represent a special hazard in relation to chronic exposure.

199. Erickson [E2] irradiated continuously, throughout gestation, mice, rats and guinea pigs at rates of 0.01 to 0.03 Gy/23 h day. Pigs were also irradiated continuously for 108 days of gestation at 0.0025 Gy/23 h day. In all species, the gonads were sampled at birth or at 6 days of age and the numbers of germ cells per organ were estimated as a function of dose. The D_0 and extrapolation numbers (n) were calculated to be as follows, on the basis of a single-hit multi-target model:

		D_0(Gy)	n
Pig	male	0.28	0.8
	female	0.27	3.2
Rat	male	2.75	0.3
	female	1.59	0.8

The low value of the extrapolation number suggests that in both males and females (but especially in the former) the germ cell response is dominated by single events. The value of 0.3 for the extrapolation number in male rats could also be attributed to heterogeneity in the composition of the irradiated cell population with respect to their sensitivity to radiation exposure.

200. After irradiation at 0.01 Gy/day throughout pregnancy, the germ cell counts were reduced to the following percentage of the controls in the species tested:

| | Total dose (Gy) | Percent of control | |
		Male	Female
Pig	1.08	1	5
Guinea pig	0.62	41	71
Rat	0.21	50	90
Mouse	0.20	71	87

These data show that the pig is by far the most sensitive species with respect to continuous irradiation during the pre-natal period, but this conclusion does not take into account the large interspecies differences in the length of the developmental period of the male and female germ cells. The paper [E2] provides useful data for the relevant comparisons, collated from other reports and from original work (references are to be found in publication [E2]). The data are summarized in Table 11.

201. Erickson's data [E2] show that in spite of the large variation of the kinetics of primitive germ stem cells in the various species, the pig remains the most sensitive species even when total doses (rather than dose rates) are used as the basis for comparison. The data also show that male germ cells are more readily killed by protracted exposure than female ones as a result of both their kinetics and of the protracted period of vulnerability. However, the data do not offer a satisfactory account of the relatively lesser susceptibility to acute than to protracted regimes of irradiation, because they may not entirely explain how the refractoriness to acute exposure of a significant segment of the primitive germ cell population might be overcome by chronic exposure. The differences shown in Table 11, and various arguments put forward in the paper, point to the need to extend consideration of this subject and of the relevant interspecies comparisons much more than has been the case so far. Sensitivity to mitotic delay, in addition to cell killing, will have to be explored further and in a systematic manner in future work.

B. OTHER MISCELLANEOUS EFFECTS

202. A number of other miscellaneous effects have also been described. Thus, for example, Swiss albino mice irradiated in utero at days 11 1/4, 14 1/4, 16 1/4 and 18 1/4 p.c. with ^{60}Co gamma rays (150 or 250 R) showed a dose-related decrease in the number of goblet cells in the crypts (and to some extent also in the villi) of the gut at 1 day and 1, 2, 4 and 6 weeks post-partum [M46]. Chajka and Lobko [C16] studied rats irradiated with x rays at 12-14 days of fetal age and investigated from day 13 to 22 the formation of the paramesonephral tracts, describing in detail disturbances in the development of the vagina.

203. Gerber and Maes [G4] investigated the radio-sensitivity of blood-forming stem cells in the bone marrow and the spleen during the fetal hepatic period (18 days p.c.) and during the post-natal and adult phases of haematopoiesis. On the basis of their capacity to produce spleen colonies in heavily irradiated transplanted mice, the stem cells isolated from the fetal liver had a D_0 of 1.29 Gy, as compared with 0.70 Gy and 0.86 Gy for the spleen and marrow cells of adult animals, respectively. Together with a decrease in the D_0 values after weaning, the percentage of cells in the S-phase and the rate of division of transplanted cells in the irradiated hosts also decreased. There was, however, no significant difference in the D_0 values between haemopoietic cells in all phases of the cell cycle and the ^{3}H-thymidine-sensitive cells in the S phase.

204. Weinberg and her group [W24, W25] described disturbances of B6D2F1 mouse and HA mouse [W33] haematopoiesis found at various times of pre- and post-natal life and induced by irradiation (0.5-3.0 Gy, ^{60}Co) of the animals at 10.5 days p.c. They consisted essentially of disruption of fetal liver cellularity, morphology and haematopoietic cell concentration extending to 14 weeks of extra-uterine age. The same authors also examined haematopoietic alterations in the beagle dog irradiated during mid-gestation at 33 days p.c. (an age corresponding approximately to that of the 10.5 day-old mouse) with 0.9 Gy from ^{60}Co gamma irradiation [W21]. Various blood indices were investigated at 42-59 days of gestation. Differences between irradiated and non-irradiated animals included a decrease of nucleated cell counts in the peripheral blood between 44 and 49 days, followed by an overshoot at later times; changes in the size and haematopoietic activity of the spleen; an overall decrease in haematopoietic functions of the fetal liver; and an increased activity of the bone marrow. The experiments left undecided whether the observed changes might be due to direct radiation damage on the migrating stem cells or to a radiation-induced defect of the intercellular interactions in the micro-environments that regulate haematopoiesis.

205. In other experiments [M2], pregnant sows were exposed to whole-body gamma radiation at rates of 1.5, 3, 9, or 20 R per day (exposures actually lasted 22-23 hours per day) for 108 days of their average gestation period of 112 days. After 3 weeks of continuous irradiation, all groups had depressed leukocyte counts which were generally related to the exposure rate. Counts remained low throughout the whole irradiation period and they did not completely recover even 3 weeks after discontinuation of exposure in post-natal life. As to the effects on the piglets, those that had been exposed to 3.2 R/day showed no effect on the leukocyte system, and those in the 7 R/day group had a moderate lymphocytopenia at birth which rapidly disappeared. This differential effect between adult and fetal animals took place in spite of the fact that the fetal leukocyte system is functionally mature during the last 5 weeks before birth.

206. To facilitate extrapolation of the above data, it should be recalled that in man the first blood cells and blood vessels are found in the extra-embryonic mesenchyme at about 18 days from conception. This

first period of haematopoiesis is succeeded and gradually replaced by blood formation within the embryo, chiefly in the mesenchyme of the liver, during the second month of development. At still later stages, starting from the 11th week on, a third period of haematopoiesis commences in the bone marrow and the lymph nodes. There is considerable overlapping between the three periods and it is only the last type of haematopoiesis that persists normally in adult life [H27]. Data obtained directly on human samples are, however, very rare. In one paper, no post-natal abnormality appeared to be associated with fetal exposure in the range of 0.01-0.03 Gy of 498 children born during 1963-1977 and examined when 5-19 years old. There were after birth 5 deaths due to accidents or acute infections, but the 493 survivors were normal in respect to stature, peripheral blood counts, mental development and, in females, menarche [L3]. In contrast, 25 children exposed in utero to diagnostic x irradiation after the 8th month of intra-uterine life to estimated doses of about 0.03-0.2 Gy showed significantly lowered leukocyte counts at 2 days and 1 year after birth [Z4].

207. Konermann [K33] reported a post-natal study of the liver of mice in which he analysed, as a function of dose and time, the growth response of the organ in animals that had been irradiated in utero. The animals were exposed to between 10 and 60 R/day during different periods of their pre-natal life, as follows: blastogenesis (1-5 days p.c.); organogenesis (6-13 days); fetogenesis (14-18 days); early embryogenesis (6-10 days); and late embryogenesis (11-15 days). In addition to weight, the content of DNA and, the ^{3}H-thymidine uptake into liver cells were followed for up to 11 weeks after birth. All irradiated animals showed a periodical increase of the proliferative liver growth, especially between the end of the first and the beginning of the second post-natal week. This proliferation decreased with the age of the irradiated conceptuses, from a clear over-compensation during blastogenesis to poor response during fetogenesis. There was also a dose dependence of the effect which (during organogenesis) was biphasic, in the sense that compensatory proliferation was small at 10 R/day, maximum at 40 R/day, and declining at 60 R/day. Overall, these responses were interpreted as attempts by the organ to attain a pre-determined normal size, but appeared to differ in many respects from the hypertrophic regenerative changes induced by post-natal liver damage. First, pre-natally induced proliferation affects, at the same time and to similar extent, both the haematopoietic and the parenchymal cells of the fetal liver, which are considered to be functionally independent components of the organ. Secondly, this compensatory growth is maximum at similar developmental stages and the maximum is not greatly dependent on the radiation dose and on the age at irradiation. Finally, radiation-induced growth stimulation of the liver appears to take place in the absence of any change or even in the presence of a decreased overall body weight.

208. About 100 beagle dogs exposed to ^{60}Co gamma radiation (270-435 R) at 55 days p.c., or at 2 days post-natal age, were examined at 7 days and at 2 and 4 years of age for effects of radiation on the kidney [J2]. Morphometric studies showed an arrest of development and maturation of the organ. For pre-natal exposure, the density of mature glomeruli was 45% less than in non-irradiated controls, while for post-natal exposure the density was only 24% less. At 2 and 4 years, a smaller reduction was observed in the same direction (37 and 32%, respectively). Glomeruli that were mature at the time of exposure underwent progressive sclerosis, characterized by proliferation of the mesangial cells and increase of the mesangial matrix, leading to a reduction of the lumen of the capillaries and the complete obliteration of many glomeruli. Thus, about 21% of the animals died from chronic kidney failure before 4 years of age: this condition was more common in male (19/58) than in female dogs (2/41), pointing to a major sex difference of unexplained origin.

209. It was also reported in the same series of experiments [L2] that an exposure of 100 R at 55 days p.c. resulted in about 80% of the animals having missing teeth, compared with about 57 and 26% in animals irradiated at 2 days p.c. or in control dogs. The upper and lower premolars were the teeth most frequently absent.

210. Developmental toxicity evaluations do not often include functional deficits, but are mostly limited to gross effects such as embryo lethality, malformations and growth disturbances. In a methodological contribution, Andrew [A7] proposed the study of developmental enzyme patterns as a means of directly evaluating the integrity of metabolic competence of developing organ systems. The full complement of enzyme activities is usually developed in mammals in a characteristic sequence: alterations from this normal pattern may occur at three periods, namely, the late fetal, early neo-natal and weaning times. The author argued that qualitative or quantitative changes in the patterns of development of one or more key enzymes in a tissue might be taken to indicate developmental toxicity. Some contributions reported along those lines in respect to radiation toxicity were already discussed in the 1977 UNSCEAR report [U2].

211. Some papers from the USSR dealt with disturbances of the enzyme levels in the liver of rats irradiated in utero. The first [S51] reported a reproducible decrease of the glucose-6-phosphatase activity observed in 21-day old fetuses that had been irradiated with 2 Gy on day 9 p.c. As was later shown, this decrease may be removed by the administration of exogenous thyroxine [K25]. The second paper [S52] reported increased tyrosine aminotransferase activity in new-born rats irradiated with 0.5 Gy on the 9th day after conception. This effect correlates with the status of the cyclic-AMP system. It was proposed that the above effects in the liver of the rat at term, following irradiation during early organogenesis, may result from changes in the amount of inductors [K25].

212. Brain weight and enzymatic activities were also investigated by Weber et al. [W8]. In an attempt to develop more sensitive end-points of damage by pre-natal irradiation, NMRI mice received a range of

doses (x rays, 0.24 to 1.9 Gy) on the 12th day of gestation. They were then sampled at various times between birth and 64 days of age to investigate the weight of their brain and the levels of acetylcholinesterase and of Na,K-ATPase in the organ. Brain weight was related to the enzyme activities in a non-linear fashion: for both enzymes there was a relatively flat dependence up to a brain weight of 350 mg (corresponding to a control age of about 17 days) and a steeper relationship as the brain weight increased. The weight of the brain was reduced in increasing proportion to dose to reach about 40% of control after the highest dose. The data were interpreted to show that, in spite of this reduction, the developmental maturation of the organ was not retarded.

C. CONCLUSIONS

213. As the growth of the anatomical structures established during the phase of major organogenesis proceeds during fetal development, fewer teratological malformations are being produced for the same radiation dose. However, more subtle changes, often documented at the microscopic level, and growth defects of the developing structures, are commonly described. During fetal development, the periods of most active growth of anatomical structures are also, in general, those that are most susceptible to radiation action. Approximate dose-effect relationships may be established for both external and internal exposures in the best documented series.

214. Among the many effects produced by external irradiation of fetal animals, those on the developing gonads have been particularly well described for a variety of animal species to a reasonable degree of quantitative detail. In the mouse, studies were made of both the inactivation of gonadal cells and the ensuing loss of reproductive performance when the animals reached sexual maturity. For external irradiation, female fertility was not appreciably affected up to 200 R of ancestral irradiation, but sterility increased conspicuously when the same exposure was delivered directly to a developing animal. Pronounced sigmoid relationships appeared to prevail for the impairment of reproductive capacity, and a good degree of inter-strain variability has been documented.

215. In the mouse, experiments on internal tritium irradiation were reported after long-term exposures from conception up to 14 days of age, as well as for single treatments delivered at various times during development. Under the first condition of exposure, the activity of tritiated water needed to cause a 50% loss of oocytes in the female gonads was estimated at about 74 kBq per ml of body water (corresponding to a uniform whole-body dose of about 0.12 Gy) with an apparently exponential relationship between absorbed dose and oocyte killing. For single injections, the late stages of organogenesis were the most sensitive in respect to loss of fertility. In both sexes, fertility was affected by doses in excess of 0.5 Gy, but male gonads tended to recover at longer times from treatment, while female fertility continued to decline.

216. In the rat, external radiation exposure resulting in doses of 1.5 Gy caused measurable male germ cell killing, which persisted long after birth without evidence of any adverse effect in the endocrine function of the gonads, or of the hypothalamo-pituitary-adrenal axis. Tritium, given as tritiated water or as organically bound tritium over many generations to developing animals, caused a loss of oocytes in the female gonads for doses of the order of 0.07 Gy. In the bonnet monkey, fractionated exposures up to a total of 2 Gy for periods of about 50 days during the latter part of pregnancy resulted in a consistent loss of oocytes, which persisted into adult life. The same is true for cows irradiated in utero at doses of 1 Gy during the phase of active mitotic division of the oogonia at 70-90 days p.c. However, there was no evidence in these animals that fertility and reproductive performance would be affected, at least over the initial period of their reproductive life.

217. Valuable interspecies comparisons of the sensitivity of the developing gonads under internal and external radiation exposure have also become available. For one species of monkey, there is evidence that the germ cells go through a highly sensitive period of short duration around the middle of the last trimester of gestation when doses from tritiated water, of the order of 0.05 Gy, might cause one-half of the oocytes to die. For external irradiation, comparisons of various species showed the existence of a wide scale of sensitivity values. It is clear that the intrinsic radio-sensitivity of the gonadal cells, together with their kinetic characteristics, determine in the various species the apparent sensitivity of the irradiated germ cells. It is necessary, therefore, to make comparisons between species, not only in respect of dose-rate, but also in terms of total dose received by the germ cells during the whole sensitivity period. When this is done, paradoxical effects such as an apparent higher response of the developing testis to protracted than to acute irradiation are found. This is indicative of the existence of phases of high sensitivity in the development of the male gonadal cells, an effect known to occur also in the adult testis. Much remains to be done to resolve and clarify these inter-species differences upon fetal irradiation.

218. A variety of miscellaneous effects have also been described for irradiation of fetal stages. The blood-forming system has been closely investigated, but detailed analysis of the radiation action is made difficult by the transition from the hepatic to the adult type of haematopoiesis which occurs before birth. Acute doses of a few tenths of Gy, or continuous exposures to a few roentgen per day, are necessary to elicit consistent changes in the blood-forming organs and the peripheral blood of the fetus. The persistence of the changes observed throughout the post-natal ages, and their significance in respect of normal haematopoiesis, are difficult to evaluate. Time- and dose-related hyperplastic reactions of the irradiated fetal liver, both in its haematopoietic and parenchymal component, have also been described. They may generally be interpreted as compensatory regeneration stimulated by the radiation-induced killing of cells. But they have a distinctly different character from the

regeneration phenomena induced by post-natal liver damage. Kidney lesions may also be induced by irradiation during the fetal stages. This damage primarily affects the capillaries and is mostly manifested by glomerulosclerosis resulting in chronic kidney failure during extra-uterine life.

219. Finally, attention should be drawn to recent attempts to develop tests of toxicity induced in irradiated fetal organs by measuring the level of enzyme activity and the development of the characteristic adult enzyme pattern. These tests are different from macroscopic or microscopic methods for scoring of malformations because they aim at documenting functional, rather than morphological, derangements from normal. While they may turn out to provide more sensitive techniques of assaying the radiation-induced damage in utero, their full methodological potential, and their relevance to clinically documented detriment, remain to be established.

V. INTERNAL IRRADIATION

220. The information available to UNSCEAR up to 1977 was insufficient for statements of general validity regarding the effect of radioisotopes taken in by the mother and irradiating conceptus. Given the chronic nature of the exposure, any evaluation of the effects and risks must be based on a precise knowledge of the dose accumulated at each particular stage in any given developmental structure, but the achievement of such a task for all nuclides and all possible conditions of administration is still far away. UNSCEAR identified a number of variables which may interact in the production of any end-effect. They are: the physical and biological characteristics of the nuclide; its chemical form; the route and the dosage schedule of administration; the kinetics of the radioactive material in the mother-fetus complex; the developmental stage at the time of treatment in relation to periods of maximum sensitivity; the species and age-related variables; and, finally, the role of maternal exposure, particularly at high doses.

221. Information in this field that has come to the attention of UNSCEAR since about 1977 has added somewhat to the previous knowledge. However, this is hardly significant compared with what is required to produce widespread generalizations relating the level of uptake of radioactive substances by the mother to the probability of effects that might be expected in the conceptus. The following paragraphs summarize the main new findings regarding the various nuclides.

222. The methodologies for the study of placental transfer have been reviewed [S16]. Moreover, factors influencing the transfer of non-radioactive substances injected into the mother have been discussed by Klinkmüller and Nau [K7] who have compiled a review of the transplacental passage of drugs through experimental observations carried out on aborted children. Some information on the placental transfer of proteins in the human species is also to be found in a paper by Dancis et al. [D2].

223. Stieve [S66, S68], Roedler [R27] and Roedler et al. [R28] reviewed experimental literature (see also a report by Ahrens et al. [A11] for a bibliographic list) and discussed the general aspects of exchange and transfer mechanisms of radioactive substances between the mother and the conceptus as they vary with the time of intra-uterine development, and the various physical and biological factors governing such transfers. It is obvious from these analyses that the need to determine experimentally the transfer coefficients and their inter-species variability prevents any straightforward extrapolation from animal to man. Examples drawn from experiments using tritium, iodine, calcium and caesium were given to illustrate the complexity of the problems involved in assessing the rate and amount of transferred radionuclides. Transplacental transfer of iron in animals and man have also been discussed [F9, T14]. Data referring specifically to tritium have been provided by Moskalev et al. [M15], and a compilation of data for the radioactive nuclides of iodine, iron, strontium and caesium has also been made available to UNSCEAR [S81].

224. Ovcharenko [O10] examined the transfer of radioactive substances from the mother to the newborn through lactation and concluded that the rate of transfer is governed by a number of factors similar to those affecting the passage across the placental barrier. In particular, he reported on an inverse relationship between the rate of transfer and the mass number of the radionuclides, in addition to a profound influence of the animal species and the body weight of the offspring. He pointed out, however, that the main factor in the amount of radioactive material passed on to the offspring through the milk is the level of radionuclide in the mother's blood.

A. EXPERIMENTAL DATA

1. Tritium

225. Yamada et al. [Y1] investigated the response of pre-implantation BC3F$_1$ mouse embryos to chronic exposures of both tritiated water or ^{60}Co gamma rays. Embryos were cultured in vitro in chemically defined media containing tritium oxide at activity levels from 3.7 to 74 MBq/ml. Taking the progression of 50% of the embryos to the blastocyst stage as the end-point for survival, the activity needed to achieve this end-point (LD$_{50}$) was found to be about 4.9, 8.5 and 16 MBq/ml for pronuclear, early 2-cell and late 2-cell embryos, respectively. In comparison with the chronic ^{60}Co treatment, the RBE of the beta radiation of tritiated water was calculated to be between 1.0 and 1.7. On the basis of other experiments on the induction of chromosomal aberrations in mouse zygotes fertilized in vitro, the RBE values for tritium were reported to be 1.8 and 1.5, relative to ^{60}Co gamma rays and to x rays, respectively [M56].

226. In another study [S18], an attempt was made to compare the outcome of tritiated water and tritiated thymidine treatments on pre-implantation mouse embryos cultured in vitro. Also in this study, the end-

point scored was the ability of the embryos to reach the blastocyst stage; tritiated thymidine was about 1000 times more effective than tritiated water in inhibiting blastocyst formation. The treatment with tritiated water was particularly effective in inhibiting the late stages of blastulation, while thymidine blocked the rapid cleavage stages. Thymidine was concentrated in the nuclei through DNA incorporation by a factor of about 1000. In very general terms, and under specific assumptions applying to the system analysed, it was concluded that there was a reasonable agreement between the dose per cell nucleus and the inhibition of blastocyst development, such that about 19 kBq/ml of tritiated thymidine corresponded to about 19 MBq/ml of tritiated water. Observations on the development of pre-implantation mouse embryos, and a discussion of effects in relation to path length and energies of the electrons emitted by ^{3}H and ^{35}S, are to be found in a paper by McQueen [M1].

227. Spindle and Pedersen [S74] investigated the effect of ^{3}H-thymidine on the development of early mouse embryos by counting the number of embryos forming blastocysts, trophoblast outgrowth, inner cell masses and differentiated primary endoderm and ectoderm. Embryos were cultured from the 2-cell stage continuously for 8 days in the presence of ^{3}H-thymidine in various concentrations. Concentrations as low as 7.4 Bq/ml reduced the percentage of embryos forming the two differentiated primary layers. At 370 Bq/ml, the embryos developing to the three post-blastocyst end-points were also reduced. Exposure of the embryos for 1 day at various developmental stages produced effects that were less severe than for continuous exposure for 3 or 8 days. The sensitivity of the embryos differed with stage: the high sensitivity of the inner cell mass to ^{3}H-thymidine, while persisting through the late blastocyst stage, declined progressively thereafter. Autoradiography experiments showed that the radiosensitivity changes of the embryos or of the inner cell mass were generally related to their capacity for incorporation of thymidine into the cell DNA.

228. Yamada and Yukawa [Y4] fertilized BC3F1 mouse oocytes in vivo or in vitro and then cultured the embryos in vitro up to the stage of blastocyst in the presence of chronic irradiation from tritiated water or thymidine, or under acute x-ray exposure in the range of 10-600 R. Taking the development of the embryo to the blastocyst stage as the end-point, the sensitivity of the embryos to the β radiation of tritiated water was confirmed as in Yamada et al. [Y1], while the LD$_{50}$ for tritiated thymidine was given as about 0.63 and 3.96 kBq/ml for pronuclear and late 2-cell embryos, respectively. The highest sensitivity to killing by acute x irradiation occurred at the beginning of the pronuclear formation.

229. Some papers dealt with tritium uptake and turnover in pregnant and fetal animals. Saito et al. [S34] exposed pregnant mice of the Heiligenberger strain to tritium in drinking water as methyl-^{3}H-thymidine at the level of 18.5 kBq/ml. The new-born animals were either nursed by their mothers that continued to drink the tritiated thymidine, or by foster mothers drinking non-radioactive water. The authors

measured in the offspring, at various ages, the incorporation of tritium into the small molecular components of the acid-soluble fraction, lipid, RNA, DNA and proteins. At the time of birth, the specific activity of the isotope in the DNA was highest in the heart and lowest in the thymus. Soon after birth, the total radioactivity per gram of tissue declined with a half-life of 2.5-2.9 days in the spleen, liver, intestine, stomach, thymus, lungs, kidney, heart and brain in the mice nursed by the non-contaminated mothers. By about 2 weeks post-partum, a slower component of tritium elimination was emerging, mainly due to the DNA-bound isotope. On the assumption that the total and DNA-bound activity is uniformly distributed in individual organs and tissues, the cumulative absorbed doses in various organs were worked out for the first 4 weeks after birth. These doses were found to be highest in the spleen (1.15 mGy) and lowest in the brain tissue (0.13 mGy). The tritium ingestion from milk in suckling animals was found to be a rather minor source for dose accumulation in the DNA-bound tritium of the cell nuclei of various organs. Similar data were also presented in another paper by the same group [S35].

230. Lambert and Phipps [L7] infused SAS/4 mice continuously during pregnancy at four activity levels, such that the new-borns would be contaminated with organically bound tritium in concentrations of 10.4-130 MBq/kg body weight. Total doses in utero were calculated to be in the four injection groups 0.15, 0.4, 0.76 and 1.72 Gy. The tritium content of various organs was measured in the mice at frequent intervals up to about 2 months of age, and again when the animals died. Full pathological investigations were performed. Early effects were seen, such as reduction of litter size, changes of the sex ratio, and neo-natal mortality, particularly at the two highest activity concentrations. These effects were judged to be more significant overall than late ones, such as a reduction of the long-term survival time which appeared in the highest activity group. There was an indication of an increased incidence of neoplastic and non-neoplastic lesions, possibly related to the intra-uterine dose; however, the significance of the various causes of death could not be judged without a full statistical analysis, which was not performed.

231. Wang and Zhao [W34] performed an experiment in which the effectiveness of β radiation from tritiated water and gamma rays from ^{137}Cs was compared in respect to their capacity to reduce cerebral development in Wistar rats. Females were injected with HTO in various concentrations on the first day of pregnancy and provided from then on with tritiated drinking water, so as to maintain the tritium concentration in body water approximately constant throughout pregnancy. The intra-uterine dose rates in the five groups of animals examined were estimated to be 0, 0.005, 0.012, 0.02 and 0.038 Gy per day. Other pregnant females were irradiated during 22 hours per day throughout gestation with a ^{137}Cs source at 7 dose rates between zero and 0.12 Gy per day. There was a good negative correlation between the size of the cerebral mass at birth and the cumulative radiation dose in the two series. Approximately the same

reduction of the brain weight was produced by 0.22 Gy of β radiation delivered over the whole pregnancy as by 0.47 Gy of gamma radiation (RBE about 2.14). At higher total cumulative doses (0.84 Gy and 1.3 Gy, respectively) the RBE was found to be lower (1.55). A significant decrease of the whole-body weight at birth was only found for cumulative gamma doses of 1.76 Gy or higher. No dose dependence was seen at lower dose levels.

232. In experiments by Lyaginskaya [L9], rats were given single intraperitoneal injections of tritium oxide (33 MBq/g) on days 4, 11 and 17 of pregnancy. This treatment was said to have resulted in fetal exposures of about 4.12, 3.00 and 2.50 Gy, respectively, by the end of the pre-natal life and 412, 420 and 478 Gy by the time of weaning. The descendants of three successive generations of the injected animals showed a reduction of life span and an increased frequency of tumours. The average life span in the various groups was as follows:

Treatment time	Life span (days)		
	First generation	Second generation	Third generation
4th day	378	394	280
11th day	556	705	288
17th day	705	735	618
Controls	910	1060	1020

Thus, the greatest reduction of life span was shown by the third-generation descendants and by the offspring of animals treated early in pregnancy. The overall tumour incidence increased in the offspring from the first to the third generation and was again highest in the offspring of animals injected on day 4.

233. Gerber and Maes [G3] raised pregnant BALB/c mice on food enriched with tritiated thymidine from the day of conception until delivery, for a total tritium intake of 4.8 MBq. At birth, and again at 4 different times up to 109 days of age, the tritium content was measured in the DNA, protein and supernatant fraction of various parenchymal organs. It was found that a total of 2.0-2.5% of the total activity in the neonatal mouse was incorporated into the DNA, while a slightly larger amount entered the proteins and lipids together. Most organs showed two metabolic components of the DNA, one with a half-life of the order of 10-20 days and another (amounting to 10-30% of the total activity incorporated into DNA) with a very slow turnover, of the order of 100 days.

234. Data along similar lines were also reported in the pig, after exposure of pregnant sows to tritiated water (about 19 and 55 MBq/liter) during pregnancy and for 43 days after birth, up to a total of 120 days [V7]. Some of the new-born pigs were left with the mother and the others were foster-fed by non-contaminated sows in order to follow the tritium oxide and organic tritium in different organs. This allowed the study of the loss of activity after birth, the metabolism of tritium under conditions of continuing exposure and the importance of uptake through milk. The turnover time of tritium oxide in the adult sow was found to be about 10 days, that in younger pigs about 8 days. There were, in addition, components of

slow turnover, amounting to less than 5% of the total. At equilibrium, the ratio of specific activity of tritium oxide in organic matter to that in tritiated water ingested was about 0.7 for body water in adult and new-born pigs and about 0.14 for organic tritium in most tissues. The ratio was higher (0.22) in the brain of the new-borns than in other tissues. The turnover times, in days, for organically bound tritium were as follows: brain, 59; muscle, 28; kidney, spleen and pancreas, 22; liver and intestine, 17. It was estimated, in conclusion, that the contribution to the integral tissue dose due to organic tritium was between 0.3 and 0.7 that from tritium oxide alone, although in the brain this contribution may equal or even exceed that from tritium oxide.

235. Carsten [C15] described a broadly based programme designed to evaluate the somatic and genetic hazards of continuous exposure to tritiated water for two generations in the mouse. The levels used were between about 11 and 110 kBq of tritium per ml of drinking water and the relative biological efficiency was obtained by comparing the effectiveness of such a treatment with that from continuous exposure to ^{137}Cs gamma. The end-points for comparison were dominant lethal mutations, chromosomal aberrations in the cells of regenerating liver, increased sister chromatid exchanges in bone marrow cells and changes in the bone marrow cell and stem-cell numbers. The RBE for HTO ingestion for all these effects was assessed to be between 1 and 2, compared with external gamma exposure.

236. A series of papers dealing with the effects of chronic exposures to tritium on brain development has been published by Zamenhof et al. [V2, Z1, Z2]. Female rats (F_0) were given tritiated drinking water (110 kBq/ml) from 60 days of age until and throughout pregnancy [Z1]. The maximum concentration of radioactivity in these animals was reached at 30 days and in the blood at 42 days after the beginning of the treatment. Under these conditions, the average dose to the cell nuclei was estimated to be 0.0078 Gy per day. The consumption of water and food and the changes of body weight before and during pregnancy in these animals did not differ from non-contaminated controls. The course of pregnancy and time of delivery were also normal. The highest specific activity in the newborn animals (F_1) was found in the nucleic acid fraction, but the bulk of radioactivity was contained in body fluids. These animals showed no sign of radiation-induced effects. The weight of the new-born animals was normal, but 60% of them had haematomas, oedemas, and subdural haemorrhages, which disappeared subsequently by the time they reached 30 days of age. No haematological changes were observed as a function of age, the only exception being a significant decrease of alkaline phosphatase. In spite of a normal brain weight, these animals had a significantly low content of DNA, protein and protein/DNA ratio in this organ. The administration of tritiated water was continued in the F_1 animals throughout weaning, adolescence, and subsequent pregnancies in the F_3, F_4 and F_5 generations. Analysis of cerebral damage in F_3-F_5 rats showed that this was not more evident than in F_2, i.e., that the effects of tritium were

not cumulative over the generations. There were, on the contrary, indications that brain damage might be less pronounced.

237. The same scheme of tritium administration was followed in other experiments by the same group [Z2]. The brains of the irradiated animals were studied at 30 and 120 days post-natally within each generation. Significant decreases were reported in weight, DNA and protein contents of some parts of the brain and the most pronouced effects were found in the diencephalon. Protein losses were more pronounced than those of DNA and the effects were overall more conspicuous at 30 than at 120 days and in the fifth than in previous generations. There was an attempt to explain these phenomena by considering the periods of maximum sensitivity of the brain structures involved, possible effects on the mothers in each generation and the capacity for repair following the radiation-induced damage to nucleic acids.

238. In other experiments [V2], female rats of 60 days of age were started on tritiated water (110 kBq/ml) and killed when 90 days old. The ovaries were excised and the oocytes removed by puncturing the follicles. Examination of the chromosomes in these cells showed that their rate of maturation was not affected by the presence of tritium. When the offspring of these females were examined at birth, the number of cells in the cerebrum was only slightly decreased as compared to controls. Other rats were exposed to tritium from 30 days before mating to 6 days after mating. This treatment was found to depress the decidual response. The offspring of this group of animals had a significantly lowered number of cerebral cells at birth. This effect was even more pronounced when exposure was continued throughout the pregnancy.

239. Finally, Radwan [R1] carried out a comparison of chronic exposure to tritiated water or organically bound tritium to study developmental (startle response, righting reflex, age at eye opening) and behavioural (diurnal and nocturnal locomotor activities) effects. Wistar rats received tritium at a concentration of 37 kBq/ml in drinking water, or at about 48 kBq/g in food, or no tritium at all for 2 generations. From the overall results, it was concluded that, for the same activity level, continuous exposure to the organically bound tritium was more damaging than that to tritiated water, despite the higher cumulative doses delivered to the brain of the animals by means of drinking water. This may mean that the higher tritium incorporation into the organic fraction of the brain after exposure to the tritiated food is responsible for the effects observed.

2. Radioactive nuclides of iodine

240. Several reports have become available concerning thyroidal exposure during developmental stages. One of them [B6] concerns the metabolism of ^{131}I in guinea-pigs during the last two weeks of gestation. The animals were killed at various times (from 5 hours to 9 days) after injection, and the blood, amniotic fluid,

thyroid glands and other tissues were sampled. Over the time indicated, the concentration of the isotope was consistently less in the blood of the mother than in that of the fetus. Moreover, concentration in the fetus was less than that in the amniotic fluid. Peak concentrations of ^{131}I in the thyroids of both the mothers and the fetuses were found at 3 days post-injection. In the fetal thyroid (per gram of tissue) the concentration was 3 times higher. The biological half-life of the nuclide in the thyroid gland was about 3 days in the fetus and about 11 days in the mother. Between 7 and 9 days post-injection, the ^{131}I in the maternal thyroid increased, and this phenomenon was interpreted to show a recycling of iodine within the pregnant animals.

241. Another group analysed the kinetics of dia-placental transfer of ^{131}I in rats fed either standard or iodine-deficient diets [S69]. Female animals were started on diets containing 41 or 320 ng of iodine per gram of food a few days after their birth. When they became pregnant, they received intravenously (on each gestation day from 17 to 20) 0.74 MBq of ^{131}I and were killed at various times (up to 24 hours) from injection. Five fetuses per female were counted for radioactivity in toto and another 5 were dissected for measurement of radioactivity in various tissues, as well as in the blood and the amniotic fluid. The ^{131}I activity concentration per gram of tissue in the fetal thyroid rose by a factor of over 1000 between day 17 and 20 of fetal age. By day 19, 35% of the radioiodine in the fetus was in the thyroid. The concentration in the fetal thyroid never exceeded that of the mother's, at least up to day 20, and it appeared to decrease from day 19 to 20. The uptake of the nuclide in the thyroid of the mothers fed the iodine-deficient diet was much higher and much more rapid than in that of the mothers kept on the standard diet. As to the uptake in the fetal thyroid, it was found to be higher at 2 hours in the offspring of the iodine deficient mothers, but by 8 and 24 hours from injection it had fallen to values lower than in the control group. These phenomena were explained on the ground that the high uptake of iodine in the thyroid of the mothers receiving a deficient diet resulted in a decreased diaplacental transfer of the nuclide available for uptake by the thyroid of the fetuses.

242. A third report [B7] is of relevance in the context of releases to the environment under normal or accidental conditions. It refers to man, and it contains calculations of the doses delivered to the thyroid glands of various age groups in the population (fetuses of 13-40 weeks of gestation, infants of 1 or 2 years, children of 5, 10, 15 years and adults), by different concentrations of inhaled or ingested iodine nuclides (^{129}I, ^{131}I, ^{132}I, ^{133}I). These calculations were carried out on the basis of assumed parameters concerning the weight of the thyroid, the biological half-life of iodine, and the amount of iodine ingested or inhaled. For the same atmospheric concentrations, the results indicate a greater fetal dose from inhalation, suggesting that the fetus is most susceptible to being affected by airborne releases of the relevant radio-nuclides. Based on data from animal studies, suggest-

ing that the thyroid sensitivity is 10-200 times higher in fetuses than in adults, the fetus was also found to be most susceptible to ingested short-lived radio-iodine. As to the longest-lived [129]I, inhalation in adults and ingested milk in the young infants are the routes likely to deliver the greatest thyroidal doses.

243. The above data [B7] combine information on age-dependent dose per unit uptake, and per unit concentration in the environment (which includes age-dependent diets and breathing rates) and age-dependent sensitivity. This information is analysed separately in another model of iodine metabolism useful for calculation of the dose to the thyroid as a function of the fetal age in the fetus and mother described by Johnson [J11]. This model, based on available human data, indicates that the doses to the fetal thyroid from radioiodine taken in by the mother range from below the dose observed in the mother's thyroid to a factor of 3, at most, above it. The composition of the diet will determine whether ingestion or inhalation is the most important pathway. As to the sensitivity of the human fetal thyroid, Johnson and Myers [J12] have argued that there is no evidence to support large differences in the effects of ^{131}I and external irradiation in post-natal human thyroids, although differences by a factor of up to 10 cannot be ruled out. Doses to the fetal thyroid from chronic radio-iodine uptake by the mother over the gestation period would not be significantly different from those to the mother's thyroid. For acute exposure at any time during pregnancy, it may be calculated [J11] that the dose to the fetal thyroid is never more than a factor of 3 higher than that to the mother's. A recent careful review of the placental transfer and fetal binding of iodine in various mammalian species, including man, contains valuable information for inter-species comparisons [S85]. This is generally in line with conclusions in [J1] and [J12].

3. Phosphorus-32

244. In experiments by Krishna et al. [K17], pregnant mice received an intraperitoneal injection of [32]P (370 kBq) at 3.5 days p.c. and were then allowed to produce offspring. The incidence of successful copulations in this group of animals, compared with that in non-injected controls, was drastically reduced, indicating that there were losses of all litters prior to implantation. There was also a reduction of the litter size at birth and at weaning, due to post-implantation mortality during the early stages of development. The weight of the litters at birth was not apparently changed by the treatment, but subsequent growth was to some extent affected. These data are qualitatively in agreement with those that would be expected from external irradiation during the pre-implantation stages of development.

245. Radiophosphorus (37 kBq/g body weight) was also injected intramuscularly into pregnant Swiss albino mice on the 7th day after fertilization, but was not found to affect substantially the development of the pituitary gland, as judged by histological tests at 18 days p.c. or 14 days of extra-uterine age. Mice

injected intraperitoneally with the same level of radiophosphorus when one day old, and autopsied at various times thereafter up to 42 days of age, showed some hypertrophy of acidophilic cells. In animals injected at 7 days, signs of cell death, followed by an increase of acidophilic cells, were found over the same time period. For injection at 14 and 21 days, a clear decrease of acidophils was found. These cells seem, therefore, the most severely affected by the injection of [32]P [D6].

4. Sulphur-35

246. Pregnant mice of the CBA strain were injected with 740 kBq of ^{35}S on 3.5 days p.c. The treatment had no effect on the mortality of the injected animals, but a slight non-significant decrease of the number of fertile matings was observed. Litter size was significantly decreased (6.4 young per female), by comparison with control animals not injected (7.5 young per female). A further loss of animals took place between birth and weaning, owing to a significant increase in the neo- and post-natal mortality of the offspring in the treated groups. The sex ratio and the whole-body weight of the young born to injected mothers were not altered with respect to non-radioactive controls [S3].

5. Selenium-75

247. Following a single administration of ^{75}Se-methionine to pregnant female rats at 11-13 days p.c., the state of the endocrine system of the progeny was evaluated at 9, 12, 18 and 26 months of age. To this effect the concentrations in blood of corticosterone, testosterone and estradiol were studied. Changes were seen to be more pronounced in the male animals [D20].

6. Fission products

248. Senekowitsch and Kriegel [S67] compared the placental transfer of fission products such as strontium, caesium, yttrium and cerium in the rat and found that the uptake by the fetus decreased from the first to the last nuclide. The mothers were injected intravenously with a standard amount of each nuclide 21 days before pregnancy, on the day of mating, and 10 or 17 days after conception. The activity concentration in the organs of the mother and the fetuses was determined on pregnancy day 19, at which time the fetal weight had a fairly large degree of variability, owing, presumably, to a very long mating period of 2 days. For each nuclide, the authors found a statistically significant positive correlation between the deposition in the fetus and its weight. Uptake also depended on the day of development and was higher the later in pregnancy administration took place. The concentration of ^{131}I in fetal organs at 8 hours post-injection showed a very large increase (by a factor of about 1000) between 17 and 20 days of intra-uterine age, particularly between days 17 and 18. Thyroid activity compared with whole-body activity was 0.44% on day 17 and it increased to 35% by day 19.

249. In work by Villiers et al. [V11], sows were chronically treated with ^{85}Sr by intraperitoneal injection twice weekly of 185 kBq, in order to follow uptake and retention in the pregnant mother and fetus. The state of pregnancy did not modify these parameters appreciably. At birth, piglets had an ^{85}Sr content amounting to about 0.5 to 1.0% of that of the delivering mother, and the radionuclide taken up in utero was only excreted very slowly. Piglets were fed after delivery by either contaminated or control sows to study uptake through the milk. Those fed by contaminated sows increased their radionuclide content by about three times before weaning, but excreted it quite rapidly thereafter, so that by about three weeks they contained the same amount of ^{85}Sr as at birth. Some aspects of the metabolism of ^{131}I in the ruminant, including pregnant and lactating animals, were also reported on by Daburon [D26].

7. Lead-203

250. At 8-18 days of gestation, pregnant mice of the C57BL strain received ^{203}Pb-nitrate intraperitoneally [D22]. The whole animals, or their excised uteri, were subjected to autoradiography or autopsied for scintillation counting of the excised organs. Lead was found in the embryonic and fetal tissues after injection at all gestational ages. On days 8-11, it appeared mainly in embryonic blood, suggesting that it was essentially incorporated into the haemoglobin of yolk-sac erythrocytes. Starting from day 12, lead was found in liver (possibly in connection with the haematopoietic function of this organ) and in the skeletal cartilage and from day 14 on in the ossified skeleton. Thus, the overall fetal concentration increased progressively with gestational age. No uptake was observed in fetal kidney, in spite of accumulation in proximal tubuli of the maternal kidney.

8. Thallium-204

251. The uptake and retention of thallium in mice during gestation was investigated by autoradiographic techniques with ^{204}Tl sulphate [O9]. About 1.85 MBq of the nuclide were injected in the peritoneum of 15-day pregnant females. Fifteen minutes after injection, the nuclide could be traced in the fetuses. The maximum fetal accumulation was seen at 2-4 hours post-injection and the minimum at the last observation time, which was 4 days after injection. Observations at 5-15 days of gestation showed that thallium crosses the placental barrier at any time. It is retained by the visceral yolk-sac placenta during early pregnancy and also by the chorioallantoic placenta and the ammnion during late gestation.

9. Transuranic nuclides

252. Although a fair amount of new information on plutonium and other transuranic compounds administered to pregnant animals has become available, this refers more to the transplacental movement and distribution of the substances rather than to the effects induced on the product of conception. In the BALB/c mouse, Weiss and Walburg [W9, W21] measured the placental transport of plutonium citrate after intravenous injection of three different concentrations of ^{239}Pu during the late stages of pregnancy. The animals were killed 48 hours post-injection for tissue preparation and analysis. The authors noted that there was an increase in the percentage of plutonium incorporated into fetal tissue with decreasing activity down to levels of 3.7 kBq per animal. This was attributed to a mass effect. This pattern of relationship was also noted for the placental tissue and was explained by the fact that a body compartment, most likely the liver, retains a greater fraction of the radioactive material at higher levels.

253. Similar and parallel experiments [W10] were also performed with americium-243 administered intravenously as citrate in various concentrations (between about 0.4 and 130 kBq/mouse) to pregnant BALB/c animals 16 days after mating. These concentrations were chosen in such a way that the number of atoms in each injected dose would be equal to the number of ^{239}Pu atoms in the study reviewed above [W21]. Forty-eight hours after injection, the concentrations of the nuclide were determined in fetuses, placentas, in the maternal femur, liver, carcass and pelt. It was found that, atom for atom, americium was incorporated into fetal tissues 10-25 times less than plutonium at similar concentrations. Here again, however, at low dose levels the average fraction incorporated into the fetuses decreased with increasing activity administered to the pregnant mothers. The same could be said for the placenta and the femur. The mass effect for americium was about a factor of 2 within the concentrations covered, that is slightly lower than that of ^{239}Pu which was nearly a factor of 4 [W21]. A scavenging effect by the maternal tissues, and particularly by the liver, was discussed as a plausible explanation.

254. The point was made, regarding these two studies [W10, W21], that extrapolations from animal to man should always be made at the low levels of environmental human exposure, which would be hundreds of times less than for the experiments reviewed. It is doubtful whether activity analyses at such extremely low levels of contamination are at all possible. However, the concept should be borne in mind that perhaps current environmental levels of the nuclides might be more readily transferred from pregnant mothers to the fetus than for the usual much higher experimental level uptakes.

255. New-born rats from dams injected with 49 kBq ^{239}Pu citrate kg^{-1} body weight 38-53 days prior to parturition contained an average of 0.008% of the maternal injected dose per neo-nate [T16]. Also in the rat Hisamatsu and Takizawa [H29] studied the placental transfer and distribution of ^{241}Am by injecting the radionuclide under the form of citrate at 15 or 18 days of gestation. The animals injected at 15 days were killed at 2, 24, 48 or 120 hours and those injected at 18 days were killed 24 hours thereafter. An autoradiographic study of the nuclide distribution in the fetus, fetal membranes and placenta showed that

the deposition in the feto-placental units increased with gestational age. Major deposition sites were the skeleton and liver, but the presence of the nuclide in the yolk sac splanchnopleure and in the exocoelom suggested also an important role of the yolk sac placenta in the transfer mechanisms. The post-natal development of rats treated with ^{241}Am was studied by Ovcharenko [O13].

256.   In the guinea-pig (outbred Harley strain), Kelman and Sikov [K5] measured the movement of ^{239}Pu in vivo at 59 to 61 days of pregnancy by perfusion of the fetal circulation, a technique which avoids the complications occurring through fetal accumulation of the nuclide. The perfusion technique also entails continuous monitoring of the pressure, heart rate, electrocardiogram, blood pressure and respiration rate of the mothers. The pregnant animals were administered trace amounts of tritiated water in order to monitor changes in the maternal blood flow to the placenta and about 1 MBq/kg of ^{239}Pu citrate intravenously. This dose of plutonium is of the order of the LD$_{50/30}$ for other species (about 740-3000 kBq/kg). Clearance of plutonium from the mother to fetus was found to be small, amounting, for example, to less than one-fifth of that for inorganic mercury. One factor that might account in part for such a low clearance is the placental blood flow of the mother, which is greatly depressed in the animals treated with plutonium.

257.   In an abstract by Andrew et al. [A8], valuable data were provided on the distribution of ^{239}Pu in the gravid baboon. Following previous evidence that, in the rat the placenta and the fetal membranes attain substantially greater concentrations of the nuclide than does the fetus, and that these observations may not be easily extrapolated to man owing to large interspecies differences, the authors chose the baboon as an experimental animal. In this species, in fact, development of the placenta is similar to that in man. Pregnant animals at various stages of gestation were administered 370 kBq/kg of monomeric ^{239}Pu intravenously. The uteri and their content were then removed surgically 24 hours later for radioanalysis and autoradiography. The mothers themselves were allowed to live an additional two to six days. The fraction of dose reaching the feto-placental unit, and the ratios of the concentrations in the fetus to those in the placenta, were found to be very similar in the rat and the baboon, when similar stages of gestation were compared. If, in addition, the morphological differences in placentation were allowed for, the autoradiographic distribution of plutonium was found to be remarkably similar in the rat and the monkey.

258.   Joshima et al. [J3] studied the effects on embryonic and fetal haematopoiesis of ^{239}Pu citrate administered intravenously to the Wistar rat (about 1.3 MBq/kg, no dose estimate available) on gestation day 9. At this time, the yolk sac begins to form the blood islands and also selectively concentrates monomeric plutonium. The injected animals were killed 5 or 10 days after injection to measure any effects in the circulating blood, yolk sac and fetal haematopoietic organs. The treatment increased pre-natal mortality and reduced maternal (but not fetal) weight gain. At both sampling times the pregnant mothers showed a decreased number of reticulocytes and leukocytes; the red blood cells were also lower at 10 days. The fetuses showed a transient decrease in the concentration of non-nucleated mature erythrocytes and changes in the distribution of cell types of the erythropoietic series, which were interpreted as disturbances in the maturation processes. The presence of plutonium also reduced the mean weight of the yolk sac and the fetal liver. In both these organs, and also in the spleen, the mean number of cells was decreased, without any shift in the distribution of the various cell classes.

259.   Kelman, Sikov and Hackett reported [K6, K23] on the effects of monomeric ^{239}Pu on the fetal rabbit. Animals at gestation days 9, 15 and 27 received 370 kBq/kg body weight of monomeric ^{239}Pu intravenously and were killed one day later; no estimate of absorbed dose was provided. Groups were also similarly injected at 9 and 15 days and killed at the 28th day of gestation. One group, injected on day 9 and killed on day 28, received a four-fold higher activity concentration. Conceptuses were examined for viability at 10, 11 and 29 days. Each fetus from litters injected at 9, 15 and 28 days, and killed on day 29, was weighed, measured and examined for sex, external abnormalities and cleft palate. Exposure to about 1.5 MBq/kg decreased fetal weight significantly, compared with that of the group receiving 370 kBq/kg, while the smaller weight losses induced by this latter activity concentration were not thought to be significant. Foetal mortality was significantly increased, except in groups receiving the lowest activity on days 9 and 15. Only 5 out of 377 fetuses examined were abnormal. This low number, and the lack of any pattern in the induction of malformations, made any association between their incidence and the exposure to plutonium rather unlikely. Subtle alterations, which could not properly be classified as malformations, were detected in the skeleton of the exposed litters and there was a general retardation of the skeletal development in the group receiving the highest activity of plutonium.

260.   Ovcharenko and Fomina [O6] reported on the effects of ^{237}Np oxalate administered intravenously to rats. They found an increased pre-implantation mortality in females. The progeny of these rats receiving 11-185 kBq/kg showed a decrease in the rate of production of red blood cells after gamma irradiation, together with a prolongation of the period of narcosis after administration of hexanol.

B.   CONCLUSIONS

261.   Although a number of new contributions regarding the effect of internal irradiation on the mammalian conceptus have appeared since the matter was last reviewed by UNSCEAR [U2], the information gathered is not systematic in regard to the nuclides tested, their chemical form, the route and schedule of administration, and the kinetics of transfer and metabolism of the substances from the mother to the feto-placental complex. Complete dose-effect relation-

ships are seldom reported. Also, data regarding various animal species, developmental stages at treatment, and type of effects scored, are very sporadic. As a consequence, any attempt to extrapolate between nuclides, doses, species, developmental stages or any other major physical or biological variable appears premature. From the long list of nuclides for which scattered information is available, three stand out as having received somewhat better attention: tritium, iodine-131 and plutonium-239. The fact that these also happen to be, potentially, among the most important for human exposure under normal or accidental conditions is probably the reason for the interest they have received. It does not mean, however, that the information available for them is very satisfactory.

262. For tritium, many contributions refer to irradiation during the pre-implantation stages in vitro. In the culture medium, activity concentrations of tritium oxide of the order of 4-16 kBq/ml have been shown to stop the progression of 50% of the zygotes to the blastocyst stage, the variability between these values being due in large part to the developmental stage of the early embryo at irradiation. Embryo sensitivity generally decreases with increased differentiation. Tritium in the form of thymidine is about 1000 times more effective in producing such effects than tritiated water. Tritium oxide and tritiated thymidine also act differently on various developmental stages. Tritium is metabolized by the embryo and its organs according to different kinetics: the loss of the radionuclide per gram of tissue in the new-born after uptake in utero shows a fast component with a half-life of a few days followed by slower components linked to the metabolism of the organically bound isotope. This has been established in both the mouse and the pig. The dose received by cells in each tissue is therefore governed by the level of tritium in the body fluids and by the specific cell kinetic and metabolic pattern of each tissue. Whole-body doses of the order of 1 Gy or less from tritium have been reported to produce changes in litter size, sex ratio, and neo-natal mortality in the mouse. They also cause increased tumour incidence and changes in the life span. Sustained levels of tritium in the drinking water of pregnant rats at concentrations of about 100 kBq/ml produced in the offspring some biochemical sign of cerebral damage (low DNA and protein content), although the weight of the brain was normal. Continuous administration of tritiated water over 5 generations showed no sign of cumulative effects. Other patterns of tritium dosage at similar concentrations also produced evidence of brain defects which could be followed well into post-natal life. There is evidence that organically bound tritium is more damaging than tritiated water for the same administered activity. The RBE for a variety of end-points (dominant lethal mutations, chromosomal aberrations, chromatid exchanges, alterations in bone marrow cells) following HTO ingestion in the mouse, compared with external gamma rays from ^{137}Cs, was assessed to be between 1 and 2.

263. Many of the experiments using radioactive iodine appear directed to clarify the relationship between the amount of activity administered to the dam and its route of uptake, on the one hand, and the level of iodine in the fetal tissues, particularly in the thyroid, on the other. The transplacental transfer of radio-iodine as a function of time from the uptake by the mother has been studied in rats and in the guinea-pig. So have the relative concentrations in the blood of the mother and of the fetus and in the amniotic fluid, and the relative uptake in the mother's and offspring's thyroid. They have also been estimated in man on the basis of some assumed parameters of uptake and metabolism. As a result of using simplifying calculations, it has been provisionally concluded from these data that for acute exposure at any time during pregnancy the dose to the thyroid of the fetus is never more than three times higher than that of the mother. For chronic uptake over the whole gestation period these doses would not significantly differ from each other.

264. Experiments on ^{239}Pu contamination of pregnant mice have shown that the proportion of this nuclide incorporated into the fetal tissues tends to be relatively higher (a factor of 4, as a maximum) with activity concentrations decreasing down to about 3.7 kBq per animal. Although atom for atom, ^{243}Am is incorporated 10-25 times less efficiently than plutonium at similar concentrations, the average fraction of administered activity incorporated into the fetus decreases also for this nuclide with increasing mass of the nuclide to the pregnant mother, by a factor of about 2. The presence of such effects should be borne in mind when assessing the uptake of environmental levels of transuranic nuclides, which are orders of magnitude lower than the experimentally tested levels.

265. Comparisons of the distribution of ^{239}Pu in the mother and fetus in the rat and the baboon have shown that when similar developmental stages are compared, and morphological differences in the placenta of the two species are allowed for, the distribution of the nuclide is very similar. While existing data are insufficient for precise estimates, no clear tendency of plutonium to concentrate into the fetus has been documented. There appears to be, on the contrary, some tendency of the placenta and fetal membranes to take up the plutonium that might otherwise be transferred to the fetus. Experiments on the effects of plutonium are relatively less common than those on its distribution. However, some haematological changes have been documented in the rat at about 1.3 MBq/kg of ^{239}Pu citrate administered on gestation day 9. Fetal weight loss and mortality (but not malformations) were significantly induced by concentrations of monomeric ^{239}Pu in the range of 1 MBq/kg administered to pregnant rabbits.

266. There appears to be an urgent need to enlarge the data base for the nuclides of most practical importance with respect to uptake, distribution in the feto-placental complex, and possible effects in the offspring, over a larger variety of radioactive chemicals and a wider range of nuclide concentrations. The importance of correlating effects to tissue doses rather than intake activities should also be emphasized. In addition to providing much needed information of potential value under conditions of normal operation and accidental exposure to radiation sources, such

new data might contribute to bringing about generalized conclusions on dose-response relationships for pre-natal internal exposure to radioactive nuclides.

VI. THE ROLE OF MODIFYING FACTORS

267. The present chapter deals with physical, chemical or biological factors that have been shown to modify the radiation response of pre-natally irradiated mammals. It focuses on radiation type and energy and the effects of combined actions, including radioprotective and radiosensitizing treatments.

A. RADIATION QUALITY

268. The insufficiency of information concerning the effect of radiation quality and dose rate, in the context of teratogenic damage and pre-natal irradiation effects in general, was pointed out by UNSCEAR in its previous review of the subject [U2]. It was concluded at the time that the data only allowed some speculation about RBE factors in respect of irradiation in utero. However, this knowledge was compatible with the notion that higher RBE factors applied to the more densely ionizing radiation and to low-LET dose protraction, as compared with high-dose-rate and low-LET radiation. UNSCEAR called specifically for a systematic exploration of this area, and over the past few years new information has in fact been produced. This information is reviewed below, according to the various types of radiation tested.

1. Neutrons

269. In experiments by Molls et al. [M33], pre-implantation mouse embryos in the G_2 phase of the 2-cell stage were exposed in vitro to either x rays (240 kV) or fast neutrons (average energy, 7 MeV). At various times thereafter (up to 63 hours post-irradiation and growth in culture), these embryos were scored for the number of cells per embryo and the number of micronuclei per cell. Both radiations did induce the formation of micronuclei at very low doses, and the kinetics of induction was found to depend on radiation dose and the length of the division delay during the first and second cell cycle after irradiation. New micronuclei were appearing even after the third and later post-irradiation mitoses, in accordance with the notion that radiation-damaged cells do not all die at the first post-irradiation division. The number of micronuclei per cell at 39 hours post-irradiation appeared to follow an essentially linear increase with the dose of x rays and a convex upward response with the dose of neutrons. An x-ray dose of 0.06 Gy was sufficient to double the average number of micronuclei per cell of the control embryos; 0.03 Gy of neutrons produced a 6-fold increase over the control values.

270. Cairnie et al. [C3] reported on teratogenic and embryolethal responses in CF_1 mice irradiated in the Janus reactor at the Argonne National Laboratory in the United States. At this facility the mean energy of the neutron spectrum was approximately 0.8 MeV; thermal neutrons and gamma rays contributed less than 1% and less than 3%, respectively, of the absorbed dose within the mice. Neutron effects were compared with those of ^{137}Cs or ^{60}Co gamma rays. Irradiation took place at 3, 5, 8 and 11 days p.c. Doses were 1, 1.5, 2.0 and 3.0 Gy for gamma rays and 0.25, 0.5, 1.0, 1.5 and 2.0 Gy for neutrons. Offspring were examined on day 17 of pregnancy for the incidence of resorptions and dead or viable fetuses. Live fetuses were also scored for gross external abnormalities and body size. The same types of responses were observed for neutrons and gamma rays. For lethal effects and malformative effects considered as a single class, the RBE in terms of average absorbed dose to the embryo was estimated to be 2.9 (the corresponding ratio in terms of kerma in free air was 2.5). Taking the average number of abnormalities per fetus as the end-point, the findings also pointed to an RBE of between 2 and 3. The highest incidence of abnormalities was obtained for irradiation on day 11, when malformations of the limbs were especially frequent. Approximate values of RBE estimated for those abnormalities that were sufficiently numerous were in the range of 2 to 3, usually closer to 3. It was pointed out that these RBE values were consistent with other values for effects dependent on cell killing in vitro and in vivo which, for the particular radiation sources used, were between 2.2 and 4.

271. Although no comparison between different types of radiation was involved, Vogel [V3, V4] exposed female Sprague-Dawley rats on pregnancy day 18 to single whole-body doses (0.2 to 1.5 Gy) of fission neutrons of 1.2 MeV average energy (neutron/gamma dose ratio approximately 7, dose median LET approximately 50 keV/μm). A dose of 0.2 Gy caused a small decrease of body weight lasting from birth to weaning. During this period, 9% of irradiated rats died, compared with 4% of the controls. After 0.5 Gy, about 24% of the irradiated animals died within the same period, with a more profound body weight loss of the survivors. One Gy caused about half of the rats to die within 24 hours of birth and over three-quarters before weaning, with a large and significant loss of weight in the survivors. No survivor among 95 rats receiving 1.5 Gy was left within 2 days of birth. The neutron LD_{50} from birth to weaning was estimated to be 0.75 Gy. Organ weight changes were followed between birth and 1 week of age and they showed an overall decrease of the measured values in irradiated animals. The most significant weight loss was found in the CNS and in the testis one month after neutron exposure. These effects were thought to be directly induced in the irradiated fetuses and not secondarily through irradiation of the mother.

272. Di Majo et al. [D7] compared the effects of fission-spectrum neutrons (zero to 0.465 Gy, average energy ~0.4 MeV, gamma contamination ~12.5% of total dose) with those of x rays (250 kV, 0-2.0 Gy at 0.13 Gy/min). The end-points scored included embryo lethality, weight reduction and teratogenic effects (gross malformations and minor anomalies). The

animals used were F_1 hybrids of C57Bl and C3H mice, irradiated at 7.5 days p.c. They were scored for the above effects at 18.5 days p.c. Mortality curves found for both radiations were highly curvilinear, with a lower "threshold" for neutrons than for x rays. The ratio of x-ray to neutron doses (1.4 and 0.47 Gy, respectively) to produce 20% mortality was approximately 3. The loss of mean fetal weight was approximately linear with increasing dose of both radiations, and the ratio of the slope regressions gave an RBE of 3.2 ± 0.8, as an average over the dose range tested. Highly curvilinear relationships with dose were observed for major malformations after x-ray irradiation, with thresholds of the order of 1 Gy. Dose relationships for neutrons, however, showed no apparent thresholds, so that the RBE of neutrons was very dependent on neutron dose. The equal effectiveness dose ratio estimated at 7% incidence of severe external malformations was 2.4, increasing to about 3.4 if other, more common, head abnormalities were also included.

273. Preliminary studies of dose-response relationships for developmental damage in the CNS of the mouse after pre-natal exposure to x rays, fast neutrons and ^{131}I were also reported [K41]. RBE values following x-ray or neutron exposures were established in relation to a number of morphological parameters such as the thinning of cortical plate, corpus callosum and fimbria hippocampi. They were shown to vary between 3 and 4, according to different times and effects. The studies included analyses of neuronal branching defects by computerized micro-video techniques, as a function of dose. There was evidence that "thresholds" existed in the region of 0.1 Gy for such types of structural damage.

274. The effects of a single whole-body dose of 0.5 Gy of neutrons (peak energy about 3 MeV) on mortality and body and brain weight in $(DBA_2 \times C57BL/6)F_1$ hybrid mice were described by Antal and Vogel [A10, V9]. Radiation was delivered at 17 ± 2 days p.c. This treatment caused a significant increase of death within two weeks after birth, from a level of about 12% in the control animals to about 41% in irradiated ones. The average birth weight showed a 15% reduction in the irradiated mice. This weight loss was not recovered until 6 months after birth. Brain weight at 3 weeks of age was 30-35% less in the irradiated mice. Early mortality and brain weight loss were not seen in mice irradiated at 1-7 days from birth. The significance of these data, particularly in regard to timing, was discussed in relation with the induction of severe mental retardation of children exposed in utero to the atomic bomb explosions. The authors' opinion is that the time of most active neuroblast proliferation is, in both species, the most vulnerable period for radiation exposure.

2. Helium ions

275. In a series of papers, Ward and his group [W2-W6] reported extensively on the effects induced by irradiation in utero by a helium ion beam generated in a synchro-cyclotron. By suitable ridge

filtration, doubly charged 530-MeV monoenergetic helium ions were modified into a heterogenous beam with an extended Bragg peak, delivering essentially a uniform radiation dose at a depth of 4-10 cm in water. This allowed animals to be exposed rather uniformly from a lateral direction. The LET spectrum was such that at 8 cm about 10% of the dose was due to tracks of LET higher than 20 keV/μm; and about 1% to tracks of LET higher than 100 keV/μm. Cobalt-60 gamma rays were used as the standard radiation for comparison.

276. In the first experimental series [W2, W4], Sprague-Dawley rats were exposed on gestation day 8 under aerobic or hypoxic (95% helium and 5% oxygen) conditions in the dose interval of 2-12 Gy. The uterine content was examined on gestation day 20 for live and dead fetuses, resorption sites, weight and gross morphological abnormalities. The number of corpora lutea served as an index of the number of ovulations, and embryonic survival was expressed as a per cent of live fetuses over the number of corpora lutea. The results may be summarized as follows:

Survival (%)	RBE		Oxygen enhancement ratio		Oxygen effect gain
	Aerobic	Hypoxic	Helium ions	Gamma rays	
50	1.0	1.2	1.7	2.2	1.2
10	1.1	1.4	1.5	2.0	1.3

Thus, the high-LET component of the helium ion beam had a negligible effect on the RBE under aerobic conditions, but lowered the effective oxygen enhancement ratio of the beam by about 25% relative to that of the gamma rays. Helium ions were significantly more effective than gamma rays in stunting fetal growth under hypoxic and aerobic conditions (1.5 and 1.7, respectively) and in producing gross morphological abnormalities under aerobic, but not under hypoxic, conditions. In fact, at 10% incidence of abnormal fetuses, the equal effect ratios were about 1.7 and 1 under oxygenated and hypoxic conditions, respectively.

277. In another paper [W3], the embryonic survival was examined in rats exposed to split doses of radiation delivered in two fractions at 5 and 6 days p.c. Helium ions, which showed a single-dose RBE (with respect to ^{60}Co gamma rays) of 1.0, had a split-dose RBE of 1.5, in accordance with expectation if the killing curves for helium ions had a smaller shoulder than that of gamma rays.

278. Finally [W5, W6], Sprague-Dawley rats were exposed to 0.5-6.0 Gy of ^{60}Co gamma rays, or to extended Bragg peak helium ions, on days 3-10 of pregnancy, and the uterine content was examined on pregnancy day 20 for scoring of resorptions and dead or live fetuses. The number of dead fetuses was referred to the number of corpora lutea to calculate the percentage of killing. The sex of the fetuses was also scored. For gamma irradiation, the LD_{50} in utero ranged from 1.4 Gy on day 3 to 5.15 Gy on day 6 of gestation. For helium ions, the values ranged from 1.7 on day 10 to 4.9 Gy on day 6. Day 6 (the time of implantation) was the most resistant stage for both radiations, while the early organogenesis period (days

9 and 10) was found to be the most sensitive. In spite of the variation of radiosensitivity over a factor of 3 to 4 during the period of development examined, the magnitude of the fluctuations at the various times was essentially the same for both radiations, so that the RBE of helium ions with respect to gamma rays was, on average, 1.0 during the whole period. A consistent feature in irradiated litters was the preponderance of male fetuses among the survivors, for which no explanation is available.

3. Negative π mesons

279. In experiments by Michel and collaborators [M4], mouse embryos in the pronuclear-zygote stage (gestation day zero) were irradiated with either 140-kV x rays or negative pions to a dose of 0.135 Gy. The animals were examined when they reached the fetal stages on gestation day 13. The developmental effects scored included intra-uterine death, retardation of growth and incidence of malformations. Significant decreases in the percentage of normal implantations were obtained with π mesons at the peak and with x rays. The effect of the pions at the plateau was less important. Irradiation with peak pions was found to be more effective than with x rays, by a factor of about 1.7.

B. COMBINED ACTIONS

1. Various chemical substances

280. Most of the data published since 1977 on the combined effects of radiation and other agents, taking as end-points various types of damage to embryonic systems, have been obtained by treatment of the very early stages of development and in vitro culture of the treated embryos. General aspects of the interaction between radiation and chemicals during pre-natal development were discussed in annex L of the 1982 UNSCEAR report [U5] and were reviewed by Streffer [S17, S36].

281. The same author and his group have used extensively the in-vitro culture of the early mouse embryo to test a number of substances in combined-treatment experiments. Following the order of publication, they reported on the interaction between ionizing radiation and lead [M31, V6], actinomycin D [M29, S19], phenols [M27], sodium nitrite [M16], cadmium [M28], ethidium bromide [M29], 2,4-dinitrophenol [M19], sodium sulfite [M43] and caffeine [M43].

282. The combined effects of these substances with x rays were studied, taking as end-points the development of 2-cell mouse embryos to hatching of blastocysts, the cell proliferation kinetics in these embryos, and the formation of micronuclei as an index of cytogenetic damage. The substances were usually added to the culture medium directly before x irradiation. Additive effects were found for all these end-points when x rays were combined with most

chemical substances. This was the case for phenol, p-nitrophenol, 2,4-dinitrophenol, sodium nitrite, sodium sulfite, 2,4,6-trinitrobenzene sulfonate and ethidium bromide.

283. A supra-additive (synergistic) effect was observed with the combination of x rays and actinomycin D, cadmium chloride or lead chloride on one of the parameters. Only with very high concentrations of caffeine did a supra-additive effect occur on the three parameters. The supra-additive effects were generally seen under conditions when recovery processes after irradiation were inhibited. Of special importance is the finding that comparatively low concentrations of lead chloride [M31] and of actinomycin D [S17, S36] induced such potentiation of the radiation effects.

284. In the field of combined actions, a few other scattered observations have also been reported. Sikov and Mahlum [S12] found that the intravenous administration of 5.5 kBq of ^{239}Pu, which by itself was ineffective, to pregnant rats at either 8.5 or 9.0 days p.c. increased synergistically the teratologic and embryo-cidal effects of trypan blue injected intraperitoneally (70 mg/kg) at these times of gestation. Trypan blue is itself a teratogen in the rat, at least up to 11 days p.c. [B29].

285. Yuguchi [Y2] treated pregnant ddN mice at 7 days p.c. with x rays (100 or 150 R) with or without ultrasound at 1.5 or 3.0 W/cm^2 (1 MHZ) for 5 minutes. The gross appearance of the offspring and the histology of their eyes were examined on the 18th day of gestation. The author found an enhancement of the embryolethal effects of 150 R by the highest dosage of ultrasound and an enhancement of the teratogenic effects of 100 R, also by the highest dosage. The histopathogenesis of the ocular abnormalities was carefully described in these experiments. The sensitivity periods in fetal mouse retina by the combined action of the cytostatic drug 5-azacytidine and x rays were investigated by Schmahl and Török [S6].

286. Sadovskaya et al. [S76] and Rantseva [R22] investigated the reproductive function and physical development of the progeny of non-inbred irradiated white mice. Females were exposed every other day to fractionated long-wave x radiation (10.2 keV) for 31 and 82 fractions (five of which were administered after mating with non-irradiated males) at doses of 0.13 or 0.26 Gy per fraction. From the number of offspring, the coefficient of reproduction and the body weight of the new-born, these treatments were apparently ineffective. However, if under the same conditions of irradiation an SHF treatment (ppm 5 MW cm^{-2}, 20 minutes per session) was also jointly administered, there was a tendency towards a reduction in fertility and a decrease in body weight, as compared with the effects of the two treatments given alone [L8].

287. Kusama and Yoshizawa [K37] reported briefly on intra-uterine death, malformations, body weight and sex ratios of mice exposed to 1 or 2 Gy of gamma radiation and 1 or 2 mg cortisone (administered in this order) on the 7th day of embryonic age. A dose of 1 Gy of x rays given alone produced no higher

mortality than that in the control, but a higher frequency of exencephaly, while both end-points were found to be higher after 2 Gy. Cortisone alone did not significantly alter any of the end-points scored. On the contrary, the combined-action groups showed rates of mortality and malformation which were twice as high as those induced by the same dose of radiation given alone, an observation implying a synergistic interaction.

288. In another series of experiments [K38], the same authors exposed pregnant ICR mice on their 7th day of gestation to various doses of gamma radiation (0.5, 1.0 and 2.0 Gy) and of caffeine (0.1, and 0.25 mg/g body weight). The drug in the combined-action groups was administered immediately after the appropriate radiation dose. Controls with no treatment, and with radiation or caffeine alone at the same doses, were also included. The end-points scored on the fetuses after killing of the pregnant mothers at 18 days of gestation were the same as in the previous series [K37]. Intra-uterine mortality increased as a function of dose following a highly curvilinear shape (upper concavity). There was no effect when caffeine was given alone, but the combination of radiation and caffeine resulted in a synergistic effect on mortality. A synergistic effect was also found in respect of the incidence of malformations both minor (polydactylia, micromelia, short tail) and serious (hydrocephaly, exencephaly, parietal hernia, cleft palate and lip). For induction of gross malformations, the dose-effect relationships for radiation alone or in combination were highly curvilinear. Body weight reduction was thought to be a good indicator of the growth-retarding effect of the treatments, but showed no signs of synergistic interaction. Finally, the sex ratio of live fetuses in the different treatment groups was not significantly different from control.

289. After showing that pre-conception exposure of ICR mice increased the incidence of anomalies and of tumours (mainly lung adenomas) in the offspring of treated mice [N4], Nomura [N13] tested tumorigenesis by irradiation in utero, followed by chemical treatment with urethane. Pregnant mice of this same strain were exposed to x rays (a single dose of 0.36 Gy) every second day between zero and 16 days of gestation. Neo-natal mice were also similarly irradiated within 1 day of birth and, in addition, other pregnant females received 1.59 Gy on gestation day zero. When 21 days old, the mice received subcutaneously 5 μM of urethane per gram body weight and were killed 5 months afterwards for scoring of tumours and malformations. Tumours were mostly papillary lung adenomas. Survival of the animals was decreased with irradiation on day zero, and body weight decreased with irradiation on days 4-10, and particularly on day 12 of gestation. Irradiation in utero alone did not change the natural tumour incidence. Irradiation on days 0-4 and 8, followed by administration of urethane, increased the number of tumours per animal, compared with both irradiation alone or urethane alone. It was speculated that unidentified events, induced by irradiation in the embryos and persisting through a large number of cell generations, may render the cells more susceptible to the post-natal treatment with urethane.

Such events may be similar to those recently described in cells transformed in vitro by x rays and discussed in annex B to the present report.

290. In a short letter, Kinner-Wilson et al. [K42] reported on 2707 children who died in 1972-1977 of various malignancies, including leukaemia, and had been exposed in utero to various types of drugs and to x rays, separately or jointly. These children were matched to 2298 control non-exposed cases. The increase in relative risks for "all drugs" and for radiation given jointly were significantly (P < 0.001) increased above the level of action of the agents given alone. When the drugs were divided into separate groups, only for two of the three groups (namely "sedatives" and "other unspecified drugs"), but not for the third ("hormones"), was there a significant association. In the view of the authors, these results cannot be attributed to artifact. The association could, in principle, be explained on one (or more) of the following mechanisms: an effect of the illnesses requiring the drug treatment; a true causal effect of the treatment(s); or an association between the drugs and another non-identified risk factor. Results are too preliminary to allow a choice among the mechanisms proposed.

2. Radioprotective and radiosensitizing treatments

291. Although part of the larger subject of radiation-drug interaction, the effects of radioprotective and radiosensitizing substances are traditionally treated separately. A number of reports have appeared on these subjects since the last UNSCEAR review [U2]. Radioprotective effects on embryonic systems were mainly studied by a group of research workers in India; radiosensitizing substances were mainly investigated in Switzerland.

(a) Radioprotective treatments

292. The drug 2-mercaptopropionyl glycine (MPG), a —SH radioprotector, was used in the studies by Dev and her group. A variety of end-points were used to assess the protective action, including organ and whole-body weight changes and functional tissue effects. Pregnant Swiss albino mice were exposed to gamma rays (250 R) at 14.25, 16.25 and 18.25 days of gestation. The post-partum weight of the offspring was remarkably improved by pre-irradiation treatment of the mothers with 20 mg/kg body weight of MPG. Of the three ages tested, the earliest was the most sensitive [D4]. Similar observations were made on mice receiving 150 R [D19] and 50 R [D5] at the same times p.c.

293. In another series [G9], pregnant Swiss albino mice at 11.5 days p.c. were injected intraperitoneally with a single dose of about 5.6 MBq of ^{131}I per mouse. Other mice received MPG (20 mg/kg) 30 minutes before the ^{131}I and daily on each subsequent gestation day until parturition. Finally, a third group of mice was similarly treated with distilled water. The body

weight of the litters born to these animals was checked, starting on the day of birth and for 6 weeks thereafter. Organ weights of the animals at 6 weeks were also obtained. MPG afforded a modest degree of protection against loss of total body weight, and marginal protection in regard to the weight of brain, kidney, testis, spleen, thymus and liver.

294. As to tissue effects, 50 R of gamma radiation from ^{60}Co, given at days 14.25, 16.25 or 18.25 resulted in a depression of the leukocyte count of the young 1 or 2 weeks after birth, with recovery by the 4th week. Treatment of the mothers with MPG (20 mg/kg) 15-30 minutes before irradiation significantly reduced the leukocyte depression at 1 or 2 weeks of age [G7]. In other experiments [G13] mice were irradiated in utero at 14.5, 16.5 and 18.5 days p.c., with or without pre-treatment of the mothers with 20 mg/kg body weight of MPG. Doses of ^{60}Co gamma rays were 0.5, 1.5 and 2.5 Gy. Male animals were killed when 6 weeks old and the weight of their testes or the total number of spermatids in tubule sections were assessed. The radiosensitivity of the testes was found to increase with increasing fetal age. There was also some protection by MPG of the testes according to both end-points scored, but the amount of protection was variable and not evaluated over a large range of doses.

295. Palyga et al. [P13] irradiated embryonic (1-14 days p.c.) and fetal (15-23 days p.c.) rats while the pregnant mothers breathed a hypoxic gas mixture containing 10% oxygen and 90% nitrogen. A single dose of 2.0 Gy was used. Judging by the incidence of still-born, and by the per cent survival 30 days after birth, the treatment afforded a reliable degree of protection against lethality.

296. Turakulov et al. [T9] studied, in pregnant dogs, rabbits and rats the specific activity and biological effects of potassium iodide in various combinations with potassium perchlorate, as a prophylactic treatment for the protection of the thyroid gland against the effects of radioactive iodine during pregnancy. They reported that a combination of the two drugs in doses of 0.5 and 300 mg/kg, administered at any time during pregnancy, is biologically harmless and shows a high protective effect.

(b) Radiosensitizing treatments

297. The hypoxic cell sensitizer misonidazole was used by Michel and collaborators in interaction studies with low- and high-LET radiation. In one report [M5, M6], pregnant NMRI mice on the 8th day p.c. received intraperitoneally various doses of the drug (from 200 to 1000 mg/kg body weight). Single doses of 0.01 Gy of 140-kV x rays and 15-MeV electrons were given. The end-points investigated were embryonic and fetal death, malformations, and growth retardation as scored at 13 or 18 days p.c. Growth retardation was assumed to be present when the fetal weight was more than two standard deviations below the average control weight. Treatment with the drug

alone at 670 or 1000 mg/kg was toxic to 13-day-p.c. embryos, while doses of 200 mg/kg were only marginally effective. On 18-day-old fetuses the drug alone (670 mg/kg) significantly increased the number of malformed living fetuses. X irradiation produced an insignificant decrease in the frequency of normal fetuses, while electron irradiation produced a marked increase of resorptions. The first observation is not surprising in view of the low doses given, but is apparently in contrast with the latter. As to combined actions, they were thought to be "at least additive" in the case of electrons and "synergistic" for the x rays. But whether the same observations might hold at other doses and times remains to be confirmed. Similarly, the differential effect of misonidazole in regard to x rays or electrons remains to be explained.

298. Michel et al. [M35] also reported on the combined effects of misonidazole with negative pions (0.125-1 Gy) or 200-kV x rays (0.125-1.5 Gy). Mouse embryos on the 8th gestation day were irradiated, with or without application of the drug, 30 minutes before exposure. The fetuses were examined on day 13 for lethality, growth disturbances or the presence of malformations. No significant killing effect was seen for either radiations in the dose range up to 1 Gy; however, the drug alone or in combination led to some lethality. Growth retardation was significantly present at 1 Gy and in combined treatments at lower doses. Multiple severe malformations and severe retardation were seen when a dose of 0.5 Gy was combined with misonidazole. The frequency of teratogenic effects (all included) was significantly higher at all doses for both the x-ray- and negative-pion-treated animals when irradiation took place after the administration of the radiosensitizer. There was, overall, a synergistic enhancement of radiation effects by the combined treatment, the extent of which varied as a function of the radiation dose and quality and also according to the induced effect.

299. In other experiments [M14], pregnant mice of strains F/A and NMRI were exposed to 0.01 Gy of whole-body pion- or x-irradiation at day 8 of gestation. Lucanthone (Miracil D), a known radiosensitizer in various biological systems, was administered intraperitoneally 30 minutes before irradiation at 35 or 70 mg/kg. Five days after treatment, the fetuses were observed for developmental anomalies (growth retardation, micro-ophthalmia, exencephaly). In both strains of mice, it was found that radiation produced a significant increase in the incidence of abnormal fetuses compared with non-irradiated fetuses. The effectiveness of negative pions (peak irradiation) was higher than for x rays with respect to the production of teratogenic effects, the RBE being between 1.7 and 1.9. The application of Lucanthone increased the number of damaged fetuses and led to various degrees of sensitization, depending on the mouse strain and dosage used. Differences between strains in respect of the incidence of malformations were explained by the possible slight difference of developmental stages at the time of treatment. A similar explanation was given for the strain differences found in the same mouse strains irradiated with 0.135 Gy in association with Lucanthone [M50].

300. Preliminary data were also reported by Balla et al. [B39] on the interaction between x rays (0.01 Gy) and the cytotoxic drug vindesine (injected intraperitoneally at 0.35 mg/kg 1 hour prior to irradiation) in mice on the 9th day of gestation. The end-points scored at 4, 12 and 24 hours after irradiation were mitotic activity and cell death in the neuroblasts of the optic vesicle. Results at 4 hours showed potentiation of the x-ray effects by a factor of 1.8, based on cell necrosis.

C. CONCLUSIONS

301. Knowledge of the effect of radiation type and energy in modifying the response of pre-natally irradiated animals is still insufficient, particularly in comparison with similar information related to other non-stochastic effects. However, for irradiation with fast neutrons of various energies, data are now available on the induction of cell killing and production of micronuclei in the early embryos; for embryolethal and teratogenic effects in mice; and for lethal effects and body or brain weight loss in rats. By comparison with the effects of x or gamma rays, in no case did neutrons show an RBE higher than 10 at the doses used, down to about a tenth of a gray of neutrons, irrespective of the neutron energy, dose range, developmental stage at irradiation and time at scoring of the effects. In most cases reported, the RBE values were actually lower than 5, although the values may vary to some extent for different types of lethal or developmental effects or malformations. Peaks of maximum sensitivity related to the stage of development of the various anatomical structures occur at the same time for neutrons as for low-LET radiation, but quantitative information is inadequate to state whether the amplitude of the sensitivity oscillations is consistently higher or lower than for low-LET radiation. Moreover, experience is too limited to recognize definite changes of the RBE as a function of dose, although somewhat higher values could be expected at low doses, judging from the form of the dose-induction relationships of the radiations under comparison in some of the experiments.

302. Information on the shape of dose-effect relationships for various end-points and on possible changes of this shape with radiation quality is, however, insufficient. This makes it difficult to predict whether, at doses of the order of 1 mGy or lower, the values of the RBE might increase appreciably, as is the case for many other non-stochastic end-points. There is still no information on the joint effect of LET and dose rate, dose fractionation, and state of oxygenation of the fetal or embryonic tissues, that would make it possible to extend to effects in utero generalizations known to be valid for other effects at the cell or tissue level in adult animals. For example, a lower sparing effect of fractionation with high-LET radiation, as compared with that of low-LET, has not been documented for systems developing in utero. Similarly, data are insufficient to say whether the RBE of different radiations is higher under anoxic than under well oxygenated conditions for a number of end-points in utero. At the same time, however, there is no indication that the developing conceptus may behave, in respect of these major radiobiological variables, in a manner that is grossly at variance with that to be predicted on the basis of adult mammalian systems.

303. A series of papers has reported rather extensively on the effects induced by pre-natal irradiation with 530-MeV monoenergetic helium ions. This radiation was slightly, but consistently, more effective than gamma rays in stunting fetal growth under hypoxic or well oxygenated conditions and in producing gross morphological anomalies under aerobic exposure. Dose splitting over 24 hours (for the same total dose administered) resulted in higher RBE values. The radiosensitivity of the embryo and fetus to killing in utero over days 3-10 of pregnancy showed oscillations within a factor of three to four but on average the RBE of helium ions with respect to gamma rays over the whole period considered was 1. Thus, there were no major features to be gained from these experiments in respect to sensitivity periods, effects of oxygen, or effects of fractionation that would not be in accordance with expectations from basic radiobiological knowledge of gamma ray and helium ion dose-effect relationships for cellular effects. An RBE value of 1.7 for peak π mesons was reported for irradiation of pronuclear-zygote mouse embryos scored at day 13 of pregnancy for a variety of developmental effects.

304. The technique of in vitro irradiation and culture of early mouse embryos has been used extensively in recent years to test for combined actions with a variety of substances added to the culture medium. In general, this technique produces information that is more valuable for general toxicological than for radiobiological purposes. However, additive effects were reported for the majority of substances tested, including phenol, p-nitrophenol, 2,4-dinitrophenol, sodium nitrite and sulfite, 2,4,6-trinitrobenzene sulfonate and ethidium bromide. In other cases, for some combinations of radiation-drug dosage or for some of the end-points scored, synergistic effects were described. This applied to drugs such as actinomycin D, cadmium and lead chloride, and caffeine. The wider significance of the findings in respect of the very low environmental levels of some of these substances, and of later stages of development, remains to be fully clarified. For exposures during the stage of major organogenesis, synergistic effects of radiation administered in conjunction with trypan blue, cortisone, caffeine, urethane, ultrasound and high frequency radiation were also reported in single instances. More systematic studies would be needed to substantiate these observations for a wider range of doses and effects.

305. Clear evidence has been gathered of a radioprotective action for the drug 2-mercaptopropionyl glycine for a number of effects at the tissue or whole-body level in pre-natally irradiated mice. On the other hand, misonidazole, a hypoxic cell sensitizer, has been shown to potentiate the action of radiation when administered in combination with low- and high-LET radiation and for a variety of teratological and developmental end-points. The same was true of another known radiosensitizer, miracil-D, which showed

different degrees of potentiation, depending on the strain of mice, the dosage used and the type of malformation scored.

VII. TUMOUR INDUCTION

306. This chapter contains separate reviews of information on animals and on man. It will not attempt to discuss the general problem of mechanisms of tumour induction by radiation, which has been considered by UNSCEAR on many occasions and most recently in annex B to the present report. It is not known at present whether the same mechanisms underlying tumour induction in adult animals apply to mammals irradiated in utero: knowledge of these mechanisms is not sufficiently advanced to allow separate analysis of carcinogenesis in adult and developing animals. The reader is therefore referred to annex B for an extended treatment of tumour induction mechanisms which, at least in relation to basic radiobiological aspects, are also assumed for the time being to apply to tumours induced by irradiation in utero. The subject of malignancy induction following pre-conception exposure is discussed in annex A to the present report (chapter VI, section A).

A. DATA FROM ANIMALS

307. Data on the relative susceptibility to tumour induction of animals irradiated before or after birth, which had appeared up to 1977, were already reviewed by UNSCEAR in annex I of its 1977 report [U2]. While noting the relative scarcity of such data, UNSCEAR had concluded that pre-natal irradiation of animals seemed to affect the growth and differentiation of tissues rather than their malignant transformation. The types of tumours induced by radiation in adult animals vary considerably with species and strains, and this was shown to be true for irradiation in utero as well. Up to the time of the 1977 review, there was no evidence, however, that pre-natal irradiation of experimental animals in utero could be more carcinogenic than irradiation of young or adult animals. The following text updates that review with recently published data. It also examines other reports not included in the previous analysis.

308. Carcinogenesis following pre-natal exposure, particularly in experimental animal systems, was reviewed by Sikov [S46]. In his paper, he emphasized the methodological difficulties of working on pre-natal animals, and discussed the likelihood of an increase in tumour incidence following exposure in utero being statistically significant at low doses with the group size normally used for such studies. He also drew attention to the need to consider patterns of effects and modifications of tumour spectra to avoid missing important effects. On the other hand, his paper illustrated the difficulties of increasing the doses to produce unequivocal evidence of effects, because irradiation of pre-natal stages may produce morphological and physiological effects in several tissues at doses that would not be considered high when working with adult animals. As a consequence, there is a narrow range of doses to show radiation carcinogenesis in pre-natal animals, which is a limiting condition for obtaining precise dose-response relationships.

309. Valuable methods of studying radiation oncogenesis in cell culture have been developed in recent years and are increasingly being used. Some of them rely on the use of embryonic cells exposed in utero and then tested for transformation in vitro. Such methods would allow, in principle, comparisons of susceptibility between cells of various fetal ages, of carcinogenic responses in vitro and in vivo [B18, B19, B20], and of interaction studies between radiation and various inducing and promoting agents. All this could be done taking as an end-point an effect such as cell transformation, which is thought to be closely related to in vivo carcinogenesis. There are, at the moment, some unsettled methodological points and difficulties in understanding the precise relationships between transformation in vitro and carcinogenesis in vivo. When these difficulties are resolved, cell transformation may emerge as a very useful tool to study the mechanisms of carcinogenesis in pre-natal stages. At the moment, however, it appears from an extensive review of the field [B31] that no significant contributions are being published along the lines suggested above.

1. The mouse

310. Rugh, Duhamel and Skaredoff [R18] working on small groups of CF1 mice exposed to x rays (100 R) at each day between fertilization and 18 days p.c. found that the tumour incidence in the offspring was not statistically increased by pre-natal irradiation, although it was higher among the females, whether irradiated or not. From these experiments, the evidence for any increase in tumorigenesis was on the whole equivocal, and it appeared that the long-term sequelae of embryonic and fetal irradiation related more to growth and total body weight (permanent stunting) rather than to tumour induction.

311. Agarwal et al. [A1] reported on the radiation dosimetry of an experiment in which a range of doses (0.1 to 2 Gy) was given at 10 or 18 days p.c. to mice in utero (strain not specified). Their paper is almost entirely confined to the physical aspects of the experiments and refers only to an increased incidence of lymphoma and breast and lung carcinoma.

312. In the experiments of Friedberg et al. [F4] pronuclear zygotes of mouse strain CD-1, randomly bred, were irradiated in utero by fast neutrons (0.15 Gy). Animals that survived up to 30 days of extra-uterine life were then kept and observed until their natural death, recording the cumulative mortality distribution, the percentage incidence of the principal neoplastic diseases and the mean age at death for each tumour class. The differences found between irradiated and sham-irradiated animals of the same sex were not found to be statistically significant.

313. Sasaki et al. have published a series of studies on carcinogenic effects induced in mice by irradiation at various intra-uterine stages. In the first of these studies [S1], (C57BL/6 × WHT)F₁ mice were exposed (200 R) at 12 or at 16-18 days p.c. and examined throughout their extra-uterine life for the induction of degenerative diseases, growth retardation and the presence of tumours. For irradiation at the middle intra-uterine stages, the prevailing effects to be observed were growth retardation, several congenital malformations and amyloid degeneration. Tumours were not in excess over non-irradiated controls in this group of mice, but there was a significant decrease of incidence of lymphoreticular, lung and uterine tumours. Lung, pituitary gland and ovarian tumours were significantly enhanced after irradiation at the late fetal stages; liver and skin tumours were only slightly increased, thymic lymphoma was not.

314. In another study [S2], data were published on mice of the same strain irradiated at 17 days p.c. (150 or 300 R), within 24 hours of birth (400 R) or at 5 weeks of age (400 R). Overall, the susceptibility to tumour induction increased with age, in the order from pre-natal to neo-natal to young-adult mice; however, the most remarkable changes were found in the spectrum of tumours produced. An excess of pituitary, pulmonary and hepatocellular tumours developed in mice irradiated in utero, but lymphoreticular neoplasms and myeloid leukaemia were not induced. For irradiation in the neo-natal stage, thymic lymphoma, pituitary, ovarian, harderian gland, but particularly hepatocellular tumours were found in excess. Exposure at the juvenile age resulted instead in a higher incidence of ovarian and harderian gland neoplasms. The complex of these findings points to the conclusion that the age-dependence of susceptibility to radiation carcinogenesis differs for different organs and tissues. The high susceptibility of peri-natal mice to x-ray-induced hepatocellular carcinogenesis found in this series was also specifically discussed in another paper [S71] and was deemed to be related to the high frequency of liver cell mitosis at the time of, or after, x irradiation.

315. Two studies by the same group are so far only available in an abstract. In the first one [S28], groups of B6WF₁ mice were exposed to 200-kVp x rays (150, 300 or 600 R) at 17 days p.c. The incidence of lymphocytic neoplasms was compared with that shown by mice irradiated at 1, 7, 35 and 195 days of age. Exposure in the late fetal stages produced significantly higher rates of such tumours, reaching about 23% after 600 R. Susceptibility to the tumours was lower in the fetal than in neo-natal and suckling mice, but not lower than in the young adult mice. Data on the breakdown of various classes of lymphocytic tumours were also reported. In the second study [S27] B6C3F₁, animals were exposed to x rays at 17 days p.c. and at days 1, 7, 35 and 105 (300 R). Animals were killed when 800 days old for study of kidney and cerebellar damage and of tumour incidence. The carcinogenic response at the fetal stage was far lower than that of neo-natal mice and the tumour spectra were very similar. In early post-natal life lymphocytic, liver and pituitary tumours developed with high incidences,

while myeloid leukaemia and harderian gland tumours were most elevated when irradiation took place at 35 and 105 days of age.

316. The results of other experiments by the same group are still in press [S72]. These experiments were carried out on B6C3F1 mice irradiated at 17 days p.c., within 24 hours of birth and at 15 weeks of age. Doses of 1.9, 3.8 and 5.7 Gy of ¹³⁷Cs gamma rays were used. Gross and histological pathology were performed on the animals at death, but data were not corrected for competing death causes. Overall, tumour incidence in irradiated animals was not significantly higher than in controls, which had themselves about 90% tumour incidence. However, late fetal animals were found to be particularly prone to pituitary tumours, which were statistically higher than in controls and had the longest latent period of all induced neoplasms. After 1.9 and 3.8 Gy, given at 17 days p.c., the incidence of tumours of the lung was significantly higher than in controls. Malignant thymic and non-thymic lymphoma was also in excess and appeared after shorter latent periods in fetal mice given 5.7 Gy; however, the susceptibility was higher in early post-natal than in pre-natal mice. The latter animals also showed a higher incidence of liver tumours than the controls, but not higher than that of neo-natal animals. Overall, the tumour susceptibility of mice irradiated in the late fetal and in the neo-natal periods was similar, but young adults were little, if at all, susceptible to the induction of pituitary, lung and liver neoplasms. The young adults were, however, more susceptible to myeloid leukaemia and to tumours of the harderian gland.

317. In order to investigate the question of the high susceptibility to radiation-induced tumours in pre-natal animals, Schmahl and collaborators [S32] set up experiments with a 2-stage carcinogenesis model. The irradiation of the NMRI mice in utero (3 daily doses of 0.8 Gy on pregnancy days 11-13) was regarded as a possible initiating stimulus, the promoting treatment being represented by the skin application of the phorbol ester TPA (12-O-tetradecanoylphorbol-13-acetate). Mice were treated with the promoter between 12 and 26 weeks of their post-natal life and observed for another 70 weeks for development of skin neoplasms. In spite of some differential effects in regard to distinct diseases, the overall conclusion was that the TPA treatment did not result in a higher tumour yield (either of the skin or of internal organs such as marrow, lung, liver, ovary) than that observed after pre-natal x irradiation alone. This result, which is at variance with other observations in adult rodent skin, was attributed to the dysplastic nature of the skin after pre-natal irradiation, which fails to respond to TPA as does normal fetal and newborn mouse skin. A decrease in the synthesis of prostaglandin induced by pre-natal irradiation would be responsible for the altered susceptibility to TPA.

318. In another series of experiments by the same group [S33] pregnant NMRI mice were subjected to fractionated x irradiation during late organogenesis (11-13 days of gestation), during the early fetal period (14-16 days) or during both periods (11-16 days).

Various fractionation schemes, with total doses ranging from 2.4 to 7.2 Gy, were tested and the offspring were followed for 39 months for the presence of ovarian tumours. With daily doses of 3 × 1.2 Gy, applied either in late organogenesis or in the early fetal period, a significant increase in the number of tumours was observed, mostly tubular adenomas, with about 20% between luteomas and granulosa cell types. Lower doses appeared ineffective. Autoradiographic observations on fetal ovaries 1 or 6 days after irradiation during late organogenesis showed a depression of the proliferation rate which was thought to be correlated with the relatively low susceptibility to tumour induction during this period. There was a sharp increase in the frequency of ovarian tumours following daily doses of 6 × 0.8 Gy or 6 × 1.2 Gy on days 11-13. Ovarian cysts were also found and they reached the highest incidences in animals treated with doses of 3 × 1.0 Gy or 3 × 1.2 Gy on days 11-13. The lowest cyst frequencies were seen in animals receiving doses for 6 consecutive days, which had the highest incidence of ovarian tumours.

319. Kusama and Yoshizawa [K24] reported on a comparison of the carcinogenic action of ^{137}Cs gamma rays on male and female C57BL/6J mice between the fetal (15 day p.c., 1 Gy), or post-natal age (30 days of age, 1 or 4 Gy). Autopsies were performed at death; tumour incidence rate, average latent period and composition of the tumour spectra were the biological end-points scored. There was no difference in the gross tumour incidence between control and irradiated mice, whether irradiation took place before or after birth. Different methods for adjustment of the data for competing risks were applied and it was concluded that the Kaplan-Meyer method was appropriate for the purpose. Under such conditions of analysis, the incidences of thymic lymphoma and breast tumours in all irradiated groups (fetal or post-natal) were found to be similar to those of the control mice. Reticular tissue neoplasms, on the other hand, showed a consistently decreased incidence in all irradiated groups, with little evidence of any special trend of the pre- as opposed to post-natal mice.

320. Pre-natal x irradiation of NMRI mice on the 12th day of gestation was reported by Schmahl to induce both dysplastic and neoplastic disorders [S65]. Dysplastic changes (see also [S62] and [S63]) include hypotrichosis, alopecia and skin ulcerations, appearing at 2-4 months of age in about one-quarter of the mice receiving 0.5-2.0 Gy. As to neoplastic changes, their incidence in the irradiated mice appeared to be generally lower than in controls, but the various classes of tumours showed a different behaviour. For example, the incidence of leukaemia (after correction for competing causes) was decreased at all doses below the normal incidence of the non-irradiated mice. By contrast, lung tumours (both benign and malignant), ovarian (see also [S33]) and liver tumours were increased, with a peak incidence at 1 Gy. Under the condition of the experiments, this dose was shown to be the most effective for tumour induction. The liver appeared to be the most sensitive organ, both for irradiation alone and in experiments using the tumour-promoting agent phorbol ester TPA.

321. Covelli et al. [C9] reported on experiments designed to investigate the role of age and LET on the susceptibility to radiation carcinogenesis and life shortening. Graded single doses of x rays (250 kV, 0.5-7.0 Gy) or attenuated fission neutrons (average energy, 0.4 Mev, 0.09-2.14 Gy) were administered to BC3F1 mice of both sexes in utero at 17 days p.c., or to male animals aged 3 or 19 months. Irradiation of 3-month-old animals caused a measurable dose-related degree of life shortening associated with a higher incidence and rate of appearance of radiation-induced tumours. Irradiation during the pre-natal ages or at 19 months, did not produce significant shortening of life after both x-ray and neutron irradiation; there was, however, a significantly higher incidence of solid tumours and reticulum cell sarcoma. The high variability of control values in the incidence of neoplastic diseases, particularly of the reticular cell tumour, and the differential carcinogenic action of x rays and neutrons in animals irradiated in utero, do not allow precise conclusions about the overall comparative susceptibility of mice irradiated at different ages. It is quite evident, however, that the changes in the tumour spectrum are much clearer effects than the overall shift of tumour incidence between animals irradiated at various ages.

322. Baserga et al. [B36] studied tumour induction in CxA F_1 mice after exposure to radioactively labelled thymidine. Variables analysed were: the age of the animals at exposure (including 15-17 days p.c. fetuses, newborn animals and adults at 2, 6 and 12-14 months of age); the magnitude of the thymidine dose and the manner of dose fractionation (between about 7.5 and 370 kBq per gram body weight delivered as single doses or in 6 fractions over 8 days); and the effect of ^{14}C-thymidine, as compared to ^{3}H-thymidine. Only malignant tumours were considered and there were no appreciable differences between mortality rate and tumour incidence between the two sexes. The data showed that both types of thymidine produced shortening of life span and an excess of tumours; that tumour incidence was dose-related and greater in animals injected as young adults than later in life; and that tumour incidence was also significantly above the spontaneous level in animals treated in the fetal stage. The small number of tumours seen, and the fact that the experiments reported did not extend until spontaneous death of the animals, preclude any meaningful comparison of tumour incidence between different ages at irradiation in this series.

323. The leukaemogenic effects of ^{32}P given intra-peritoneally as NaPO$_4$ were studied in 3-5-months-old BALB female mice and in animals of both sexes between 11 and 15 days p.c. [H17]. After contamination, animals were observed until spontaneous death or were killed when leukaemia was diagnosed; in any case the experiments were terminated when the animals were 2 years old. Autopsy examinations were performed and leukaemia (including leukaemia proper, lymphosarcoma and reticulum cell sarcoma) was diagnosed microscopically. Lack of separation between various types of leukaemias diminishes the usefulness of this study. In adult females, a significantly elevated incidence of leukaemia was seen, but the dose depen-

dence over the range of activities of ^{32}P administered (about 1.5 to 4.5 MBq per animal) was not significant. In females exposed as fetuses the incidence of leukaemia was also significantly increased, and the females appeared definitely more susceptible than males. Furthermore, there was a negative correlation with the dose in females (over the range of about 90 kBq to 3.3 MBq per animal), while in males no such correlation was documented. These differences were attributed to the fact that ^{32}P at the doses given affects ovarian development and disturbs an interaction with oestrogens in leukaemogenesis. Comparison of the incidence of leukaemia showed that female animals treated as adults were approximately as susceptible as when injected as fetuses.

324. Between the years 1971 and 1982, Rönnbäck published a series of papers [R4, R10-R14] (also collected and jointly commented in a thesis [R5]) in which he described the effects of ^{90}Sr irradiation on the fetal ovaries of CBA mice. In none of these papers was there information on the actual doses absorbed in the fetal ovaries. However, it has recently been estimated [R26] that the effects of 11.1 kBq ^{90}Sr given to the pregnant mother would correspond approximately to those seen after doses to fetal ovaries of 0.010-0.013 Gy, given continuously over 4 days, from the 18th day of gestation to the 2nd day of extrauterine life.

325. In short, it is shown in this series of experiments [R5] that the time for administration of the radionuclide to the pregnant mothers is a very important factor in determining the final degree of injury to the ovaries of the fetuses. When the number of germ cells remaining in the ovaries was scored at 56 days of extra-uterine age, it was found that the later during pregnancy that ^{90}Sr had been administered, the worst was the degree of injury to be seen, the maximum of effect being found for contamination at 19 days p.c. The earliest maturation stages, i.e., the "naked" oocytes, were in all cases the most sensitive cells. An activity-effect relationship was established in the range of 11-370 kBq ^{90}Sr given to the pregnant mother, and it was found that the fraction of germ cells remaining in the ovaries decreased linearly as a function of logactivity. The slope of the curve, however, remained the same, whether the damage was scored at 28, 56 or 84 days of age. Considering that there is a pronounced natural decrease of the number of oocytes as a function of age in untreated control mice, this observation indicates that the rate (as a function of dose) at which the germ cells decrease in the irradiated ovaries is independent of their initial number. A statistically significant reduction of naked oocytes was seen in these experiments after about 11 kBq ^{90}Sr.

326. In parallel with the short-term morphologically recognizable damage, long-term functional and carcinogenic effects were also assessed in these experiments by testing the reproductive capacity and the incidence of ovarian tumours in the mice contaminated in utero. Reproductive performance over a period of 7 months was tested by standard methods over the range of 46-740 kBq ^{90}Sr given to 19-day pregnant mothers. Only starting from 320 kBq were there signs of

impaired fertility. The signs were quite obvious at 740 kBq, the rate of pregnancy being significantly reduced. The total number of litters and of offspring per female, and the reproductive period, started to decline at 185 kBq and were significantly affected at 370 kBq. It should be noted, for the sake of comparison, that at 185 kBq only 25% of the oocytes and follicles remained in the ovaries at the beginning of the mating period and that, 7 months later, at the end of it, the ovaries were essentially depleted of germ cells.

327. Tumour incidence was observed in the ovaries of 10-month-old animals that had been contaminated as fetuses with ^{90}Sr activities in the range of 46-740 kBq. Eighty-three out of 104 animals showed interstitial fibrosis, cysts and proliferation of the germinal epithelium. Different types of ovarian tumours (1 granulosa cell, 2 cystic adenomas, 18 tubular adenomas) were also found in these animals. There was a direct relationship between the frequency of animals showing proliferation and "down growth" of the germinal epithelium into the ovarian parenchyma and the frequency of animals having tubular adenomas, but tumours were not found until about 14% of the animals had shown downgrowths. Stimulation of the follicle-depleted gonads by gonadotropic hormones might be an important factor in the proliferative phenomena leading ultimately to the production of tumours.

328. Another paper by Walinder and Rönnbäck [W30] added more information on the induction of thyroid and pulmonary tumours in CBA mice, given pre-natally ^{131}I and whole-body x irradiation at 18-19 days of gestation. This paper gave emphasis to the role of cellular proliferation as a tumour-enhancing factor, particularly by comparison with proliferation in the adult mouse. It confirmed that tumour frequency was higher and latency shorter in the thyroid of the pre-natally irradiated animals than in the adults. Lung tumours were not more frequent in pre-natally irradiated mice than in non-irradiated ones, although their latent period was significantly shorter. Cell killing was found to be more pronounced in the thyroids of mice irradiated as adults than in animals exposed to the same doses in their fetal life. Therefore, the loss of cells' reproductive capacity leading to a lower tumour incidence was held to be less important for pre- and neo-natal thyroid carcinogenesis, than for carcinogenesis in mature glands. It was pointed out, however, that many other factors, in addition to cell proliferation, may determine the final incidence of tumours: for example, cells in the organs of the fetal and the adult animal could be at various stages of differentiation. This condition, among others, would of course make comparisons across ages extremely difficult.

2. The rat

329. Sikov and Lofstrom [S13, S46] treated Sprague-Dawley rats with x rays (20 or 100 R on day 10 and 50 or 185 R on day 15 of gestation). Later in the animals' life they observed decreases in growth and longevity that were exposure-related. The incidence of mammary

tumours in female animals given the highest exposure at 15 days was decreased. However, there was a shortening of the latent period in tumours developing in irradiated rats, as opposed to those appearing in the controls. An exposure of 50 R produced a tumour rate almost identical with that in the controls, with a greater tendency towards the presence of multiple tumours in tumour-bearing animals. Tumours of other sites were not appreciably increased. After 185 R, the gonads were atrophic, and this suggested an association between the decreased incidence of mammary tumours and the ovarian changes at this level of exposure.

330. Wegner and Graul [W17] irradiated (180-kV x rays, 1 Gy) Wistar rats in utero on the 9th day p.c. and followed them after birth for the appearance of malformations and tumours. About 40% of the animals showed brain or eye malformations and 10% developed tumours (as compared with a spontaneous rate of 3.4%) mostly of the malignant type, although benign mammary tumours were also observed. Animals bred through the second generation had no malformations, no significant decrease of life expectancy and no increased tumour incidence. In other experiments [W18], animals of the same strain were exposed (270 R) on the 18th day p.c. There was a high incidence of microcephaly and microophthalmia and genital hypoplasia in both sexes. In males, the incidence of tumours (total and malignant) was increased significantly above the control level, but it appeared to be slightly lower in these animals than in other animals exposed post-natally. In females, the incidence of mammary tumours was markedly decreased by pre-natal exposure, while it increased in rats exposed after birth. Other tumours of the genital tract (uterus, ovary) were reduced by pre-natal as compared with post-natal exposure. When all genital tumours were excluded, the incidence of other malignancies was slightly greater in females exposed post-natally than pre-natally.

331. The experiments by Strel'tsova and Pavlenko-Mikhailov [S48] were carried out on outbred white rats irradiated during the pre-implantation period (7 days p.c., 240 animals), during late organogenesis (14 days p.c., 105 animals) and during the fetal period (19 days p.c., 120 animals). The methods for counting stages in development are not specified in the paper. A single dose of 1 Gy of ^{60}Co gamma rays was administered in all cases. The animals, together with some controls, were followed in time to study tumour appearance. The results reported refer to 219 test and 53 control animals dying between 200 and 600 days of age. About 17% of the control animals developed tumours during this time, as compared with about 65% of the animals irradiated during early organogenesis, late organogenesis (63%) and the fetal period (43%). Animals irradiated at 14 days p.c. developed tumours up to 400 days of life, while in the other two test groups tumours only appeared between 120 and 180 days of life. Male animals irradiated at 7 days p.c. showed tumours of the mammary gland and bones, while the females irradiated at the same time showed ovarian and bone tumours, which were not observed in control animals.

332. Kalter et al. published a series of papers on the interaction of ethylnitroso-urea (ENU) and x rays administered in utero in respect of the oncogenic response of rats. In a first series of experiments [W7] pregnant Sprague Dawley rats received 2 Gy of x irradiation on days 15 or 16 p.c., and 10 mg/kg ENU one to four days later. Controls only irradiated or only injected with ENU were also set up. By the 15th month post-exposure, about 17% of the offspring exposed to both agents pre-natally developed neurogenic tumours, as opposed to 62% of those exposed to ENU alone, or to no tumours at all in those exposed only to radiation. The first signs of tumours appeared later in animals exposed to the combined treatment. In order to probe deeper into this antagonistic action, in a second experimental series [K1, K2], rats were irradiated on day 16 with a range of doses from 0.05 to 2.5 Gy and received ENU (10 mg/kg intraperitoneally) on day 20 of gestation. The frequency of animals surviving beyond 4 weeks of age that developed tumours in the course of their entire life span was inversely related to the dose of x rays. Thus, ENU alone caused about 69% of animals to develop tumours; 0.25 Gy + ENU, 46%; and 2 Gy + ENU, 15%. The mean time for the appearance of neurogenic tumours and the mean number of tumours for each affected animal were unrelated to tumour frequency. Analysis of the rate of tumour appearance indicated that the initiation, rather than the promotion, stages of tumour induction could be responsible for the reduced frequency. Killing of target cells, probably glioblasts, was not in itself entirely sufficient to explain the results.

333. The subject of the interaction between radiation and ENU was also taken up in another paper by Schmahl and Kriegel [S82]. In their experiments, single and combined treatments were administered to Wistar rats with the chemical alone or after x-ray doses of 0.5-1.5 Gy. Animals were in the 13th day p.c., at which time both agents may induce brain malformations and ENU, alone or in combination, may produce brain tumours. The possible correlations between the teratological and the carcinogenic end-points were investigated by a histopathological analysis of the type and degree of malformations, and the distribution patterns of tumours in the forebrain. The existence of a correlation was shown not only by the simultaneous occurrence of both effects in the same brains, but also by a higher tumour multiplicity (mostly gliomas) in the malformed brains and their preferential location in the subependymal layer, which was also the most heavily malformed structure. Another effect of irradiation, the occurrence of heterotopic neuronal nodules called "rosettes", which is only apparent at doses above 1 Gy, correlated negatively, however, with the occurrence of gliomas. In view of the authors, this explains the substantially decreased incidence of gliomas following combined treatments involving doses in excess of 1.0 Gy, and also the consistent multiplicity of tumours, in spite of their decreased frequency.

334. Cahill and his group studied neoplastic and life-span effect after chronic exposure to tritium. In a first paper [C1], Sprague-Dawley rats were exposed to equilibrium levels of tritiated water during pregnancy

and up to parturition. Four different levels of the radionuclide resulted in cumulative whole-body doses of about 0.066, 0.66, 3.3 and 6.6 Gy. The animals at the two higher dose levels showed, throughout their life span, an increased incidence of mammary fibroadenomas. Data were not such as to allow the definition of a precise dose-response curve; they were, however, not incompatible with linearity. Increasing doses of radiation shortened the time for the onset of mammary fibroadenoma. A second paper [C2] reported that the offspring of the animals exposed in utero to doses up to 0.66 Gy showed no effect with respect to the overall incidence of neoplasia, to incidence rate, or to age at onset of mammary fibroadenomas. Females exposed to 3.3 or 6.6 Gy were sterile and had lower rates of mammary fibroadenomas than did controls. At 6.6 Gy females showed a lower incidence of overall tumours. Regardless of dose, females had a significantly higher incidence of neoplasia and a longer life span than males.

335. In another set of experiments, Berry et al. [B37] attempted to induce bone tumours in the offspring of Sprague-Dawley rats by treating pregnant mothers (16, 18 or 20 days p.c.) with ^{32}P (about 37 or 110 kBq per gram body weight). Fetal tissues were judged to be resistant to irradiation since no increased frequency of tumour was found in the treated animals. However, naturally-occurring tumours showed a clear tendency to appear earlier in post-natal life in the treated animals. On this basis, it was concluded that transplacental exposure of rats to ^{32}P provided no evidence of enhanced oncogenic effects in the fetus.

336. Other experiments were reported by Schmahl and Kollmer [S31, S64] on the carcinogenic effect of ^{90}Sr injected into pregnant rats at 18 days p.c. (3.7 or 5.5 MBq per rat). The radionuclide accumulated in the ossification centres of the skull of fetal animals to deliver a dose which was calculated to be between 0.6 and 1.2 Gy (over the entire life span) within the bone surfaces. Approximately 50% of this dose was delivered within a week of the injection of the nuclide. The offspring of the treated animals were examined at autopsy and pathologically. They had an incidence of pituitary tumours which was, as compared with non-treated control animals, about 10 times higher in the males and three times higher in the females. In about 6% of treated animals, metastasizing meningeal sarcomas were seen, and in 2%, pituitary adenomas and meningeal sarcomas occurred simultaneously.

337. Sikov et al. [S47, S54, M40] injected intravenously into adult, weanling, new-born and 19-days-p.c. rats ^{239}Pu cytrate in different amounts, adjusted in such a way as to deliver radiation doses of approximately 0.07, 0.23 and 0.7 Gy to these animals' femurs during the first 10 days after injection. Doses to the various age groups were markedly different. Most of the dose to the younger animals was absorbed within the first few months. Weanlings and adults received a more prolonged and substantially higher cumulative exposure. The animals were observed until their natural death, but the experiment was terminated after 30 months. The survival times of rats exposed post-natally became progressively shorter as the dose increased, but no life shortening was seen in animals

exposed pre-natally. Bone tumour incidence increased in all exposed groups, irrespective of age. Younger rats appeared to be less sensitive on an administered-dose basis, but were perhaps more sensitive on a cumulative-dose basis. A biphasic cumulative dose-incidence relationship with a maximum at about 0.25 Gy and a drop at 0.8 Gy was seen in animals exposed pre-natally, but it is not clear how much of this phenomenon may be true or spurious (for example, owing to confounding maternal effects). Pre-natally exposed rats cross-fostered to non-injected females, in order to ensure that they would only be exposed while in utero, had the highest incidence of bone tumours, even higher than that of rats remaining with the injected mothers. This result was probably related to the high dose given to the dams, which affected their capacity to care for the offspring. The site of radiation-induced tumours also varied as a function of age: in the younger animals, most tumours arose in the head or in the vertebrae; in the adults and weanlings, they were mostly in the extremities, with only a few in the vertebrae or other places. It was concluded that the younger animals were probably more susceptible per unit dose than the adults. It is clear, however, that this susceptibility is also a function of the rate of dose delivery and therefore is not easily defined.

338. Two abstracts reported on the late effects of ^{131}I in Fisher rats. The first [C20] regarded animals exposed in utero to concentrations of Na ^{131}I ranging from 4 kBq to 3.7 MBq during days 16-18 of pregnancy. Two months post-partum, the animals showed an alteration of immunological reactions (cell-mediated immune response and antibody-dependent cell-mediated cytotoxic response) to the carcinogen 1,2-dimethyl-hydrazine, suggesting that the original peri-natal exposure produced a persistent altered reaction to the chemical. The second abstract [L11] reported on a higher immunological response of the male animals exposed in utero, which was 1.7 times that of the female offspring.

339. Sikov et al. [S80] exposed groups of 50 to 80 pre-natal, new-born, weanling and adult rats to various levels of ^{131}I and scored their thyroids microscopically at death or at 30 months of age for the presence of tumours. These were commonly C-cell type in control animals and follicular in the exposed ones. Doses were estimated by radioanalysis in the thyroids of the various groups. When given post-natally the ^{131}I increased tumour incidence significantly in the range of 1 Gy, but led to a further decrease down to control levels after doses of 20 Gy or greater. When given pre-natally (from 17 days on), the ^{131}I produced a higher incidence of tumours at all dose levels of 0.4, 4.25 and 34 Gy. The form of the dose-response relationships was characterized by a peak at intermediate doses in the two older groups, but was progressively increasing with dose in the two groups exposed perinatally.

3. The dog

340. Preliminary data are also gradually becoming available for the dog irradiated in utero. In one report

[P7], 4 groups of 120 beagles were irradiated with gamma rays from ^{60}Co in the late fetal period (55 days p.c.) or soon after birth (2 days of age) with 20 or 100 R delivered over a constant time of 10 minutes. The morbidity and mortality of these animals was followed over 2 years and compared with that of 450 control dogs and of other dogs exposed to the same dose levels at other ages. Three of the 240 dogs at the 100 R level and 1 of the 240 at the 20 R level died with tumours within the observation time, while in controls and animals exposed at other ages, no tumours were observed . No tumour would be expected to appear by chance in irradiated dogs.

341. An abstract published in 1978 [B4] updated the experience to 5 years post-exposure and concluded that of 20 dogs developing tumours, 19 had been irradiated. The experiments were not sufficiently advanced to draw significant conclusions as to the role of age as a factor in radiation injury. Another report [B28] gave evidence that the incidence of lymphoma in the irradiated dogs, especially those exposed at 55 days p.c., was considerably higher than that in the controls or than that expected in a random canine population. Final results of these series, as well as of another series on beagle dogs receiving continuous whole-body irradiation [S29, S30], will not be available for a few years.

342. Experiments by Momeni [M41] were aimed at studying the incidence of bone sarcoma and myelo-proliferative disorders as a function of dose rate and time in beagle dogs fed diets containing ^{90}SrCl (in equilibrium with ^{90}Y) from mid-gestation to 1.5 years of age. Median incidence time and standard deviation of the distribution were calculated for the tumours at each level of administered activity. For primary osteosarcoma, this time increased from 2.8 years of age for animals receiving 1.3 MBq ^{90}Sr/day to 12.6 years for those receiving about 1.50 kBq ^{90}Sr/day. Although very valuable for extrapolation of the carcinogenic effect to low doses and dose rates, these data do not lend themselves to a comparison of susceptibility to tumour induction in the pre- as opposed to post-natal ages.

B. DATA FROM MAN

343. One of the most important sources of information about the induction of tumours in children irradiated pre-natally is the so-called Oxford Survey of Childhood Cancer. Data from this series were first reported in 1956 [S44] by Stewart and her colleagues. These authors confirmed in 1958 [S23] that the mothers of children who died from leukaemia or other malignant diseases remembered having been subjected to abdominal or pelvic x rays during the related pregnancy with a frequency that was higher than that of the mothers of control children who had not developed cancer. This finding stimulated much interest. For a description and history of the Oxford Survey see Steward [S22]. Soon other reports followed and the experience accumulated up to 1961 [F6, K21, K28, M39, P9, S23, S44, S45] was summarized by UNSCEAR [U3] as in Table 12.

344. In its 1964 report [U3] UNSCEAR reviewed other data that had appeared up to that time [L5, C12, M22, M25, W16]. It pointed out that, as established by MacMahon [M22], the joint maximum likelihood estimate of the relative risk factors in all the surveys reported was 1.4, with 95% confidence limits of 1.2 to 1.6. On that basis, UNSCEAR concluded that, although accurate dose estimates were not available, irradiation of fetal tissues could give rise to a greater risk per unit dose than post-natal irradiation, possibly by a factor as high as 5. It pointed out at the same time, however, that it was difficult to separate such leukaemogenic effect of radiation from other possible etiologic factors connected with the reason that had prompted the radiological examination of the conceptus in utero.

345. Further data on the carcinogenic risk of irradiation in utero were reviewed again in the 1972 UNSCEAR report [U4]. The papers by Graham et al. [G11], Jablon and Kato [J4] and Stewart and Kneale [S24, S26] were specifically examined. The report drew attention to the discrepancy between the negative data from Hiroshima and Nagasaki and those from irradiations performed for medical reasons. It also discussed the difficulties of deriving precise estimates of risk from cohort (rather than from case control) studies, because the cancer risk in children less than 10 years of age is rare (of the order of 10^{-4}) and cohort studies of sufficient size are therefore difficult to carry out. The report concluded that children born of mothers irradiated during pregnancy seemed to have an increased risk of cancer in their early age. The estimate put forward at the time, most likely in excess, was of the order of $2 \ 10^{-3} \text{ Gy}^{-1}$ a^{-1} over a 10-year period, in the range of 0.002 to 0.2 Gy. However, the possibility could not be ruled out that the associations found (or at least part of them) could be related to factors other than irradiation itself.

346. In 1977, UNSCEAR again examined the problem of the carcinogenic risk of irradiation in utero, on the basis of other data by Mole [M23], Newcombe and MacGregor [N3], Holford [H16], Stewart and Kneale [S24], Jablon and Kato [J4], and Kato [K20]. The analysis led to the conclusion that the risk, per unit absorbed dose, of fatal malignancies induced by fetal irradiation could be in the region of $2\text{-}2.5 \ 10^{-2} \text{ Sv}^{-1}$. Half of these malignancies could be attributed to leukaemia and one quarter to tumours of the nervous system.

347. Subsequently, the Committee on the Biological Effects of Ionizing Radiation (BEIR) [C13] examined the literature available up to 1980 on the subject of radiation carcinogenesis in utero. In essence, it concluded that an association existed between intra-uterine irradiation and childhood cancer, but it recognized that such an association could be attributed, to some extent, to factors involved in the selection process for submitting the pregnant mothers to radiodiagnostic examinations. Strong support for a causal relationship came from twin data from the Oxford series, while weak support for a selection effect came from the ascertained relationship between pre-natal irradiation and neo-natal health and from

the relationship between neo-natal health and later, clinically detectable cancer. The BEIR Committee, on the basis of adjusted data from the Oxford Survey estimated the relative risk of cancer after exposure in utero relative to irradiation after birth to be 5.0 for the first-trimester exposure and about 1.5 for the remaining intra-uterine life. The period at risk appeared to be within the first 12 years of post-natal life for haemopoietic tumours and within 10 years for other solid tumours. The risk coefficients were estimated to be at 2500 excess fatal leukaemias and 2800 excess fatal cancers of other types per million children, year and gray.

348. MacMahon [M52] later reviewed the conclusions of the BEIR Committee report on this subject, adding some useful considerations. According to this author, there is no doubt about the existence of a relationship between exposure in utero and subsequent likelihood of developing a malignancy within the first 10 years of life. The relative risk associated with pre-natal exposure is of the order of 40 to 50% over non-exposed children. A number of variables (medical, sociological, methodological) have clearly been identified which tend to confound the association, but even correcting the data on their account would not be sufficient to justify the association quantitatively. The most difficult problem is that of establishing whether the association is causal or by chance. On the one hand, it is difficult to prove that this may not have been due to characteristics of the mothers, the children, or the pregnancy, that may also have been associated with a tendency of the children to develop a malignancy. On the other hand, no such characteristics have been found. There is, in favour of a direct causality, the observation of Mole [M23] on single and twin pregnancies, but this is based on a re-interpretation of the same series. Against a causal relationship there are, however, cogent data from Hiroshima and Nagasaki and from experimental animals. According to MacMahon [M52] it is biologically implausible that fetal doses in the region of a small fraction of a Gy should increase the relative cancer risk by 40 or 50% within 10 years of age while doses in excess of 1 Gy should fail to do so over longer periods of time, as pointed out by Jablon and Kato [J4]. There is, further, [M52], the constancy of the relative risk over all categories of malignancy, which is not in agreement with evidence on radiation carcinogenesis [U2] indicating a remarkable degree of variability between tissues and ages in their response to radiation. Finally, on the question of the alleged dose-response relationship, MacMahon [M52] argues that data analysis as a function of dose is based on the acceptance of the causal nature of the association, which he is inclined to doubt in the case at hand. Given the difficulty of finding new material for independent analyses, MacMahon is also inclined to regard this issue, important as it may be, as an unresolved curiosity which will gradually fade into medical history, giving rise, in the process, to more confusion than understanding.

349. The references given thus far, on which previous conclusions have in large part been founded, are the most relevant to the point at issue but they by no

means exhaust the long list of papers published on this subject, even before the last UNSCEAR review. Other references should also be kept in mind to complete the publications available up to about 1977 [A9, B11, B22, B32, D14, D15, G2, G10, G12, J8, L6, M26, O5, S22, S25, S39, S41, S42, W15]. What follows updates information published since then.

1. Atomic bomb survivors

350. The most recent report on the mortality experience of children exposed in utero to the atomic bombs refers to the period 1945-1976 [K4]. The study sample included 1293 children (1074 exposed at Hiroshima and 219 at Nagasaki) whose status and causes of death were obtained from Japanese family records and death certificates. Doses in utero were estimated by two different groups: one at the Oak Ridge National Laboratory in the United States, the other at the National Institute of Radiological Sciences in Chiba, Japan. The methods used by the two groups were slightly different, but the tissue doses obtained were almost identical and correlated well with the T65 dose, although they were lower by about 40%. (These doses will, however, be subject to revision at some later stage.) Total deaths up to 1976 numbered 203, and the mortality ratio increased linearly with T65 and tissue dose in both cities. The dose-related mortality ratio varied, however, with age at death: it increased with dose for those dying under 1 year of age, particularly for those dying within 1 month of birth; it showed no increase at 1-9 years of age; and an increase was again suggested after 10 years of age. Analysis of the data as a function of trimester of exposure showed a significant increase of mortality ratio with dose only for children exposed in the third trimester.

351. Mechanical injury received by the mother was insufficient to provide an explanation for the excess in early infant death. Birth order and birth weight could not have seriously affected the relationship between mortality and exposure. Precise information about the causes of death was not available for 55 of the 203 deaths, and these 55 occurred almost exclusively within a year of birth. This circumstance did not allow a fine breakdown of causes of death. The following, however, were analysed: perinatal death, which was found to increase with dose; and cancer death (2 leukaemias and 3 solid tumours of the digestive organs), which was not found to be related to dose, even when additional samples defined only in 1960 were analysed. There was no statistically significant evidence of an excess in cancer death among individuals irradiated in utero. However, the sample size and the number of deaths were too small to reach a firm conclusion.

352. A further report by Ishimaru et al. [I3] is of relevance. These authors studied the incidence of leukaemia in a sample of 3636 children (including controls and exposed in utero) in the two cities. Exposed were those whose fetal doses were between 0.01 and 0.49, and in excess of 0.5 Gy. The crude annual incidence rates for exposed and controls in

both cities during 1945-1979 are shown in Table 13. During the 34-year follow-up period, 3 leukaemia cases were identified, 2 in the control groups, and 1 in the group exposed between 0.01 and 0.49 Gy. It was calculated that, in order to show any statistically significant effect of radiation, 7 cases of leukaemia would have to occur among the 705 irradiated subjects included in the sample. Thus, there appears to be no excess risk for the exposed children. This is in agreement with previous findings [J4, K4] in this series.

353. In 1974, Mole [M23] used a radiobiological argument to show that the discrepancy between the observations from Japanese children exposed to atomic radiation in utero and medically irradiated British children could be the result of an artefact, since the killing of potentially transformed cells, particularly at the highest doses, might be responsible for the low rate of tumour induction observed in the Japanese series. Using reports from the early 1970s [J4, K20], and correcting the tumour induction data according to an exponential cell killing function, Mole showed (under a number of qualifying assumptions) that the true induction rate per unit dose might have been three to four times higher than that actually found, thus bringing the results of the Japanese series much closer to those of the Oxford series. In the meantime, new information has been produced [K4] which extends the observation period up to 1976 in Japan, always with negative conclusions. Mole's reasoning was also based on old dosimetric data that are currently under revision. His conclusions, therefore, will have to be verified against the new dosimetry (particularly the doses to the fetus) to see whether they retain their validity.

2.   Medical exposures

354.   The present study reviews only the contributions that have appeared since the last UNSCEAR report on the subject [U2]. Kneale and Stewart returned to the analysis of the Oxford Survey with two more papers published in 1976. The object of the first paper [K9] was to discover whether the excess of fetal irradiation histories associated with development of early neoplasms could be an artefact due to the association between obstetric radiography and other birth factors of etiologic importance. To this end the authors applied the Mantel-Haenszel procedure, which permits identification of separate effects of associated factors in retrospective surveys, to analyse the effects on childhood cancer of social class, maternal age, birth order, and fetal irradiation. A further objective was to test whether these conditions might also have similar effects on other childhood cancers than reticulo-endothelial-system (RES) neoplasms. The new analysis showed that all these factors did exert independent effects on RES neoplasms and all, except sibship position, independently influenced cancers other than leukaemia. However, the degree of these joint associations could not account for the fact that radiation exposure in utero, under the conditions tested, is associated with a higher risk of developing juvenile cancer.

355.   The second paper [K19] addressed several different points and led to a number of conclusions. There was no statistically significant proof of a dose-effect relationship, but only suggestions, that the risk of developing juvenile cancer did increase in proportion to the number of radiographic films used. In view of the retrospective character of the survey, of the variability in the number of films used and their exposure in different places and over a long period, this evidence may not be very reliable. There was also a suggestion of a higher susceptibility to cancer induction for children irradiated in the first trimester. There were relatively fewer cancer cases among children with abnormal radiological findings than among other x-rayed children, owing, presumably, to a positive association between several ante-natal conditions and early non-cancer death. There were also relatively fewer cancer cases for recent than for remote exposures, probably due to a progressive lowering of film doses between 1940 and the time of reporting.

356.   In 1981, Totter and MacPherson [T2] published a critical review of the data in the Oxford Survey, in order to re-examine the evidence in favour of a causal relationship between fetal irradiation and cancer development. This review was based on a number of arguments. First, the authors showed that the greater frequency of x-ray examinations reported among the cancer cases than among the non-cancer cases decreased with time between 1946 and 1963. This observation had been made before by others [B22, S24, S26], but, according to Totter and MacPherson [T2], had not been given the appropriate weight. In particular, the alleged risk had not been placed in a context relative to the natural risk of cancer induction. Secondly, the authors pointed out the striking discrepancy between the Oxford experience and that of Hiroshima and Nagasaki, also repeatedly noted in the past [J4, K4] and confirmed by the most recent findings [I3, K4].

357.   Thirdly, Totter and MacPherson [T2] criticized the method used in Stewart's work of separating the "radiogenic" and "idiopathic" cases of cancer from the overall cancer cases. In their view, this method assumes that the idiopathic cases have the same likelihood of being irradiated as the general population and, therefore, as the control. Such an assumption would be acceptable if it could be shown that: (a) the irradiation of the mothers took place at random; and (b) the characteristics of the idiopathic cases were sufficiently close to those of the control population. In order to test for (a), irradiated and non-irradiated controls were compared for a number of traits (described in [B22]), adjusted for the purpose of identifying the mothers most likely to have problems during pregnancy or selecting the most affluent families. The analysis showed consistent differences among the irradiated and non-irradiated controls treated as two populations. From these, Totter and MacPherson concluded that the choice of irradiating the pregnant mothers was not made at random. To test for (b), the cases developing tumours were compared with tumour-free controls and then shown to be significantly different from the controls in respect of a variety of population characteristics (social class, urban or rural residence, sibship, age and

medical history of the mother, etc.). The differences were thought to be significant and taken as evidence against the assumption that the idiopathic cases would be irradiated with the same frequency as control cases.

358. Fourthly, Totter and MacPherson [T2] criticized the dose-response curves of Stewart [B22, S24] that show an excess risk of childhood malignancy, increasing as a function of the number of films used in the pre-natal x-ray examinations. They pointed out that the Oxford series only demonstrated a difference in frequency of pre-natal x rays between the groups developing and not developing cancer. Under such circumstances, the greater risk caused by the irradiation procedure may only be inferred on the unproven assumption that the normal x-ray frequency in the cancer group is the same as is the non-cancer one. Furthermore, the notion of excess risk as defined by Stewart (the relative risk minus 1), presupposes zero risk for zero dose and therefore assumes that any value greater than zero for each number of x-ray films may be attributed to the x-ray exposure. Finally, the excess risk in Stewart's work is not related to dose, but to the number of films used in the x-ray examination, which is not a good measure of dose because this number was never known with any accuracy. Furthermore, the dose per film varied consistently with time and, therefore, by pooling exposures received at different dates, different doses per film would be indiscriminately mixed.

359. In an expanded treatment of the Oxford data published in another paper [T6], Totter showed that the dose-response relationship claimed by Stewart and Kneale [S24] could be duplicated or improved upon by substituting random numbers in place of the actual numbers found in the survey. According to Totter [T6], the claimed dose-response relationship would be the result of a statistical fault in the use of "excess risk", due to the fact that the highest exposures are received by the smallest number of persons. Therefore, data points with the greatest relative error are multiplied by the reciprocal of the lowest frequency which is itself expected to have a large error. The numbers resulting would thus carry the greatest, and not the least, weight in an ordinary regression analysis.

360. Commenting on the correlation—as opposed to causation—between in utero exposure and subsequent increased risk of malignancy, Burch [B13] pointed out the impossibility of excluding that the medical conditions prompting the selection of cases to undergo obstetric radiology might themselves be associated with an enhanced occurrence of childhood malignancy. He stressed the lack of supporting evidence from the Hiroshima and Nagasaki studies, and pointed out that an independent analysis of the age of onset of childhood malignancies, as found in the Oxford series [B34], cast doubt on the validity of the causal association.

361. Bross's hypothesis, that leukaemia risk from obstetric radiology could be increased by the presence of genetic factors that also enhanced the risk of certain indicator diseases, was tested on the Oxford childhood cancer cases by Kneale and Stewart [K10]

who analysed the interaction of pre-natal irradiation and post-natal diseases in children developing tumours. The authors studied about 6000 cases born between 1953 and 1962 who died before 12 years of age, together with matched controls. Reticular system neoplasms (3199 cases) and other solid tumours (2803 cases) were studied, together with matched controls (6002). Those that had developed a serious infection prior to death were evaluated separately. The data showed that there was a significant association (at the 5% level) between the two variables (cancer and infection) in those which were x-rayed, but not in the non-irradiated controls. Respiratory infections (pneumonia, bronchitis, tonsillitis) were the diseases mainly responsible for the effect. The data are compatible with both the hypothesis of an early damage to the immune system caused by radiation, or that of an earlier origin and termination of the non-irradiated than irradiated cancer cases. Contrary to Bross' interpretation, it is suggested that the relatively low frequency of infections among the non-x-rayed cases might be an artefact caused by an earlier development of immune system faults in the x-irradiated cases.

362. In a short letter [B35], Burch commented on Mole's findings [M23] that there is a similar excess of leukaemia and solid cancers in singleton and twin births, in spite of their different rates of radiological examination. He pointed out that calculations of death rates for leukaemia and solid tumours during the first 10 years of life, combining irradiated and non-irradiated singletons, on the one hand, and irradiated and non-irradiated twins, on the other, result in a slightly, but not significantly, lower rate in the latter. Considering that 50% of twins were irradiated in utero (as opposed to only 10% of singletons), which would lead one to expect a 20% higher rate in twins, the finding cannot easily be reconciled with the view that tumour incidence is causally related to radiation exposure. Burch further pointed out that Mole's estimates [M23] are affected by such wide error limits that they cannot legitimately be used to support the idea of the causal relationship. He concluded, therefore, that, although it may be prudent to act as though ante-natal exposure may increase the carcinogenic risk, the validity of the phenomenon has not been scientifically proved.

363. Einhorn [E6] observed that cell proliferation and differentiation are most active during embryonic life, but cancer is rarely seen to occur after irradiation at these stages. On the other hand, human embryos become susceptible to tumour induction after the period of major organogenesis, particularly in those tissues that have a late development and are still immature at birth. The author suggested that these phenomena might be explained on the assumption that the regulators influencing development, which are most active during the embryonic life, might be the same ones that control cancer induction during that developmental period.

364. In its 1964 report [U3] UNSCEAR already reviewed a study by MacMahon [M25] on 734,243 children born and discharged alive in 1947-1954 in 37

maternity hospitals in the north-east areas of the United States. The frequency of intra-uterine exposure of the entire child population was estimated by reviewing the records of a 1% systematic sample (7242 singleton children). Abdominal or pelvic irradiation was found to have taken place in 770 of these children's mothers, corresponding to 10.6% of the reviewed sample. It was ascertained, by review of death and birth certificates, that 584 children born in the study population had subsequently died of cancer. The pregnancy and delivery records of 569 cases were inspected. Out of 556 children dying of cancer that had been born of single pregnancies, 85 (15.3%) had been exposed in utero to diagnostic x rays. The higher frequency of pre-natal x rays in these cancer cases, compared with the rest of the sample (10.6%), was found to be statistically significant. Data were corrected for indirect associations with birth order and other complicating variables, and the final adjusted cancer mortality risk was found to be about 40% higher in the in-utero-irradiated than in the non-irradiated members of the test population. The excess of neoplasms found applied equally to leukaemia, tumours of the CNS and other neoplasms. The excess cancer mortality of the exposed children was most marked at the ages of five to seven years (with a relative risk of about 2.0) and apparently exhausted by the age of 8 years. There was a small non-significant trend toward a higher mortality in the most heavily irradiated children, but no significant variation of the risk was found with the intra-uterine age of children.

365. Monson and MacMahon [M53] reported recently on an extension of their previous study [M25]. The new paper includes data for five additional hospitals and extends the period of coverage of birth and death. It is based on cancer deaths occurring between 1947 and 1967 among 1,429,400 children born between 1947 and 1960 in 42 maternity hospitals. It excludes children born of multiple pregnancies or dead in the delivery hospitals. Out of this study sample, through a search of death certificates, 1342 children were identified who died from cancer before the age of 20. The birth records of these children, and of a 1% sample of the total population, were reviewed in order to determine which of the children had received irradiation in utero through irradiation of the mother's abdominal region. Since pre-natal x-ray exposure may be associated with many causes of childhood death, in addition to cancer death, the authors followed the x-ray experience of other children who died from causes other than cancer. This control sample included children born in 17 hospitals during the study period, who died after 3 months of age in 1950, 1955, 1960 or 1965. The risk ratio for leukaemia between the 1% sample and the study sample was 1.48, that is, very similar to the 1.5 found in the earlier analysis [M25]. On the other hand, the risk ratios for cancer of the CNS and other cancers were appreciably lower (1.16 and 1.14) by comparison with those found in the previous study (respectively, 1.6 and 1.4). In view of the similarity of the risk ratios, all solid tumours were combined in the subsequent analysis.

366. The excess of leukaemia cases in children with a history of x-ray exposure (over the selected cases

based on the 1% sample) was only evident between 2 and 7 years from birth, whereas the excess of solid tumours occurred between 2 and 9 years. Thus, further analysis was limited only to children who died before their 10th birthday. The maximum likelihood risk ratio (MLR) for leukaemia was essentially the same in the initial study (1.48) [M25] and in the extension (1.58) [M53]. For solid tumours, the MLR was 1.45 in the initial study and 1.06 in the extension. The overall total MLR for leukaemia of 1.52 and for solid tumours of 1.27 are not significantly different when directly compared (P = 0.4). In order to evaluate other possible confounding factors, the frequency of x-ray exposure of children in the 1% sample was examined according to selected characteristics, together with the incidence rate of cancer for the same characteristics. This analysis showed that factors such as birth order, sex, birth weight, year of birth and abnormality of pregnancy (acting alone or in association) could confound the correlation between x rays and cancer, being associated with both in the same direction. On the other hand, race, pay status and previous fetal loss were potential negative confounding variables, in the sense that children with more exposure had developed less cancer. Maternal age and religion were not consistently associated with x-ray exposure or cancer risk and could not, therefore, have confounded the data.

367. Correction for each of the potential confounders brought about little change in the risk ratio. There was, at the same time, no indication that the overall association between cancer and x irradiation was present only in a limited sub-population of the whole sample. When the number of x-ray examinations observed among children with cancer was compared with those expected according to the year of birth, an excess of x rays was observed from 1947 through 1957 for leukaemia, but only for the period 1951-1954 for solid cancer. However, no reason for this clustering of the excess was identified. Children developing leukaemia did not appear to have received a higher rate of examination with x rays until the third trimester, but children developing other solid tumours had a higher rate of examination also during the first and second trimesters. Although no information was available on the actual doses received, there was no suggestion of a crude dose-response relationship, based on the type of examination.

368. From a discussion of possible sources of ascertainment bias, related to the facts that the record search was not blind and that there was some loss of information between the first and the second assessment, no evidence appeared that these conditions might have introduced any significant bias in the association between x-irradiation and cancer. It was concluded, therefore, that these new data were in overall agreement with other data pointing to a risk ratio of malignancy associated with pre-natal exposure to x rays of about 1.5. There is, therefore, no question in the mind of the authors as to the significance of their findings, but they believe that the relationship shown is not causal. This view is argued on the basis of the absence of confirmatory evidence from the experience of Hiroshima and Nagasaki, and from

experience in experimental animals. The authors point out that searches for variables that may have confounded the association have failed to identify any factor that might be of sufficient weight to explain the data. There may be, in principle, as suggested by Totter and MacPherson [T2], some kind of generalized greater access to medical care among fetuses that will eventually develop cancer, but such a hypothesis is difficult to test experimentally.

369. In a review article [D23], Doll outlined the main features of the Oxford Survey and discussed some of its difficulties. These included: (a) the possible bias introduced by incorrect reporting of previous x-ray history by the mother of a child who later developed cancer; and (b) the possibility that the association shown in the Survey might be a secondary one, due to the fact that some unidentified factor might be the cause of both the higher tendency to develop a tumour and of the higher probability of prenatal x-ray exposure. Doll was satisfied that the first issue was not likely to have influenced the results to any appreciable degree. As to the second one, although recognizing that it may be impossible to overcome it in any observational study, Doll believes that it is unlikely for three reasons: first, the failure to identify such a factor, in spite of intensive searching; second, the allegedly good relationship between number of x-ray exposures and the increase in excess risk (an argument which has, however, been challenged by Totter [T2, T6]); and, third, Mole's evidence on twins [M23] (although this, while in agreement with the later data of Harvey et al. [H23], is not accepted by MacMahon [M55] as a definitive proof).

370. Shiono et al. [S11] reported on a prospective study of 55,908 women participating in a collaborative perinatal project in the United States. They examined the x-ray exposure history of 145 mothers whose children developed neoplasms up to 7 years of age, and of 290 matched control mothers whose children developed no tumours. Of the 145 tumours under study, 40 were malignant and 105 benign. For x-ray exposure during pregnancy the relative risk values were 1.09 (P = 0.526) and 0.94 (P = 0.635) for malignant and benign tumours, respectively. Corresponding values for exposure before pregnancy were 2.61 (P = 0.021) and 1.07 (P = 0.475). For pre-conception exposure, there was no dose-response relationship of statistical significance in the groups of mothers whose children developed either benign or malignant tumours. For pre- and post-conception exposure combined, there was a suggestion that the relative risk could be higher for malignant neoplasms, but the significance of probability value was borderline. For benign tumours, the values of relative risk were not significantly different from 1.

371. Taken together, the data [S11] were thought to be consistent with an increased risk of malignant neoplasms among children whose mothers had been exposed to x rays before and during pregnancy, with a somewhat higher relative risk estimate for pre-conception exposure. There was no significant association between exposure and development of benign tumours. The data were interpreted according to the model of

Knudson [K26], who postulated that certain tumours might be the results of two mutational events which could be in the form of either two somatic mutations or of one transmitted germinal mutation followed by one somatic mutation. According to this hypothesis, any agent that would increase the rate of mutation in germinal cells would be expected to enhance the risk of tumours. In addition, owing to the time factor involved in the accumulation of mutations, tumours (such as retinoblastoma) caused by a germinal plus somatic mutations would be expected to arise in early ages.

372. Salonen [S56] carried out a study on pre- and perinatal factors in childhood cancer, based on tumour registry data in Finland during the years 1959-1968. The immediately preceding baby born in the same maternal health centres from which the test cases had been drawn provided the control data. The number of test-control pairs of children included in the final analysis was 972. For all these pairs of children, information was sought concerning the parents, the pregnancy, the events at birth and the post-natal health, in order to compare the outcome of control and test children histories. Comparisons were carried out in terms of the total number of tumours and of leukaemias, brain and other tumours. There was no significant correlation between cancer and a number of potential etiological factors such as parental factors (ages of parents, mother's blood group, duration of marriage, social class of the family), pregnancy factors (numbers of deliveries or of pregnancies, pre- or post-mature delivery, use of drugs) or child factors (date of delivery, birth weight, vaccinations). As to leukaemia induction, the risk ratio in the group that had been irradiated in utero with pelvic radiology was 1.9, with an upper confidence limit of 6.7 at the 2% level. However, 5% of the mothers carrying children that developed leukaemia underwent pelvic radiography, as opposed to 3.7% of the mothers of non-leukaemic children. Therefore, owing to the rare occurrence of intra-uterine irradiation, the group was too small to render the increase of the risk ratio statistically significant.

373. A new study on childhood cancer in twins exposed pre-natally has recently been published [H23]. It is a case-control study, involving over 32,000 twins born in Connecticut, United States, from 1930 to 1969 and followed to 15 years of age. The twins were investigated for a possible relationship between pre-natal x-ray exposure and childhood cancer and leukaemia. By concentrating on twins, rather than singleton births, it was hoped to reduce the chance of a medical selection bias, since twins were often exposed to x rays for diagnostic purposes, more so, in any case, than for any other medical condition. By matching the records of a twin and a tumour registry, 31 childhood cancers were selected for study (11 in boys and 20 in girls) and each of these cases was matched with 4 twin controls. Evidence for x-ray exposure and for other factors affecting pregnancy, delivery and maternal health was collected from a number of other sources. Abdominal exposure of the mother was particularly sought. It was estimated that the dose to the fetus from such procedures ranged

from 0.0016 to 0.04 Gy, with an average of 0.01 Gy per examination. All but one exposure occurred in the third trimester. The relative risk was taken as a measure of the association between radiation exposure and childhood cancer. Twelve out of 31 (39%) of the cases and 28 out of 109 controls (26%) were found to have been exposed pre-natally. The crude relative risk associated with pre-natal exposure was calculated to be 1.8 (0.8-4.2 were the 95% confidence limits). When adjusted for all the potentially confounding factors, the relative risk was 1.4-1.9. The adjusted risk for leukaemia was 1.6 (0.4-6.8) and for other childhood cancer 3.2 (0.9-10.7). In addition to pre-natal exposure, low birth weight was the only variable that appeared to increase the cancer risk. It has been suggested [D24], and accepted as a likely explanation [H26], that post-natal exposure of low-weight children might be responsible for such an effect. These data [H23], showing an overall 2.4 risk of childhood cancer associated with pre-natal exposure, are in agreement with the results from the Oxford series [S23] and the U.S. study [M53] and with the twin data as examined by Mole [M23]. In the view of the authors, they provide further evidence, though based on small numbers, that low-dose pre-natal irradiation may indeed increase the risk of childhood cancer.

374. MacMahon, however, in an editorial published at the same time [M55] questioned this conclusion on three different accounts. First, the small number of cases involved (31 twins with cancer), which is barely enough to give statistical significance to the excess risk of 2.4 found in the study. Second, the assumption that twins were only exposed on account of their being twins, and not also for other reasons, among which might have been the elusive factor operating in singletons (as well as, perhaps, in twins) which makes irradiated children more prone to develop cancer in childhood. Third, the possibility, mentioned in the paper, that natural cancer incidence may be lower in twins than in singleton babies. If this is true, and if twins are irradiated more often than children born single having a higher cancer risk, twins should, in fact, have a higher cancer incidence. The series may, however, have been too small to document any difference. It should also be mentioned that this latter argument may lose much of its validity because in the study by Harvey et al. [H23], mono- and di-zygotic twins were pooled and there is no a priori reason to think that these two classes may have the same natural incidence of cancer, an issue also taken up by Waight [W31]. In conclusion the new study [H23] does not seem to provide any firmer evidence in favour of a causal association between pre-natal exposure and childhood cancer.

375. Preliminary data showing a non-significantly elevated risk of malignancy in children exposed to ante-natal diagnostic radiation among 555 childhood cancer cases in Great Britain have also been reported recently [H30]. Although the relative risk of developing leukaemia or lymphoma over the first 14 years of life was 1.33 (C.I. 0.85-2.08) among exposed (as compared to non-exposed) children, it was 5.57 (C.I. 1.72-18.09) for children developing such malignancies within 2 years of age. It has already been pointed out

[E8] that with the small number of cases involved when statistics are broken down, the possiblity arises of calculating a large number of relative risks and finding one "significant" purely by chance. Further analysis of this series will have to await a fuller account of the findings.

376. A summary of the relative risks of leukaemia found in studies of pre-natally exposed children since the 1964 report of UNSCEAR is given in Table 14.

C. CONCLUSIONS

1. Data from animals

377. Even though more relevant data have appeared since the 1977 UNSCEAR review, it remains difficult to provide overall conclusions on the subject of tumour induction in pre-natally irradiated animals, in comparison with irradiation of post-natal ages. It is, perhaps, appropriate to underline the difficulties hindering an overall judgement, because their discussion may help to point out the reasons why conclusions should be prudent.

378. First, there is the natural variability between species and strains with respect to the number and types of tumours arising in intact animals and the different susceptibility of various tumour types to radiation. Given this background variation, it is difficult to project information across species for the overall tumour induction or for the susceptibility to given tumour types. This objective is rendered even more difficult by the fact that information is rarely available over a large range of doses and an adequate number of animals. It should be stressed that generalizations based on only a few dose groups may be misleading, because information collected so far points to the existence of dose-induction relationships of complex forms. Just as in adult systems, curves going through a maximum, and then decreasing with increasing doses, have been documented in animals irradiated in utero. There is every reason to suspect that the placement of such maxima in respect to the dose axis and their relative height may vary with different animal species and tumour types, and to expect that, as a first approximation, wide extrapolations between species may be unwarranted.

379. Some experiments have convincingly documented differences between sexes in the susceptibility to tumours by irradiation in utero, not only in respect of tumours of the reproductive organs (or known to be dependent on the action of sexual hormones) but also in respect of neoplastic diseases, such as those of the haemolymphopoietic system, for which such dependencies are not very strong in the adult. The concomitant action of radiation on the developing reproductive and hormonal systems may to some extent be related to such differential actions. There are also indications that differential effects may be present for radiation of low- and high-LET, the latter being considerably more effective for carcinogenesis of animals in utero. Data on such matters are few and preliminary, however.

380. The notion that radiation may be consistently more carcinogenic when delivered to animals in utero than to adult animals is not easy to document on the evidence currently available: but, here again, comparisons should only be made with great circumspection. It is not a straightforward procedure to compare the results obtained from animals early in development with those obtained from animals in full maturity, because the target cell responsible for the induction of some tumour types may not yet be present in embryonic or fetal animals. Under such conditions, comparisons of induction rates may be of little value. Furthermore, for given histotypes, the target cells, even if already present, may be in various stages of differentiation, a condition which could reflect, to an unknown extent, on the final incidence of tumours produced. Finally, in view of the other radiation effects induced in developing animals (growth disturbances, malformations, killing), the dose "window" over which the carcinogenic action can be analysed is rather narrow. This adversely affects the significance of the results, because the number of animals available for analysis of tumour induction may be reduced by the concomitant presence of such effects.

381. All the above considerations apply both to external and internal irradiation. In the latter case, however, comparative estimates of tumour susceptibility between in utero and adult animals are further affected by the fact that the rate of dose delivery to the sensitive structures may be substantially different and the dose delivered to the target cells (particularly in case of tissues such as the bone) may have a biologically different meaning when delivered at various developmental stages. The structures into which the dose is absorbed, the rate of delivery and the total integration times are, in the case of internal irradiation, of overwhelming importance for meaningful assessments.

382. Under these conditions, conclusions applying to one tumour type could not easily be extended to other tumours or to all tumours. This further reinforces the notion that extrapolations in such matters should be extremely guarded and generalizations very cautious. Taking into account these numerous pitfalls, the evidence reviewed does not convey an overall impression of a significantly higher susceptibility to the induction of tumours of animals irradiated in utero. This conclusion, based on a review of all or specific tumour types, is also in accordance with the conclusions of a previous UNSCEAR review [U5]. This showed that irradiation in utero of mice produces less marked life-shortening than irradiation during post-gestational ages, or even no life-shortening at all, particularly for irradiation of the early embryo. Similarly, experience with the rat showed a doubtful effect of radiation in inducing life-shortening, and, in any case, an effect not substantially different from that produced by similar doses given soon after birth. This conclusion is also based on the assumption, exhaustively discussed and accepted [U5], that radiation-induced life shortening, at doses below the lethal range, is mainly attributable to the appearance of extra tumours.

383. Given the above reservations, it appears that the majority of cases analysed in terms of total tumour rates points to a lower, rather than a higher, susceptibility to tumour induction of the developing animals. What is most convincingly borne out from the data is that irradiation in utero produces a different spectrum of tumours than does post-natal irradiation of young or old animals. This observation is in line with the general belief that the histogenesis of the cell lines, which are the probable targets for tumour induction, proceeds at different times and rates in the developing mammal. Accordingly, one should not expect to find the same types and rates of neoplastic transformation for irradiation of the embryonic, fetal and adult stages. Furthermore, changes in tumour spectra between animals irradiated pre- and post-natally differ for different species. This is in agreement with the notions that the rate of organ and tissue formation is very dependent on the species and that each has a characteristic pattern of naturally occurring tumours.

2. Data from man

384. Data on the induction of tumours by pre-natal irradiation in man may be divided into two groups: those obtained from the survivors of the atomic bombs at Hiroshima and Nagasaki, and those derived from medical exposures. The most recent reports on the Japanese survivors have continued to show no evidence of excess cancer death among individuals irradiated in utero at the time of the explosions. Although the sample size and the number of deaths involved in this survey up to now are too small to allow firm statements, the doses received are sufficiently large, particularly in comparison with those delivered in the course of obstetric examinations, to give weight to the general conclusion. For leukaemia, in particular, a second independent report confirmed the absence of an excess risk in a sample of over 700 irradiated subjects. It is of course possible that when the atomic bomb survivors irradiated in utero will reach the older ages at which cancer normally appears, they might show higher incidence rates, as compared to non-exposed controls.

385. The Oxford Survey, the largest survey on children exposed for medical reasons while still in utero, has continued to stimulate controversial discussion. On the one hand, the group involved in the survey from its very origin have refined the analysis of the data and shown the existence of a number of factors of social and medical relevance that could affect the association between exposure in utero and proneness to develop cancer in childhood. These factors could not have been of such weight to render the association statistically non-significant.

386. On the other hand, critics of the Oxford series tend to believe that there may have been some selection of the mothers undergoing radiological examination during pregnancy. They point to differences between the social and medical conditions of children developing tumours and those not developing them, the differences being such that, for the traits

examined, the children could be considered to belong to different populations. Criticism has also been expressed of the analysis of the dose-response relationship and the way the doses (or their equivalent expressions) were defined for the purpose. Other analyses of the Oxford series data tended to disprove the causality of the association between x-ray exposure and tumour induction. According to these analyses, it is impossible to exclude that medical or other conditions leading to the selection of cases undergoing pre-natal radiology might themselves be associated with the increased occurrence of malignancy in childhood.

387. One strong argument in favour of a causal relationship between pre-natal irradiation and childhood cancer was the finding of a similar excess of leukaemia and solid tumours in children born of single or twin pregnancies, in spite of the fact that the children in the latter category had a much higher rate of radiological examinations. This argument has, however, been challenged on statistical grounds because the numerical estimates on which it had been based could be affected by such wide error limits as to render the comparisons meaningless.

388. Additional independent evidence for an association has come from the extension of a survey already reported in 1962, based on about 1.5 million children of whom more than 1300 developed cancer before the age of 20. The new study confirmed in part the previous findings for leukaemia, pointing out a 50% higher risk of developing this disease among children irradiated in utero than among non-irradiated children. In part, however, it modified previous conclusions regarding incidence of solid tumours, lowering the relative risk in the exposed population to about 15% higher than the controls from a previous value of 50%. The study also analysed and confirmed the existence of confounding variables that could potentially enhance or reduce the association between in utero irradiation and the likelihood of developing cancer. At the same time, it pointed out that correcting for such factors would be insufficient to explain. the excess risk in the irradiated children. Overall, therefore, these conclusions are in reasonable agreement with those from the Oxford series. Other, smaller series have given essentially non-significant answers.

389. The experience concerning the carcinogenic action in man of irradiation in utero thus appears paradoxical in many respects. On the one hand, a prospective study on children exposed to relatively high doses from the atomic explosions has consistently failed, over the years, to reveal any increased risk [J4, K4, I3]. On the other hand, two larger, independent, retrospective studies carried out in Great Britain [S44] and in the United States [M25, M53] have consistently shown an increased risk of developing leukaemia and solid tumours in children exposed for medical reasons to much lower doses. The magnitude of the leukaemia risk is evaluated at about 50% higher than in non-exposed children, and that for solid tumours possibly somewhat less. None of the critics of these findings have denied the existence of such an apparently increased risk: they have rather been inclined to explain the finding on the ground of faulty methodo-

logy, or to deny, on various grounds, the causality of the association between exposure and malignancy.

390. The methodological defect of the Oxford series would consist, according to Totter [T6], in the use of the "excess risk". This notion is faulty, because: (a) it is based on the assumption that the frequency of x-ray examinations is similar in both the leukaemic and the non-leukaemic children; (b) it presupposes that the risk is zero for zero dose; and (c) it is based on imperfect "dose" estimates. There is also a statistical difficulty in the use of "excess risk", owing to the fact that the data points with the largest errors are given the greatest weight in the analysis. These criticisms, however, could not apply to the United States series, which uses the methodology of the maximum likelihood risk ratio as a summary statistic, and yet comes quite independently to very similar conclusions.

391. Other critics have tended to deny the causality of the association shown in the Oxford and New England series by providing evidence that the populations of children who will or will not develop malignancies are different in respect of a number of medical and socio-economic characteristics [T2]. The existence of confounding factors that could affect the association between exposure and increased risk is a well established fact, one to which the researchers themselves in the Oxford [K9] and New England [M53] series have given much attention. In both cases, the conclusion is that correcting for such factors is insufficient to disprove the significance of the association, which must therefore be accepted as sound observational evidence. Differences between the two sets of children who may or may not eventually develop a malignant disease imply that some characteristics of the mothers, of the children themselves, or of their relationship during pregnancy may have prompted a different rate of radiological examination of the two populations. These characteristics, rather than the exposure itself, could be associated with the induction of tumours. It is, of course, impossible to prove that this may not have happened, but it must also be recognized that none of the factors examined so far has been shown to be responsible for the association and it is difficult to suggest other factors for further examination [M52].

392. Other arguments in favour of a causal relationship have been proposed by Mole [M23] who examined the excess of leukaemia and cancer in children born of single or twin pregnancies and observed that, in spite of the higher rate of radiological examination of the twins, they had a similar excess of leukaemia and cancer. If valid, this would be an internally consistent proof of the causality, but Mole's calculations have been challenged [B35] on the ground that the risk in twins could actually be lower than in singletons and, in any case, the errors affecting the estimates are too large to be conclusive in either sense. Proportionality between risk and exposure might be another indirect proof of the causality, but the difficulties of assessing the doses precisely have been long recognized [S24, S26, B22, T2] and these cast doubt on the foundations themselves of the dose-response analysis.

393.   In summary, therefore:

(a) The finding of a positive association between exposure in utero and subsequent development of leukaemia and cancer during childhood, in the Oxford and New England series is in contrast with the absence of any such correlation in the Japanese series;

(b) The fact that higher doses are involved in the Japanese than in the other two series is a further cause for concern, as radiobiological effects are usually expected to follow some positive function of dose. The different nature of the exposures, and the fact that the Japanese series is prospective, and the other two retrospective, do not help in resolving the difference;

(c) It is also difficult to explain why high doses given at Hiroshima and Nagasaki soon after birth show their carcinogenic potential only many years after exposure, while the relatively smaller doses involved in medical exposure in utero seem to exhaust their potential within the first 10 years after exposure;

(d) The Oxford and the New England series are at variance with data from experimental animals, which are, in the vast majority, essentially negative in terms of a higher carcinogenic risk of pre-natal exposure. Nothing can be said as to whether the change in the overall tumour spectrum, often found in experimental animals irradiated pre- or post-natally, may also apply to man, because the epidemiological series have not been followed long enough. It may, of course, be possible that, considering all malignancies that will be expressed up to the death of the human cohorts irradiated in utero and the attendant detriment, pre-natal irradiation might result in less overall detriment for the same dose than post-natal exposure;

(e) On radiobiological grounds, the constancy of the relative risk of irradiation in utero over the whole spectrum of malignancies appears to be in contrast with the well known variability of different tumour histotypes to the carcinogenic action of radiation. This observation could be due to chance, or to the short observation period of the medical irradiation series, and could still be modified with longer follow-up, but it remains, at the present state of knowledge, unexplained;

(f) The constancy of the relative risk also implies proportionality between natural and radiation-induced malignancies over all developing tissues (at least up to the present stage of follow-up) which is by no means a common experience for irradiation of adult systems;

(g) Similarly implausible on embryological and radio-biological grounds is the observation of a higher relative risk of leukaemia for exposure during the first trimester (than during the last two) when it is known that adult haemopoiesis has not yet begun and target cells to be transformed into leukaemic cells have not presumably differentiated.

394.   It is, in the last analysis, the joint consideration of the findings described, and their evaluation in the light of all the above-mentioned inconsistencies, that may determine acceptance or rejection of the causality of the relationship, because data, to be credible, should fit into an overall logical framework accounting for all of them, and not for only a few. It is interesting to note, in this respect, that the authors involved in the Oxford series favour the causal nature of the association, while those involved in the New England series reject such a notion. In the view of UNSCEAR, the important consideration is the existence of the association. For the Committee's own purposes to neglect the matter until (and if) it is given some plausible explanation would be unacceptable because, if the association exists, it could, to some extent, affect the estimates of radiation burden in man. Under the circumstances, the only possible course of action is to recognize the association and to assume its causal nature, keeping in mind, however, that its true nature remains unresolved because the data do not fit into an overall logical picture of radiation carcinogenesis as it is currently understood. It is to be hoped that further, independent data will help to resolve the existing discrepancies, although it appears unlikely that direct evidence will ever be produced for lack of suitable material to study. In choosing this course of action, UNSCEAR wishes to stress that acceptance of the causality of the association is assumed simply on account of prudence for any relevant practical consequences. On purely scientific grounds, in fact, the issue should either be dismissed for lack of scientific coherence or should be left undecided, pending further new evidence. UNSCEAR, although its functions are only those of a body assessing data on their scientific merit, is not insensitive to the practical consequences of its deliberations. Thus, it believes that not to include the potential harm of exposures in utero (whatever it may be) in the total balance of radiation risks would unduly weight scientific orthodoxy against the practical needs of safety. The Committee will, of course, be ready to modify this position on the strength of any new scientific evidence that might be forthcoming.

VIII.   RISK ESTIMATES

A.   GENERAL

395.   Quantitative risk estimates for radiation damage after exposure in utero are of considerable importance for their possible practical implications. An early expression of the absolute amount of risk likely to occur under these circumstances is to be found in the 1969 UNSCEAR report [U1]. This stated that, in respect of severe mental retardation associated with a reduced circumference of the skull, an estimate of the risk coefficient derived from observations in Japan, with high acute doses in excess of 0.5 Gy, might be set at about $10^{-1} \, Gy^{-1}$, averaged over the gestation period. The report stressed the uncertainties involved in extrapolating such a value to smaller doses, in the absence of suitable human data and with insufficient knowledge of the underlying mechanisms. The 1977

UNSCEAR report [U2] endorsed this provisional value, again underlining the limitations under which it had been derived and the difficulties involved in extrapolating it to other exposure conditions. The report also pointed out that a survey of the available human experience, with doses in the region of 0.01-0.2 Gy, had given negative or inconclusive answers. They could only be of indirect value in excluding the possibility that, at such doses, the human embryo might be 10 times more sensitive than implied by the incidence of malformations at higher doses.

396. The 1977 report [U2] was criticized in a paper by Mole [M36] as being an inaccurate account of facts which could convey the impression that radiation exposure of the human embryo in its early stages could be positively harmful and thus might engender apprehension about the relevant risk. The paper in question is a complex one. It comprises a text aimed at setting risk in perspective (particularly with respect to the normal risk of handicaps at the end of a normal pregnancy), in view of a reconsideration of the so-called 10-day rule, and an appendix setting out in detail the criticisms of the UNSCEAR report and the arguments on which the main conclusions rest.

397. While recognizing that the discussion of experimental findings could in each instance be extremely detailed, UNSCEAR believes that this should not be the specific purpose of its assessments, which aim at overall evaluations of specific fields. It believes that the assessment of developmental effects of irradiation in utero, on the basis of the evidence available in 1977 [U2], should not be modified on account of the criticisms raised. It also believes, however, that the most recent findings in this field, and the widespread attention they have commanded, have made the field a particularly worthy subject for further study and review.

398. In other papers [M9, M10], Mole discussed, and rejected, the notion that the very early human conceptus (0-14 days) is an especially radiosensitive organism. This notion, he found, was derived from too-facile generalizations based on laboratory animal experiments, without due consideration for the specificity of human development. First, he examined the most recent evidence on small head size and mental retardation from Hiroshima and Nagasaki [O3] to show that the distribution of cases, as a function of the week of gestation at the time of exposure, is incompatible with the hypothesis that the earliest stages of pregnancy are the most sensitive in regard to impairment of mental function. This should, of course, be expected on the ground that embryo killing (either pre- or post-implantation) and malformations, and not mental retardation, are the types of damage expressed by irradiation at the early stages.

399. Mole then underlined [M9, M10] the good correlation, originally pointed out by Dobbing and Sands [D12], between the period of rapid proliferation of neuroblasts in the developing human CNS between about 10 and 18 weeks of pregnancy (8-16 weeks after fertilization) and the clustering of mental retardation cases at around the same time in the Japanese

experience. This observation (which had been previously overlooked by workers in radiation biology and by the 1977 UNSCEAR report) is indeed very valuable because it correlates precisely cellular events in the human brain with radiation-induced functional damage. It is, however, in line with the general notion that the sensitivity of a given structure is highest at the time of its maximum growth, an observation repeatedly documented for many structures in experimental animals and to which the human experience would be expected to conform.

400. Mole further discussed [M9, M10] the significance of malnutrition in connection with the Japanese experience, pointing out that food shortage before, and particularly after, the bombing might have been responsible for an unusually high control level of mental retardation and might, if so, have led to an over-estimate of the effect of irradiation (under the hypothesis of a combined action). Mole also discussed points such as: the effect of excluding 2 cases of Down's syndrome in the irradiated subjects and 1 case of encephalitis in infancy in the control subjects; the difficulties with the definition of microcephaly as diagnosed at Hiroshima and Nagasaki; the lack of correlation between small head size and mental retardation; the effect of perinatal mortality; and the lack of other data on morphological abnormalities in the Japanese series. The author also reviewed other series, to show the relative infrequency of major developmental malformations as commonly understood.

401. In that part of the paper [M9] which refers to observations on laboratory animals, Mole stressed that species intercomparison should only be carried out with due regard for the timing and duration of developmental events. This conclusion is quite acceptable when actual times or rates of induction are discussed (which was never the case in the 1977 UNSCEAR report [U2]) but not when projections across species are so general as simply to point out the good correlation, found in various species, between stages of organogenesis of structures and their sensitivity to irradiation.

402. Finally, Mole discussed [M9] the mechanisms of morphological and functional damage following irradiation in utero, pointing out the distinction that should be made between "malformations" resulting from failure of embryonic organization and having clear teratogenic connotations and "maldevelopment" resulting from cell depletion distributed randomly throughout an irradiated tissue. Mental retardation would belong to this second class of damage. Difficulties in the definition of malformations and growth disturbances, and the frequent association of various types of damage, were discussed at length in the 1977 UNSCEAR report [U2]. In the light of the above definitions, Mole believes there is no evidence in the human species to show that radiation is an efficient teratogen.

403. When teratogenic effects are described, a distinction is often made between malformations and growth disturbances, even though it is recognized that

the two effects are often associated. In a paper by Spiers [S15], the hypothesis is developed that growth retardation and teratogenic effects may not be independent end-points of common causes. Evidence for this is drawn from epidemiological observations on some human congenital malformations in twins; from multiple as opposed to single malformations; and from the association between malformations and growth retardations in patients with Down's syndrome and in children from normal and diabetic mothers. On the basis of analyses carried out on such data, it is argued that growth retardation may represent a state of increased susceptibility to congenital malformations in the sense that they will be more likely to occur when the overall growth rate of the fetus is grossly disturbed. A more recent paper by Tchobroutsky et al. [T13] has pointed to a high correlation between fetal defects and early growth delay observed by ultrasound, thus confirming that growth retardation may constitute a state of increased susceptibility to the occurrence of congenital malformations.

404. In another paper [M21], Mole discussed the latest evidence from Japan, emphasizing the good agreement between embryological and radiological findings in man and the absence of any record of maldevelopment other than mental retardation. This paper also contained a valuable review of case reports in the literature, pointing to mental retardation as the most significant category of damage in the human species. As to experimental observations, the paper accepted that pre-implantation irradiation of the conceptus leads to a dose-dependent reduction of surviving normal individuals, while irradiation during the period of major organogenesis causes a great variety of visible malformations. In pointing out the differences between findings in man (where true malformations are uncommon) and in other animals (where teratological damage is prevalent), the paper suggests that a slower rate of cell division of the human embryo might be the reason for such differences.

405. The fact that in man growth disturbances, small head size and mental retardation are the predominant effects of acute exposure during pregnancy was also noted by Brent [B25-B27]. This is at variance with data in experimental animals [U2] in which malformations of different organs and structures are a common finding after comparable doses. According to Brent, there may be various explanations for such differences. First, development of the CNS in man proceeds throughout gestation and well into the neonatal period [D12, H14], while other organ systems develop over a much shorter time. For example, in man organogenesis may last from the 2nd to the 8th week of gestation, corresponding to about 5% of the whole pregnancy, while in the rat it may last from day 9 to 13, corresponding to 20% of pregnancy [P11]. Secondly, the manner of exposure is usually different in animal and human populations. In the first case, exposure is often aimed at inducing specific malformation by selective irradiation at certain times, while in man exposure has usually occurred at random and has therefore been relatively more likely during the fetal stages when sensitivity of the developing brain remains high.

406. In 1977, the International Commission on Radiological Protection (ICRP) [I4], in the context of a general attempt to develop an index of harm applying to a working population for radiation protection purposes, provided some estimates of risk during various stages of pregnancy and for various types of effects. In summary, the risk of lethality (before implantation or in utero) for irradiation during the pre-implantation stages was estimated, by extrapolation from data in rodents, to be of the order of 10^{-3} a^{-1} for exposure of a female working population at the rate of 1 Sv a^{-1}, weighted over the 8 days pre-implantation during which this risk was assumed to operate. (This rate of exposure was taken simply for comparative purposes.) For all malformations occurring after exposure at the same rate during the period of major organogenesis (assumed to last for 17 weeks during pregnancy) the risk was set at 10^{-3} a^{-1} Sv^{-1}. The risk of inducing a fatal childhood malignancy was set at $2.3 \ 10^{-2} Sv^{-1}$. On the assumption that the risk of fatal malignancy in females (allowing for breast cancer) is $1.5 \ 10^{-2} \ Sv^{-1}$, that the fetus is exposed for an average period of 7 months during which the mother remains at work at the rate of 1 Sv a^{-1}, and that the average number of births per year per woman is 0.065, it was further calculated that the average risk of inducing a fatal childhood malignancy would be about 6% of that in the adult member of a female working population.

407. In 1979, Mole [M36] addressed the problem of quantitative risk estimates and produced the following figures. For mortality after exposure to x or gamma irradiation in the 1-4 months embryo or fetus, 0-1 additional cases per 1000 births after a tissue dose of 0.05 Gy low-LET radiation; for mental retardation in adolescence, 0-25 additional cases per 1000 liveborn after 0.5 Gy tissue dose (0-1 case after 0.05 Gy); and for malignant diseases before the 10th birthday, about 50 excess cases per 1000 of all live births after 0.5 Gy tissue dose (about 5 cases after 0.05 Gy). Such estimates, derived from evidence concerning brief exposures, would not be expected to be strongly influenced by dose protraction because most of the risk is attributable to cancer production. Scaled down to 0.01 Gy of low-LET radiation on a linear non-threshold hypothesis, the overall risk would lie in the range of zero to 10^{-3} cases, which should be compared with the natural probability of occurrence of serious handicaps in average pregnancies, which was estimated to be upwards of $3 \ 10^{-2}$.

408. Brent [B25, B27] discussed the risk estimates from irradiation in early life. He stated that, since, contrary to most other teratogens or embryopathic agents, radiation has an effect on the developing embryo which is direct and not mediated through maternal metabolism and placental transfer, one may extrapolate the results of irradiation experiments with pregnant mammals to the human more readily than with any other teratogen. However, in view of the numerous differences pointed out in the developmental pattern and in the response of man and other mammals, UNSCEAR believes that great caution should be exercised in such extrapolations, especially

for the more quantitative projections. Moreover, risk estimates ultimately to be applied to humans for practical purposes should essentially be derived from human experience, carefully adapted to the special situation to which exposure applies.

409. In order to estimate risk, Brent summarized, in tables, the effects of acute exposures at 1 Gy and at 0.1 Gy or less, on various developmental stages of the rat and mouse (displayed in relation to corresponding human gestation periods). He then extrapolated from them the minimum doses to produce lethality, malformations, growth retardation and other effects in the human embryo, as in Table 15. Brent's conclusion from these data is that the hazard of exposure in the range of diagnostic roentgenology is extremely low when compared with spontaneous risks in human pregnancy. Tubiana [T4] estimated that a dose of 0.02 Gy to a fetus could induce, at the most, the risk of 1 case of cancer in 2000 children.

410. Kameyama [K22] addressed the problem of risk to the human embryo and fetus by simple extrapolation to humans from observations on the lowest effective doses in experiments with rats and mice, warning, however, about the danger of such straightforward projections. In a general review of the field, he estimated the lowest doses for non-stochastic effects in the mammalian embryo and fetus to be as follows (figures given in Gy to the relevant tissues): for resorption of pre-implantation embryo, 0.05; for acute cytological changes, 0.05-0.1; for minor skeletal anomalies, 0.05; for malformations, 0.15-0.20; for histogenetic and functional disorders of the CNS, 0.20-0.25; and for impaired fertility, 0.20-0.25. From these data, Kameyama concluded that the risk of non-stochastic effects of diagnostic irradiation of children in utero, for doses which are normally less than 0.01 Gy and up to 0.02 Gy as a maximum, would be extremely low, and probably negligible, given the appropriate control measures. It should be noted that carcinogenic and mutagenic effects are specifically excluded from these estimates, although these effects, according to other evaluations, constitute the major portion of the overall risk.

411. Russell [R8] discussed the problem of critical periods in the course of development. Although her contribution has mainly methodological value, it does contain observations of very general importance, particularly regarding the role of sensitive stages in the estimate of the attending risks. It points out, for example, that to consider the embryo as a whole, without defining the sensitivity of its cell subpopulations in the course of time, is a simplification that may produce a loss of sensitivity in the detection of risks, i.e., in an under-estimation of it. Conversely, extrapolation of the risk from single short-term exposures, carried out during high susceptibility stages, to protracted exposures, may lead to over-estimation of the risk because a given effect which can readily be induced with an optimum dose at a well defined stage of development may not be visible at all at other stages, even those occurring in close proximity to the critical periods.

B. EFFECTS AND PERIODS OF MAXIMUM SENSITIVITY

412. Before attempting any quantitative estimate, it is necessary to examine the nature of the risk under discussion and the time periods in human development over which such risk might apply. The effects that have been identified in the preceding discussion as relevant to human irradiation are reviewed below. For exposure during the pre-implantation phases, animal data (particularly in rodents) have documented pre-implantation death. As discussed in the 1977 UNSCEAR report [U2] this is more readily apparent in polytocous animals and may appear as death of single individuals (inferred from a dose-related decrease of the average number of implants) or as death of whole litters (documented by a dose-related increase of sterile matings). There are no data that might suggest the presence of such an effect in man. This is probably due to the fact that it is difficult to observe. Pre-implantation loss would actually be likely to result only in a missed menstruation, an event of such minor clinical consequence that it is hardly necessary to account for it. However, there is every reason to expect that a sufficiently high dose of radiation received by a pre-implanted human embryo would entail a definite probability of death: the question is, what magnitude should be assigned to this risk? In vivo data from the mouse, which were discussed in the 1977 report [U2] (and which have not been contradicted by the latest evidence on embryos irradiated and cultured in vitro, discussed in chapter II) point to a net increment of pre-implantation embryonic loss coefficient of the order of 1 Gy^{-1}. (For the purpose of the present study, the exposure unit R will be taken to give an absorbed dose of 0.01 Gy, a procedure that is not likely to underestimate the risk.) Evidence in rodents reviewed in the 1977 report [U2] is not incompatible with non-threshold dose relationships for irradiation during the pre-implantation stages. The same could be said for the in vitro data reviewed in chapter II. As to the length of the period over which such a risk could remain in effect, it might extend as a maximum over the first two weeks from fertilization.

413. In man, the phase of major organogenesis may be taken to last approximately from the 2nd to the 8th week after fertilization. Earlier in the present study, attention was called to the fact that, contrary to what happens for other mammalian species (e.g., rodents), where the relative duration of organogenesis over the whole period of pregnancy is longer, there is little or no evidence in the human that malformations in the teratological sense are to be seen. This may mean that: (a) the observations available for irradiation during organogenesis are too few; or (b) that exposures were too low; or (c) that grossly malformed fetuses are eliminated in the course of further development; or (d) that the human species behaves differently from other mammalian species in the sense that radiation during organogenesis may not result in gross teratological damage. The first of these alternatives is certainly true: the shortage of human data concerning irradiation of major organogenesis stages was pointed out in chapter III. The probability may not be excluded that a wider data base, or higher doses,

might have provided evidence in the positive sense. The other alternative, that grossly malformed fetuses are lost, is actually a well ascertained fact: as pointed out in chapter I, the incidence of malformed embryos decreases as a function of their increasing age. The phenomenon is to be seen as a result of a progressive elimination of embryos and fetuses carrying malformations that are too severe to be compatible with further development in utero or extra-uterine life. As to the human species being an exception to the general behaviour of other mammalian species, in the sense that it does not respond to irradiation during the phases of major organogenesis with induction of teratological defects, this alternative is hardly credible. As pointed out before, the lack of teratological effects, compared with maldevelopment of the CNS, may be justified on different grounds: for example, the much longer duration of CNS development in man over the time for organogenesis of other body structures.

414. It may be asked whether, for the purpose of risk estimation, the lack of data on teratological damage in man (compared with the relatively more common occurrence of CNS lesions) is sufficient reason to discard the possibility that such damage might occur at all. UNSCEAR believes that it is not, and will assume accordingly that such damage might occur during the 3rd to 8th week post-conception. Since the number of body structures that could be damaged is roughly similar for all mammals, irrespective of their body size, one could assume, if one considers together malformations of all types, that the ratio of malformed to normal fetuses per unit dose seen in animals may be taken as an expression of the risk of malformation induction per unit dose over the period in question for man. Therefore, for UNSCEAR's purposes, it will be assumed that the risk of an absolute increase of malformed fetuses of the order of $5 \ 10^{-1} \ Gy^{-1}$ (see paragraph 95) in animals might apply to the human species as well, over the period from 2 to 8 weeks post-conception. This must be interpreted as an upper value. (Here again the exposure unit R is taken to give an absorbed dose of 0.01 Gy on the average over all embryonic structures.) It is actually possible that the most severe of these conditions may never be seen in man, because they are aborted in early stages of development. It must be emphasized that using data derived from experimental animals on the assumption of linearity, and projecting these data to man, is likely to result in an upper estimate of risk, not only because radiation-induced teratological defects are not seen at low doses in humans, but also because the existence of a threshold may not be excluded in any species.

415. Data in animals have shown [U2] that as development of the embryo proceeds, the dose needed to kill the embryo becomes greater and the form of the dose-response relationships becomes increasingly sigmoid. For the purpose of UNSCEAR's estimates, doses resulting in death of the embryo post-implantation are too high to be considered in the present context. They would not be relevant to the exposure of the population, but only to exposure of pregnant women under accidental conditions. The evaluation of such cases is clearly beyond the scope of the present exercise, which aims at providing estimates of general validity for the exposure of the whole population, or large population groups, under controlled exposures. Death of the embryo in utero during embryonic or fetal stages (or death during post-natal life as a consequence of exposure in utero), therefore, is not considered further here.

416. The number of children classified as severely mentally retarded is increased by exposure in utero. From the data discussed in III. B, it appears reasonable to assume that the risk coefficient for low-LET radiation over the period 8-15 weeks is $4 \ 10^{-1} \ Gy^{-1}$ and over the period 16-25 weeks, $10^{-1} \ Gy^{-1}$. Before 8 weeks the risk is apparently zero and after 26 weeks the risk is very low.

417. Growth disturbances and other effects have also been shown to occur for exposure during the fetal period. Quite aside from the clinical significance of a reduction in body size in the absence of other clinical signs (which is indeed doubtful), it is difficult to express growth disturbances per unit dose and it is therefore impossible to provide a value of the risk for such graded effects. As for those effects on the developing gonads, which result in reduction of the reproductive capacity, it has been shown that distinctly sigmoid relationships prevail for these effects, so that it may be assumed that they may not be observed at doses of one tenth of a Gy or less. Accordingly, no attempt will be made to estimate the risk for these effects.

418. The last type of effects to be discussed is the induction of leukaemia and other solid tumours. Reasons have been given in chapter VII for assuming the existence of a causal relationship between pre-natal irradiation and induction of malignancy, in spite of the fact that, on purely scientific grounds, the supporting information is not entirely convincing. At face value, data show that the risk of developing a malignancy after irradiation in utero at doses of the order of 0.01 Gy is fully expressed within the first 10 years of life and is increased by about 50% over the normal rate. The risk may be estimated, according to a previous UNSCEAR analysis [U2] to be of the order of $2 \ 10^{-2} \ Sv^{-1}$. Some evidence indicates [C13, M36] that the risk during the first trimester might be substantially higher than that for the last two trimesters. The relevant data appear unconvincing, however; constancy of the risk throughout pregnancy is therefore assumed in the following discussion.

C. RISK ESTIMATES

419. The risk estimates given in the preceding section relate to effects of different nature and severity. Therefore, they cannot be easily compared or aggregated. They should be viewed in the light of a number of qualifications, as follows:

(a) The risk estimates have been specified as if the dose relationships for the relevant effects were linear, although, as previously discussed, many dose-effect relationships for the most complex functional non-stochastic effects have actually been shown to be curvilinear (concave upwards). The estimates are therefore likely to be in excess by some unknown factor, particularly at the very low doses.

(b) The risk estimates have been derived by using data on acute irradiation at high, rather than low, dose rates and apply therefore to this irradiation condition. Basic radiobiological considerations suggest that projection of these estimates to low-dose rate low-LET irradiation could cause these estimates to be lowered by some factor, at least for those effects that are characterized by curvilinear dose-response relationships. It has, however, been argued [M36] that no modification of the risk would occur in the case of tumour induction, which is regarded as a process initiated in a single cell. If this were true, the overall reduction of incidence due to low-dose rate would thus depend on the relative importance of cancer induction and other harmful conditions.

(c) Overall, for small doses, the detriment calculated from the risk estimates given in the previous section appears rather small, in comparison with the natural prevalence of malformations at birth which has been taken in chapter I section C to be of the order of $6 \cdot 10^{-2}$. For example, a dose to the conceptus of 0.01 Gy delivered over the whole pregnancy would add a probability of health effects (mortality and induction of malformations, severe mental retardation, leukaemia and other solid tumours) in the liveborn of less than 0.002 to the natural probability of 0.06 of a new-born child being seriously handicapped. In addition, it should be kept in mind that when radiation is delivered acutely, not all the above risks will operate jointly; on the other hand, for radiation delivered chronically, for reasons developed in point (b) above, the risk would be expected to be lower.

IX. CONCLUSIONS

420. As a follow-up to its 1977 study [U2], UNSCEAR has undertaken a revision of data pertaining to the effects and risks of pre-natal irradiation. The revision has taken into account data in human embryology, particularly of the CNS, which were either unavailable or not sufficiently well established at the time of the previous study; new information derived from experimental animal systems; and re-evaluated dosimetric and medical data on children exposed before birth during the explosions at Hiroshima and Nagasaki. All this called for a new assessment of a field that has attracted much attention over the last few years. In addition to covering such effects as tumour induction by pre-natal irradiation, this new revision aims to provide a consideration in depth of the human data and attempts to quantify the risk to man by irradiation in utero.

421. Data derived from human material have been helpful in mapping out, with increasing precision, developmental events that are of importance in the context of radiobiology. Research on morphological embryology is yielding an accurate description of human developmental stages at the same time that new techiques of observation in vivo are establishing a good correlation between descriptive morphology and body size in embryos and fetuses. The histogenesis and development of certain structures, such as the CNS, which are particularly susceptible to radiation damage at pre-natal stages, are also becoming better known at the biochemical level. Through biochemical, histological and cell kinetic analysis, the main events in the development of the brain structures are being followed; and the overall process of brain maturation is emerging as a long sequence of phenomena lasting well into the post-natal stages of development.

422. In primates, new techniques of cell labelling have allowed the reconstruction, to a remarkable degree of precision, of the kinetics leading to the formation of the cerebral cortex. It has been established that cell division, cell migration and cell maturation in a tightly arranged sequence of time and events are involved in the formation of the brain cortex. The time of most active division of undifferentiated neuronal cells is the most sensitive to the radiation insult in man. This is in good agreement with what had previously been ascertained in experimental animals. Radiation-induced disturbances of cell division, migration and maturation invariably result, through various mechanisms, in a loss of neuronal function. This loss may not be repaired by other neuronal cells, which are unable to divide, or by glial cells, which have no neuronal function.

423. After irradiation, congenital anomalies of other body structures, besides those of the CNS, are uncommon in man, but very common in experimental animals. The apparent discrepancies have been discussed, and reasons and explanations given. The relevant findings must be taken as warnings against any indiscriminate attempt to project to man results obtained in animals. Any such projection must take into account the embryological peculiarities of each species. Extrapolations, particularly of the more quantitative findings, are, in principle, unjustified.

424. Congenital malformations in the human species may be classified, according to their etiology, into those of simple genic origin (about 6% of all malformations scored at birth), those having a complex multifactorial origin (about 50%), those due to chromosomal defects (about 5%) and those known to be associated with a variety of environmental factors (about 6%). For about one-third of all malformations seen at birth, therefore, no apparent cause can at present be identified. Children malformed at birth are the survivors among a greater number of malformed embryos and fetuses who have died at some stage of intra-uterine development. If malformations are scored in grown-up children, the incidence is, again, higher than at birth. Total incidence figures are highly dependent on the method of scoring; the size of sample; diagnostic criteria; ethnic and genetic background; age and parity of the parents; and seasonal, geographical and socio-economic conditions. The same is true for the various classes of malformations. As a convenient average for its assessments, UNSCEAR has adopted a

natural figure of about 6% of newborn children being affected by anomalies that may seriously reflect on their viability and physical well being.

425. No new data have appeared on the effects of irradiation in man during the pre-implantation stages. There have been, however, many new findings on in vitro irradiation and culture of rodent embryos. A generally decreasing sensitivity to killing of pre-implanted embryos, as a function of time and complexity of development, has been confirmed by these new data. There are also ample oscillations of sensitivity in relation to the various phases of the cell cycle during the earliest segmentation divisions. From the whole of these data, killing of single embryos, or of entire litters in polytocous animals, emerges as the most important effect of pre-implantation irradiation. For rodent irradiation in vitro and in vivo, doses of the order of 0.1 Gy or less have been reported to have a significant effect on embryonic and fetal mortality.

426. Recent data on the irradiation of experimental animals during the stages of major organogenesis have added significant details to previous conclusions of UNSCEAR [U2], but have not changed them drastically. It remains true that the effects resulting from irradiation of experimental animals during this phase are mostly the teratological ones, accompanied by growth disturbances of the various body structures or of the whole body. There is a pronounced time dependence for each class of malformation, because the period of maximum sensitivity of any one structure coincides with the time of its most active proliferation and differentiation. For each specific type of malformation, particularly those of the skeleton and of the CNS for which new data have been gathered, sigmoid dose-response relationships are usually found. A wealth of data on the pathogenesis of malformations in the CNS has been of help in understanding how the radiation damage to the developing neuronal cells might be translated into functional CNS damage, through the disturbance of division, migration and intercellular connection of the irradiated neurons.

427. Sensitivity to radiation damage in the human CNS starts at the borderline between the end of organogenesis (8 weeks after conception) and proceeds well into the conventional fetal stages, up to 25 weeks. An important step forward in the analysis of this effect and the attendant risk has been made possible through a review of dosimetric and clinical data on children irradiated in utero during the atomic explosions at Hiroshima and Nagasaki. It has been confirmed that some of these children have developed clinically severe mental retardation and the incidence of this condition has been analysed as a function of post-conceptional time at irradiation and as a function of the dose received by the embryos, according to the most recently available dosimetric evaluations. Mental handicap is not seen in children irradiated up to 8 weeks from conception, is at a maximum between 8 and 15 weeks when neuronal proliferation is most active and decreases to lower values between 16 and 25 weeks, when glial cell proliferation and neuronal synaptogenesis occur. The number of children classified as severely mentally retarded is increased by radiation exposure in utero. The excess number of mentally retarded in the dose range (0.04-2 + Gy) is apparently linear with dose at 8-15 weeks, with an average risk coefficient of $4 \cdot 10^{-1} \text{Gy}^{-1}$; it is, on the other hand, concave upwards at 16-25 weeks with a coefficient of the order of 10^{-1}Gy^{-1}. There is an indication that, in addition to these extreme mental handicaps, other less prominent functional brain deficits might be present in children irradiated in utero. While not all aspects of these findings may be explained on the basis of present radiobiological knowledge, their significance is thought to be high, particularly in respect of the quantitation of the attendant risk.

428. For irradiation of animals during the fetal stages, a variety of effects have been described, but those on the developing gonads have been particularly well documented, both at the anatomical level and also in respect of the ensuing loss of reproductive capacity when animals irradiated in utero reach the fertile age. Although the form of the dose-effect relationships for loss of germ cells may (at least under some conditions) appear to be exponential, pronounced sigmoid relationships with dose appear to prevail for impairment of reproductive capacity, with a fair degree of inter-strain and inter-species variability. Doses of a few tenths of a gray as a minimum, are necessary to elicit observable fertility changes in various animal species. Other effects induced by fetal irradiation have been described for the haemopoietic system, the liver and the kidney. Such effects all occur at fairly high radiation doses.

429. The effects of internal irradiation of the mammalian conceptus are greatly influenced by the nuclides tested, their chemical form, the route and schedule of administration, and the kinetics of transfer and metabolism of the radioactive substances from the mother to the fetus through the placenta. Information on all these aspects, for all nuclides, is far from complete and only a few nuclides appear to have received some attention. Tritium has been investigated in relation to its different chemical forms, its metabolism, the type of effects induced as a function of dose, and its relative biological effectiveness by comparison with external gamma exposure. Radio-iodine has been studied in respect of its kinetic behaviour following acute or protracted exposures, through a comparison of the uptake in the mothers' or fetus' thyroid. Plutonium distribution and incorporation in various organs of the mother and the fetus have also been studied in three different mammalian species in an attempt to compare the findings among species. The available evidence does not show a preferential tendency of actinides to concentrate in the embryo and fetus. There appears to be a need to enlarge the data base for the nuclides of importance, particularly in regard to their uptake, distribution and effects over an adequate range of concentrations and tissue doses.

430. Radiation effects in the mammalian conceptus may be modified to different degrees by a number of factors. Among these factors, the type and energy of radiation have been investigated. Relative biological

effectiveness (RBE) values in the region of about 5 for fast neutrons and helium ions (as compared with gamma radiation) have been reported, with a clear indication that the actual values could vary according to the types of effects scored and the dose level. An increase of RBE with decreasing radiation dose has not been convincingly shown, but may be expected from the shape of the dose-response relationships reported so far. Information on the interplay of LET, the oxygen effect, and dose-rate or fractionation has not been found to be very abundant for effects in utero, although there is no reason to suspect that the developing conceptus may behave differently from adult mammalian systems in respect of these major radiobiological parameters.

431. In the field of combined actions, ionizing radiation has been found, in isolated instances, to behave synergistically with some chemical agents, ultrasound or high-frequency radiation. More thorough and systematic studies would be required, however, to substantiate these reports over a wider range of doses and effects. Radioprotective and radiosensitizing drugs have also been tested in combination with radiation; the results indicate that the developing tissues are roughly similar to adult ones in their response to these substances.

432. UNSCEAR has analysed and assessed a large body of literature on tumour induction following in utero irradiation of experimental animals. It has identified a number of weak points in these contributions which make it difficult to draw overall conclusions, particularly for a comparison of the carcinogenic action of radiation in pre- as opposed to post-natal stages. The species, strain and sex variability, the lack of extended dose-response analyses, the different stages of organ histogenesis and differentiation, the variable types and dosages of radiation, as well as objective methodological and technical difficulties, may affect any such straightforward comparison. However, there is no good evidence of a significantly higher susceptibility to tumour induction of pre-natal animals. On the contrary, the data point to a lower susceptibility upon irradiation in utero. In any case, the most striking effects are on the spectrum of the types of tumours developed after irradiation of pre- or post-natal ages, rather than on the incidence rate of all tumours.

433. Data on tumour induction by pre-natal irradiation in man come from two different major sources. On the one hand, the survivors of the atomic explosions at Hiroshima and Nagasaki, who were exposed while still in utero, have continued to show, upon successive reviews, no evidence of excess cancer. On the other hand, two much larger retrospective surveys in children exposed in utero on account of medical indications have consistently shown an excess of tumour and leukaemia cases over the first 10 years of post-natal life, which may be estimated to be roughly 50% above the natural incidence for the doses involved in those studies. A number of social and medical factors have been identified that may affect the association between irradiation in utero and proneness to develop cancer in childhood. However,

these factors are not of sufficient weight to explain the association entirely. Other reasons have been discussed which render the results of the different series difficult to reconcile.

434. The authors involved in the analysis of the two retrospective surveys described disagree about the causal association between irradiation in utero and the likelihood of developing leukaemia and cancer. UNSCEAR believes that the important consideration in these matters is the existence of the association, which has been firmly established. As to the causal relationship, to deny it on the ground that such positive evidence does not agree with the experience in Japan or the data in animals would mean putting undue weight on scientific considerations over the practical need of allowing for any possible risk. Therefore UNSCEAR accepts, provisionally, the causal nature of the association, for practical purposes, but emphasizes that this is simply on account of prudence and not on any scientific grounds. UNSCEAR will follow these matters and be ready to modify its position on the strength of any new evidence.

435. UNSCEAR has attempted to work out quantitative risk estimates for a number of radiation-induced effects in utero (mortality and induction of malformations, mental retardation, tumours and leukaemia) and to attribute the risk to the period of pregnancy over which it applies. Under a number of qualifying assumptions, it is possible to conclude that, for the small doses likely to be encountered in practice, the overall risk is relatively small (no more than 0.002 for the liveborn at 0.01 Gy) in relation to the natural incidence of malformations in non-irradiated individuals, which is of the order of 0.06 in the human species.

X. RESEARCH NEEDS

436. At various points in the preceding text attention has specifically been drawn to areas where there is a lack or substantial limitation of information that might enable full understanding and assessment of the data in man on which risk estimates should be based. In other cases such limitations have been implied in discussing the difficulties of deriving sufficiently firm generalizations. It appears useful to summarize such research needs, in the hope that they might be considered when planning future work.

437. Any occasion to collect information directly from the human species should of course be pursued with the highest priority. This applies first of all to observations on radiation effects on embryos or fetuses irradiated in utero, although it appears that the material available for further studies is rather limited. In this respect, re-examination and updating at suitable intervals of children exposed for medical reasons would still be useful to search for possible long-term effects of radiation. Similarly useful and very important is the analysis of mental and physical development, school performance and other functional tests on the survivors

of the atomic explosions irradiated in utero, in order to complete the picture with the more subtle and less conspicuous effects of irradiation that may have affected these subjects.

438. The need for more detailed quantitative information applies equally to normal human development, as a necessary background for the study of radiation-induced effects. There is a need for a fine description and timing of the landmarks of human development during the embryonic and fetal stages, the variability in the occurrence of such landmarks as a function of time, and of ethnic and other characteristics. Attention and support to institutions whose scope is to describe such developmental events is important, because this knowledge is fundamental to many branches of the medical and biological research.

439. In view of the limited amount of information that may be obtained directly on human subjects, the use of models of radiation effects in utero will continue to be of paramount importance for the understanding of mechanisms and the projection of effects and risks. Although all models may be useful in different respects, depending on the answers required from them, it is to be expected that research on small mammals (rodents in particular) may be more suitable for the study of mechanisms, while research on higher mammals (primates) may be more interesting for extrapolation of the effects to man. In both cases, it is the consequences of small doses (below about 0.1 Gy of low-LET and correspondingly lower doses of high-LET radiation) that should be particularly studied. This implies designing and testing of techniques which may be sensitive to such small doses, while retaining significance and value for predictive purposes.

440. In very general terms, considering the large sample size needed, models in rodents are probably more useful for the analysis of dose- and time-effect relationships, the study of repair effects, the analysis of variability inter- and intra-species, the analysis of combined modalities of treatment, the comparative effects of radiation of different types and energy and different patterns of radiation exposure. Comparative studies on different species should also be useful in the analysis of the time sequence of various radiation-induced phenomena as they correlate with the occurrence and the duration of developmental events in each particular species.

441. It should be realized that, particularly in the case of the development of nervous system and radiation effects thereon, the size of the structures to be analysed and the duration of the phenomena involved make it preferable to use primate species for more meaningful extrapolations to man. The same may be said for the study of somatometric growth of the body and brain and for the analysis of higher nervous functions in such animals. There is also a need to correlate in these animals morphological with functional effects by making use of modern techniques of behavioural analysis. However, financial and other limitations involved in this type of research should be recognized.

442. It is also important to realize that it is no longer possible to view the brain as a single organ, but to analyse the developmental events and radiation-induced changes systematically in the different structures of the brain, to apply the newest neurobiological and neurochemical techniques, to move from the study of effects such as cell death to the migration of cells, synaptogenesis, and the fine tuning of cellular and histological interactions.

443. In order to obtain much needed information of potential value under normal and accidental conditions of exposure to internal radiation sources, there is an urgent need to enlarge the data base on the metabolism and effects in utero of radionuclides, especially of those having practical importance, over a wide range of chemical forms and activity concentrations. Such studies should be carried out in relation to tissue dose, rather than intake concentrations, in order to facilitate generalized conclusions on dose-response relationships. More generally, better estimates of the actual doses absorbed by the fetus at various representative pre-natal ages could be very useful.

444. Finally, there is a need for inter-species comparisons of the radiation response of developing germ cells in various animals and both sexes for acute and long-term exposure.

T a b l e   1

Approximate time of the beginning and end
of the major developmental periods in some mammalian species
(days p.c.)
[U2]

Species	Pre-implantation	Major organogenesis	Fetal period
Hamster	0-5	6-12	13-16.5
Mouse	0-5	6-13	14-19.5
Rat	0-7	8-15	16-21.5
Rabbit	0-5	6-15	16-31.5
Guinea-pig	0-8	9-25	26-63
Dog	0-17	18-30	31-63
Man	0-8	9-60	60-270

<u>Correlations between menstrual age and crown-rump length</u>
according to [S55] or [J9]

Menstrual age		Crown-rump length according to [S55]	Crown-rump length according to [J9] a/
Weeks	Days	(mm)	(mm)
9	63	31	24
10	70	40	33
11	77	50	43
12	84	61	53.5
13	91	74	66
14	98	87	82.5
15	105	101	99.5
16	112	116	117
17	119	130	135
18	126	142	151

a/ This study was based exclusively on fetuses obtained
from artificially induced abortions.

T a b l e   3

<u>Regression coefficients for fetal organ weights</u>
[B14]

Organ	N	Coefficients a/			Standard error of estimate
		a (10^{-2})	b (10^{-4})	c (10^{-6})	
Brain	71	14.828	-0.126	-	6.127
Liver	75	6.097	-0.421	0.032	4.919
Lung	76	3.777	-0.286	0.016	3.475
Kidney	78	0.857	-0.016	0.003	0.842
Heart	76	0.592	0.029	-0.002	0.498
Thymus	76	0.073	0.042	-0.002	0.417
Thyroid	70	0.035	0.074	-	0.048
Pancreas	71	0.085	-0.002	-	0.118
Adrenal	76	0.478	-0.033	0.002	0.384
Spleen	75	-0.001	0.046	-0.003	0.244

a/ Coefficients for the polynomial regression formula
$y = ax + bx^2 + cx^3$ where x is body weight and
y is organ weight.

T a b l e   4

Developmental stages in human embryos
[08]

Carnegie stage	Pairs of somites	Length (mm)	Age a/ (days)	Age b/ (days)	Features
1				1	Fertilization
2			1.5-3	2- 3	From 2 to about 16 cells
3			4	4- 5	Free blastocyst
4			5-6	5- 6	Attaching blastocyst
5		0.1-0.2	7-12	7-12	Implanted although previllous
5(a)		0.1	7-8		Solid trophoblast
5(b)		0.1	9		Trophoblastic lacunae
5(c)		0.15-0.2	11-12		Lacunar vascular circle
6		0.2	13	13-15	Chorionic villi; primitive streak may appear
6(a)					Chorionic villi
6(b)					Primitive streak
7		0.4	16	15-17	Notochordal process
8		1.0-1.5	18	17-19	Primitive pit; notochordal and neurenteric canals
9	1- 3	1.5-2.5	20	19-21	Somites first appear
10	4-12	2 -3.5	22	22-23	Neural folds begin to fuse; two pharyngeal bars; optic sulcus
11	13-20	2.5-4.5	24	23-26	Rostral neuropore closes; optic vesicle
12	21-29	3-5	26	26-30	Caudal neuropore closes; three pharyngeal bars; upper limb buds appearing
13	30- ?	4-6	28	28-32	Four limb buds; lens disc; otic vesicle
14		5-7	32	31-35	Lens pit and optic cup; endolymphatic appendage distinct
15		7-9	33	35-38	Lens vesicle; nasal pit; anti-tragus beginning; hand plate; trunk relatively wider; cerebral vesicles distinct
16		8-11	37	37-42	Nasal pit faces ventrally; retinal pigment visible in intact embryo; auricular hillocks beginning; foot plate
17		11-14	41	42-44	Head relatively larger; trunk straighter; nasofrontal groove distinct; auricular hillocks distinct; finger rays
18		13-17	44	44-48	Body more cuboidal;elbow region and toe rays appearing; eyelids beginning; tip of nose distinct; nipples appear; ossification may begin
19		16-18	47.5	48-51	Trunk elongating and straightening
20		18-22	50.5	51-53	Upper limbs longer at bent elbows
21		22-24	52	53-54	Fingers longer; hands approach each other, feet likewise
22		23-28	54	54-56	Eyelids and external ear more developed
23		27-31	56.5	56-60	Head more rounded; limbs longer and more developed

a/ According to [012] for stages 11-23; miscellaneous sources for stages 1-10.
b/ According to [J14].

Table 5

Birth prevalences of all isolated common congenital abnormalities
per 1000 total births, based on a WHO study
[S38]

ICD code [W28]	Congenital anomaly	Average	Minimum	Source of data a/	Maximum	Source of data a/	Comments
740	Anencephalus and similar anomalies	1.1	0.1	LL	4.5	BE	Obvious territorial cluster in the
741.0	Spina bifida	0.8	0.1	M	4.2	BE	British Isles
742.0	Encephalocele	0.1	0.0	X	0.7	AL	
	Neural tube defects	2.0	0.6	C	9.0	BE	
745.0-747.9*	Congenital cardio-vascular malformations	6.1	3.2	BI	18.5	G	Very heterogeneous category. Various types should be evaluated separately
745.3-4*	Ventricular septal defect	1.7	0.4	BI	3.3	LE	
749.1-2	Cleft lip and/or cleft palate	1.0	0.0	ME CT	1.6	J	Ethnic differences: African: ~ 0.4 European: ~ 1.0 Oriental: ~ 1.9
750.5*	Congenital hypertrophic pyloric stenosis	2.0	0.1	SI	3.3	A	Ethnic differences: African: ~ 0.5 European: ~ 2.0 Oriental: ~ 0.4
752.5	Undescended testicle	1.2	0.0	X	12.2	BO	Diagnosis depends on time of birth and post-natal age
752.6*	Hypospadias	2.8	0.4	S	4.3	R	There are common minor variants
754.3	Congenital dislocation of hip	0.3	0.0	X	3.2	BO	Increasing trend owing to neo-natal screening
754.5-754.6	Varus, valgus and other deformities	2.7	0.4	C	20.9	PA	Very heterogeneous category. Various types should be evaluated separately
754.53*	Structural talipes different types equinovarus	1.3	1.0	S	3.0	L	
755.0	Polydactyly	1.1	0.0	ME	6.2	P	Obvious ethnic cluster
758.0	Down's syndrome	0.8	0.0	AL, CT	3.9	LL	Decreasing trend
550.1*	Congenital inguinal hernia	18.1	10.2	N	130.0	E	Not included in chapter XIV of the ICD

a/

A	Aberdeen, United Kingdom	LE	Leiden, The Netherlands
AL	Alexandria, Egypt	M	Manila, Philippines
BE	Belfast, United Kingdom	MA	Madrid, Spain
BI	Birmingham, United Kingdom	MC	Mexico City, Mexico
BO	Bogota, Colombia	ME	Melbourne, Australia
C	Calcutta, India	N	Newcastle, United Kingdom
CT	Cape Town, South Africa	P	Pretoria, South Africa
E	Edinburgh, United Kingdom	PA	Panama
G	Greenland	R	Rochester, United States of America
H	Hong Kong	S	Sweden
J	Johannesburg, South Africa	SI	Shiraz, Islamic Republic of Iran
K	Kuala Lumpur, Malaysia	SP	Sao Paolo, Brazil
L	London, United Kingdom		
LL	Llubljana, Yugoslavia	X	Several centres

Table 6

Birth prevalences of all isolated common congenital abnormalities
per 1000 total births based on a Hungarian study
[C18]

ICD Code [W28]	Congenital anomaly	Average	Etiology a/	Comments
740	Anencephalus and similar anomalies	1.1 (0.8)	MTM)	A decreasing trend in recent years (shown
742.0	Encephalocele	0.2 (0.2)	MTM)	in parentheses)
	Neural tube defects	2.9 (1.9)	MTM)	
745.0- 747.9	Congenital cardiovascular malformations	10.6	H	Result of population screening
745.3-4	Ventricular septal defect	2.1	MTM	In a proportion of cases, spontaneous closure occurs
749.1-2	Cleft lip and/or cleft palate	1.0	MTM	-
750.5	Congenital hypertrophic pyloric stenosis	1.5	MTM	Only operated cases
752.5	Undescended testicle	3.6	MTM	After third month. This figure is ~ 35 in males at birth
752.6	Hypospadias	2.2	MTM	Trend is increasing
754.3	Congenital dislocation of hip	28.0	MTM	Only treated cases, i.e., without true abnormality
754.5- 754.6	Varus, valgus and other deformities of feet	3.0	M	Mainly postural deformities
754.53	Structural talipes equinovarus	1.3	MTM	A true abnormality
755.0	Polydactyly	0.3	G	Not a common abnormality in Hungary
758.0	Down's syndrome	1.2	C	Verified by chromosomal analysis
550.1	Congenital inguinal hernia	11.4	MTM	Only operated cases

a/ C = chromosomal; G = genic, at least some part; H = heterogeneous;
M = maternal; MTM = multifactorial threshold model; i.e., polygenic
disposition interacting with a variety of environmental factors.

Table 7

Birth prevalences of some isolated moderately frequent congenital abnormalities per 1000 total births

ICD Code [W28]	Congenital anomaly	Average	Minimum	Source of data a/	Maximum	Source of data a/	Hungarian study [C18]	Etiology b/
742.3	Congenital hydrocephalus	0.6	0.2	MC	2.0	AL	0.8	H
749.0	Cleft palate	0.2	0.0	X	0.5	ME	0.4	MTM (?)
750.3	Oesophageal atresia and stenosis and/or tracheo-oesophageal fistula	0.1	0.0	X	0.5	SP	0.2	U
751.2	Atresia and stenosis of large intestine, rectum and anal canal	0.2	0.2	ME CT	0.6	K	0.2	U
753.1	Cystic kidney	0.03	-		-		0.1	G_1
755.1	Syndactyly	0.2	0.0	X	0.7	J	0.3	G_2
755.3-5	Reduction deficiencies of limb	0.2	0.0	HP	1.8	SP	0.4	H
756.6	Anomalies of diaphragm	0.1	-		-		0.2	MTM
756.7	Exomphalos	0.1	0.0	X	0.5	MA	0.2	MTM

a/ Abbreviations explained in the footnote a/ to Table 5.
b/ G_1 = genic, at least type I and II; G_2 = genic, at least some part; H = heterogeneous; MTM = multifactorial threshold model.

Table 8

Percentage distribution of congenital anomaly groups
(modified from [V8])

Group of congenital anomalies	Authors a/							
	A	B	C	D	E	F	G	H
	Total birth prevalence							
	1.4	1.5	1.3	2.8	3.8	2.2	8.5	7.4
Central nervous system	26.3	13.3	21.0	11.6	5.7	7.7	8.5	4.2
Cardiovascular system	7.2	7.0	5.9	8.7	10.9	19.2	10.2	11.0
Cleft lip and palate	11.6	10.8	9.5	8.8	6.3	7.9	3.2	2.0
Alimentary system	5.4	4.9	4.1	8.7	7.4	7.9	7.3	3.8
Genito-urinary system	18.2	7.2	2.0	7.8	15.7	12.4	13.6	12.7
Limbs	27.2	53.0	38.0	35.9	36.8	28.1	39.2	41.2
Down's syndrome	3.5	3.6	6.5	-	5.7	6.3 b/	1.4	1.6

a/ A = Büchi, 1950 (reference given in [V8];
 B = Stevenson et al., 1958 (reference given in [V8];
 C = Stevenson, 1966 (reference given in [V8];
 D = Klemetti, 1966 (reference given in [V8];
 E = Villumsen, 1970 [W8];
 F = Trimble and Doughty, 1974 [T10];
 G = Myriantropoulos and Chung, 1974 [M45];
 H = Czeizel and Sankaranarayanan, 1984 [C19].
b/ All chromosomal aberrations.

T a b l e 9

Incidence of severe mental retardation in individuals
exposed pre-natally to the atomic bombing of Hiroshima and Nagasaki a/

Data for the two cities have been combined and the cases distributed
by gestational age at exposure and fetal absorbed dose,
based on the T65 revised dosimetry b/

(Source of data: [04])
[This table is taken from I11]

Ages	Dose categories (Gy) c/				
	> 0.01	0.01-0.09	0.10-0.49	0.50-0.99	1.00+
Cities combined					
All gestational ages					
Subjects	1085	292	169	34	19
Retarded	9	4	4	6	7
Percent	0.8	1.4	2.4	17.6	36.8
0-7 weeks					
Subjects	210	55	26	2	2
Retarded	1	0	0	0	0
Percent	0.5	0.0	0.0	0.0	0.0
8-15 weeks					
Subjects	257	69	50	13	9
Retarded	2	3	4	4	6
Percent	0.8	4.3	8.0	30.8	66.7
16-25 weeks					
Subjects	312	86	45	15	5
Retarded	2	1	0	2	1
Percent	0.6	1.2	0.0	13.3	20.0
26+ weeks					
Subjects	306	82	48	4	3
Retarded	4	0	0	0	0
Percent	1.3	0.0	0.0	0.0	0.0

a/ Note that the frequency distribution by gestational age in this Table is slightly inconsistent with that given in [03] due to differences in grouping; these differences have little effect on the risk estimates. The data for the two cities are separately presented elsewhere [03, 04].

b/ The tissue gamma dose is taken to be equal to 0.42 times the gamma kerma plus 0.077 times the neutron kerma, the tissue neutron dose to be equal to 0.14 times the neutron kerma, and the total tissue dose to be the sum of the two individual tissue doses.

c/ The mean doses within these dose categories over all gestational ages are 0, 0.04, 0.23, 0.72, and 1.61 Gy, respectively.

T a b l e   10

The relationship of mental retardation to absorbed fetal dose

(Source of data: [O4])
[This table is taken from I11]

Gestational age	Cities combined					
	a	s_a	b (Gy^{-1})	s_b (Gy^{-1})	Deviance	P
All gestational ages	0.768	0.253	0.174 a/	0.041	3.78	0.29
8-15 weeks	0.917	0.567	0.404 a/	0.078	1.11	0.77
16-25 weeks	0.601	0.415	0.101	0.059	3.25	0.36
Relationship of mental retardation to dose: 'controls' excluded						
8-15 weeks	2.189	2.242	0.378 a/	0.089	0.61	0.74
16-25 weeks	0.409	1.055	0.106	0.068	3.20	0.20
Relationship of mental retardation to dose: 'controls' combined						
Pooled control	0.863	0.278	0.406 a/	0.077	1.11	0.77

The deviance, which is a measure of the goodness-of-fit of the model to the data, has three or two degrees of freedom depending upon whether the zero dose group is or is not included in the modeling; the P value is the probability (two tailed) of exceeding the deviance by chance under the null hypothesis. a is the estimated number (intercept) of cases of mental retardation (per 100 individuals) in the zero dose group and s_a its standard error; bD is the increase in the frequency of mental retardation, with dose D, expressed in grays (100 rad); and s_b is its standard error. Note that with the binomial distribution the deviance takes the form $2\{\text{Sum } z \ln(z/\hat{Q}) + \text{Sum } (n-z) \ln[(n-z)/(n-\hat{z})]\}$ where the z's are the observed values, $\hat{Q}$ the estimates of the p's under the complete model, that is when the p's are all different and match the data completely, and the $\hat{z}$'s are the estimates of the p's under the fitted model.

a/ Significant at the 0.001 level.

T a b l e   11

Approximate length of the oogenetic period in the female a/ and approximate life span of gonocytes in the male b/ for selected mammalian species
(Data from [E2])

Species	Sex	Days	References as quoted in the original publication [E2]
Mouse	male	14	Erickson [E2] (1978)
	female	5	Peters (1970)
Rat	male	17	Huckins and Clermont (1968)
	female	6	Beaumong and Mandl (1962)
Guinea pig	male	50	Erickson [E2] (1978)
	female	25	Ioannon (1964)
Pig	male	158	Erickson (1964)
	female	77	Black and Erickson (1968)
Bovine	male	340	Erickson and Martin (1972)
	female	100	Erickson (1966)
Monkey	male	~1000	Van Wanegen and Simpson (1954)
	female	100	Baker (1966)
Man	male	~3500	Charney et al. (1952)
	female	120	Baker (1963)

a/ Time in days from the formation of the germinal ridge to the end of significant mitotic activity of the oogonia.
b/ Time in days from the formation of the germinal ridge to the appearance of the first differentiated spermatogonia.

Table 12

Relative leukaemia risk in retrospective studies
of children dying of leukaemia
after diagnostic irradiation in utero
[U3]

Age of leukaemics (years)	Years of deaths for leukaemics	Percentage of mothers receiving abdominal irradiation during pregnancy		Relative risk (95% limits in parentheses)	Ref.
		Leukaemics	Controls		
< 10	1953-1955	96/780 (12.3%)	117/1.638 (7.1%)	1.8 (2.4-1.4)	[S23]
< 10	1951-1955	20/70 (28.6%)	48/247 (19.4%)	1.7 (2.9-0.8)	[F6]
?	1955-1956	37/150 (24.7%)	24/150 (16.0%)	1.7 (3.7-1.0)	[K21]
?	1955-1956	34/125 (27.2%)	27/125 (21.6%)	1.4 (2.5-0.7)	[K21]
?	1950-1957	72/251 (28.7%)	58/251 (23.1%)	1.3 (2.0-0.9)	[K21]
?	1946-1956	5/55 (9.1%)	8/55 (14.5%)	0.6 (2.0-0.2)	[K28]
< 20	1940-1957	3/65 (4.6%)	3/65 (4.6%)	1.0 (12.0-0.6)	[M39]
< 20	1940-1957	3/65 (4.6%)	7/93 (7.5%)	0.6 (2.4-0.1)	[M39]
< 20	1940-1957	3/65 (4.6%)	2/82 (2.4%)	1.9 (40.0-1.1)	[M39]

Table 13

Crude annual incidence rate of leukaemia
among children exposed in utero and controls, 1945-1979
[I3]

		Fetus total dose (Gy)				Total
		Not in city	0	0.01-0.4	> 0.5	
Subjects		2306	625	620	85	3636
Person-years		72444	19403	19078	2255	113180
Leukaemia cases		1	1	1	0	0
Rate (10^{-5})		1.38	5.15	5.24	0.00	2.65
90% confidence limit	Upper	6.55	24.46	24.87	–	6.85
	Lower	0.07	0.27	0.27	–	0.72

T a b l e   14

Relative risk of leukaemia in pre-natally exposed children: summary of most recent studies a/

Study source		Years of incidence	Relative risk	Reference
United States		1947-1960	1.52 b/	[M53]
United States,	white	1947-1967	2.88	[D15]
	black	1947-1967	0.00	[D15]
United Kingdom		1943-1965	1.48 b/	[S24]
Finland		1959-1968	1.90	[S56]
Hiroshima/Nagasaki		1945-79	2.15 c/	[K4, I13]
United Kingdom, twins		1943-1965	2.20 b/	[M23]
United States, twins		1930-1969	1.60 d/	[H23]
United Kingdom		1980-83	1.33	[H30]

a/ Most cases and excess risks reported here occurred before the age of 10.
b/ Significant at 0.5% level or better.
c/ Relative risk from Japan was calculated from 1 case of leukaemia in 21,333 person-years at risk in irradiated groups compared with 2 cases in 91,847 person-years in control groups (Table 13) [I3]; the difference is not statistically significant.
d/ In this series, the relative risk of solid tumours was a non-significant 3.2; other series have found values less than the relative risk for leukaemia.

T a b l e   15

Estimation of the acute LD/50 dose, minimal malforming doses, cell depleting dose, and doses for the human embryo based on compilation of mouse, rat, and human data
[B27]

Age	Approximate minimal lethal dose (Gy)	Approximate LD/50 (Gy)	Minimum dose for recuperable growth retardation in adult (Gy) a/	Minimum dose for recognizable gross malformation (Gy)	Minimum dose for induction of genetic, carcinogenic and minimal cell depletion phenomena
Day 1	0.10	0.7-1.0	No effect	No effect	Unknown
Day 14	0.25	1.4	0.25	-	Unknown
Day 18	0.50	1.5	0.25-0.50	0.25	Unknown
Day 28	> 0.50	2.2	0.50	0.25	Unknown
Day 50	> 1.00	2.6	0.50	0.50	Unknown
Late fetus to term		3.0-4.0	0.50	> 0.50	Unknown

a/ Estimates for maximum dose effective in reducing body weight. Specific organs or measurements may be more or less sensitive.

REFERENCES

A1 Agarwal, Y.C., P. Ayappan, and A.V. Santhamma. Carcinogenic effect of radiation on the mouse embryo; physical aspects of radiation dosimetry. Strahlentherapie 150: 618-623 (1975).

A2 Aldeen, K.A.M. and G. Konermann. Effects of acute x-irradiation on the pre-implantation embryos and on the implantation reaction in the mouse. Radiat. Environm. Biophys. 15: 47-55 (1978).

A3 Alexandre, H.L. Effects of x-irradiation on pre-implantation mouse embryos cultured in vitro. J. Reprod. Fertil. 36: 417-420 (1974).

A4 Alexandre, H. Correlation between cytological and morphogenetic effects of acute x-irradiation of pre-implantation mouse embryos cultured in vitro. J. Reprod. Fertil. 53: 399-402 (1978).

A5 Andersen, A.C. and A.G. Hendrickx. Fractionated x-irradiation damage to developing ovaries of the bonnet monkey (Macaca radiata). p. 50-52 in: UCD-472-123 (1976).

A6 Andersen, A.C., A.G. Hendrickx and M.H. Momeni. Effects of pre-natal fractionated x-ray exposures on the ovary of the bonnet monkey. Radiat. Res. 67: 526 only (1976).

A7 Andrew, F.D. Techniques for assessment of teratogenic effects: developmental enzyme patterns. Environm. Health Perspect. 18: 111-116 (1976).

A8 Andrew, F.D., R.L. Bernstine, D.D. Mahlum et al. Distribution of plutonium-239 in the gravid baboon. Radiat. Res. 70: 637-638 (1977).

A9 Ager, E.A., L.M. Schuman, H.M. Wallace et al. An epidemiological study of childhood leukemia. J. Chron. Dis. 18: 113-132 (1965).

A10 Antal, S. and H.H. Vogel. Neuroblast destruction in mouse and man after neutron irradiation in utero. p. 77-88 in: Effects of prenatal irradiation with special emphasis on late effects. EUR-8067 (1984).

A11 Ahrens, E., U. Mahn, S. Howe et al. Plazentalokalisation und diaplazentare Passage von Radionukliden. ISH-24 (1983).

A12 Altman, J. Postnatal development of the cerebellar cortex in the rat. I. The external germinal layer and the transitional molecular layer. J. Comp. Neurol. 145: 353-398 (1972).

A13 Altman, J. Postnatal development of the cerebellar cortex in the rat. II. Phases in the maturation of the Purkinje cells and of the molecular layer. J. Comp. Neurol. 145: 399-464 (1972).

A14 Altman, J. Postnatal development of the cerebellar cortex in the rat. III. Maturation of the components of the granular layer. J. Comp. Neurol. 145: 465-541 (1972).

A15 Antal, S. and Z. Fülöp. Histological studies in developing brain after 0.5 neutron irradiation in utero. p. 141-153 in: Radiation Risks to the Developing Nervous System. Gustav Fischer, Stuttgart, 1986.

A16 Antal, S., A. Fonagy, Z. Fülöp et al. Decreased weight, DNA, RNA and protein content of the brain after neutron irradiation of the 18-day mouse embryo. Int. J. Radiat. Biol. 46: 425-433 (1984).

B1 Balla, I., C. Michel and H. Fritz-Niggli. Cellular damage and recovery of the early developing mouse eye following low dose irradiation. I. X rays on day 8 of gestation. Experientia 37: 1105-1106 (1981).

B2 Balla, I., C. Michel and H. Fritz-Niggli. Cellular damage and recovery of the early developing mouse eye following low dose irradiation. II. X rays on day 9 of gestation. Experientia 39: 95-96 (1983).

B3 Balla, I. and C. Michel. Cellular damage of the eye-anlage following x-irradiation of the mouse embryo. p. 59-64 in: Developmental Effects of Prenatal Irradiation. Gustav Fischer, Stuttgart, 1982.

B4 Benjamin, S.A., R.W. Thomassen, G.M. Angleton et al. Effect of whole-body irradiation during prenatal and early postnatal development in the beagle dog. Radiat. Res. 74: 514 only (1978).

B6 Book, S.A. ^{131}I uptake and retention in fetal guinea pigs. Health Phys. 32: 149-154 (1977).

B7 Book, S.A. Age-related variation in thyroidal exposures from fission-produced radioiodines. p. 330-343 in: Developmental Toxicology of Energy-Related Pollutants (D.D. Mahlum et al., eds.). DOE Symposium Series No. 47, CONF-771017 (1978).

B8 Brizzee, K.R., K.R. Baskin, B. Kaack et al. Congenital anomalies and neuron and dendritic spine loss in the cerebral cortex and hippocampus of newborn squirrel monkeys following 200 rads prenatal irradiation. p. 219-231 in: Developmental Effects of Prenatal Irradiation. Gustav Fischer, Stuttgart, 1982.

B9 Brizzee, K.R., J.M. Ordy and A.N. D'Agostino. Morphological changes of the central nervous system after radiation exposure in utero. p. 145-173 in: Developmental Effects of Prenatal Irradiation. Gustav Fischer, Stuttgart, 1982.

B10 Brizzee, K.R., J.M. Ordy, B. Kaack et al. Prenatal cobalt-60 irradiation effects on early postnatal development of the squirrel monkey offspring. p. 204-227 in: Developmental Toxicology of Energy-Related Pollutants. (D.D. Mahlum et al., eds.). DOE Symposium Series No. 47, CONF-771017 (1978).

B11 Bross, I.D.J. and N. Natarajan. Risk of leukemia in susceptible children exposed to preconception, in utero, and postnatal irradiation. Prev. Med. 3: 361-369 (1974).

B13 Burch, P.R.J. Does fetal irradiation cause childhood malignancies? Brit. J. Radiol. 51: 146 only (1978).

B14 Burdi, A.R., M. Barr and W.J. Babler. Organ weight patterns in human fetal development. Human Biol. 53: 355-366 (1981).

B15 Berry, M. and A.W. Rogers. The migration of neuroblasts in the developing cerebral cortex. J. Anat. 99: 691-709 (1965).

B17 Bornhausen, M., A. Burgmeier, A. Matthes et al. Effects of prenatal treatment with ionizing radiation and/or heavy metal compounds on the conditioned behaviour of rats. p. 309-312 in: Developmental

Effects of Prenatal Irradiation. Gustav Fischer, Stuttgart, 1982.

B18 Borek, C., C. Pain and H. Mason. Transformation of embryo cells x-irradiated in utero and assayed in vitro: qualitative and quantitative aspects. Radiat. Res. 67: 628 only (1976).

B19 Borek, C., C. Pain and H. Mason. From uterus to petri dish: the neoplastic transformation of hamster embryo cells irradiated in utero and assayed in vitro. Nature 266: 452-454 (1977).

B20 Borek, C. and C. Pain. From uterus to petri dish: transformation in utero and in vitro. Radiat. Res. 70: 649-650 (1977).

B22 Bithell, J.F. and A.M. Stewart. Prenatal irradiation and childhood malignancy: a review of British data from the Oxford Survey. Br. J. Cancer 31: 271-287 (1975).

B25 Brent, R.L. Effects of ionizing radiation on growth and development. Contr. Epidem. Biostatist. 1: 147-183 (1979).

B26 Brent, R.J. Radiation teratogenesis: fetal risk and abortion. p. 223-252 in: Biological Risks of Medical Irradiation. Am. Inst. Physics, New York, 1980.

B27 Brent, R.L. Radiation teratogenesis. Teratology 21: 281-298 (1980). This paper was also printed as [B26].

B28 Benjamin, S.A., G.M. Angleton, L. Bishop et al. Hematopoietic neoplasms and related disorders in beagles irradiated during development. Radiat. Res. 87: 505 only (1981).

B29 Beck, F. Model systems in teratology. Brit. Med. Bull. 32: 53-58 (1976).

B30 Berry, M. and J.T. Eayrs. The effects of x-irradiation on the development of the cerebral cortex. J. Anat. 100: 707-722 (1966).

B31 Borek, C. Radiation oncogenesis in cell culture. Adv. Cancer Res. 37: 159-232 (1982).

B32 Bloom, A.D., S. Neriishi and P.G. Archer. Cytogenetics of the in utero exposed of Hiroshima and Nagasaki. Lancet 7558: 10-12 (1968).

B34 Burch, P.J.R. The biology of cancer. A new approach. MTR, Lancaster, 1976.

B35 Burch, P.J.R. Radiation hazards. Brit. J. Radiol. 54: 697 only (1981).

B36 Baserga, R., H. Lisco and W. Kisieleski. Further observations on induction of tumors in mice with radioactive thymidine. Proc. Soc. Exptl. Biol. Med. 110: 687-690 (1962).

B37 Berry, C.L., J. Amerigo C., Nickols et al. Transplacental carcinogenesis with radioactive phosphorus. Hum. Toxicol. 2: 49-62 (1983).

B38 Berry, M. and J.T. Eayrs. Histogenesis of the cerebral cortex. Nature 197: 984-985 (1963).

B39 Balla, I., C. Michel and H. Fritz-Niggli. Mitotic alterations and cell death in the early eye promordia of mice by Vinderine (VDS) and x rays. p. 351-364 in: Radiation Risks to the Developing Nervous System. Gustav Fischer, Stuttgart, 1986.

B40 Bornhausen, M. Analysis of behavioural changes induced by pre-natal irradiation. p. 283-292 in: Radiation Risks to the Developing Nervous System. Gustav Fischer, Stuttgart, 1986.

C1 Cahill, D.F., J.F. Wright, J.H. Godbold et al. Neoplastic and lifespan effects of chronic exposure to tritium. I. Effects on adult rats exposed during pregnancy. J. Natl. Cancer Inst. 55: 371-374 (1975).

C2 Cahill, D.F., J.F. Wright, J.H. Godbold et al. Neoplastic and lifespan effects of chronic exposure to tritium. II. Rats exposed in utero. J. Natl. Cancer Inst. 55: 1165-1169 (1975).

C3 Cairnie, A.B., D. Grahn, H.B. Rayburn et al. Teratogenic and embryolethal effects in mice of fission-spectrum neutrons and gamma rays. Teratology 10: 133-139 (1974).

C5 Coffigny, H. and C. Pasquier. Etude chez le rat adulte des effets d'une irradiation pre- ou post-natale de 150 rads. p. 48-51 in: CRSSA-RA (1976).

C6 Coffigny, H., C. Pasquier and J.P. Dupouy. Adrenal activity of adult rats irradiated with 150 rads during fetal life. p. 237-243 in: Developmental Toxicology of Energy-Related Pollutants (D.D. Mahlum et al., eds.). DOE Symposium Series No. 47, CONF-771017 (1978).

C7 Coffigny, H., C. Pasquier, G. Perrault et al. Study in adult rats of the effects of irradiation with 150 rads at different stages during gestation and the neonatal period. Effect on the development of the genital organs. p. 207-220 in: Late Biological Effects of Ionizing Radiation, Vol. II. IAEA, Vienna, 1978.

C9 Covelli, V., V. Di Mato, B. Bassani et al. Influence of age on life shortening and tumor induction after x-ray and neutron irradiation. Radiat. Res. 100: 348-364 (1984).

C10 Cerda, H., K.J. Johanson and K. Rosander. Radiation-induced DNA strand breaks and their repair in the developing rat brain. Int. J. Radiat. Biol. 36: 65-73 (1979).

C11 Carter, C.O. Genetics of common single malformations. Brit. Med. Bull. 32: 21-26 (1976).

C12 Court-Brown, W.M., R. Doll and A.B. Hill. Incidence of leukemia after exposure to diagnostic radiation in utero. Brit. Med. J. 5212: 1539-1545 (1960).

C13 Committee on the Biological Effects of Ionizing Radiation (BEIR). The effects on populations of exposure to low levels of ionizing radiation. National Academy Press, Washington, D.C., 1980.

C14 Commission of the European Communities. Concerted action on registration of congenital abnormalities. Executive report on pilot years 1979-1981. Supplement on pilot years 1979-1981. Report XII.26.83 (1983).

C15 Carsten A.L. "TRITOX", a multiple parameter evaluation of tritium toxicity. p. 117-142 in: Effects of prenatal irradiation with special emphasis on late effects. EUR-8067 (1984).

C16 Chajka, E.N., P.I. Lobko. Disturbances in the vagina development of the white rat offspring under the effect of x-ray irradiation. Arkh. Anat. Gistol. Embryol. 84: 73-81 (1983).

C17 Cowan, W.M., J.W. Fawcett, D.D.M. O'Leary et al. Regressive events in neurogenesis. Science 225: 1258-1265 (1984).

C18 Czeizel, A. and G. Tusnády. Etiological studies of isolated common congenital abnormalities in Hungary. Akadémiai Kiadó, Budapest, 1984.

C19 Czeizel, A. and K. Sankaranarayanan. The load of genetic and partially genetic disorders in man. I. Congenital anomalies: estimates of detriment in terms of years of life lost and years of impaired life. Mutat. Res. 128: 73-103 (1984).

C20 Cole, D.A., R.H. Stevens, P.T. Liu et al. Radiation recall of a perinatal iodine-131 exposure in rats. p. 103 in: Abstracts of Papers for the 32nd Annual Meeting of the Radiation Research Society, Florida, 1984.

C21 Campbell, S. and J.M. Pearce. Ultrasound visualization of congenital malformations. Brit. Med. Bull. 39: 322-331 (1983).

C22 Campbell, S. and P. Smith. Routine screening for congenital abnormalities by ultrasound. p. 325-329 in: Prenatal Diagnosis. The Royal College of Obstetricians and Gynecologists. London, 1984.

D1 Deroo J., G.B. Gerber and J. Maes. Biogenic amines, amioacids and regional blood flow in rat brain after pre-natal irradiation. p. 211-220 in: Radiation Risks to the Developing Nervous System. Gustav Fischer, Stuttgart, 1986.

D2 Dancis, J., J. Lind, M. Oratz et al. Placental transfer of proteins in human gestation. Am. J. Obst. Gynecol. 82: 167-171 (1961).

D3 Das, G.D. Experimental analysis of embryogenesis of cerebellum in rat. II. Morphogenetic malformations following x-ray irradiation on day 18 of gestation. J. Comp. Neurol. 176: 435-452 (1977).

D4 Dev, P.K., S.M. Gupta, P.K. Goyal et al. Radioprotective effect of MPG (2-Mercaptopropionylglycine) on the post-natal growth of mice irradiated in utero. Strahlentherapie 157: 553-555 (1981).

D5 Dev, P.K., S.M. Gupta, P.K. Goyal et al. Protection from body weight loss by 2-Mercaptopropionylglycine (MPG) in growing mice irradiated in utero with gamma radiation. Experientia 38: 962-963 (1982).

D6 Dev, P.K. and P.N. Srivastava. Effects of radiophosphorus on the developing endocrine glands of Swiss albino mice. Strahlentherapie 157: 418-426 (1981).

D7 Di Majo, V., E. Ballardin and P. Metalli. Comparative effects of fission neutrons and x irradiation on 7.5-day mouse embryos. Radiat. Res. 87: 145-158 (1981).

D8 Dobson, R.L. and M.F. Cooper. Tritium toxicity: effect of low-level HOH^3 exposure on developing female germ cells in the mouse. Radiat. Res. 58: 91-100 (1974).

D9 Dobson, P.L., C.G. Koehler, J.S. Felton et al. Vulnerability of female germ cells in developing mice and monkeys to tritium, gamma-rays and polycyclic aromatic hydrocarbons. p. 1-14 in: Developmental Toxicology of Energy-Related Pollutants (D.D. Mahlum et al., eds.). DOE Symposium Series No. 47, CONF-771017 (1978).

D10 Domon, M. Cell cycle dependent radiosensitivity in two-cell mouse embryos in culture. Radiat. Res. 81: 236-245 (1980).

D11 Domon, M. Radiosensitivity variation during the cell cycle in pronuclear mouse embryos in vitro. Cell Tissue Kinet. 15: 89-98 (1982).

D12 Dobbing, J. and J. Sands. Quantitative growth and development of human brain. Arch. Dis. Child. 48: 757-767 (1973).

D13 Dobbing, J. The later development of the brain and its vulnerability. p. 565-577 in: Scientific Foundations of Pediatrics (J.A. Davis and J. Dobbing, eds.). William Heinemann Medical Books, London, 1974.

D14 Diamond, E.L. and A.M. Lilienfeld. A prospective study of the relationship of fetal irradiation to leukemia. Acta Unio Internationalis Contra Cancrum 20: 1169-1171 (1964).

D15 Diamond, E.L., H. Schmerler and A.M. Lilienfeld. The relationship of intra-uterine radiation to subsequent mortality and development of leukemia in children. Am. J. Epidemiol. 97: 283-313 (1973).

D16 Drumm, J.E. and R. O'Rahilly. The assessment of prenatal age from the crown-rump length determined ultrasonically. Am. J. Anat. 148: 555-560 (1977).

D17 Dobbing, J. and J. Sands. Head circumference, biparietal diameter and brain growth in fetal and postnatal life. Early Human Development 2: 81-87 (1978).

D18 Dobbing, J. and J. Sands. Vulnerability of developing brain. IX. The effect of nutritional growth retardation on the timing of the brain growth-spurt. Biol. Neonate 19: 363-378 (1971).

D19 Dev, P.K., B.P. Pareek, S.M. Gupta et al. 2-Mercaptopropionylglycine protection against growth-inhibiting effects in in-utero irradiated mice. Acta Anat. 112: 249-253 (1982).

D20 Dedov, V.I. and T.A. Noretz. State of the endocrine system and offspring of rats administered ^{75}Se-selenomethionine. Radiobiologiya 22: 409-412 (1982).

D21 Dobbing, J. The pathogenesis of microcephaly with mental retardation. p. 199-212 in: Effects of prenatal irradiation with special emphasis on late effects. EUR-8067 (1984).

D22 Danielsson, B.R.G., L. Dencker and A. Lindgren. Transplacental movement of inorganic lead in early and late gestation in the mouse. Arch. Toxicol. 54: 97-107 (1983).

D23 Doll, R. Radiation hazards: 25 years of collaborative research. Brit. J. Radiol. 54: 179-186 (1981).

D24 De Swiet, M. Prenatal x-ray exposure and childhood cancer in twins. New Engl. J. Med. 312: 1574 only (1985).

D25 Dobson, R.L., T.C. Kwan and T. Straume. Tritium effects on the mouse ovary: oocyte killing, fertility loss, and genetic implications. p.231-232 in: Tritium Radiobiology and Health Physics (M. Matsudaira et al., eds.). NIRS-M-52 (1985).

D26 Daburon, F. Quelques aspects du métabolisme de l'iode chez les ruminants. Revue des Magasins Vétérinaire 119: 323-356 (1968).

E1 Easterly, C.E. An examination of birth anomalies in the counties surrounding the Oak Ridge nuclear facilities. Health Phys. 37: 817 only (1979).

E2 Erickson, B.H. Interspecific comparison of the effects of continuous ionizing radiation on the primitive mammalian stem germ cells. p. 57-67 in: Developmental Toxicology of Energy-Related Pollutants (D.D. Mahlum et al., eds.). DOE Symposium Series No. 47, CONF-771017 (1978).

E3 Erickson, B.H. and R.A. Reynolds. Oogenesis, follicular development and reproductive performance in the prenatally irradiated bovine. p. 199-205 Vol. II. in: Late Biological Effects of Ionizing Radiation. IAEA, Vienna, 1978.

E5 Erzurumlu, R.S. and H.P. Killackey. Critical and sensitive periods in neurobiology. Curr. Topics Developm. Biol. 17: 207-237 (1982).

E6 Einhorn, L. Are there factors preventing cancer development during embryonic life? Oncodev. Biol. Med. 43: 219-229 (1983).

E7 Edwards, M.J. Unclassified mental retardation. Lancet 8129: 928 only (1979).

E8 Ennis, J. and C.R. Muirhead. X-rays in pregnancy and risk of childhood cancer. Lancet II: 1185 only (1985).

F2   Fischer, D.L. and M. Smithberg. In vitro and in vivo x-irradiation of pre-implantation mouse embryos. Teratology 7: 57-64 (1972).

F4   Friedberg, W., G.D. Hanneman, D.N. Faulkner et al. Fast neutron irradiation of mouse embryos in the pronuclear-zygote stage: mortality curves and neoplastic diseases in 30-day postnatal survivors. Proc. Soc. Exptl. Biol. Med. 151: 808-810 (1976).

F6   Ford, D., J.C.S. Paterson and W.L. Treuting. Fetal exposure to diagnostic x-rays, and leukemia and other malignant diseases in childhood. J. Natl. Cancer Inst. 22: 1093-1104 (1959).

F8   Friede, R.L. Dating the development of human cerebellum. Acta Neuropath. 23: 48-58 (1973).

F9   Fohmann, A. and F.E. Stieve. Diaplazentarer Transfer von Radioeisen bei Tier und Mensch. ISH-15 (1982).

G2   Gibson, R.W., I.D.J. Bross, S. Graham et al. Leukemia in children exposed to multiple risk factors. New Engl. J. Med. 279: 906-909 (1968).

G3   Gerber, G.B. and J. Maes. Incorporation and turnover of tritium in neonatal mice and their mothers after feeding tritiated thymidine during pregnancy. Health Phys. 40: 755-759 (1981).

G4   Gerber, G.B. and J. Maes. Radiosensitivity of hemopoietic stem cells during fetal and early postnatal development. p. 175-180 in: Developmental Effects of Prenatal Irradiation. Gustav Fischer, Stuttgart, 1982.

G7   Goyal, P.K., S. Kumar and P.K. Dev. Modification of postnatal leucocyte count in Swiss albino mice after gamma irradiation in utero by MPG (2-Mercaptopropionylglycine). Radiobiol. Radiother. 22: 304-308 (1981).

G8   Granroth, G. Defects of the central nervous system in Finland. IV. Associations with diagnostic x-ray examinations. Am. J. Obst. Gynecol. 133: 191-194 (1979).

G9   Gupta, S.M., P.K. Goyal and P.K. Dev. Weight changes in mice after intrauterine treatment with MPG (2-Mercaptopropionylglycine) against ^{131}I-irradiation. Experientia 37: 898-899 (1981).

G10   Gehan, E.A. Relationship of prenatal irradiation to death from a malignant disease. Biometrics, March: 239-244 (1972).

G11   Graham, S., M.L. Levin, A.M. Lilienfeld et al. Preconception, intra-uterine and postnatal irradiation as related to leukemia. Natl. Cancer Inst. Mono. 19: 347-371 (1966).

G12   Gunz, F.W. and H.R. Aktinson. Medical radiations and leukemia: a retrospective survey. Brit. Med. J. 1: 389-393 (1964).

G13   Goyal, P.K. and P.K. Dev. Radioresponse of fetal testes of mice and its modification by MPG (2-Mercaptopropionylglycine). Strahlentherapie 159: 239-241 (1983).

G14   Glazunov, I.S. and N.Ya. Tereshcenko. The functional state of the children's nervous system in remote periods after radiation impact. The S.S. Korsakov Journal of Neuropathology and Psychiatry 68: 1438-1445 (1968).

G16   Gilmore, D.H. and M.B. McNay. Spontaneous fetal loss rate in early pregnancy. Lancet 1: 107 (1985).

H2   Hayashi, Y., K. Hoshino and Y. Kameyama. Effect of low dose x-ray irradiation on genesis and differentiation of the cerebral cortex. 10. Early changes of undifferentiated nerve system cells of the mouse exposed in utero on the 13th day. Kankyo Igaku Kenkyusho Nenpo 29: 172-174 (1978) (in Japanese).

H3   Heinzmann, U. Radiation-induced dysplasia of the third cerebral ventricle in the mouse. p. 71-78 in: Developmental Effects of Prenatal Irradiation. Gustav Fischer, Stuttgart 1982.

H4   Hoshino, K., Y. Hayashi, Y. Ito et al. Effect of low dose x-ray irradiation on genesis and differentiation of the cerebral cortex. 9. Observation of the cerebral cortex construction in the mouse exposed in utero on the 13th day. Kankyo Igaku Kenkyusho Nenpo 29: 169-171 (1978) (in Japanese).

H5   Hudson, D.B., T. Valcana and P.S. Timiras. Monoamine metabolism in the developing rat brain and effects of ionizing radiation. Brain Res. 114: 471-479 (1976).

H9   Hayashi, Y. and Y. Kameyama. Early pathological changes of mantle cells of the telencephalon by lowdose x-irradiation in mouse embryos and fetuses. Cong. Anom. 19: 37-46 (1979).

H10   Hayashi, Y., K. Hoshino and Y. Kameyama. Effects of low-dose x-irradiation on the developing brain in mice. J. Radiat. Res. 20: 16 only (1979).

H11   Hayashi, Y., K. Hoshino and Y. Kameyama. Effects of low-dose x-irradiation on the developing brain in mice. J. Radiat. Res. 22: 48-49 (1981).

H12   Hoshino, K., Y. Hayashi and Y. Kameyama. Effect of low-dose x-irradiation on the developing brain in mice. J. Radiat. Res. 21: 30 only (1980).

H13   Hoshino, K., Y. Hayashi and Y. Kameyama. Effects of low-dose x-irradiation on the developing brain in mice. J. Radiat. Res. 22: 48 only (1981).

H14   Howard, E., D.M. Granoff and P. Bujnovszky. DNA, RNA and cholesterol increases in cerebrum and cerebellum during development of human fetus. Brain Res. 14: 697-706 (1969).

H15   Hicks, S.P. and C.J. D'Amato. Effects of radiation on development, especially of the nervous system. Am. J. Forensic Med. Path. 1: 309-317 (1980).

H16   Holford, R.M. The relation between juvenile cancer and obstetric radiography. Health Phys. 28: 153-156 (1975).

H17   Holmberg, E.A.D., C.D. Pasqualini, E. Arini et al. Leukemogenic effect of radioactive phosphorus in adult and fetally-exposed BALB mice. Cancer Res. 24: 1745-1748 (1964).

H18   Hoshino, K. and Y. Kameyama. Effects of low-dose x-irradiation in utero on the development of cortical architecture of the brain in mice. Environ. Med. 27: 29-34 (1983).

H19   Heinzmann, U. X-ray induced dysplasia in the developing telencephalic choroid plexus of mice exposed in utero. Teratology 26: 39-52 (1982).

H20   Harlap, S., P.H. Shiono and S. Ramcharon. A life table of spontaneous abortions and the effects of age, parity and other variables. p. 145-158 in: Human Embryonic and Foetal Death (I.H. Porter and E.G. Hook, eds.). Academic Press, N.Y., 1980.

H21   Hook, E.B. Prevalence of chromosomal abnormalities during human gestation and implications for studies of environmental mutagens. Lancet II: 169-172 (1982).

H22   Hook, E.B. Human teratogenic and mutagenic markers in monitoring about point sources of pollution. Environ. Res. 25: 178-203 (1981).

H23   Harvey, E.B., J.D. Boice, M. Honeyman et al. Prenatal x-ray exposure and childhood cancer in twins. New Engl. J. Med. 312: 541-545 (1985).

H25 Heinzmann, U., W. Abmayr and H. Kriegel. Energy metabolism and functional activity in the developing x-ray induced hydro-microcephalus. p. 155-166 in: Radiation Risks to the Developing Nervous System. Gustav Fischer, Stuttgart, 1986.

H26 Harvey, E.B. and J.D. Boice. Prenatal x-ray exposure and childhood cancer in twins. New Engl. J. Med. 312: 1575 only (1985).

H27 Hamilton, W.J., J.D. Boyd and H.W. Mossman. Human embryology. Fourth edition. The Williams and Wilkins Company, 1978.

H28 Hoshino K. and Y. Kameyama. Cell cycle and radiosensitivity of matrix cells in the telencephalon of 13-day mouse fetuses. J. Radiat. Res. 25: 28 only (1984) (Abstract).

H29 Hisamatsu S. and Y. Takizawa. Placental transfer and distribution of americium-241 in the rat. Radiat. Res. 94: 81-88 (1983).

H30 Hopton, P.A., P.A. McKinney, R.A. Cartwright et al. X-rays in pregnancy and the risk of childhood cancer. Lancet II: 773 only (1985).

I1 Inouye, M. Malformation of the cerebral cortex of rats caused by embryonal exposure to x rays. Kankyo Igaku Kenkyusho Nenpo 29: 175-178 (1978) (in Japanese).

I2 Ishikawa, H. Mental retardation occurring in embryos exposed in utero to the atomic bomb (Hiroshima) after 30 years follow-up study. Seishin Igaku 20: 1179-1187 (1978).

I3 Ishimaru, T., M. Ichimaru and M. Mikami. Leukemia incidence among individuals exposed in utero, children of atomic bomb survivors and their controls; Hiroshima and Nagasaki, 1945-79. RERF TR-11-81 (1981).

I4 International Commission on Radiological Protection. Problems involved in developing an index of harm. ICRP Publication 27. Pergamon Press, Oxford, 1977.

I5 International Commission on Radiological Protection. The evaluation of risks from radiation. Health Phys. 12: 239-302 (1966).

I6 Inouye, M. Cerebellar malformations in prenatally x-irradiated rats: quantitative analysis and detailed description. Teratology 20: 353-364 (1979).

I7 Inouye, M. and Y. Kameyama. Cell death in the developing rat cerebellum following x-irradiation of 3 to 100 rad: a quantitative study. J. Radiat. Res. 24: 259-269 (1983).

I8 Ilina, K.P. The question of the effect of exposure to radiation in the case of x-ray examinations of pregnant women. p. 72-73 in: Radiation Health Evaluation of Exposure to Radiation in X-ray Examination. Leningrad, 1972.

I9 International Clearinghouse for Birth Defect Monitoring System. Annual Reports 1980, 1981, 1982. Also: Flynt, J.W. and S. Hay. International Clearinghouse for Birth Defects Monitoring System. Contrib. Epidem. Biostatist. 1: 44-56 (1979).

I10 Inouye M. and Y. Kameyama. Long-term neuropathological consequences of low-dose x-irradiation on the developing cerebellum. J. Radiat. Res. 27 (in print) (1986).

I11 International Commission on Radiological Protection. Developmental effects of irradiation on the brain of the embryo and fetus. ICRP publication 50 (in preparation) (1986).

I12 Ishimaru, T., R. Nakashima and S. Kawamoto. Relationship of height, body weight, head circum-ference and chest circumference at age 18 to gamma and neutron doses among in utero exposed children, Hiroshima and Nagasaki. RERF TR-19-84 (1984).

I13 Ichimaru, T., T. Ishimaru, M. Mikami et al. Incidence of leukaemia in a fixed cohort of atomic bomb survivors and controls. Hiroshima and Nagasaki, October 1950-December 1978. RERF TR-13-81 (1981).

J1 Jacquet, P., L. de Clerq and G. Kervyn. Studies on the sensitivity of the mouse egg to low doses of x-irradiation. p. 51-57 in: Developmental Effects of Prenatal Irradiation. Gustav Fischer, Stuttgart, 1982.

J2 Jaenke, R.S., R.D. Phemister, D. Davis et al. Progressive renal glomerular injury in the perinatally-irradiated beagle. Radiat. Res. 67: 525-526 (1976).

J3 Joshima, H., P.L. Hackett and M.R. Sikov. Effects of ^{239}Pu on hematopoiesis in prenatal rats. Radiat. Res. 70: 622 only (1977).

J4 Jablon, S. and H. Kato. Childhood cancer in relation to prenatal exposure to atomic bomb radiation. Lancet II: 1000-1003 (1970).

J5 Jensen, K.F. and J. Altman. The contribution of late-generated neurons to the callosal projection in rat: a study with prenatal x-irradiation. J. Comp. Neurol. 209: 113-122 (1982).

J6 Jensh, R.P., I. Weinberg and R.L. Brent. Teratologic studies of prenatal exposure of rats to 915-MHz microwave radiation. Radiat. Res. 92: 160-171 (1982).

J7 Jordaan, H.V.F. Development of the central nervous system in prenatal life. Obstet. Gynecol. 53: 146-150 (1979).

J8 Jablon, S. Comments on "The carcinogenic effects of low level radiation. A re-appraisal of epidemiologists methods and observations". Health Phys. 24: 257-258 (1973).

J9 Jakobovits, A., L. Iffy, M.B. Wingate et al. The rate of early fetal growth in the human subject. Acta Anat. 83: 50-59 (1972).

J10 Jacquet, P., G. Kervyn and D. de Clercq. In vitro studies on the radiosensitivity of the mouse zygote. p. 19-29 in: Effects of prenatal irradiation with special emphasis on late effects. EUR-8067 (1984).

J11 Johnson, J.R. Fetal thyroid dose from intakes of radioiodine by the mother. Health Phys. 43: 573-582 (1982).

J12 Johnson, J.R. and D.K. Myers. Is ^{131}I less efficient than external irradiation at producing thyroid cancers? A review. p. 289-301 in: Biological Effects of Low-level Radiation. IAEA, Vienna, 1983.

J13 Jensen, K.F. and H.P. Killackey. Subcortical projections from ectopic neocortical neurons. Proc. Natl. Acad. Sci. (U.S.A.) 81: 964-968 (1984).

J14 Jirásek, J.E. Development of the genital system and male pseudohermaphroditism. John Hopkins Press. Baltimore, 1971.

J15 Jacquet P. and S. Grinfeld. Données récentes sur la sensibilité de l'embryon aux rayonnements ionisants au cours des premiers stades de son développement. Rev. Quest. Scientif. 156: 343-369 (1985).

K1 Kalter, H., I. Ormsby and J. Warkany. X-ray dose-related reduction of ENU-induced transplacental tumor frequency in rats. Teratology 21: 48A only (1980).

K2 Kalter, H., T.I. Mandybur, I. Ormsby et al. Dose-related reduction by prenatal x-irradiation of the transplacental neurocarcinogenicity of ethylintrosourea in rats. Cancer Res. 40: 3973-3976 (1980).

K3 Kameyama, Y., K. Hoshino and Y. Hayashi. Effects of low dose x-radiation on the matrix cells in the telencephalon of mouse embryos. p. 228-236 in: Developmental Toxicology of Energy-Related Pollutants (D.D. Mahlum et al., eds.). DOE Symposium Series No. 47, CONF-771017 (1978).

K4 Kato, H. Mortality of in-utero children exposed to the A-bomb and of offspring of A-bomb survivors. p. 49-60 Vol. I, in: Late Biological Effects of Ionizing Radiation. IAEA, Vienna, 1978.

K5 Kelman, B.J. and M.R. Sikov. Plutonium movement across the hemochorial placenta of the guinea pig. Placenta, Suppl. 3: 319-326 (1981).

K6 Kelman, B.J., M.R. Sikov and P.L. Hackett. Effect of monomeric ^{239}Pu on the pregnant and fetal rabbit. Teratology 21: 48A only (1980).

K7 Klinkmüller, K.D. and H. Nau. Drug transfer to the embryo, fetus and neonate. p. 253-265 in: Developmental Effects of Prenatal Irradiation. Gustav Fischer, Stuttgart, 1982.

K8 Knauss, G. Dose-response relationships of embryonary radiation damage for example in the mouse skeleton after antenatal exposure to x-radiation. Thesis, University of Freiburg Medical Faculty, 1980.

K9 Kneale, G.W. and A.M. Stewart. Mantel-Haenszel analysis of Oxford data. I. Independent effects of several birth factors including fetal irradiation. J. Natl. Cancer Inst. 56: 879-883 (1976).

K10 Kneale, G.W. and A.M. Stewart. Interaction of prenatal irradiation and postnatal disease in the aetiology of childhood cancers. p. 337-344 in: Developmental Effects of Prenatal Irradiation. Gustav Fischer, Stuttgart, 1982.

K11 Konermann, G. Periodical compensation responses of the mouse brain in the course of postnatal growth following fractionated irradiation during embryogenesis. Strahlentherapie 153: 399-414 (1977).

K12 Konermann, G. Consequences of prenatal radiation exposure on perinatal and postnatal development: morphological, biochemical and histochemical aspects. p. 237-250 in: Developmental Effects of Prenatal Irradiation. Gustav Fischer, Stuttgart, 1982.

K13 Konermann, G. and I. Schwald. The formation of tigroid substance during post-natal maturation of the brain of mice after pre- and peri-natal x-irradiation. Radiat. Environ. Biophys. 18: 197-220 (1980).

K14 Korogodin, V.I. and Yu. V. Korogodina. Disorganization of the cerebellar cortex structure of rats caused by gamma-irradiation during differentiation. Radiobiologyia 18: 59-69 (1978).

K17 Krishna, M., D.N. Ebenezer, P. Ramchander et al. Effect of maternally administered phosphorus-32 on pre- and post-natal mortality and development in mice. Indian Soc. Nucl. Techn. Agric. Biol. Newsl. 2: 27-29 (1973).

K18 Ku, K.Y. and P. Voytek. The effects of U.V. light, ionizing radiation and the carcinogen N-acetoxy-2-fluorenylacetamide on the development in vitro of one- and two-cell mouse embryos. Int. J. Radiat. Biol. 30: 401-408 (1976).

K19 Kneale, G.W. and A.M. Stewart. Mantel-Haenszel analysis of Oxford data. II. Independent effects of fetal irradiation. J. Natl. Cancer Inst. 57: 1009-1014 (1976).

K20 Kato, H. Mortality in children exposed to the A-bombs while in utero, 1945-1969. Am. J. Epidemiol. 93: 435-442 (1971).

K21 Kaplan, H.S. An evaluation of the somatic and genetic hazards of the medical uses of radiation. Am. J. Roentgenol. 80: 696-708 (1958).

K22 Kameyama, Y. Low-dose radiation as an environmental agent affecting intrauterine development. Environmental Medicine 26: 1-15 (1982).

K23 Kelman, B.J., M.R. Sikov and P.L. Hackett. Effects of monomeric ^{239}Pu on the fetal rabbit. Health Phys. 43: 80-83 (1982).

K24 Kusama, T. and Y. Yoshizawa. The carcinogenic effects of fetal and postnatal radiation in female mice. J. Radiat. Res. 23: 290-297 (1982).

K25 Kuzin, A.M., L.V. Slozhenikina, L.A. Fialkovskaya et al. On the mechanism of a radiation-induced change in enzymic differentiation during development. Radiat. Environm. Biophys. 21: 206-216 (1983).

K26 Knudson, A.G. Germinal and somatic mutations in cancer. p. 287-303 in: Genetic epidemiology (N.E. Morton and C.S. Chung, eds.) Academic Press, New York, 1978.

K27 Kobyletzki, D. and J. Gellen. Zur Vorhersage des embryonalen Entwicklungszustandes beim Menschen. Arch. Gynak. 209: 293-304 (1970).

K28 Kjeldsberg, H. Relationships between leukemia and x-rays. T. Norske Laegerforen. 77: 1052-1053 (1957).

K29 Kakushina, E.A. and L.A. Plodovskaya. The effects of x rays on the fertility of irradiated animals. p. 111-119 in: Influence of ionizing radiation during pregnancy on the condition of the fetus and newborn offspring. Moscow, 1960 (in Russian).

K30 Kameyama, Y. Factors in manifestation of developmental abnormalities of the central nervous system by environmental agents. J. Toxicol. Sci. 8: 91-103 (1983).

K32 Kalter, H. and J. Warkany. Congenital malformations. Etiologic factors and their role in prevention. New Engl. J. Med. 308: 424-431 and 491-497 (1983).

K33 Konermann, G. Periodische Kompensationsreaktionen im Verlaufe des postnatalen Wachstums von der Leber der Maus nach fraktionierter Röntgenbestrahlung während der Embryogenese. Strahlentherapie 152: 550-576 (1976).

K34 Konermann, G. Die Prämyelinsynthese und Hirnmyelinisierung bei der Maus nach fraktionierter Röntgenbestrahlung im pränatalen Alter. Strahlentherapie 156: 51-64 (1980).

K35 Kiyono, S., M. Seo and M. Shibagaki. Effects of environmental enrichment upon maze performance in rats with microcephaly induced by prenatal x-irradiation. Jap. J. Physiol. 31: 769-773 (1981).

K36 Konermann, G., B. Metzger and E. Roser. Postnatal development of the CNS after prenatal irradiation. p. 61-76 in: Effects of prenatal irradiation with special emphasis on late effects. EUR-8067 (1984).

K37 Kusama, T. and Y. Yoshizawa. Embryonic effects on mice of radiation in combination with adrenocortical hormone. J. Radiat. Res. 24: 17 only (1983).

K38 Kusama, T. and Y. Yoshizawa. The synergistic effects of radiation and caffeine on embryonic development in mice. J. Radiat. Res. 25: 225-233 (1984).

K39 Kline, J., Z. Stein, M. Susser et al. Environmental influences on early reproductive loss in a current New York City study. p. 225-240 in: Human Embryonic and Foetal Death (I.H. Porter and E.G. Hook, eds.) Academic Press, N.Y., 1980.

357

K40 Kerr, G.D. Organ dose estimates for the Japanese atomic bomb survivors. Health Phys. 37: 487-508 (1979).

K41 Konermann, G. Brain development in mice after pre-natal irradiation: modes of effect manifestation; dose-response relationships and the RBE of neutrons. p. 93-116 in: Radiation Risks to the Developing Nervous System. Gustav Fischer, Stuttgart, 1986.

K42 Kinnier-Wilson, L.M., G.W. Kneale and A.M. Stewart. Childhood cancer and pregnancy drugs. Lancet II: 314-315 (1981).

L1 Lu, B. Survey of hereditary ophthalmopathies and congenital ophthalmic malformations in high-background areas. Chin. J. Radiol. Med. Prot. 2: 58-59 (1983) (in Chinese).

L2 Lee, A.C., G.M. Angleton and J.C. Simpson. Relative frequency of missing teeth in beagles exposed to cobalt-60 gamma rays during periods of growth and development. Radiat. Res. 67: 525 only (1976).

L3 Li, R., W. Xiao, S. Dou et al. A follow-up study of 498 children exposed to in utero diagnostic x-radiation. Chin. J. Radiol. Med. Prot. 5: 179-182 (1985) (in Chinese).

L4 Leck, I. Descriptive epidemiology of common malformations. Brit. Med. Bull. 32: 45-52 (1976).

L5 Lewis, T.L.T. Leukemia in childhood after antenatal exposure to x rays. Brit. Med. J. 5212: 1551-1552 (1960).

L6 Lilienfeld, A.M. Epidemiological studies of the leukemogenic effects of radiation. Yale J. Biol. and Med. 39: 143-164 (1966).

L7 Lambert, B.E. and M.L. Phipps. The long-term effects of tritium incorporated in utero. p. 143-158 in: Effects of prenatal irradiation with special emphasis on late effects. Report EUR-8067 (1984).

L8 Liberman, A.N., I.E. Bronshtein, M.S. Sakovskaya et al. p. 10-11 in: Proceedings of the 4th All-Union Symposium "Industrial Hygiene and the Biological Effect of Electromagnetic Waves of Radio Frequency". USSR Academy of Medical Sciences, Moscow, 1972.

L9 Lyaginskaya, A.M. Current problems of the action of ionizing radiation on the foetus. p. 122-131 in: Biological Effects of Small Doses of Radiation. (Y.I. Moskalev, ed.) Moscow, 1983.

L10 Larsell, O. The morphogenesis and adult pattern of the lobules and fissures of the cerebellum of the white rat. J. Comp. Neurol. 97: 281-356 (1952).

L11 Liu, P.T., R.H. Stevens, D.A. Cole et al. Late effects of iodine-131 in utero exposure: toxicological effects in first generation of rats. p. 101 in: Abstracts of Papers for the 32nd Annual Meeting of the Radiation Research Society. Florida, 1984.

M1 MacQueen, H.A. Lethality of radioisotopes in early mouse embryos. J. Embryol. Exptl. Morphol. 52: 203-208 (1979).

M2 McFee, A.F., F.H. Cross and M.N. Sherrill. Hematopoietic recovery of pigs after chronic prenatal irradiation. p. 244-253 in: Developmental Toxicology of Energy-Related Pollutants (D.D. Mahlum et al., eds.). DOE Symposium Series No. 47, CONF-771017 (1978).

M3 Meadows, A.T., J. Gordon, D.J. Massari et al. Declines in IQ scores and cognitive dysfunctions in children with acute lymphocytic leukaemia treated with cranial irradiation. Lancet 8254: 1015-1018 (1981).

M4 Michel, C., H. Blattmann, I. Cordt-Riehle et al. Low dose effects of x-rays and negative pions on the pronuclear zygote stage of mouse embryos. Radiat. Environm. Biophys. 16: 299-302 (1979).

M5 Michel, C. and H. Fritz-Niggli. Teratogenic and radiosensitizing effects of misonidazole on mouse embryos. Brit. J. Radiol. 54: 154-155 (1981).

M6 Michel, C., H. Fritz-Niggli, I. Cordt-Riehle et al. Radiosensitization in embryonic development: the interaction of misonidazole and low radiation doses. p. 287-292 in: Developmental Effects of Prenatal Irradiation. Gustav Fischer, Stuttgart, 1982.

M7 Miller, J.F., E. Williamson, J. Glue et al. Fetal loss after implantation. A prospective study. Lancet: 554-556 (1980).

M8 Michel, C. and H. Fritz-Niggli. Induction of developmental anomalies in mice by maternal stress. Experientia 34: 105-106 (1978).

M9 Mole, R.H. Consequences of pre-natal radiation exposure for post-natal development. p. 127-144 in: Developmental Effects of Prenatal Irradiation. Gustav Fischer, Stuttgart, 1982.

M10 Mole, R.H. Consequences of pre-natal radiation exposure for post-natal development. A review. Int. J. Radiat. Biol. 42: 1-12 (1982).

M11 Molls, M. and C. Streffer. Micronucleus formation and chromosomal aberrations after irradiation of 2-cell mouse embryos in G_2-phase. Radiat. Res. 87: 493 only (1981).

M12 Molls, M., C. Streffer and N. Zamboglou. Development of x-irradiated 2-cell mouse embryos in relation to micronucleus formation and G_2-delay. p. 65-70 in: Developmental Effects of Prenatal Irradiation. Gustav Fischer, Stuttgart 1982.

M13 Molls, M., U. Weissenborn and C. Streffer. Irradiation of mouse embryos in pronucleus and 2-cell stage: dependence of micronuclei formation and cell proliferation upon DNA amount and cell cycle phase. Strahlentherapie 158: 504-512 (1982).

M14 Michel, C. and H. Fritz-Niggli. Radiation damage in mouse embryos exposed to 1 rad X-rays or negative pions. Fortschr. Röntgenstr. 127: 276-280 (1977).

M15 Moskalev, Yu. I., A.M. Lyaginskaya and A.G. Istomina. Tritium oxide transfer through placenta, its intake with milk and biological action of tritiated water on the fetus. p. 245-251 in: Tritium (A.A. Moghissi and M.W. Carter, eds.). Messenger Graphics, Las Vegas, 1973.

M16 Müller, W.U., C. Streffer and C. Fischer. Combined treatment of pre-implantation mouse embryos in vitro with sodium nitrite and x rays. Radiat. Environ. Biophys. 20: 187-194 (1982).

M17 Mullenix, P., S. Norton and B. Culver. Locomotor damage in rats after x-irradiation in utero. Exp. Neurol. 48: 310-324 (1975).

M19 Müller, W.U., C. Streffer and N. Zamboglou. The combined treatment of preimplantation mouse embryos cultured in vitro with x-rays and 2,4-Dinitrophenol. p. 203-298 in: Developmental Effects of Prenatal Irradiation. Gustav Fischer, Stuttgart, 1982.

M20 Miller, R.W. and W.J. Blot. Small head size following in utero exposure to atomic radiation, Hiroshima and Nagasaki. ABCC-TR-35-72.

M21 Mole, R.H. Human experience of radiation damage following pre-natal exposure: its interpretation and implications. p. 213-227 in: Effects of Prenatal Irradiation with Special Emphasis on Late Effects. EUR-8067 (1984).

M22 MacMahon, B. and G.B. Hutchison. Prenatal x ray and childhood cancer: A review. Acta Unio Internationalis Contra Cancrum 20: 1172-1174 (1964).

M23 Mole, R.H. Antenatal irradiation and childhood cancer: causation or coincidence? Br., J. Cancer 30: 199-208 (1974).

M25 MacMahon, B. Prenatal x-ray exposure and childhood cancer. J. Natl. Cancer Inst. 28: 1173-1191 (1962).

M26 Miller, R.W. Relation between cancer and congenital defects: an epidemiologic evaluation. J. Natl. Cancer Inst. 40: 1079-1084 (1968).

M27 Müller, W.U., C. Streffer and N. Zamboglou. Effects of a combined treatment with x-rays and phenols on pre-implantation mouse embryos in vitro. Radiat. Environm. Biophys. 19: 247-258 (1981).

M28 Müller, W.U., C. Streffer and U. Kaiser. The combined treatment of pre-implantation mouse embryos in vitro with cadmium ($CdSO_4$, CdF_2) and x rays. Arch. Toxicol. 51: 303-312 (1982).

M29 Müller, W.U. and C. Streffer. Influence of actinomycin-D or ethidium bromide on the radiation risk in mouse embryos at the pre-implantation stage in vitro. Strahlentherapie 158: 630-636 (1982) (in German).

M30 Moore, G.W., G.H. Hutchins and R. O'Rahilly. The estimated age of staged human embryos and early foetuses. Am. J. Obstet. Gynecol. 139: 500-506 (1981).

M31 Molls, M., A. Pon, C. Streffer et al. The effects of lead and x-rays, alone or in combination, on blastocyst formation and cell kinetics of pre-implantation mouse embryos in vitro. Int. J. Radiat. Biol. 43: 57-69 (1983).

M32 Molls, M., C. Streffer, B. Fellner et al. Development of cytogenetic effects and recovery after irradiation of preimplantation mouse embryos. p. 31-48 in: Effects of Prenatal Irradiation with Special Emphasis on Late Effects. EUR-8067 (1984).

M33 Molls, M., C. Streffer and N. Zamboglou. Micronucleus formation in pre-implanted mouse embryos cultured in vitro after irradiation with x-rays and neutrons. Int. J. Radiat. Biol. 39: 307-314 (1981).

M34 Molls, M., C. Streffer, D. van Beuningen et al. X-irradiation in G_2 phase of two-cell mouse embryos in vitro: cleavage, blastulation, cell kinetics and fetal development. Radiat. Res. 91: 219-234 (1982).

M35 Michel, C., I. Cordt-Riehle, H. Fritz-Niggli et al. Combined application of misonidazol and piotron pions on mouse embryos. Radiat. Environ. Biophys. 21: 155-162 (1983).

M36 Mole, R.H. Radiation effects on pre-natal development and their radiological significance. Brit. J. Radiol. 52: 89-101 (1979).

M39 Murray, R., P. Heckel and L.H. Hempelman. Leukemia in children exposed to ionizing radiation. New Engl. J. Med. 261: 585-589 (1959).

M40 Mahlum, D.D., M.R. Sikov, J.O. Hess et al. Age and carcinogenesis of ^{239}Pu. p. 43-60 in: Biological Implications of Radionuclides Released from Nuclear Industries, Vol. I. IAEA, Vienna, 1979.

M41 Momeni, M.H. Competitive radiation-induced carcinogenesis: an analysis of data from beagle dogs exposed to ^{226}Ra and ^{90}Sr. Health Phys. 36: 295-310 (1979).

M42 Minamisawa, T. and S. Sasaki. The electrocorticograms of the adult and aged mouse x-irradiated during the perinatal period. Electroencephalography and Clin. Neurophysiology 55: 73-81 (1983).

M43 Müller, W.U. and C. Streffer. Combined effects after exposure during the pre-implantation period. p. 49-60 in: Effects of Prenatal Irradiation with Special Emphasis on Late Effects. EUR-8067 (1984).

M44 Meyer, I. Skelettmißbildungen der neugeborenen Maus nach Röntgenbestrahlung in utero, unter besonderer Berücksichtigung der hyperplastischen Wachstumsphänomene am Neurokranium. GSF-1130 (1980).

M45 Myrianthopoulos, N.C. and C.S. Chung. Congenital malformations in singletons: epidemiologic survey. Birth Defect Original Article Series 10 No. 11: 1-58 (1974).

M46 Mehta, G. and P.K. Dev. Quantitative estimation of goblet cells in postnatally developing jejunum of Swiss albino mice after pre-natal irradiation. Natl. Acad. Sci. Lett. 4: 257-259 (1981).

M47 Molls, M., N. Zamboglou and C. Streffer. A comparison of the cell kinetics of pre-implantation mouse embryos from two different mouse strains. Cell Tissue Kinet. 16: 277-283 (1983).

M48 Matsuda, Y., T. Yamada, I. Tobari et al. Preliminary study on chromosomal aberrations in eggs of mice fertilized in vitro after x-irradiation. Mutat. Res. 125-130 (1983).

M49 Müller, F. and R. O'Rahilly. The first appearance of the major divisions of the human brain at stage 9. Anat. Embryol. 168: 419-432 (1983).

M50 Michel, C., M. Fritz-Niggli, H. Blattmann et al. Effects of low-dose irradiation with x rays and pimesons on embryos of two different mouse strains. Strahlentherapie 153: 674-681 (1977).

M51 Miller, R.W. Delayed effects occurring within the first decade after exposure of young individuals to the Hiroshima atomic bomb. Pediatrics 18: 1-18 (1956).

M52 MacMahon, B. Childhood cancer and prenatal irradiation. p. 223-228 in: Cancer: Achievements, Challenges and Prospects for the 1980s (J.H. Burchenal and H.F. Oettgen, eds.). Grune and Stratton, New York, 1981.

M53 Monson, R.R. and B. MacMahon. Prenatal x-ray exposure and cancer in children. p. 97-105 in: Radiation Carcinogenesis: Epidemiology and Biological Significance (J.D. Boice and J.F. Fraumeni, eds.). Raven Press, New York, 1984.

M54 McKusick, V.A. Mendelian Inheritance in Man. 6th edition. Johns Hopkins University Press, Baltimore, 1983.

M55 MacMahon, B. Prenatal x-ray exposure and twins. New Engl. J. Med. 312: 576-577 (1985).

M56 Matsuda, Y., T. Yamada and I. Tobari. Chromosomal effects of tritium in mouse zygotes fertilized in vitro. p. 193-206 in: Tritium Radiobiology and Health Physics (H. Matsudaira et al., eds.). NIRS-M-52 (1985).

M57 Müller, F. and R. O'Rahilly. Cerebral dysraphia (future anencephaly) in a human twin embryo at stage 13. Teratology 30: 167-177 (1984).

N1 Nash, D.J. and L.S. Sprackling. Reproductive function in mice exposed to ancestral and direct irradiation. p. 254-266 in: Developmental Toxicology of Energy-Related Pollutants (D.D. Mahlum et al., eds.). DOE Symposium Series No. 47, CONF-771017 (1978).

N2 Neumeister, K. Findings in children after radiation exposure in utero from x-ray examination of mothers: results from children studied after one to seven years. p. 119-134 in: Late Biological Effects of Ionizing Radiation, Vol. I. IAEA, Vienna, 1978.

N3   Newcombe, H.B. and J.F. McGregor. Childhood cancer following obstetric radiography. Lancet 2: 1151-1152 (1971).

N4   Nomura, T. Parental exposure to x rays and chemicals induces heritable tumours and anomalies in mice. Nature 296: 575-577 (1982).

N5   Nishimura, H., K. Takano, T. Tanimura et al. Normal and abnormal development of human embryos: first report of the analysis of 1213 intact embryos. Teratology 1: 281-290 (1968).

N6   Nishimura, H., T. Tanimura, R. Semba et al. Normal development of early human embryos: observation of 90 specimens at Carnegie stages 7 to 13. Teratology 10: 1-18 (1974).

N7   Neumeister, K. and S. Wässer. Langzeit-Untersuchungen an Kindern nach Strahlenbelastung in utero mit kleinen Dosen. Radiol. Diagn. 24: 379-387 (1983).

N8   Neumeister, K. and S. Wasser. Zur Problematik von Röntgenuntersuchungen in der Frühschwangerschaft. Radiol. Diagn. 24: 539-547 (1983).

N9   Neel, J.V. and W.J. Schull. The effect of exposure to the atomic bombs on pregnancy termination in Hiroshima and Nagasaki. National Academy of Sciences—National Research Council Publication No. 461. Washington, D.C., 1956.

N10   Neel, J.V. A study of major congenital defects in Japanese infants. Am. J. Hum. Gen. 10: 398-445 (1958).

N11   Neumeister, K. and S. Wässer. Findings in children after radiation exposure in utero from x-ray examination of mothers: results from children studied after one to ten years. p. 229-242 in: Effects of Prenatal Irradiation with Special Emphasis on Late Effects. EUR-8067 (1984).

N12   Neriishi, S. and H. Matsumura. Morphological observations of the central nervous system in an in-utero exposed autopsied case. J. Radiat. Res. 24: 18 only (1983).

N13   Nomura, T. Induction of persistent hypersensitivity to lung tumorigenesis by in utero x-radiation in mice. Environ. Mutagen. 6: 33-40 (1984).

N14   Nishimura, H. Prenatal versus postnatal malformations based on the Japanese experience on induced abortions in the human being. p. 350-368 in: Aging Gametes (R.J. Blandan, ed.). Karger, Basel, 1975.

O1   Ordy, J.M., K.R. Brizzee, W.P. Dunlap et al. Effects of prenatal ^{60}Co irradiation on the post-natal neural, learning and hormonal development of the squirrel monkey. Radiat. Res. 89: 309-324 (1982).

O2   Ordy, J.M., K.R. Brizzee and R. Young. Prenatal cobalt-60 irradiation effects on visual acuity, maturation of the fovea in the retina, and the striate cortex of squirrel monkey offspring. p. 205-217 in: Developmental Effects of Prenatal Irradiation. Gustav Fischer, Stuttgart, 1982.

O3   Otake, M. and W.J. Schull. In utero exposure to A-bomb radiation and mental retardation: a reassessment. Brit. J. Radiol. 57: 409-414 (1984).

O4   Otake, M. and W.J. Schull. Mental retardation in children exposed in utero to the atomic bombs: a reassessment. RERFTR-1-83 (1983).

O5   Oppenheim, B.E., M.L. Griem and P. Meier. Effects of low-dose prenatal irradiation in humans: analysis of Chicago lying-in data and comparison with other studies. Radiat. Res. 57: 508-544 (1974).

O6   Ovcharenko, E.P. and T.R. Fomina. The effect of injected ^{237}Np-oxalate on the gonads of rats and their offspring. Radiobiologiya 22: 374-379 (1982).

O7   O'Rahilly, R. and F. Müller. The first appearance of the human nervous system at stage 8. Anat. Embryol. 163: 1-13 (1981).

O8   O'Rahilly, R. Early human development and the chief sources of information on staged human embryos. Europ. J. Obstet. Gynec. Reprod. Biol. 9: 273-280 (1979).

O9   Olsen, I. and J. Jonsen. Whole body autoradiography of ^{204}Tl in embryos, fetuses and placentas of mice. Toxicology 23: 353-358 (1982).

O10   Ovcharenko, E.P. Transfer of radionuclides to descendants with the mother's milk. Meditsinskaya Radiologiya l: 71-78 (1982).

O11   O'Rahilly, R. and F. Müller. Embryonic length and cerebral landmarks in staged human embryos. Anat. Rec. 209: 265-271 (1984).

O12   Olivier, G. and H. Pineau. Horizons de Streeter et âge embryonnaire. C.R. Ass. Anat. 47: 573-576 (1962).

O13   Ovcharenko, E.P. Characteristics of the post-natal development of the offspring of female rats treated with americium-241. p. 430-438 in: Remote Consequences of Radiation Exposure (Y.I. Moskalev, ed.). Atomizdat, Moscow, 1971.

P1   Pedersen, R.A. and B. Brandriff. Radiation- and drug-induced DNA repair in mammalian oocytes and embryos. Conference on DNA repair and mutagenesis in bacteria. CONF-790676-5 (1979).

P2   Pedersen, R.A. and J.E. Cleaver. Repair of U.V. damage to DNA of implantation stage mouse embryos in vitro. Exptl. Cell Res. 95: 247-253 (1975).

P3   Philippe, J.V. Influence of ionizing radiation on fetoplacental growth in mice. Amer. J. Obstet. Gynec. 123: 640-645 (1975).

P4   Philippe, J.V. Fertility and irradiation: a preconceptional investigation in teratology. Amer. J. Obstet. Gynecol. 123: 714-718 (1975).

P5   Pietrzak-Flis, Z. Effects of chronically ingested tritium on the oocytes of two generations of rats. p. 111-115 in: Developmental Effects of Prenatal Irradiation. Gustav Fischer, Stuttgart, 1982.

P7   Phemister, R.D., R.W. Thomassen, G.M. Angleton et al. Early malignant neoplasms in dogs irradiated during the perinatal period. Radiat. Res. 70: 669-670 (1977).

P9   Polhemus, D.W. and R. Koch. Leukemia and medical radiation. Pediatrics 23: 453-461 (1959).

P11   Poswillo, D. Mechanisms and pathogenesis of malformations. Brit. Med. Bull. 32: 59-64 (1976).

P13   Palyga, G.F., R.B. Strelkov, N.N. Partskhaladze et al. On the possibility of radiation protection of the organism during the embryonal period of development by the use of a gas hypoxic mixture. Radiobiologiya 22: 542-545 (1982).

P14   Porteous, D.D. Leukemia in the AKR mouse after x-irradiation in utero. Int. J. Radiat. Biol. 4: 601-608 (1962).

P15   Pietrzak-Flis, Z. and M. Wasiliewska-Gomulka. Effects of lifetime intake of organically bound tritium and tritiated water on the oocytes of rats. Radiat. Environm. Biophys. 23: 61-68 (1984).

P16   Plummer, G. Anomalies occurring in children in utero, Hiroshima. ABCC 29-C-59 (1952).

P17 Pochin, E.E. Personal communication (1985).

R1 Radwan, I. Behavioral effects of chronic exposure to organically bound tritium and tritiated water. p. 105-110 in: Developmental Effects of Prenatal Irradiation. Gustav Fischer, Stuttgart, 1982.

R4 Rönnbäck, C. Disturbances of fertility in female mice strontium-90-contaminated as foetuses. Acta Radiol. Oncol. 20: 337-343 (1981).

R5 Rönnbäck, C. ^{90}Sr induced effects on the foetal ovary of the CBA mouse. Experimental studies on germ cells and follicular development, fertility and tumour incidence. Thesis, University of Uppsala, 1982.

R6 Rugh, R. Are mouse fetuses which survive microwave radiation permanently affected thereby? Health Phys. 31: 33-39 (1976).

R8 Russell, L.B. Utilization of critical periods during development to study the effects of low levels of environmental agents. p. 143-162 in: Measurement of Risks. (G.G. Berg and H.D. Maillie, eds.). Plenum Publishing Corp., New York, 1981.

R9 Rakic, P. Neuronal migration and contact guidance in the primate telencephalon. Postgrad. Med. J. 54: 25-40 (1978).

R10 Rönnbäck, C., B. Henricson and A. Nilsson. Effect of different doses of strontium-90 on the ovaries of the foetal mouse. Acta Radiol. Suppl. 310: 200-209 (1971).

R11 Rönnbäck, C. Effect of ^{90}Sr on ovaries of foetal mice depending on time for administration during pregnancy. Acta Radiol. Oncol. 18: 225-234 (1979).

R12 Rönnbäck, C. Effect of different ^{90}Sr doses on the microscopic structure of foetal mouse ovaries. Acta Radiol. Oncol. 19: 145-152 (1980).

R13 Rönnbäck, C. Influence of ^{90}Sr-contaminated milk on the ovaries of foetal and young mice. Acta Radiol. Oncol. 20: 131-135 (1981).

R14 Rönnbäck, C. and A. Nilsson. Neoplasms in ovaries of CBA mice strontium-90-treated as foetuses. Acta Radiol. Oncol. 21: 121-128 (1982).

R16 Russell, L.B. Irradiation damage to the embryo, fetus and neonate. p. 33-54 in: Biological Risks of Medical Irradiations (G.D. Fullerton et al., eds.) Am. Inst. Physics, New York, 1980.

R18 Rugh, R., L. Duhamel and L. Skaredoff. Relation of embryonic and fetal x-irradiation to life time average weights and tumour incidence in mice. Proc. Soc. Exptl. Biol. Med. 121: 714-718 (1966).

R19 Russell, L.B. Sensitivity of the homeotic-shift pre-screen for environmental teratogens. Teratology 19: 45a only (1979).

R20 Russell, L.B. and C.S. Montgomery. Radiation sensitivity differences within cell-division cycles during mouse cleavage. Int. J. Radiat. Biol. 10: 151-164 (1966).

R21 Roux, C., C. Horvath, R. Dupuis. Effects of pre-implantation low-dose radiation on rat embryos. Health Phys. 45: 993-999 (1983).

R22 Rantseva, E.G. Study of the reproductive characteristics of white mice upon exposure to the combined action of ionizing SHF radiation and noise. Restorative and compensatory processes in radiation injury. p. 210-211 in: Abstracts of the 8th All-Union Scientific Conference. Leningrad, TSNIIRRI, 1982.

R23 Rakic, P. Neurons in Rhesus Monkey visual cortex: systematic relation between time of origin and eventual disposition. Science 183: 425-427 (1974).

R24 Rakic, P. Normal and abnormal neuronal migration during brain development. p. 35-44 in: Radiation Risks to the Developing Nervous System (H. Kriegel et al., eds.). Gustav Fischer, Stuttgart, 1986.

R25 Reyners, H., E. Gianfelici de Reyners and J.R. Maisin. The role of the glia in late damage after prenatal irradiation. p. 117-132 in: Radiation Risks to the Developing Nervous System. Gustav Fischer, Stuttgart, 1986.

R26 Rönnbäck, C. Effects on foetal ovaries after protracted, external gamma irradiation, as compared with those from internal depositions. Acta Radiol. Oncol. 22: 465-471 (1983).

R27 Roedler, H.D. Metabolismus radioaktiver Stoffe. Report to the Ministry of Interior of the Federal Republic of Germany. 1986.

R28 Roedler H.D., A. Herzberger and A. Kaul. Biokinetics of internal emitters and absorbed dose to the human fetus. p. 446-469 Vol. 1 in: Radiation, Risk, Protection. IRPA, Berlin (West), 1984.

R29 Reyners, H., E. Gianfelici de Reyners, R. Hooghe et al. Irradiation prénatale à trés faible dose de rayons x: lésions de la substance blanche. C.R. Soc. Biol. (in publication) (1986).

S1 Sasaki, S., T. Kasuga, F. Sato et al. Late effects of fetal mice x-irradiated at middle or late intrauterine stage. Jap. J. Cancer Res. 69: 167-177 (1978).

S2 Sasaki, S., F. Sato, T. Kasuga et al. Carcinogenic effects of ionizing radiation administered at perinatal stage of mice. NIRS-R-7.

S3 Satyanarayana, R., P.P. Reddy and O.S. Reddi. Prenatal effects of ^{35}S in mice. Indian J. Exp. Biol. 15: 310-311 (1977).

S4 Schlesinger, D.M. and R.L. Brent. Effects of x irradiation during preimplantation stages of gestation on cell viability and embryo survival in the mouse. Radiat. Res. 75: 202-216 (1978).

S5 Schmahl, W. Kinetics of telencephalic neural cell proliferation during the fetal regeneration period following a single x-irradiation at the late organo-genesis stage. I. Sequential study of cell kinetics during the phase of acute events. Radiat. Environ. Biophys. 21: 19-31 (1982).

S6 Schmahl, W. and P. Török. Strahlensensible Perioden der fetalen Retina bei kombinierter Einwirkung von Azazytiden und Röntgenstrahlen in utero. p. 299-303 in: Developmental Effects of Prenatal Irradiation. Gustav Fischer, Stuttgart, 1982.

S7 Schmahl, W., L. Weber and H. Kriegel. X-irradiation of mice in the early fetal period. I. Assessment of lasting CNS deficity developing mainly in the subsequent perinatal period. Strahlentherapie 155: 347-357 (1979).

S8 Schneider, B.F. and S. Norton. Neuronal damage in chick and rat embryos following x-irradiation. Teratology 22: 303-309 (1980).

S9 Semagin, V.N. Effect of prolonged irradiation with low doses on the brain of rat embryos. Radiobiologiya 15: 583-588 (1975) (in Russian).

S11 Shiono, P., C.S. Chung and N.C. Myrianthopoulos. Preconception radiation, intrauterine diagnostic radiation and childhood neoplasia. J. Natl. Cancer Inst. 65: 681-686 (1980).

S12 Sikov, M.R. and D.D. Mahlum. Effects on the rat embryo of combined exposure to ^{239}Pu and Trypan Blue. p. 9-10 in: BNWL-1850 Pt. 1 (1974).

S13 Sikov, M.R. and J.E. Lofstrom. Increased tumour incidence following prenatal x-irradiation of the rat. p. 372-390 in: Radiation Effects in Physics, Chemistry and Biology (M. Ebert and A. Howard, eds.) North Holland, Amsterdam, 1963.

S15 Spiers, P.S. Does growth retardation predispose the fetus to congenital malformations? Lancet: 8267: 312-314 (1982).

S16 Sternberg, J. Placental transfers: modern methods of study. Am. J. Obst. Gynecol. 84: 1731-1748 (1962).

S17 Streffer, C. Some fundamental aspects of combined effects by ionizing radiation and chemical substances during prenatal development. p. 267-285 in: Developmental Effects of Prenatal Irradiation. Gustav Fischer, Stuttgart, 1982.

S18 Streffer, C., D. Van Beuningen and S. Elias. Comparative effects of tritiated water and thymidine on the preimplanted mouse embryo in vitro. Curr. Top. Radiat. Res. Quart. 12: 182-193 (1977).

S19 Streffer, C., D. Van Beuningen and M. Molls. Radiobiological investigations with the preimplanted mouse embryo. p. 175-179 in: Human Fertilization. Thieme, Stuttgart, 1978.

S21 Sidman, R.L. and P. Rakic. Neuronal migration, with special reference to developing human brain: a review. Brain Res. 62: 1-35 (1973).

S22 Stewart, A. Low dose radiation cancers in man. Adv. Cancer Res. 14: 359-390 (1971).

S23 Stewart, A., J. Webb and D. Hewitt. A survey of childhood malignancies. Brit. Med. J. June 28: 1495-1508 (1958).

S24 Stewart, A. and G.W. Kneale. Radiation dose effects in relation to obstetric x-rays and childhood cancer. Lancet 7658: 1185-1188 (1970).

S25 Stewart, A. and G.W. Kneale. Age-distribution of cancers caused by obstetric x-rays and their relevance to cancer latent periods. Lancet 7662: 4-8 (1970).

S26 Stewart, A. and G.W. Kneale. Changes in the cancer risk associated with obstetric radiography. Lancet 7534: 104-107 (1968).

S27 Sasaki, S., T. Kasuga, F. Sato et al. Age dependence of susceptibility to carcinogenic and non carcinogenic somatic effects of x rays in mice. J. Radiat. Res. 22: 39 only (1981).

S28 Sasaki, S., T. Kasuga and N. Kawashima. Induction of lymphocytic neoplasms by x irradiation at late fetal stage on mice. J. Radiat. Res. 23: 41 only (1982).

S29 Stitzel, K.A., M. Shifrine and L.S. Rosenblatt. Summary of activities in the external radiation leukemogenesis project, June 21, 1980—July 26, 1981. p. 82-93 in: UCD-472-127 (1982).

S30 Stitzel, K.A., M. Shifrine, S.L. Munn et al. Induction of leukemia by chronic irradiation, starting in utero. p. 94-98 in: UCD-472-127 (1982).

S31 Schmahl, W. and W.E. Kollmer. Radiation induced meningeal and pituitary tumours in the rat after prenatal application of strontium-90. J. Cancer Res. Clin. Oncol. 100: 13-18 (1981).

S32 Schmahl, W., H. Kriegel and E. Senft. Can prenatal x-irradiation in mice act as an initiator stimulus in a modified 2-stage Berenblum/Mottram experiment with postnatal promotion with phorbol ester TPA. J. Cancer Res. Clin. Oncol. 97: 109-117 (1980).

S33 Schmahl, W. and H. Kriegel. Ovary tumours in NMRI mice subjected to fractionated x irradiation during fetal development. J. Cancer Res. Clin. Oncol. 98: 65-74 (1980).

S34 Saito, M., C. Streffer and M. Molls. Tritium distribution in newborn mice after providing mother mice with drinking water containing tritiated thymidine. Radiat. Res. 95: 273-297 (1983).

S35 Streffer, C., M. Saito and M. Molls. Metabolism and effects of HTO and tritium-thymidine during prenatal development in mice. p. 3-19 in: Colloquium on the Toxicity of Radionuclides. Centre d'Etudes d'Energie Nucléaire. Brussels, 1964.

S36 Streffer, C., D. Van Beuningen, M. Molls et al. In vitro culture of preimplanted mouse embryos. A model system for studying combined effects. p. 381-396 in: Late Biological Effects of Ionizing Radiation, Vol. II. IAEA, Vienna, 1978.

S38 Stevenson, A.C., H.A. Johnston, M.I.P. Stewart et al. Congenital malformations: a report of a study of series of consecutive births in 24 centres. WHO, Geneva, 1966.

S39 Stewart, A. Myeloid leukemia and cot death. Brit. Med. J. 4: 423 only (1972).

S40 Schmahl, W., H. Kriegel and L. Weber. Developmental neuropathology of mouse neocortex following early fetal x-irradiation. Bibliotheca Anat. 19: 308-312 (1981).

S41 Stewart, A. The carcinogenic effects of low level radiation. A reappraisal of epidemiologists methods and observations. Health Phys. 24: 223-240 (1973).

S42 Stewart, A. and R. Barber. The epidemiological importance of childhood cancers. Brit. Med. Bull. 27: 64-70 (1971).

S43 Skidmore, F.D. An analysis of the age and size of 483 human embryos. Teratology 15: 97-102 (1977).

S44 Stewart, A., J. Webb, D. Giles et al. Malignant disease in childhood and diagnostic irradiation in utero. Lancet II: 447 only (1956).

S45 Stewart, A. Aetiology of childhood malignancies. Congenitally determined leukemias. Brit. Med. J. I: 452-460 (1961).

S46 Sikov, M.R. Carcinogenesis following prenatal exposure to radiation. Biol. Res. in Pregnancy 2: 159-167 (1981).

S47 Sikov, M.A., G.M. Zwicker, J.D. Hess et al. Late effects of perinatally administered plutonium. p. 361-374 in: Developmental Toxicology of Energy-Related Pollutants (D.D. Mahlum et al., eds.). DOE Symposium Series No. 47, CONF-771017 (1978).

S48 Strel'tsova, V.N. and Ju.N. Pavlenko-Mikhailov. On tumours arising in animals exposed to irradiation in their embryogenesis period. Vopr. Onkol. 24 (9): 25-30 (1978) (in Russian).

S49 Schmahl, W. Kinetics of telencephalic neural cell proliferation during the fetal regeneration period following a single x-irradiation at the late organogenesis stage. II. Cycle times and the size of the functional compartment of neural epithelial cells of distinct lesion districts. Radiat. Environm. Biophys. 22: 95-115 (1983).

S50 Schull, W.J. Recent estimates of risk to the human embryo and fetus. Radiat. Res. 94: 540 only (1983).

S51 Slozhenikina, L.V., A.A. Kuodyavtseva and A.M. Kuzin. Action of ionizing radiation on the induction of glucose-6-phosphotase synthesis in liver of rat embryos. Radiobiologiya 14: 489-492 (1973) (in Russian).

S52 Slozhenikina, L.V., L.A. Fialkovskaya, L.P. Mikhailets et al. Changes in the activity of tyrosine-aminotransferase after gamma irradiation at early embryogenesis and possible role of cAMP system in this process. Radiobiologiya 18: 643-647 (1978) (in Russian).

S53 Shapiro, F.B. Fertility of female mice irradiated during embryonic development and survival rate of their offspring. Doklad. Akad. Nauk. SSR 125: 921-924 (1959) (in Russian).

S54 Sikov, M.R., D.D. Mahlum, G.M. Zwicker et al. Late effects of ^{239}Pu injection in adult, weanling, newborn and fetal rats. p. 183-185 in: PNL-3300 Pt. 1 (1980).

S55 Streeter, G.L. Weight, sitting height, head size, foot length and menstrual age of human embryos. Contrib. Embryol. Carnegie Inst. 11: 147-170 (1920).

S56 Salonen, T. Prenatal and perinatal factors in childhood cancer. Ann. Clin. Res. 8: 27-42 (1976).

S57 Shibagaki, M., M. Seo, T. Asano et al. Environmental enrichment to alleviate maze performance deficits in rats with microcephaly induced by x-irradiation. Physiol. Behav. 27: 797-802 (1981).

S58 Schmahl, W., I. Meyer, H. Kriegel et al. Cartilagenous metaplasia and overgrowth of neurocranium skull after x-irradiation in utero. Virchows Arch. A. Path. Anat. and Histol. 384: 173-184 (1979).

S59 Schmahl, W., E. Senft, W. Weber et al. X-irradiation of mice in early foetal period influences dose-dependently sex ratio of offspring until weaning. Experientia 35: 541-543 (1979).

S60 Schmahl, W., L. Weber and H. Kriegel. Sexual dimorphism of mouse fetal brain lesions after x-irradiation prior to gonadal differentiation. Experientia 35: 1653-1655 (1979).

S61 Schmahl, W. and L. Weber. Sexual dimorphism in newborn mouse epithalamus after fractionated x-irradiation at late stage of organogenesis. Virchows Arch. A. Path. Anat. and Histol. 389: 43-57 (1980).

S62 Schmahl, W., E. Senft, V. Erfle et al. Dermal dysplasia, hypotrichosis and dorsal skin ulcers in adult NMRI mice after x-irradiation in utero. Virchows Arch. A. Path. Anat. and Histol. 385: 271-282 (1980).

S63 Schmahl, W. Psoriasis: is it transplacentally induced? Medical Hypotheses 6: 907-911 (1980).

S64 Schmahl, W., W.E. Kollmer, D. Berg et al. Postnatal effects on Wistar rat pituitary morphology and function after application of strontium-90 on day 18 of pregnancy. p. 329 in: Biological Implications of Radionuclides Released from Nuclear Industries, Vol. I. IAEA, Vienna, 1979.

S65 Schmahl, W. Long-term effects after prenatal irradiation. p. 89-99 in: Effects of prenatal irradiation with Special Emphasis on Late Effects. EUR-8067 (1984).

S66 Stieve, F.E. Exchange and transfer mechanisms of radioactive compounds between the mother and the developing offspring in utero. Review of the experimental literature. p. 150-181 in: Effects of Prenatal Irradiation with Special Emphasis on Late Effects. EUR-8067 (1984).

S67 Senekowitsch, R. and H. Kriegel. Diaplacental transfer and distribution of some radionuclides in fetal organs at different stages of gestation. p. 183-197 in: Effects of Prenatal Irradiation with Special Emphasis on Late Effects. EUR-8067 (1984).

S68 Stieve, F.E. Schäden durch energiereiche Strahlen während der Schwangerschaft. p. 161-187 in: Schädigende Noxen in der embryofetalen Entwicklung.

(G. Stark, ed.) Milupa A.G., Friedrichsdorf/Taunus, 1983.

S69 Senekowitsch, R., H. Kriegel, S. Möllenstädt et al. Kinetics and diaplacental transfer of ^{131}I in rats fed with either standard diet or iodine deficient diet. p. 473-476, Vol. I in: Radiation, Risk, Protection (A. Kaul, R. Neider, J. Pensko et al., eds.). Fachverband für Strahlenschutz e.V., 1984.

S70 Streffer, C., D. van Beuningen, M. Molls et al. Kinetics of cell proliferation in the preimplanted mouse embryo in vivo and in vitro. Cell Tissue Kinet. 13: 135-143 (1980).

S71 Sasaki, S., T. Kasuga, F. Sato et al. Induction of hepatocellular tumor by x-ray irradiation at perinatal stage of mice. Gann. 69: 451-452 (1978).

S72 Sasaki, S. and T. Kasuga. Life-shortening and carcinogenesis in mice irradiated at perinatal period with γ-rays. 22nd Hanford Life Science Symposium, Richland, Washington, 1983 (in press).

S73 Seo, M.L., M. Inouye, and M. Shibagaki. Effects of environmentally differential rearing upon maze performance in prenatally irradiated mice cephalic rats. Teratology 26: 221-227 (1982).

S74 Spindle, A., K. Wu and R.A. Pedersen. Sensitivity of early mouse embryos to ^{3}H-thymidine. Exp. Cell Res. 142: 397-405 (1982).

S75 Semagin, V.N. and V.V. Antipov. Compensatory possibilities of higher nervous activity in the irradiation of embryos. p. 66-101. Abstract submitted by the Delegation of USSR, Moscow, 1978.

S76 Sakovskaya, M.S., I.E. Bronshtein, A.N. Liberman et al. Experimental studies of combined x-ray and SHF radiation. p. 37-41 in: Health Evaluation of Radiation and Non-radiation Factors and their Combination. LNIIRG, Leningrad, 1976.

S77 Spranger, J., K. Benirsche, J. G. Hall et al. Errors of morphogenesis: concepts and terms. J. Pediatr. 100: 160-165 (1982).

S78 Schull, W.J. and M. Otake. Neurological deficit among the survivors exposed in utero to the atomic bombing of Hiroshima and Nagasaki: a reassessment and new directions. p. 399-419 in: Radiation Risks to the Developing Nervous System. Gustav Fischer, Stuttgart, 1985.

S79 Sasaki, S. Quantitative histological study on confusion of the cerebellar cortex architecture in perinatally irradiated mice. p. 179-189 in: Radiation Risks to the Developing Nervous System. Gustav Fischer, Stuttgart, 1986.

S80 Sikov, M.R., D.D. Mahlum, G.E. Dagle et al. Relationships between age at exposure to iodine-131 and thyroid tumor incidence in rats. p.79 in: Abstracts of Papers for the 32nd Annual Meeting of the Radiation Research Society. Florida, 1984.

S81 Strahlenexposition von Embryo und Fetus aufgrund einer Inkorporation radioaktiver Stoffe. Report from the Institut für Strahlenhygiene des Bundesgesundheitsamtes (1985).

S82 Schmahl, W. and H. Kriegel. Correlations between the degree and type of forebrain malformations and the simultaneous neuro-oncogenic properties of ethylnitrosourea after diaplacental exposure in rats, alone and in combination with x irradiation. Teratog., Carcinog., Mutagen. 5: 159-175 (1985).

S83 Schull, W.J. and M. Otake. The central nervous system and in utero exposure to ionizing radiation:

the Hiroshima and Nagasaki experience. p. 515-536 in: Epidemiology and Quantitation of Environmental Risk in Humans from Radiation and Other Agents (A. Castellani, ed.). Plenum Press, New York, 1985.

S84 Snow, M.H.L. Growth and its control in early mammalian development. Brit. Med. Bull. 37: 221-226 (1981).

S85 Stieve, F.E., G. Zemlin and I. Griessl. Plazentarer Transfer von Jod und seinen Verbindungen. Report GSF 41/85 (1985).

T1 Török, P. and G. Kistner. Reproductive performance of mice after injection of tritiated water at different embryonic development stages. p. 91-96 in: Developmental Effects of Prenatal Irradiation. Gustav Fischer, Stuttgart, 1982.

T2 Totter, J.R. and H.G. MacPherson. Do childhood cancers result from prenatal x-rays? Health Phys. 40: 511-524 (1981).

T3 Tribukait, B. and E. Cekan. Dose-effect relationship and the significance of fractionated and protracted radiation for the frequency of fetal malformations following x-irradiation of pregnant C3H mice. p. 29-35 in: Developmental Effects of Prenatal Irradiation. Gustav Fischer, Stuttgart, 1982.

T4 Tubiana, M. The problems raised by the irradiation of pregnant women. Effects of ionizing radiations on the embryo and foetus. Bull. Cancer 66: 155-174 (1979).

T5 Tabuchi, A., T. Hirai, S. Nakagawa et al. Clinical findings on in utero exposed microcephalic children. ABCC-TR-28-67.

T6 Totter, J.R. Some observational bases for estimating the oncogenic effects of ionizing radiation. Nucl. Safety 21: 83-94 (1980).

T7 Török, P., W. Schmahl, I. Meyer et al. Effects of a single injection of tritiated water during organogenesis on the pre-natal and post-natal development of mice. p. 241-253 in: Biological Implications of Radionuclides Released from Nuclear Industries, Vol. I. IAEA, Vienna, 1979.

T8 Tamaki, Y. and M. Inouye. Avoidance of and anticipatory response to shock in prenatally x-irradiated rats. Physiol. Behav. 22: 701-705 (1979).

T9 Turakulov, Y.K., L.A. Ilin, A.M. Lyaginskaya et al. The application of potassium iodide in combination with potassium perchlorate for the purpose of protecting against radioactive iodine during pregnancy. p. 19. Information Bulletin No. 305, Uzbek SSR Branch of the Academy of Sciences, Tashkent, 1983.

T10 Trimble, B.K. and J.H. Doughty. The amount of hereditary disease in human population. Ann. Hum. Genet. 38: 199-223 (1974).

T11 Timmermanns, R., J. Maes, J. Deroo et al. Serotonin receptors, vascular functions and lipids in rat brain after pre-natal irradiation. p.221-230 in: Radiation Risks to the Developing Nervous System. Gustav Fischer, Stuttgart, 1985.

T12 Tanaka, H., S. Iwasaki, H. Suzuki et al. Biochemical analysis of cerebrum of fetal rat x-irradiated in utero. Content and composition of DNA, superoxide dismutase and lipid peroxide. p. 231-244 in: Radiation Risks to the Developing Nervous System. Gustav Fischer, Stuttgart, 1985.

T13 Tchobroutsky, C., G.L. Breart, D.C. Rambaud et al. Correlation between fetal defects and early growth delay observed by ultrasound. The Lancet I: 706-707 (1985).

T14 Takahashi, S., Y. Kubota and O. Matsuoka. Placental transfer of iron-59 in rats after intravenous injection of 59-Fe-irondextran at near term. J. Radiat. Res. 24: 137-147 (1983).

T15 Tanimura, T., T. Nelson, R.R. Hollingsworth et al. Weight standards for organs from early human fetuses. Anat. Res. 171: 227-236 (1971).

T16 Taylor, D.M. Mobilization of internally deposited plutonium from the rat by pregnancy and lactation. Int. J. Radiat. Biol. 38: 357-360 (1980).

U1 United Nations. Report of the United Nations Scientific Committee on the Effects of Atomic Radiation. Official Records of the General Assembly, Twenty-fourth session, Supplement No. 13 (A/7613). New York, 1969.

U2 United Nations. Sources and Effects of Ionizing Radiation. Report of the United Nations Scientific Committee on the Effects of Atomic Radiation to the General Assembly, with annexes. United Nations sales publication E.77.IX.1. United Nations, New York, 1977.

U3 United Nations. Report of the United Nations Scientific Committee on the Effects of Atomic Radiation. Official Records of the General Assembly, Nineteenth session, Supplement No. 14 (A/5814). United Nations, New York, 1964.

U4 United Nations. Ionizing Radiation: Levels and Effects. Report of the United Nations Scientific Committee on the Effects of Atomic Radiation, with annexes. United Nations sales publication E.72.IX.17 and 18. United Nations, New York, 1972.

U5 United Nations. Ionizing Radiation: Sources and Biological Effects. United Nations Scientific Committee on the Effects of Atomic Radiation, 1982 Report to the General Assembly, with annexes. United Nations sales publication E.82.IX.8. United Nations, New York, 1982.

U6 Ujeno, Y. Epidemiological studies on disturbances of human fetal development in areas with various doses of natural background radiation. I. Relationship between incidences of Down's syndrome or visible malformation and gonadal dose equivalent rate of natural background radiation. Arch. Environ. Health 40: 177-180 (1985).

U7 Ujeno, Y. Epidemiological studies on disturbances of human fetal development in areas with various doses of natural background radiation. I. Relationship between incidences of hidatidiform mole, malignant hidatidiform mole, and chorionepithelioma and gonadal dose equivalent rate of natural background radiation. Arch. Environ. Health 40: 181-184 (1985).

V2 Van Marthens, E. and S. Zamenhof. The effects of short term and chronic exposure to tritiated drinking water on pre- and post-natal brain development. p. 97-103 in: Developmental Effects of Prenatal Irradiation. Gustav Fischer, Stuttgart, 1982.

V3 Vogel, H.H. Neutron irradiation of rat embryos in utero. Radiat. Res. 70: 621-622 (1977).

V4 Vogel, H.H. Neutron irradiation of rat embryos in utero. p. 267-280 in: Developmental Toxicology of Energy-Related Pollutants (D.D. Mahlum et al., eds.). DOE Symposium Series No. 47, CONF-771017 (1978).

V5 Various Authors. Human malformations. Brit. Med. Bull. 32: 1-94 (1976).

V6 Van Beuningen, D., C. Streffer, M. Molls et al. Kombinationswirkung von Blei und ionisierender

Strahlung auf die Proliferation von Sangerzellen (Mäuseembryonen in vitro). p. 117-125 in: Risiken und Nutzen der Strahlentherapie bösartiger Tumoren. Georg Thieme Verlag, Stuttgart, 1978.

V7 Van Bruwaene, R., G.B. Gerber, R. Kirchmann et al. Tritium metabolism in young pigs after exposure of the mothers to tritium oxide during pregnancy. Radiat. Res. 91: 124-134 (1982).

V8 Villumsen, A.L. Environmental factors in congenital malformations. A prospective study of 9006 human pregnancies. FADLs Forlag, Copenhagen, 1970.

V9 Vogel, H.H. and S. Antal. Neutron irradiation of late mouse embryos (15-19 days) in utero. Radiat. Res. 98: 52-64 (1984).

V10 Van Beuningen, M., C. Streffer and D. van Beuningen. NAD-content and metabolism in the mouse embryo and developing brain. p. 245-295 in: Radiation Risks to the Developing Nervous System. Gustav Fischer, Stuttgart, 1986.

V11 Villiers, P.A., F. Daburon and J. Remy. Administration chronique de strontium-85 à la truie. Etude du passage aux produits pendant la gestation et la lactation. p. 85-100 in: Proceedings of the Fifth International Congress of the French Society for Radiation Protection, Grenoble, 1971.

W1 Ward, W.F., H. Aceto and C.H. Karp. Effect of intrauterine position on the radiosensitivity of rat embryos. Teratology 16: 181-186 (1977).

W2 Ward, W.F., H. Aceto, R. Jolly et al. RBE and OER of extended-Bragg-peak helium ions: survival and development of rat embryos. Int. J. Radiat. Biol. 30: 317-326 (1976).

W3 Ward, W.F., H. Aceto and M. Sandusky. Repair of sublethal and potentially lethal damage by rat embryos exposed to gamma rays or helium ions. Radiology 120: 695-700 (1976).

W4 Ward, W.F., H. Aceto and M. Sandusky. RBE and OER of extended-Bragg-peak helium ions: embryo survival and teratogenesis in rats. Radiat. Res. 67: 553-554 (1976).

W5 Ward, W.F., H. Aceto and M. Sandusky. Embryonic survival in rats exposed to gamma rays or helium ions on days 3-10 of gestation. Radiat. Res. 67: 69-81 (1976).

W6 Ward, W.F., H. Aceto and D. Stallard. Comparison of the teratogenic effectiveness of ^{60}Co gamma rays and extended-Bragg-peak helium ions. Radiat. Res. 70: 621 only (1977).

W7 Warkany, J., T.I. Mandybur and H. Kalter. Oncogenic response of rats with x-ray-induced microcephaly to transplacental ethylnitrosourea. J. Natl. Cancer Inst. 56: 59-64 (1976).

W8 Weber, L.W.D., W. Schmahl and H. Kriegel. Enzymatic method for the sensitive demonstration of postnatal effects caused by prenatal x-irradiation in mouse brain. p. 233-236 in: Developmental Effects of Prenatal Irradiation. Gustav Fischer, Stuttgart 1982.

W9 Weiss, J.F. and H.E. Walburg. Cross placental transfer of plutonium in mice. Radiat. Res. 70: 637 only (1977).

W10 Weiss, J.F. and H.E. Walburg. Placental transfer of americium and plutonium in mice. Health Phys. 39: 903-911 (1980).

W11 Whittingham, D.G., M.F. Lyon and P.H. Glenister. Long-term storage of mouse embryos at −196° C: the effect of background radiation. Genet. Res. 29: 171-181 (1977).

W12 Wanner, R.A. and M.J. Edwards. Comparison of the effects of radiation and hyperthermia on pre-natal retardation of brain growth of guinea-pigs. Brit. J. Radiol. 56: 33-39 (1983).

W13 Winick, M., J.A. Brasel, E. Velasco et al. Effects of early nutrition on growth of the central nervous system. Birth Defects 10: 29-36 (1974).

W15 Wells, J. and C.M. Steer. Relationship of leukemia in children to abdominal irradiation of mothers during pregnancy. Am. J. Obstet. Gynecol. 81: 1059-1063 (1961).

W16 Wise, M.E. Irradiation and leukemia. Brit. Med. J. II: 48-49 (1961).

W17 Wegner, G. and E.H. Graul. Tumoren als Spätschäden der Nachkommenschaft von Wistar-Ratten nach Ganzkörperbestrahlung am 9. Graviditätstag. Strahlentherapie 123: 609-613 (1964).

W18 Wegner, G., E. Stutz and F. Büchner. Tumoren und Mißbildungen bei der Wistar-Ratte in der ersten Generation nach Ganzbestrahlung des Muttertieres mit 270 R am 18. Graviditätstag. Beitr. Path. Allgem. Pathol. Anat. 124: 396 (1961).

W19 Weber, L. and W. Schmahl. Developmental patterns of three X chromosomal enzyme activities in the brains of female and male mice. Lack of sex-dependent reaction to a fractionated prenatal x-ray dose. Dev. Neurosci 5: 222-232 (1982).

W20 Weber, L. and W. Schmahl. Sex-dependent action of prenatal fractionated x-irradiation in the mouse. Biochemical findings. Experientia 35: 1656-1657 (1979).

W21 Weiss, J.F. and H.E. Walburg. Influence of the mass of administered plutonium on its crossplacental transfer in mice. Health Phys. 35: 773-777 (1978).

W22 Wood, J.W., K.G. Johnson and Y. Omori. In utero exposure to the Hiroshima atomic bomb: follow-up at twenty years. ABCC 9-65 (1965).

W23 Wood, J.W., K.G. Johnson, Y. Omori et al. Mental retardation in children exposed in utero, Hiroshima-Nagasaki. ABCC 10-66 (1966).

W24 Weinberg, S.R. and T.J. MacVittie. Perturbations of murine haemopoiesis of fetal neonatal and young adult mice after prenatal low-dose irradiation with cobalt-60. Experimental Haematology 10: (Suppl. 11) 158 only (1982).

W25 Weinberg, S.R. Murine neonate haemopoiesis following in utero total-body irradiation. Biol. Neonate 43: 272-280 (1983).

W26 World Health Organization. Guidelines for the study of genetic effects in human populations. IPCS International Program on Chemical Safety Environmental Health Criteria. WHO, Geneva, 1985.

W27 World Health Organization. Task Group on Prevention of Avoidable Mutational Diseases. Kiev, 1984 (in press).

W28 World Health Organization. International Classification of Diseases. Ninth Revision, Vol. II. WHO, Geneva, 1977.

W29 Weinberg, S.R., T.J. MacVittie, A.C. Bakarich et al. Haemopoiesis in the beagle foetus after in utero irradiation. Int. J. Radiat. Biol. 44: 367-375 (1983).

W30 Walinder, G. and C. Rönnbäck. Neoplastic effects after prenatal irradiation. p. 101-115 in: Effects of Prenatal Irradiation with Special Emphasis on Late Effects. EUR-8067 (1984).

W31 Waight, P.J. Prenatal x-ray exposure and childhood cancer in twins. New Engl. J. Med. 312: 1574-1575 (1985).

W32 Winick, M. Nutrition and mouse cell growth. Fed. Proc. 29: 1510-1515 (1970).

W33 Weinberg, S.R., E.G. McCarthy and T.J. MacVittie. Fetal murine hemopoiesis following in utero low-dose irradiation. J. Embryol. Exp. Morphol. 62: 37-46 (1981).

W34 Wang, Z. and S. Zhao. Response of cerebral development in fetal rats to doses of the tritiated-water beta and ^{137}Cs gamma radiation. Radiat. Prot. 5: 190-201 (1985) (in Chinese).

Y1 Yamada, T., O. Yukawa, K. Asami et al. Effect of chronic HTO β or cobalt-60-gamma radiation on preimplantation mouse development in vitro. Radiat. Res. 92: 359-369 (1982).

Y2 Yuguchi, S. Eye abnormalities in fetuses caused by simultaneous irradiation of x-rays and ultrasound. Nagoya Med. J. 24: 99-123 (1980).

Y3 Yamada, T., O. Yukawa, Y. Matsuda et al. Changes in radiosensitivity of the in vitro fertilized mouse ova during zygotic stage from fertilization to first cleavage. J. Radiat. Res. 23: 450-456 (1982).

Y4 Yamada, T. and O. Yukawa. Changes in sensitivity of mouse embryos during the pronuclear and the 2-cell stage. p. 5-7 in: Effects of Prenatal Irradiation with Special Emphasis on Late Effects. EUR-8067 (1984).

Z1 Zamenhof, S. and E. van Marthens. The effects of chronic ingestion of tritiated water on prenatal brain development. Radiat. Res. 77: 117-127 (1979).

Z2 Zamenhof, S. and E. van Marthens. The effects of pre- and post-natal exposure to tritiated water for five generations on postnatal brain development. Radiat. Res. 85: 292-301 (1981).

Z3 Zhou, J. and J. Wang. Studies of radiation effects on mouse embryos in the pre-implantation stage. Chin. J. Radiol. Med. Prot. 2: 18-20 (1982) (in Chinese).

Z4 Zhou, J. et al. Changes of leukocyte count in babies x-irradiated in utero. Chin. J. Radiol. Med. Prot. 3: 34-36 (1983) (in Chinese).